Shah's
Public Health *and* Preventive Health Care *in* Canada

Shah's Public Health *and* Preventive Health Care *in* Canada

Sixth Edition

Bonnie Fournier, RN, MSc, PhD
Associate Professor
School of Nursing
Thompson Rivers University
Kamloops, British Columbia

Fareen Karachiwalla, MD, MPH, CCFP, FRCPC

Associate Medical Officer of Health
York Region Public Health
Newmarket, Ontario;
Adjunct Assistant Professor
School of Medicine
Queen's University
Kingston, Ontario

Adjunct Lecturer
Clinical Public Health Division
Dalla Lana School of Public Health
University of Toronto
Toronto, Ontario

Founding Author & Consultant

Chandrakant P. Shah, MD, O. Ont.
Professor Emeritus
Dalla Lana School of Public Health
University of Toronto;
Honorary Consulting Physician
Anishnawbe Health Toronto
Toronto, Ontario

ELSEVIER

VP Education Content: Kevonne Holloway
Content Strategist (Canada Acquisitions): Roberta A. Spinosa-Millman
Director, Content Development: Laurie Gower
Content Development Specialist: Martina van de Velde
Publishing Services Manager: Deepthi Unni
Project Manager: Manchu Mohan
Design Direction: Amy Buxton

Printed in Canada

Last digit is the print number: 9 8 7 6 5 4 3 2 1

Working together
to grow libraries in
developing countries

www.elsevier.com • www.bookaid.org

ABOUT THE AUTHORS

Dr. Bonnie Fournier is a registered nurse and an associate professor in the School of Nursing at Thompson Rivers University, Kamloops, British Columbia, Canada. Her career has spanned more than 20 years and includes nursing in areas such as mental health, community health, and global health with a focus on addressing health inequities through policy approaches, community building, and community-based participatory research. Dr. Fournier has taught undergraduate and graduate nursing in Canada and the Middle East and has had the privilege of teaching community health representatives in the Northwest Territories. In 2008, she was recognized for outstanding achievements early in her career with the Horizon Award from the University of Alberta. Her research is focused on population health interventions using arts-based methods (photovoice, theatre, art, storytelling, dance) to advance health equity for children and youth whose lives are affected by stigma, poverty, and geography. She is a principle investigator on several Tri-Agency grants, including a Project Grant from CIHR to reduce HIV stigma in Ugandan school-children using local traditional knowledge and arts-based methods.

Dr. Fareen Karachiwalla is a physician practising Public Health & Preventive Medicine as well as family medicine in Ontario. She currently works as Associate Medical Officer of Health for the Regional Municipality of York, where her broad responsibilities include providing leadership and strategic direction to the Control of Infectious Diseases Division and Public Health Branch. She holds a faculty appointment at both Queen's University and the University of Toronto, where she teaches, lectures, and acts as a field supervisor for public health physicians in training. Her most recent professional and academic accomplishments include supporting the creation of the Overdose Prevention Site in Kingston, Ontario; leading a local health agency to develop a vision on health equity; and initiating a review of organizational best practices to enhance equity in the workplace.

Fareen is a strong advocate for health equity issues in her community, and her main passions include healthy public policy, intersectoral collective impact, and achieving equity within organizational structures.

Fareen completed her Public Health & Preventive Medicine residency program at the University of Toronto, her Master's in Public Health degree (with a focus on health systems and policy) at Johns Hopkins University, and Family Medicine training at St. Michael's Hospital in Toronto. She continues to practise Family Medicine part time with the Inner City Health Associates in Toronto, working primarily with refugees and undocumented migrants, as well as inner-city populations facing homelessness and complex mental health and addictions issues. During her postgraduate medical training at the University of Toronto's Public Health & Preventive Medicine program, Dr. Karachiwalla received the honourable C.P. Shah research award for her mixed-methods research in the care of transgendered people.

Dr. Chandrakant Shah, Professor Emeritus, Dalla Lana Faculty of Public Health at the University of Toronto, was a practising physician, a public health practitioner, and an advocate for improving the health and well-being of marginalized groups in Canadian society. He was a professor in the Department of Public Health Sciences, University of Toronto, from 1972 to 2001. He was instrumental in developing the Endowed Chair in Aboriginal Health and Wellbeing at the University, the first of its kind in Canada. He held cross-appointments in the departments of Health Policy, Management and Evaluation, Paediatrics, Family and Community Medicine in the Faculty of Medicine and in the Faculties of Social Work and Nursing at the University of Toronto. He was a staff physician at the Anishnawbe Health Toronto from 2001 to 2016 and is now Honorary Consultant. At present, he is also Board Member and Secretary Treasurer of the Anishnawbe Health Foundation.

He is the recipient of the **John Hastings Award** (1997) from the Faculty of Medicine for his excellent services to the University of Toronto and communities. In 1999, he received the highest award of the Canadian Public Health Association, the **R. D. Defries Award and Honorary Life Membership**, for his contribution to furthering medical education in public health as well as his advocacy for disadvantaged populations such as the homeless, unemployed, and poor. He is the recipient of the **Eagle Feather**, the highest award given by First Nations House at the University of Toronto for his lifetime work with the aboriginal community, and particularly for developing an annual *Visiting Lectureship on Native Health* program series. He received the **25th Anniversary Race Relations Award** from the Urban Alliance on Race Relations in 2000 for his work in creating racial harmony; a **Certificate of Recognition** by the City of Toronto Public Health Department for outstanding commitment and dedication towards the pursuit of Access and Equity at the University of Toronto in 2001; an **Honorary Life Membership** from the Ontario Medical Association in 2002 and designation of **Senior Member** from the Canadian Medical Association in 2003 for his lifetime devotion to improving the health of Canadians and particularly the marginalized population; a **Lifetime/Outstanding Achievement Award in 2005 by Indo-Canada Chamber of Commerce** for his lifetime work for improving the health and wellbeing of Indigenous people, homeless, unemployed, and other marginalized groups as well as his contribution to public health education in Canada; the **Order of Ontario** in 2005 by the Government of Ontario for being a pioneer in public health education in Canada and in developing innovative health care programs and being an advocate for Indigenous Peoples, the homeless, the unemployed, and children living in poverty; the **Outstanding Physicians of Ontario** in 2007 by the Council of the College of Physicians and Surgeons of Ontario; the **2010 J. S. Woodsworth Award** by the New Democratic Party of Ontario for outstanding Commitment and Excellence in the Fight for the Elimination of Racial Discrimination, particularly for Indigenous People, through his teaching, research, clinical service, and advocacy work; **The Queen Elizabeth II Silver Jubilee Medal**, 2012 Government of Canada; **The Canadian Race Relation Foundation, Award of Excellence**: Honourable Mention in Best Practice Award, 2012 for Aboriginal Cultural Safety Awareness Initiative; **Association of Ontario Health Centers, 2014 Health Equity Award** for Aboriginal Cultural Safety Awareness Initiative; the **Ontario Ministry of Health and Long Term: Minister's Medal Honouring Excellence in Health Quality and Safety, Individual Champion 2014** for his initiative on educating Ontario's Health Sciences Students in Colleges and Universities in the area of Indigenous Cultural Safety; and the **Gujarat Gaurav (Pride of Gujarat, India) Award** by Gujarat Public Affairs Council of Canada in 2016. He has been listed in *Who's Who in Canada* from 1995–2019 and in Wikipedia.

In 1987, the University of Toronto established an annual award and a scholarship in his name, **The C.P. Shah Award**, to be granted to the Public Health and Preventive Medicine Resident for their best work in the field of public health. In July 2001, the university also established **The Queen Elizabeth II/C.P. Shah Graduate Scholarships in Science and Technology**, which will fund $15,000 per year for a doctoral stream student in Public Health Sciences. In 2007, the C.P. Shah Alumni Award of Excellence in Public Health was established, to be awarded annually to the outstanding alumnae of Dalla Lana Faculty of Public Health.

REVIEWERS

John P. Crawford, MSc, PhD (Path), DC, FCCSS(C)
Chiropractor and Athletic Injuries Specialist
Associate Professor
Canadian Memorial Chiropractic College
Toronto, Ontario

Genevieve Currie, RN, MN
Professor
School of Nursing
Mount Royal University
Calgary, Alberta

Natalie Frandsen, RN, MN
Assistant Teaching Professor
University of Victoria
Human and Social Development, School of Public
    Health & Social Policy
Victoria, British Columbia

Shawn N. Fraser, PhD
Professor
Faculty of Health Disciplines
Athabasca University
Athabasca, Alberta

Brenda J. Gamble, PhD
Associate Dean, Accredited Health Programs
Associate Professor
Faculty of Health Sciences
Ontario Tech University
Oshawa, Ontario

Ian Johnson, MD, MSc, FRCPC
Associate Professor
Dalla Lana School of Public Health
University of Toronto
Toronto, Ontario

Dr. Yuri Kagolovsky, MD, MSc, PhD, CHIM
Professor
School of Health & Life Sciences and Community
    Services
Conestoga Institute of Technology and Advanced
    Learning
Kitchener, Ontario

Christina Murray, RN, MN, PhD
Associate Professor
Faculty of Nursing
University of Prince Edward Island
Chalottetown, Prince Edward Island

M. Helena Myllykoski, RN, NP, MHSc, MN
Associate Professor
School of Nursing and Midwifery
Mount Royal University
Calgary, Alberta

Maisam Najafizada, PhD
Assistant Professor
Faculty of Medicine
Memorial University of Newfoundland
St. John's, Newfoundland

Kent V. Rondeau, PhD
Associate Professor
Faculty of Extension
University of Alberta
Edmonton, Alberta

Jennifer Shea, PhD
Assistant Professor of Aboriginal Health
Division of Community Health & Humanities
Faculty of Medicine
Memorial University
St. John's, Newfoundland

Bridget V. Stirling, RN, MPH, PhD
Assistant Professor
University of Calgary (Qatar Campus)
Doha, Qatar

Lawrence W. Svenson, PhD, FRSPH
Associate Professor
Division of Preventive Medicine
Faculty of Medicine and Dentistry
University of Alberta
Edmonton, Alberta

Janis M. Wegerhoff, RN, MN
Adjunct Professor
School of Nursing
Faculty of Health and Social Development
University of British Columbia (Okanagan Campus)
Kelowna, British Columbia

Michelle (Hogan) Yoksimovich, RN, MScN, PhD, COHN
Professor
Brock University–Loyalist College Collaborative
  Nursing Program
Belleville, Ontario

The fifth edition of this book, published in 2003 and often referred to as the "blue book," became a foundational text for students in medicine and public health. This new edition, revised, expanded, and illustrated in greater detail, is now aimed at a wider audience and should be of value both to professionals across the health sector and to students in nursing, allied health, public health, and medicine. Additionally, the title has changed from *Public Health and Preventive Medicine* to *Shah's Public Health and Preventive Health Care*. This change reflects the text's broader scope, with a focus on health promotion, prevention, the social determinants of health, and health equity. In honour of Dr. Shah, the founding author of the previous five editions and consultant on the sixth edition, the book title acknowledges his major contributions as a leader, teacher, and mentor in the field of public health and preventive health care.

The purpose of this book is to help readers learn about their roles as health care professionals, administrators, or policy makers by understanding the extent of health and disease in Canada and the functions and challenges of our health care system. It is also intended for members of the general public who are interested in participating in the ongoing debate on these issues by providing the fundamentals about the health and health care of Canadians. It is critical for all readers, regardless of their discipline or role, to understand the immense role that social and political forces have in shaping health and health care. It is only with this knowledge that a true multidisciplinary and holistic approach can be taken to understand issues lying at the root of the health inequities experienced in Canadian society and take action on such issues to create health for all. In this new edition, we emphasize action strategies to address health inequities that health professionals, administrators, or policy makers can implement. It is our belief that understanding is not enough, and that knowing what to do and how to take action must also be included in any public health textbook.

Much has changed since the fifth edition was published in 2003. Perhaps one of the most significant developments in the past decade was the establishment of the Truth and Reconciliation Commission (TRC) and its *Calls To Action* aimed at addressing the legacy of residential schools and moving towards reconciliation between Indigenous and non-Indigenous people of Canada. There is a growing recognition that reconciliation involves everyone. The TRC's calls to action in the area of health emphasize the need for students and professionals to be culturally competent, to understand Indigenous health issues (including the history and legacy of residential schools), and to recognize the value of Indigenous healing practices. In keeping with this goal, our sixth edition has included a chapter focused specifically on Indigenous health and has highlighted examples of Indigenous-led action and practice challenges in all areas of preventive health.

Just as reconciliation involves everybody, this book takes the view that efforts to enhance health equity and achieve health for all are the responsibility of all sectors of society and should be community led and strengths based. The addition of two new authors, Dr. Fournier (who holds a nursing degree and has more than 20 years of experience as a professor in academia) and Dr. Karachiwalla (who holds a medical degree with a range of experience in both primary care and public health practice), emphasizes the need for those with differing but complementary backgrounds to work together, share perspectives, and bridge the gap between academia and practice.

ACKNOWLEDGEMENTS

We sought a diverse group of reviewers and would like to specifically thank them. In addition, we thank Kathy Zhang for her support on a range of chapters and Marina Afanasyeva for her expertise in the area of occupational health.

We would like to acknowledge all the work that the editorial and publication teams did to support the Sixth Edition, specifically Martina van de Velde and Roberta Spinosa-Millman at Elsevier, who provided guidance, support, and patience.

NEW FEATURES IN THE SIXTH EDITION

This edition has been extensively revised. Examples have been updated using current Canadian and international research and statistics:

- NEW figures and fully revised tables to better illustrate complex concepts
- NEW chapter on **Indigenous health**
- NEW chapter on **mental health and substance use**
- NEW chapter on **groups experiencing health inequities**
- Learning tools in each chapter include the following:
  - **Learning Objectives** guide students in knowing what they should learn from the content.
  - **Chapter Outlines** provide an overview of the structure and content of each chapter.
  - **Key Terms** list the chapter's most important terms; they are identified at the beginning of each chapter and then boldfaced where they are introduced and defined within the chapter.
  - Themed boxes:
    - **Case Study** boxes present hypothetical patient scenarios relating to concepts discussed in the text, providing opportunities for students to reflect on content and how it can be applied to practice.
    - **Research Perspective** boxes present areas of research on specific topics discussed in the chapter, to provide further perspective for students.
    - **In the News** boxes provide examples of how specific health care topics and issues have been covered by the media.
    - **Interprofessional Practice** boxes highlight collaborative practice and the roles of various members on the health care team.
    - **Clinical Example** boxes provide examples of how tools and policies may look in clinical practice settings.
    - **Real-World Example** boxes provide examples of how specific concepts and policies discussed in the text have been applied in health care.
    - **Evidence-Informed Practice** boxes apply the latest research findings in public health and community health.
    - **Critical Thinking Questions** and **Exercises** for each major section in a chapter encourage students to reflect on specific topics, develop problem-solving skills, and consider how they might address current health care issues in practice.
- **Chapter summaries** provide a summary of the key points highlighted in each chapter.
- **Key Websites** direct students to tools and resources they can use in their practice.
- **References** have been thoroughly updated and are presented in APA format.

LEARNING SUPPLEMENTS FOR INSTRUCTORS AND STUDENTS

The sixth edition also features an Evolve website with additional resources for instructors and students, available at http://evolve.elsevier.com/Canada/Shah/publichealth/, and includes the following learning aids:

Evolve Instructor Resources

- Answer Guidelines for the in-text Critical Thinking Questions and Exercises
- Image Collection of the full-colour images from the text for use in lectures
- TEACH lesson plans with electronic resources organized by chapter to help instructors develop and manage the course curriculum. This exciting resource includes the following:
  - Objectives
  - Teaching Focus
  - Key Terms
  - Student and instructor resource listings
  - Detailed chapter outlines
  - Teaching strategies with learning activities
- Test Bank in ExamView software, allowing instructors to create new tests; edit, add, and delete test questions; sort questions by category, cognitive level, difficulty, and question type; and administer and grade online tests
- PowerPoint slides, organized by chapter, to assist instructors with lectures

Evolve Student Resources

- Glossary of all key terms from the text
- Review Questions to help review student understanding of the mains concepts discussed in each chapter

CONTENTS

Canada, which was founded on unceded Indigenous lands having the largest land mass second to Russia, with more than 100 comprehensive land claims and self-government negotiations established, is geographically and contextually diverse. Spread across 10 provinces and three territories, Canada's population reached 36 million in 2016, with two of three people (66%) living within 100 km of the southern Canada–United States border, an area that represents about 4% of Canada's territory (Statistics Canada, 2017). Additionally, approximately 18% of Canada's population lives in rural or remote communities dispersed throughout 95% of Canada's territory (Statistics Canada, 2017).

Canada is described as a federation governed by a parliamentary democratic system based on a British-style parliamentary system. The parliament consists of an elected House of Commons and an appointed Senate. The head of government is the prime minister. Under the Canadian Constitution, the federal government has relatively minimal power in the delivery of health and social services, with few exceptions. The provincial and territorial governments bear the principal responsibility for a broad range of social policy programs and services, including the majority of publicly financed and administered health services. Municipal and local governments also play a key role in the health of Canadians through improving the social, economic, and built environments. Municipalities adopt and implement healthy public policies (bylaws) to create or enhance the physical and social aspects of the environment where people live, learn, work, and play. Municipal bylaw examples include zoning that limits the location of fast food restaurants in school zones, establishing smoke-free recreational spaces, regulating idling control, and harm-reduction zoning that allows for needle exchanges or methadone clinics. Table I.1 outlines health responsibilities at the three levels of government (see Chapter 13 for a historical review).

The last statement in the Canadian Constitution, which states ". . . Peace, Order & Good Government," reflects how Canadians view government's role in "public good." By and large, Canadians want and expect their government to be involved when it comes to their health and well-being, their environment, the air they breathe, and the water they drink, and they want to have a social security network when they are unemployed, disabled, or retire. This can be seen in Canadians' firmly held values about their health care, which are reflected in decades of polling data. In data from 1985 to 2002, for example, what mattered most to Canadians was our health care system. Canadians are proud of their health care system and supportive of the Canada Health Act, but they are also very worried about the future of the system (Mendelsohn, 2002). Although they are extremely proud of their system, they are constantly vigilant that it stays responsive to their future needs.

The strategic and service delivery plans of the provinces and territories all share two common goals. The first goal is improving overall population health, including optimal health and well-being, through health promotion and disease prevention policies and increasing mindfulness of the social determinants of health. The second goal is improving health system performance, focusing on the accessibility (especially of primary care services), quality, safety, and effectiveness of health services. Most strategic plans also emphasize the sustainability of a publicly funded system through ensuring value for money.

Improving the health of Canadians means ensuring that our health system is efficient and provides the highest quality of care. The World Health Organization (WHO) defines health systems as "all the activities whose primary purpose is to promote, restore or maintain health" (WHO, 2000, p. 5; WHO, 2016). Health systems therefore include both *health care services* provided to individuals and groups and *public health services* and *policies* (Table I.2). Health care services include preventive, diagnostic, therapeutic, rehabilitative, and palliative care services targeted to individuals or specific population groups.,

Public health is defined as "the organized efforts of society to keep people healthy and prevent injury, illness and premature death" (Government of Canada, 2008). As evidenced by this definition, public health activities are much broader than the health care system and most often consist of the following key functions: population health assessment, surveillance, disease and injury

TABLE I.1   Federal, Provincial, and Municipal Health Responsibilities

Federal	Provincial	Municipal or Local

• Canadian Health Transfer Payments
• Health research
• Data collection
• Public health and health protection
• Funding, administration, and delivery of services to:
  • First Nations and Inuit
  • War veterans
  • Members of the Canadian Forces and the Royal Canadian Mounted Police
  • Inmates of federal penitentiaries
	• Funding, administration, and delivery of health care:
	  • Hospitals
	  • Physician remuneration
	  • Drug plans
	  • Long-term care
	  • Home care
	  • Mental health
	  • Other health services
		• Waste and waste management
		• Water
		• Social services
		  • Housing
		• Parks, recreation, culture
		• Bylaws for healthy public policy (e.g., environment, transportation)

TABLE I.2   Public Health versus Health Care

	Public Health	Health Care
Target	Population	Individual patient
Tools for assessment	Epidemiology, biostatistics	Diagnostic imaging, laboratory results
Relationship between practitioner and client	Indirect	Direct
Emphasis	Promotion and prevention	Treatment

prevention, health protection, health promotion, and emergency preparedness. Public health activities focus on health determinants that apply to the entire population (Canadian Institute for Health Information [CIHI], 2014). The goal of the public health system is to keep people out of the health care system. Key differences between the public health system and the health care system are listed in Table I.2.

Improving the health of the population while responding to people's legitimate expectations and protecting them against the cost of ill health through a variety of activities is the role of health systems, including public health (WHO, 2016). Strengthening health systems leads to improved health.

Although public health activities are broadly defined, this book focuses on public health efforts that relate to health care and the Canadian health system at large. It focuses primarily on public health work common to Canadian public health agencies (including ensuring healthy physical and social environments), with a clear recognition however, that almost all levels of government and all sectors of society (including arts, economics, and so on) influence the health of Canadians. When possible, these examples are drawn out to reinforce this notion.

TEXT ORGANIZATION

This sixth edition of *Shah's Public Health and Preventive Health Care in Canada* provides an introductory overview that is geared toward undergraduate students in various health disciplines, as well as others who are interested in knowing about Canadian health and health care system. The first three chapters provide an overview of the prevailing concept of what is meant by the terms health and disease, disability, determinants of health, and strategies to improve health, followed by commonly used tools to measure health and commonly used health indicators.

The understanding of health care and the public health system described earlier grounds this sixth edition of the text with a recognition that good information is required to make better decisions and ultimately will lead to better health outcomes for Canadians. Therefore, we have chosen to adopt the Canadian Institute for Health Information's (CIHI) Health System Performance Measurement Framework (HSPMF), which has four distinct quadrants (foci) (Fig. 1.1), as the basis for the following chapters in this text. The HSPMF is a well-accepted national model. Building on the CIHI–Statistics Canada

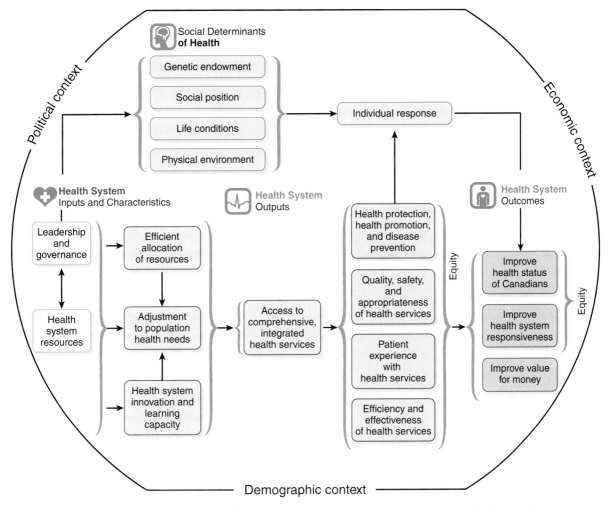

Fig. 1.1 Health System Performance Measurement Framework. (From Canadian Institute for Health Information [2012]. *A Performance Measurement Framework for the Canadian Health System* (p. iv). Ottawa: Author. Retrieved from https://secure.cihi.ca/free_products/HSP-Framework-ENweb.pdf.)

Health Indicators Framework, which is internationally recognized, the HSPMF not only classifies performance information but also transforms it into an actionable framework, offering analytical and interpretive dimensions that can be used to manage and improve health system performance.

In line with the WHO's conceptual framework of the determinants of health, the CIHI model reflects the influential nature of political (e.g., government of the day, democratic tools), economic (e.g., country level resources and ideas about wealth distribution), and demographic (e.g., aging, new immigrant, Indigenous populations) factors on health. According to this model,

the health system is divided into four interrelated quadrants: (1) Health System Inputs and Characteristics, (2) Health System Outputs, (3) Health System Outcomes, and (4) Social Determinants of Health. The four quadrants of the framework are linked together in a causal chain, symbolized by the arrows that connect the quadrants and illustrate the nature of the expected relationships among the quadrants.

In the book, before we can look at the outputs and outcomes of the health system, it is essential that students learn some basic knowledge regarding the concept of health and disease in modern society, measurement of health, how different health indices are derived, and how one can achieve health for all. These concepts are discussed in Chapters 1 to 3.

The focus is always on the end goal of producing better outcomes within a high-performing health system. Within this framework, performance is viewed as a dynamic process in a constant state of change:

1. *Social Determinants of Health*: Within the framework, there is an acknowledgement that individuals are profoundly influenced by where they live, learn, work, grow, and play. This quadrant includes the factors that are outside of the health system and influence a population's health behaviour. As shown in the framework, individual responses to health system outputs are impacted by structural factors of social determinants of health, which are social position, life condition, physical environment, and genetic endowment. These factors shape individuals' and families' socioeconomic positions, such as income and social status, education, gender, and ethnicity. Structural factors can also impact biological, material, psychosocial, and behavioural factors, which are collectively referred to as "intermediary determinants of health." Subfactors of the intermediary determinants of health include:

   a. Biological: genetic endowment, aging processes, and sex-related biology
   b. Material: characteristics of neighbourhoods, homes, workplaces, and the physical environment
   c. Psychosocial stress, sense of self-control, social support networks
   d. Behavioural: physical exercise, diet, substance use, and nutrition

These intermediary determinants of health can influence an individual's health both positively and negatively. Measuring the intermediary determinants of health is essential to understand what shapes population health and health inequality. Although it is imperative to recognize that social determinants of health play an important role in population and public health, having an efficient health system could allow resources to be reallocated to other governmental sectors such as education (e.g., prenatal education and early childhood education to prevent low birth weights and child obesity) and social services (e.g., home health care, rehabilitation, and community support).

We address the various aspects of the social determinants of health in Chapters 1 and 5.

2. *Health System Outcomes*: This quadrant corresponds to three inherent goals of the Canadian health system: improve health status of Canadians, improve health system responsiveness, and improve value for money.

   a. The goal of improving the health status of Canadians is subdivided into the following three elements:
      i. Health conditions, which are health problems and changes of health status, such as diseases and injuries. These conditions can be measured in the population by prevalence rate, incidence rates, or condition-specific mortality rates.
      ii. Human functioning, which is the general health status and functioning capacity of the population, associated with the consequences of illness. It can be measured by potential years of life lost or healthy life expectancy.
      iii. Well-being, which is the level of physical, mental, and social well-being of individuals. It can be measured by examining material conditions, quality of life, and sustainability of well-being over time.

   b. Improving health system responsiveness means the health system must provide services to improve population health in a way that satisfies the needs and expectations of the people it serves. This goal also implies an equitable distribution of health status and system responsiveness across different socioeconomic cohorts.

   c. Improving value for money indicates the level of achievement of health system outcomes in relation to the resources used. The term "value" in the framework pinpoints the ability of the health system to balance the allocation of resources to obtain the best health outcomes, such as health status, health system responsiveness, and equity for the resources used.

These three goals are also referred to as the three performance dimensions under the health system outcomes quadrant. The dimension of equity is applied to the first two dimensions.

These dimensions are discussed in Chapters 5 through 12.

3. *Health System Inputs and Characteristics*: This quadrant represents the internal components of the health system. The internal components are considered to be prerequisites of health system performance; they influence performance directly and are viewed as levers of health system performance improvement.

As shown in the framework, the internal components are leadership and governance, efficient allocation of health system resources, adjustment to population health needs, and health system innovation and learning capacity.

These areas are discussed in Chapters 13 through 17.

4. *Health System Outputs*: This quadrant contains dimensions relating to characteristics of the health services produced by the health system. It can be divided into two components. The first component represents the capacity of the system to deliver high-quality services, such as health promotion and disease prevention, to the population in an equitable way. The second component reflects the quality attributions of health services: person centred, safe, appropriate and effective, and efficiently delivered. The two components of this quadrant contain five dimensions of performance: (1) access; (2) health protection, promotion, and disease prevention; (3) quality, safety, and appropriateness of health services; (4) patient experience; and (5) efficiency. The outputs discussed in this quadrant include all outputs from the provision of health services via different health sectors: primary, acute, community, promotion, and prevention. The attainment of outputs from these care sectors impacts the success of health system outcomes.

These dimensions of performance are discussed in Chapter 15.

LIMITATIONS OF THE TEXT

As indicated, this text covers a very large number of topics, and many of these topics could easily become a text unto themselves. However, because the information in the text is intended to be introductory in nature, a more in-depth analysis of each topic can be done through course assignments, whereby students could analyze their own province or territory for local solutions.

REFERENCES

Canadian Institute for Health Information. (2014). *Population health and health care*. Retrieved from https://secure.cihi.ca/free_products/CIHI_Bridiging_Final_EN_web.pdf.

Government of Canada. (2008). Chapter 2: The Chief Public Health Officer's report on the state of public health in Canada 2008—What is public health? Retrieved from https://www.canada.ca/en/public-health/corporate/publications/chief-public-health-officer-reports-state-public-health-canada/report-on-state-public-health-canada-2008/chapter-2a.html.

Mendelsohn, M. (2002). *Canadians' thoughts on their health care system: preserving the Canadian model through innovation*. Saskatoon, SK: Commission on the Future of Health Care in Canada.

Statistics Canada. (2017). *Population size and growth in Canada: Key results from the 2016 Census*. Retrieved from https://www150.statcan.gc.ca/n1/daily-quotidien/170208/dq170208a-eng.htm.

World Health Organization. (2000). *The world health report 2000. Health systems: Improving performance*. Retrieved from http://www.who.int/whr/2000/en/whr00_en.pdf?ua=1.

World Health Organization). (2016). *Strategizing national health in the 21st century: A handbook*. Geneva: WHO. Retrieved from https://www.who.int/healthsystems/publications/nhpsp-handbook/en/.

PART 1

Achieving Health For All

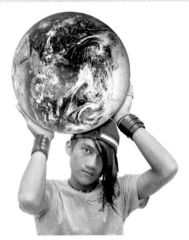

Fleying/Canstockphoto.com

The primary determinants of disease are mainly economic and social, and therefore its remedies must also be economic and social. Medicine and politics cannot and should not be kept apart.
Geoffrey Rose, *The Strategy of Preventive Medicine*

Social injustice is killing people on a grand scale.
Commission on Social Determinants of Health

The "health for all" movement began in the early 1980s, when the World Health Assembly adopted a Global Strategy for Health for All by the Year 2000. The movement did not mean an end to disease and disability but that resources for health would be evenly distributed and essential health care would be accessible to everyone. However, nearly 40 years later, we are still working toward "health for all."

For health care professionals, it is vital to understand what makes people healthy. Public health practice is an approach to maintaining and improving the health of populations that is based on attention to human rights, evidence-informed policy and practice, and addressing the underlying determinants of health. The foundation of all public health activities are the concepts of social justice and health equity, which relate to taking action on the social determinants of health (Canadian Public Health Association [CPHA], 2017).

Part I of this book deals with the foundational concepts of population and public health and includes a focus on health and disease, the social determinants of health, health promotion, inequalities, inequities, and social justice. A synopsis of the methods and strategies used in determining the factors that influence health and disease is discussed and then, subsequently, how we can address these factors to improve health is covered. This section provides evidence that what determines our health goes beyond traditional health care to the social and economic influences in our society. Canada has led the world in this regard since publishing the Lalonde Report in 1974 and Ottawa Charter for Health Promotion in 1986.

Foundational Concepts in Population and Public Health

Additional resources are available online at http://evolve.elsevier.com/Canada/Shah/publichealth/

OBJECTIVES

- Define population health and understand the history as it relates to health promotion.
- Describe and differentiate among various concepts of health, disease, and illness.
- Name and describe three views of health.
- Describe the range of factors that determine the health of a population.
- Define and differentiate among the concepts of health inequality, health inequity, and social justice.
- Describe the Public Health Core Competencies.
- List the reasons public health ethics differs from biomedical ethics.
- Apply a framework of public health ethics to a population health intervention.

CHAPTER OUTLINE

KEY TERMS

activity limitation
behavioural model of health
biomedical model of health
built environment
determinants of health
disability
disease
epidemiological triangle
etiology
germ theory of disease

gradient
health
health promotion
illness
illness behaviour
impairment
inequalities
inequities
intermediary determinants of health

noncommunicable diseases (NCDs)
participation restriction
population health
primary health care (PHC)
social determinants of health
social justice
socioenvironmental model of health
structural determinants of health

INTRODUCTION

In Canada, many diseases, particularly **communicable diseases** (i.e., conditions that are infectious in nature or are transmitted person to person or between animals and people; Seeberg & Meinert, 2015), have been controlled with the advent of better living conditions, the availability of antibiotics, new technology (see Chapter 18), and public health interventions, such as immunization and universal health care. Mortality in the population has been drastically reduced, and life span has increased. However, **noncommunicable diseases (NCDs)** (i.e., conditions that are not transmissible between people and are more often chronic in nature, such as heart disease or cancer; Seeberg & Meinert, 2015) have emerged as important health concerns and are more prevalent in specific populations.

In this chapter, we review the foundational concepts of public health and population health to set the groundwork for the remaining chapters in Part I. We discuss the concepts of health, disease, social determinants of health, health promotion, inequality, inequity, and social justice. We conclude the chapter with a discussion of public health competencies and public health ethics because they should be considered critical in the planning of population health strategies and interventions.

POPULATION HEALTH

A Brief History

The Public Health Agency of Canada (PHAC) defines **population health** (PH) as "an approach to health that aims to improve the health of the entire population and to reduce health inequities among population groups" (PHAC, 2012). Population health approaches explicitly consider how societal influences and the determinants of health exert a profound influence on health and well-being throughout the life cycle. The outcomes or benefits of a population health approach, therefore, extend beyond improved population health outcomes to include a sustainable and integrated health system, increased national growth and productivity, and strengthened social cohesion and citizen engagement.

Population health builds on a long tradition of public health and health promotion. However, the concept was derived from the work of the Canadian Institute for Advanced Research (CIAR) (Evans & Stoddart, 1990), which defined health in terms of epidemiological indicators and focused on determinants of disease and death rather than strategies for change. Shortly after the publication of the CIAR model of population health, the Canadian government adopted and adapted it. In 1994, a federal, provincial, and territorial advisory committee on population health was created. Several Canadian documents were published that focused on population health but included a much broader definition of health than the CIAR model, such as *Strategies for Population Health: Investing in the health of Canadians*, *Population Health Promotion: An Integrated Model of Population Health and Health Promotion* (Hamilton & Bhatti, 1996; see Chapter 3), *Taking Action on Population Health: A Position Paper for Health Promotion and Programs Branch Staff* (Health Canada, 1998), and *Population Health—Putting Concepts into Action* (Zollner & Lessof, 1998). The Health Promotion Directorate was replaced by the Population Health Directorate in 1995, and 2 years later, the federal Cabinet adopted the population health approach to guide health policy. It wasn't until 2004 that health promotion surfaced again within the federal government, with the creation of an internal Center for Health Promotion based in the Public Health Agency of Canada branch. The term *population health promotion* is being used to describe both health promotion and population health and reflects a shift in how health is defined, as will be discussed in the next section (Box 1.1).

Definitions of Health

This section focuses primarily on definitions and notions of health and disease and explores theories of disease causation. The various definitions and views of

---

BOX 1.1   Canada's Role in Health as a Basic Human Right

The Senate Subcommittee on Population Health was established in 2007 with the aim of examining and reporting on the social determinants of health in the Canadian population. It also investigated the effects of social determinants of health on existing health disparities and inequities. In June 2009, the Subcommittee submitted *A Healthy, Productive Canada: A Determinant of Health Approach* to the Senate, in which it clearly stated the premise that health is a basic human right (Senate Subcommittee on Population Health, 2009). Good health for all is a responsibility of society as a whole and is a prerequisite for individuals and communities to function well.

health are significant because how you define health dic-tates the strategies you will use to promote health and prevent disease.

The World Health Organization (WHO) consti-tution, formed in 1946, states: "the enjoyment of the highest attainable standard of health is one of the fun-damental rights of every human being without dis-tinction of race, religion, political belief, economic or social condition" (WHO, 1946). We have a right to health; therefore, we have a right to all of the prereq-uisites of health. Health is multidimensional: it is not merely the presence or absence of disease but also has social, psychological, and cultural determinants and consequences. In 1948, the WHO defined health as "a complete state of physical, mental and social well-being and not merely the absence of illness" (WHO, 1946). In 1986, the WHO developed a new definition of health (see Exercise 1.1). However, there are still predominant views of health that continue to impact the approaches taken to achieve health for all.

Three Views of Health

There are different ways to view health, which can be organized into three major theories or approaches: bio-medical, behavioural (lifestyle), and socioenvironmen-tal (Labonte, 1993).

EXERCISE 1.1: Comparing and Contrasting Definitions of Health from the World Health Organization

In 1986, the WHO introduced a new definition of health as "the ability to identify and to realize aspirations, to satisfy needs, and to change or cope with the environ-ment. Health is therefore a resource for everyday life, not the objective of living. Health is a positive concept emphasizing social and personal resources, as well as physical capacities."

Compare and contrast the WHO's 1986 definition with its original 1946 definition. What are some key differences?

Biomedical View of Health. Just as definitions of health have changed over time, so have theories about the nature and causes of disease. Recently, the role ascribed to social and psychological factors in the causal processes leading to disease has received increasing attention. Underlying much of what con-stitutes medical practice is the biomedical model. This has its roots in the 17th century, a time when mind and body were seen as separate entities, the body being a physical entity activated by mental processes. According to this view, the body is akin to a machine, which can be corrected when things go wrong by procedures designed to repair damage or restore functioning. Thus, the model focuses on the causes and treatment of ill health and disease in terms of biological cause and effect. This approach ignores the part played by social, psychological, spiritual, and economic factors in disease onset and recovery.

A critical assessment of the history of disease reveals that major communicable diseases, such as tuberculosis and cholera, began to decline long before the introduction of effective therapy. Improvements in sanitation, nutrition, and general living conditions are now thought to be important factors in reducing the mortality resulting from these scourges (Prüss-Üstün & Neira, 2016). Second, the evaluation of the factors underlying today's major causes of death and disability has been illuminating. For example, motor vehicle collisions, which constitute the major cause of death and potential years of life lost in young adults, are largely the result of risk-taking behaviours and the broader socioeconomic and psychosocial factors that influence such behaviours. Deaths caused by motor vehicle collisions cannot be reduced by traditional forms of medical treatment but require behavioural changes, such as increased caution, sobriety, the use of seatbelts, and changes in the conditions that lead to that behaviour (e.g., social norms; laws affecting access to alcohol; engineering in cars, such as stan-dard inclusion of seatbelts, rearview cameras, field disturbance sensors). Therefore, a concept of health must include other factors in addition to traditional curative medicine.

Behavioural (Lifestyle) View of Health. The down-fall of the **biomedical model of health** is that it does not adequately emphasize or expand upon all the other influencers of health—including people's day-to-day behaviours, shaped by their environments (political, economical, and social). The **behavioural model of health** posits that people's behaviours are primarily what cause disease and that solutions to improve health include working on changing people's behaviours (e.g., getting them to stop smoking or to eat healthier). This theory is limited by the fact that it does not account for the larger influencers on people's behaviours day to day, such as their environment (and how easy or difficult it is for them to engage in health-promoting behaviours such as eating well and exercising).

Socioenvironmental View of Health. The **socioenvironmental model of health** is a more comprehensive theory and is the one embraced in this book. According to this model, health is seen more holistically as the product of one's environment (political, economic, and psychosocial). These determinants of health influence one's behaviour; thus, achieving good health for all means not only focusing on individual level behaviour change but also on policy change, advocacy, and community development and mobilization in multiple different sectors to improve health (Public Health Ontario [PHO], 2014a).

According to this socioenvironmental definition, **health** is "the ability to identify and to realize aspirations, to satisfy needs, and to change or cope with the environment. Health is therefore a resource for everyday life, not the objective of living. Health is a positive concept emphasizing social and personal resources, as well as physical capacities" (CPHA & WHO, 1986). Measures of health must incorporate these distinct dimensions of human experience. What determines health is more than simply factors relating to biology or genetics. Health encompasses social and political concerns and the relationship of individuals to their environment. The **determinants of health**, a concept that is very instrumental to public health, are defined as the conditions in which people are born, grow, live, work and age (WHO, n.d.-a). From this perspective, health is the responsibility not only of the traditional health care sector but also of all the sectors, institutions, and organizations that may influence the well-being of individuals and communities. In infectious or communicable diseases, the influence of other sectors in the control of disease and prevention of epidemics is recognized (e.g., trade policies, housing regulations, restaurant

inspection); nonetheless, there remains much to do in acknowledging the roles of nonhealth sectors in the prevention and control of NCDs. To enjoy the "highest attainable standard of health," inequities must be reduced.

Health Inequalities

At the heart of our modern-day health issues, such as NCDs, are **inequalities** in health. Inequalities are differences in health status among population groups defined by specific characteristics and can be empirically determined, such as differences between males and females. It is important to note that the terms "health inequalities'" and "health **inequities**" are often used interchangeably; however, they are different, and it is important to clarify their differences because they reflect different perspectives on the "causes" of health outcomes, indicating different solutions. *Health inequality*, for example, is a higher incidence of disease X in group A compared with group B of population P. If disease X is randomly or equally distributed among all groups of population P, then there is no presence of health inequality in that population. Although health inequality is an empirical concept, easily determined by epidemiological data, health inequity, on the other hand, is a normative concept. *Health inequity* refers to inequalities in health that are deemed to be unfair or unjust. It could be argued that most of the health inequalities across class and ethnicity are unjust because they reflect an unfair distribution of the underlying social determinants of health (e.g., educational opportunities, safe working conditions).

Some social groups have markedly better health than others, with lower death rates and less illness and disability. For example, in Canada, poorer health outcomes exist among populations living in poverty, persons living with disabilities, LGBTQ2S+ individuals, Indigenous peoples, persons living in rural and remote communities, and immigrants and refugees, to name a few (Senate Subcommittee on Population Health, 2009). (Some of these groups and the health inequities they experience are discussed further in Chapter 6.) Differences in health can also be connected to geographic location, race or ethnic origin, and employment status.

There are now documented statistical links between health and socioeconomic position (Williams, Priest,

BOX 1.2 Is Rising Inequality Responsible for Greater Stress, Anxiety, and Mental Illness?

Wilkinson and Pickett (2019) argue in their book, *The Spirit Level*, that inequality creates greater social competition and divisions, which in turn foster increased social anxiety and higher stress and thus greater incidence of mental illness, dissatisfaction, and resentment. And that leads to coping strategies—drugs, alcohol, and addictive behaviours such as shopping and gambling—which themselves generate further stress and anxiety. This book builds on their previous work which demonstrated that income inequality affects everyone in society. Their analysis shows that people at all levels of the social hierarchy do better in more equal societies.

& Anderson, 2016; Lago et al., 2017; PHAC, 2018b). At each rung up the income ladder, Canadians have less sickness, longer life expectancies, and improved health. Data from other countries have also shown a clear inverse relationship between socioeconomic position (income level, education level, and status and position in society) and a wide range of health indicators, including acute and chronic illness rates, days of restricted activity, psychiatric symptoms, high blood pressure, height, obesity, low birth weight, prematurity, ability to conceive, and self-perceived health (PHAC, 2018b). Moreover, there is evidence to show that these differences have widened over the past 4 decades despite universal access to health care in many developed countries, demonstrating that that there are more powerful determinants for health than the health care system (Box 1.2).

Explanations for Socially Produced Inequalities in Health. A number of explanations account for the association between socioeconomic position and health. In 1977, the United Kingdom government created a working group to investigate the relationship between social position and health and produced the *Black Report*, which summarized the evidence about the relationship between occupation and health. It showed that those who were classified as unskilled manual workers (social class V) consistently had poorer health status than those who were classified as professionals (social class I). The report clearly documented the link between social

position and health. Explanations for this abound and include the following:

- **Natural and social selection:** The social gradient in health is caused by those who are already unhealthy moving down the socioeconomic scale, but those who are healthy move up the socioeconomic scale (Cundiff, Boylan, Pardini, & Matthews, 2017).
- **Materialist and structuralist explanations:** Groups at the lower end of the socioeconomic scale lack adequate financial and other resources to maintain their physical and psychological well-being and to protect themselves from hazardous physical or social environments. The argument against the materialist explanation is that the relationship between income and health status follows a **gradient**, with each successively lower income grouping having successively lower health status. In general, the lower an individual's socioeconomic position, the worse their health. There is a social gradient in health that runs from the top to the bottom of the socioeconomic spectrum. The social gradient in health means that health inequities affect everyone.
- **Neomaterialist mechanism:** This ascribes the gradient in health status across income levels to individuals at each income level having, for example, less well-balanced diets, less adequate housing, more exposure to hazardous working conditions or environmental toxins than individuals at the next highest income level, and less access to social infrastructure (Lynch & Kaplan, 1997).
- **Cultural and behavioural explanations:** Individuals are less healthy because they consume health-damaging substances such as tobacco and alcohol at higher rates, have diets high in sugars and fats and low in fibre, are less likely to exercise regularly, and make less use of preventive health services (Allen et al., 2017). Building on these explanations Marinko, Shi, Starfield, and Wulu (2003) articulated six explanations using a micro and macro approach (Table 1.1).

Inequities and Social Justice

The systematic differences in inequalities are referred to as health inequities when they are avoidable, unnecessary, and unfair (Dahlgren & Whitehead, 1991), which are rooted in a value orientation of social justice (WHO, 2008). **Social justice** can be defined as "the fair distribution of society's benefits, responsibilities, and their

TABLE 1.1 Explanations of Income Inequalities

Explanation	Description of Income Inequality
Psychosocial (micro): social status	The experience of living in social settings of inequality forces people constantly to compare their status, possessions, and life circumstances with those of others, engendering feelings of shame and worthlessness among the disadvantaged, along with chronic stress that undermines health.
Psychosocial (macro): social cohesion	Income inequality erodes social bonds that allow people to work together, decreases social resources, and results in low trust and civic participation, greater crime, and other unhealthy conditions.
Material (micro): individual income	Income inequality means fewer economic resources among the poorest, resulting in lessened ability to avoid risks, treat injury or disease, or prevent illness
Materialist (macro): social disinvestment	Income inequality results in less investment in social and environmental conditions (safe housing, good schools) necessary for promoting health among the poorest.
Statistical artifact	The poorest in any society are usually the sickest. A society with high levels of income inequality has high numbers of poor and consequently has more people who are sick.
Health selection	People are not sick because they are poor. Rather, poor health lowers one's income and limits one's earning potential.

Adapted from Murray, M., & Marks, D. F. (2008). Challenging social inequalities in health (Table 1, p. 5). From R. Crane (Ed.), *Handbook of families and poverty.* London: Sage. Based on Marinko, J. A., Shi, L., Starfield, B., & Wulu, J. T. (2003). Income inequality and health: A critical review of the literature. *Medical Care Research and Reviews, 60,* 334–347, 407–452.

consequences. It focuses on the relative position of one social group in relationship to others in society, as well as on the root causes of disparities [inequalities] and what can be done to eliminate them" (Canadian Nurses Association, 2006, p. 7).

A growing body of research has shown that the systematically unequal distribution of power, prestige, and resources (economic and social) creates health inequities and affects where individuals work, live, learn, and play (Raphael, 2008). Political and economic forces, also known as political economy, suggest that inequities exist because of the production and distribution of wealth, the relative political power of social classes, and the extent to which society relies extensively on market control of the distribution of resources—neoliberal ideology (Raphael & Bryant, 2006). Social democratic nations create the conditions necessary for health. These conditions include equitable distribution of wealth and progressive tax policies that create a large middle class; strong programs that support children, families, and women; and economies that support full employment (Navarro & Shi, 2001).

Public policies, such as labour policies, employment policies, provision of social safety nets, and the degree of availability of health and social services determine the distribution of resources and thus create systematic differences in health, which are avoidable by reasonable action and are unfair and unjust (WHO, 2008). Public policy decisions made by governments are themselves driven by a variety of political, economic, and social forces, constituting a complex space in which the relationship between politics, policy, and health works itself out (WHO, 2008). Any serious effort to reduce health inequities will involve changing the distribution of power within society to the benefit of disadvantaged groups. Developing strategies that lead to a more just and healthy society are needed. Raphael and Bryant (2006) call on health promoters and population health researchers to "get political" and recognize the importance of political and social action in support of health (see Chapter 3).

Spirituality and Health

Spirituality also represents a deviation from conventional ways in how health and health care are conceptualized. Spirituality encompasses the practices, beliefs, and values that a person holds concerning his or her place in the cosmos. Spirituality is a fundamental part of being human, and to one degree or another, all humans tend to search for meaning and purpose in their lives, as well as connectedness to others, themselves, and the world around them (the core parts of spirituality). Spirituality can exist in the context of organized religion or not. Regardless, over the past couple of decades, the importance of spirituality to health and health care has been recognized and written about more. Specifically, more clients interfacing with the health care system have a desire to include spiritual dimensions in their care, and this inclusion of spirituality has been known to improve client outcomes, as well as client-centeredness (Puchalski, Blatt, Kogan, & Butler, 2014). Achieving high spiritual well-being positively impacts quality of life. The mechanisms through which it does so are likely multifold. One way in which having high spiritual well-being is thought to influence health is that spirituality helps promote good coping mechanisms (e.g., when people face significant life stressors) and fosters feelings of being emotionally supported (Fabbris et al., 2017). Its impact on health may be through a psychoneurohumoral mechanism that reduces stress and through social connectedness, which increases one's social network. The spiritual model incorporates a holistic approach in which healing plays a central role.

Healing is different from treatment. Treatment focuses on discrete physical abnormalities to mitigate them or cure the body. Healing applies to *all* dimensions of a person's existence; correcting a physical abnormality is but one aspect of a healing approach. In healing, how an illness affects the psychological and spiritual dimensions of the affected person's life must be considered.

Examples of spiritual practices can include mindfulness, meditation, and yoga—all of which are more commonly being embraced by North American society (Jain, Khatri, & Jamadar, 2015). Meditation has been shown to have positive benefits. In a recent study of medical students, for example, the practice of meditating twice a day for 15 minutes for a couple of months improved self-esteem, as well as anxiety levels (Jain et al., 2015). Mindfulness is an approach that highlights the importance of focusing one's attention on the here and now. Mindfulness has shown positive results when it comes to improving the well-being of people with type 2 diabetes, mental health conditions such as depression, and HIV, likely through reducing the production of stress hormones and improving control over one's emotions (Sadipun, Dwidiyanti, & Andriany, 2018). The practice of yoga, which encompasses a broad range of techniques, such as breathing, meditation, and self-knowledge,

> **BOX 1.3   Spirituality and Living Longer and Healthier Lives**
>
> Research by Shah (2003) reported that 43,000 deaths annually could be blamed on poor spiritual beliefs. There are health benefits from being a spiritual person, such as reduced stress, and evidence that spirituality promotes healthy lifestyles and increases social connectedness. Spirituality can also lessen the need for pleasure-seeking and risk-taking behaviours such as drinking, smoking, material gain, or promiscuous sex.

among others, has increased dramatically in the population. It, too, has been shown to improve spirituality and be beneficial for health conditions, such as postmenopausal symptoms, low back pain, cancer, and heart disease (Park, Braun, & Siegel, 2015) (Box 1.3).

Disease and Illness

The strength of this broad definition of health is that it includes psychosocial as well as biophysical dimensions. **Disease** refers to abnormal, *medically* defined changes in the structure or functioning of the human body; **illness** (or sickness) refers to the *individual's experience* or *subjective perception* of lack of physical or mental well-being and consequent inability to function normally in social roles.

The International Classification of Functioning, Disability and Health (ICF) is a framework developed by the WHO to classify and measure health and disability at the individual and population level. The ICF defines disability quite broadly, positing that disability results from an interaction between people with a certain health condition (e.g., cerebral palsy), personal factors (e.g., attitude, motivation, self-esteem), and environmental factors (e.g., social supports, accessible transport). They use **disability** as an umbrella term to encompass three concepts: impairment, activity limitations, and participation restrictions (WHO, 2018a). **Impairment** is defined as any loss or abnormality of psychological, physiological, or anatomical structure or function. **Activity limitation**, on the other hand, occurs when a person is challenged in performing a certain task or action. Finally, **participation restriction** occurs when a person cannot be involved in a specific domain of life (e.g., employment). Activity limitation, participation restriction, and impairment all result from factors related to the health condition, person, and environment

(WHO, n.d.-b). This definition really highlights the importance of a person's surroundings for shaping whether or not they are considered to have a disability. In this definition, a person with cerebral palsy who lives in a community with lots of social supports, a lack of discrimination in employment and other domains of life, and an accessible infrastructure may have very few limitations when it comes to activities and participation in day-to-day roles compared with a person with the same physiological impairments who lives in an environment where they cannot easily get around (because of inaccessible sidewalks and buildings, for example) or they face a range of discriminatory attitudes when it comes to work or personal relationships.

These conceptual distinctions point to the many ways in which a person's environment influences their health. For example, individuals with paraplegia can better participate in the workforce if they can access the building in which they work, or if they can work from home via electronic devices. Similarly, providing income assistance to people living with disabilities (which many provinces and territories do) allows such people who may be unable to participate in the workforce to secure housing, healthy foods, and other basic necessities. Societal interventions such as these help to create conditions that support meaningful integration of individuals with activity limitations or restricted participation in society. The community health and population health models that are described in a later section and the conceptual model of health indicators described in Chapter 4 take similar approaches to the multidimensionality of health.

Theories of Disease Causation

The **germ theory of disease** emerged at the end of the 19th century. Although the idea that disease was caused by a communicable agent had existed since the 16th century, it was verified only in the late 19th century. Louis Pasteur and Robert Koch showed that these agents (germs) were living organisms that enter the body via food, water, or air. From this theory emerged the doctrine of specific **etiology**: the idea that each disease has a single and specific cause.

The germ theory suggests that many diseases are caused by the growth and reproduction of specific microorganisms within a host body. However, this is usually not true because we are exposed to a lot of different organisms every day yet rarely get sick. So, it is incorrect

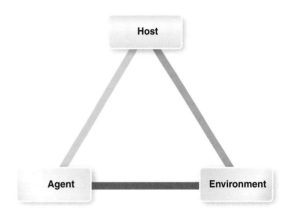

Fig. 1.1 The epidemiological triangle.

to designate an organism or any other noxious agent as the sole cause of disease.

From an epidemiological point of view, an agent (e.g., transmissible organism) is necessary but not sufficient because suitable conditions for the host and the environment must also be present for disease to develop (Virtual Campus for Public Health, n.d.). The **epidemiological triangle** in Fig. 1.1 shows the interaction among agent, host, and environment. The agent may be chemical (e.g., lead), biological (e.g., bacteria), or physical (e.g., violence); host factors may be genetic or acquired and influence susceptibility to disease; environmental factors may be biological, social, or physical and may affect exposure and susceptibility. Thus, all diseases are multifactorial and may be preventable by changing factors specific to the host, environment, or agent (if possible). Successful control of diseases usually requires action on multiple points of the epidemiological triangle.

Although the epidemiological triad has most often been applied to communicable diseases, it has also been used to explain and address phenomena such as injuries. For example, applying the epidemiological triangle to mortality caused by motor vehicle collisions may help us not only to understand some of the factors that increase the chance of death but also the ways in which we can intervene as a society to address it. In this example, the agent can be considered the vehicle. Vehicles that are much older, which may not have a good brakes or tires, can be more prone to accidents. Hosts (or drivers) are more prone to collisions if they have consumed alcohol or cannabis, and the road or broader environment may also have a significant impact on collision rates. For example, roads that have very few lights can result in more nighttime accidents.

CRITICAL THINKING QUESTION 1.2: What strategies or interventions would you use to address disease or promote health for each view of health (biomedical, behavioural, and socioenvironmental)?

CONCEPTUALIZATIONS OF THE SOCIAL DETERMINANTS OF HEALTH

There have been many conceptualizations of the social determinants of health over the past 40 years. Concern for the social determinants of health is not new and has been traced back to the mid-1800s, when the living conditions were known to be the primary determinant of health (see Raphael & Bryant, 2006, for a historical perspective). Traditionally, health care providers in hospitals have been concerned primarily with diagnosing and treating existing disease in individuals. The quantity and quality of their services are widely seen as the main factor in deciding if a population is healthy or not. Thus, in health care, the biomedical model has been the most prominent perspective, followed by the behavioural model, for teaching people how to live healthy lifestyles so as to prevent disease. However, this view has been challenged by more comprehensive concepts of health, such as the socioenvironmental model. The impetus for this broader view arose in the 1970s when educating the public to improve health was not necessarily focused on changing behaviours and improving health, especially among populations that were experiencing health inequities (see Chapter 6).

In 1974, the Lalonde Report, titled *A New Perspective on the Health of Canadians*, was released in Canada. This report fundamentally changed the view that the health care system was the most important factor in determining health status to advocating for the importance of investing resources beyond health services to improve the health of a population. In this report, Marc Lalonde, Minister of Health, outlined four elements that determine the health of Canadians (termed the health field): human biology, environment, lifestyle, and the health care organization (Lalonde, 1975). During this pivotal time, there was a new emphasis on community health arising from a change in social values also reflected in

several provincial reports that provided a supportive environment for this fundamental change (Ontario 1970, 1974; Quebec, 1970; Nova Scotia, 1972; Manitoba, 1972) as well as federal reports (Government of Canada, 1969, 1973). A common thread among these reports was that changes were needed in the Canadian health care system to shift from expensive acute care hospital to less costly home care and community care that focused on health promotion and maintenance.

In Canada, the health field concept was slow to take hold, however. Criticisms abounded, including about how lifestyle and environment were conceptualized in the report because it implied that individuals are to blame for the poor choices that led to their poor health, with little or no emphasis on the factors at the community and societal levels that influence health (Labonte & Penfold, 1981). Regardless of the limitations of the health field concept, however, the Lalonde report received worldwide attention and influenced a return to **primary health care (PHC)** at the Alma Ata Conference in 1978.

The Alma Ata declaration reaffirmed that health is a holistic concept (not just the mere absence of disease) and that health is a fundamental human right for all. The Alma-Ata declaration also drew attention to the gross inequities in health that exist between people and highlighted the importance of PHC, which was defined as "essential health care based on practical, scientifically sound, and socially acceptable methods and technology made universally accessible to individuals and families in the community through their full participation and at a cost that the community and country can afford to maintain at every stage of their development in the spirit of self-reliance and self-determination" (WHO, 1978, p. 2). PHC is based on five principles: accessibility, public participation, health promotion, appropriate technology, and intersectoral collaboration, which are underpinned by social justice and equity in health, with a focus on the population, community, and individuals. Central to the declaration was the notion that not only is health important for social and economic development but also that social and economic development is key to achieving health for all. Additionally, this achievement requires the participation of multiple sectors of society—not only health care—as well as the participation and involvement of community members in health care organization and planning (WHO, 1978). These basic tenets are central to the idea of health promotion and continue to be seen in that light.

Broadly, the determinants of health can be organized into four groups: (1) physical environment; (2) psychosocial environment; (3) lifestyle, behavioural, and modifiable risk factors; and (4) access to health services. We will discuss these determinants first and then look at to the social determinants of health.

The Physical Environment

Factors in the physical environment include the quality of air, water, and soil; the safety of food, drugs, and other products that humans consume or are exposed to; the physical handling and disposal of waste; the control of excessive noise; and the control of animal and insect vectors that can transmit diseases, for example (see Chapters 10 and 11). The physical environment is both outdoors and indoors and can affect human health directly (e.g., by exposure to potentially hazardous agents such as chemicals or radiation) or indirectly (e.g., by global warming, which is predicted to diminish food production). A major challenge is the development of economic production methods that sustain a healthy environment (sustainable development) as a legacy for our children.

The **built environment**—often defined as the manmade physical surroundings we encounter day to day (including buildings, parks, road systems, and other infrastructure)—has an impact on our health. It can include aspects of both the physical and psychosocial environment (discussed further later in this chapter). The built environment has been shown to influence rates of physical activity, healthy eating, injuries, socialization, and mental health, among others. How we design our spaces is, therefore, critical to addressing issues such as loneliness, obesity, and even equity. For example, public parks and more green spaces for people to gather in can promote social interactions, as well as exercise opportunities. The presence of things such as bike lanes and well-connected bus routes can promote active transportation, encouraging people to walk, bike, or take public transportation to work and to school.

CRITICAL THINKING QUESTIONS 1.3

1. How might the interventions described (e.g., public parks and spaces, bike lanes) affect health equity?
2. What other features in the built environment might help to increase physical activity? What features might help to promote healthy eating?

The Psychosocial Environment

The psychosocial environment, which includes things such as our relationships, how we deal with stress, social support, and social networks, has a major impact on health. For example, researchers have focused on specific factors that predispose an individual to illness, such as bereavement, social mobility, migration, cultural change, income, unemployment, and work hazards (Drydakis, 2015; Schnall, Dobson, Rosskam, & Elling, 2018; Griep et al., 2016; Kivimäki et al., 2015; Frost, Lehavot, & Meyer, 2015). Research has applied a systematic approach to the assumptions that life changes, particularly those involving some form of loss, are stressful and render an individual vulnerable to health problems because of that stress (Lovallo, 2015). However, whether life stress leads to some form of illness can depend on the presence of one or more mediating factors. Personality characteristics, coping styles, and the presence of social support are the main variables shown to influence an individual's response to life stress. Social support can provide a sense of belonging and intimacy and can help people to be more competent and self-efficacious. A meta-analytic review of eligible studies from 1980 to 2014 indicated that social isolation, loneliness, and living alone were associated with an increased likelihood of mortality rates of 29%, 26%, and 32%, respectively (Holt-Lunstad et al., 2015).

This is a complex area conceptually and methodologically, but current research indicates that an individual's social circumstances, particularly social support, frequently exert a significant influence over health status (see In the News box). This is discussed further in Chapter 5.

Lifestyle, Behavioural, and Modifiable Risk Factors

Lifestyle involves aspects of individuals' behaviour and surroundings that they control; however, as just discussed, it must take into account that behaviour is influenced by the social, physical, and economic environment in which people live and work. Healthy living involves "making positive choices that enhance your personal physical, mental and spiritual health" (PHAC, 2018c) but a person is much more able and empowered to make these positive choices when they have an adequate income, employment, education, and social support, for example.

🌐 IN THE NEWS

The Loneliness Epidemic and Mainstream Media

Dr. Vivek Murthy, a former Surgeon General of the United States, helped raise the profile of loneliness as an important determinant of health. Large international newspapers, including *The New York Times* and *The Washington Post*, ran headlines using phrases such as "loneliness kills" and "the loneliness epidemic," drawing attention to what Dr. Murthy describes as the rise in rates of loneliness among people of all ages and walks of life and the link between loneliness and the risk of an earlier death (which he equates to the risk of premature death when smoking 15 cigarettes a day). Furthermore, in January 2018, the United Kingdom appointed a Minister for Loneliness—the first ever of its kind—to further the discussion and better assess the impact of loneliness on health in Britain (McGregor, 2017; Yeginsu, 2018).

The use of mobile phones is also having an influence on the loneliness epidemic. According to a study of university students, using a mobile phone for more than 1 hour per day was associated with higher loneliness scores than those who used their phone less than 1 hour per day (Tan, Pamuk, & Dönder, 2013).

CRITICAL THINKING QUESTION 1.4: Are there other factors that could be driving the loneliness epidemic where you live?

While communicable diseases like tuberculosis and cholera used to be the main causes of death, today NCDs are responsible for about 70% of deaths worldwide. Although NCDs are commonly perceived to be an issue predominantly in high-income countries, it is actually low- and middle-income countries (LMICs) that face the brunt of the burden, with nearly 90% of deaths resulting from NCDs occurring in LMICs. The global community has recognized four major lifestyle or behavioural risk factors as being particularly important to address the growing burden of NCDs: tobacco use, unhealthy diets, physical inactivity, and deleterious alcohol consumption (WHO, 2018b). These are discussed in greater detail in Chapter 5.

Access to Health Services

Accessibility is one of the principles of the PHC and can play a role in determining health. Access to health services refers to the ability of individuals or groups to obtain the services they need and is regarded as an important determinant of health. Indigenous populations in Canada, for example, do not have equitable access to health services (this is discussed in more detail in Chapter 7).

Improving access means reducing barriers to accessing care for underserved groups. Examples of reducing barriers include providing patients with bus fare and child care services to make it easier for them to attend appointments; documenting language preferences of patients, identifying language skills of practitioners, and providing interpreter services; extending clinic hours and locating clinics close to where people live and work; offering a welcoming and culturally safe practice environment (described further in Chapter 6); and creating opportunities to provide health care services beyond the clinic or hospital walls, such as outreach to local schools or by partnering with community groups and religious organizations (University of Chicago, 2011).

Social Determinants of Health Frameworks

In Canada, there are predominately two frameworks of the social determinants of health that have been widely adopted: The Public Health Agency's (social) determinants of health and Raphael's (2016) social determinants of health. The comparisons with other frameworks and conceptualizations can be seen in Table 1.2, and the Public Health Agency's determinants are explained in Table 1.3. For an example of how governments are addressing the social determinants of health, refer to the Interprofessional Practice box.

The Canadian government continues to recognize that there are many factors that influence health. The PHAC lists 11 determinants of health (summarized in Table 1.3) that are known to influence both health and health equity. Within those determinants are the **social determinants of health**, a more specific group of factors (education, income, and employment, for example) that relate to a "person's place in society" (PHAC, 2018a).

Health Promotion as Another Tool for Addressing the Social Determinants of Health

Subsequent to the Lalonde Report, Jake Epp, Minster of Health and Welfare Canada, released the document *Achieving Health for All: A Framework for Health Promotion* (Epp, 1986) at the First International Conference on Health Promotion, held in Ottawa in 1986. The Epp report identified inequities in health as one of the

TABLE 1.2 Conceptualizations of the Social Determinants of Health

Ottawa Charter (WHO, 1986)	World Health Organization (WHO, 2003)	Raphael (2016)	Health Canada (PHAC, 2017)
• Peace • Shelter • Education • Food Income • Stable ecosystem • Sustainable resources • Social justice • Equity	• Social gradient • Stress • Social exclusion • Work • Unemployment • Social supports • Addictions • Food • Transport	• Income and income distribution • Education • Unemployment and job security • Employment and working conditions • Early childhood development • Food insecurity • Housing • Social exclusion • Social safety net • Health services • Indigenous status • Gender • Race • Disability	• Income and social status • Employment and working conditions • Education and literacy • Childhood experiences • Physical environment • Social supports and coping skills networks • Healthy behaviours • Access to health services • Gender • Culture

PHAC, Public Health Agency of Canada; *WHO,* World Health Organization.
Adapted from Raphael, D., & Bryant, T. (2006). Maintaining population health in a period of welfare state decline: political economy as the missing dimension in health promotion theory and practice. *Promotion & Education,13*(4), 236–242.

TABLE 1.3 Public Health Agency of Canada's Classification of the Determinants of Health

Determinant	Relevance
1. Income and social status	The most important determinant of health nationally. However, it is the distribution, rather than the actual amount of wealth, that is associated with healthier populations (i.e., the more evenly wealth is distributed, the better off the population is as a whole).
2. Employment and working conditions	Health status is improved with increased control over work circumstances and lower levels of stress. Unemployment is highly correlated with poorer health (described further in Chapter 12).
3. Education and literacy	Provides skills useful for daily tasks, employment (income and job security), and community participation
4. Childhood experiences	A wide range of chronic conditions seem to have their origins in fetal and infant life. Prenatal and early childhood experiences are also important in the development of coping skills and competence.
5. Physical environment	Factors in the natural environment, such as air, water, and soil quality, are key influences on health. Human-built factors such as housing, workplace, community, and road design are also important (see Chapter 11). Many of the writings from a population health perspective do not account for environmental implications.
6. Social supports and coping skills networks	The effects of social support may be as important as identified risk factors (e.g., smoking, physical activity, obesity, and high blood pressure). It is not the quantity of relations that matter but the quality.
7. Healthy behaviours	Psychological characteristics such as personal competence, locus of control, and mastery over one's life contribute to the adoption of positive health behaviours; however, the focus on personal health practices has been characterized as blaming the victims instead of societal factors.
8. Access to health services	Contributes to healthier people. However, increased expenditures on health care seems to be less successful in improving the health of Canadians.

Continued

TABLE 1.3	**Public Health Agency of Canada's Classification of the Determinants of Health—cont'd**
Determinant	**Relevance**
9. Biology and genetic endowment	The functioning of body systems and genetic endowment contribute to health status, as well as the process of development.
10. Gender	Biological differences in sex and socially constructed gender norms influence health and health service use.
11. Culture	Racism and culturally unsafe care influence the way people interact with health care systems. Cultural norms, traditions, and practices also influence health and health service use.

From Public Health Agency of Canada. (2018). *Social determinants of health and health inequalities.* Retrieved from https://www.canada.ca/en/public-health/services/health-promotion/population-health/what-determines-health.html

INTERPROFESSIONAL PRACTICE

Working Collaboratively Across Disciplines and Sectors to Address the Social Determinants of Health at the Local Level

Given that the social determinants of health lie outside public health, working intersectorally with health partners and nonhealth partners and in collaboration with communities is an essential part of the public health role for addressing health equity.

Public health organizations across Canada are creating health equity–specific staff positions as a means of increasing internal organizational capacity to address the social determinants of health. In 2012, the Ontario Ministry of Health and Long-term Care implemented a province-wide initiative to support Ontario public health units (PHUs) to address health inequities and meet the needs of locally identified priority populations. PHUs hired two new full-time equivalent public health nurse (PHN) positions (for a total of 72 new positions provincially) with social determinants of health–specific knowledge and expertise to "enhance supports to program and services needs of specific priority populations impacted most negatively by determinants of health" (Peroff-Johnston & Chan, 2012). The PHNs worked with health educators, clients, hospital administrators, dietitians, social workers, and occupational therapists to address the social determinants of health. The social determinants of health PHNs focused on populations most affected by inequities to make health equity central to the activities of public health. The program evaluation (McPherson et al., 2016) found that PHUs benefitted from the implementation of cross-organizational social determinants of health PHN positions, structurally embedding health equity as an organizational and system priority that engaged many actors internally and externally. However, the impact on local priority populations that are experiencing inequities is unknown.

CRITICAL THINKING QUESTION 1.5: Read the following report: *Learning to Work Differently: Implementing Ontario's Social Determinants of Health Public Health Nurse Initiative* (which can be found at http://nccdh.ca/images/uploads/comments/SDOH_Nurse_Study_EN.pdf).

Drawing on what you learned from this report, what specific approaches would you consider when implementing a health equity strategy in your workplace or situation?

challenges to achieving health for all. The Epp report was also criticized for emphasizing individual and community effort to address health challenges; individualizing health; and ignoring the social, economic, and political causes of behaviour and disease. However, the report continued to expand the notion of the social determinants of health being underpinned by equity. This conference led to the international community defining health promotion and developing the Ottawa Charter for Health Promotion, a framework for public health action, which has an explicit focus on the SDH and is, used even today. According to the charter, **health promotion** is defined as follows:

"the process of enabling people to increase control over, and to improve, their health. To reach a state of complete physical, mental, and social well-being, an individual or group must be able to identify and to realize aspirations, to satisfy needs, and to change or cope with the environment. Health is, therefore, seen as a resource for everyday life, not the objective of living. Health is a positive concept emphasizing social and personal resources, as well as physical capacities.

Therefore, health promotion is not just the responsibility of the health sector but goes beyond healthy lifestyles to well-being" (WHO, 1986, p. 14).

Following this landmark conference, health promotion in Canada in the 1990s faced some challenges—struggling with an undue emphasis on behavioural and lifestyle factors in shaping health and working at the individual level to promote change. Internationally, however, momentum continued, and in 1997, another major declaration on health promotion was developed: The Jakarta Declaration on Leading Health Promotion into the 21st Century (PHO, 2014b). The Jakarta Declaration represented an opportunity for the global community to come together to reinforce and recommit to the principles of health promotion work. The Jakarta Declaration placed much emphasis on the importance of poverty, urbanization, and violence as key determinants of health and called on governments to work together to empower communities, build an infrastructure for health promotion, and develop new and innovative modes of action (WHO, 1997).

Since 2000, a number of landmark global conferences have taken place in the domain of health promotion (described further in the Table 1.4), all of which reiterate the importance of the social determinants of health and emphasize foundational principles of health promotion, such as:

- Health is a fundamental human right.
- Health and inequities in health are shaped by a broad number of determinants of health (which include the political, economic, physical, and social environment).
- Although individual lifestyles and behaviours influence health, they, too, are shaped by these broader contextual factors.
- Action to improve health and health inequities requires the participation and cooperation of multiple sectors of society.

The World Health Organization's Commission on Social Determinants of Health

In 2008 in a landmark document, the WHO's Commission on Social Determinants of Health (CSDH) released its final report entitled *Closing the Gap in a Generation: Health Equity Through Action on the Social Determinants of Health*. In this report, a new model for the social determinants of health is proposed (Fig. 1.2) that outlines how **intermediary determinants of health** (those

things that affect health more directly, like adequate housing conditions and lifestyle factors such as food choices) are ultimately determined by the **structural determinants of health,** which include political, social, and economic forces, such as governance and public policy decisions.

Choices that people make about what they eat and how active they are do not just boil down to individual preferences and motivation but instead are rooted in public policies that influence how affordable and accessible these lifestyle "choices" may be. For example, policies that mandate that workers be paid adequate wages ensure that people have the means to eat healthy and engage in leisure time physical activity.

According to the revolutionary final report by the WHO, inequities in health arise because of the unequal distribution of power and wealth in societies, which makes health promoting behaviours much more feasible for some groups compared with others. As a result, the WHO challenged the global community to not only improve living, playing, and working conditions for all but also to tackle what it calls "the inequitable distribution of power, money, and resources" (National Academies of Sciences, Engineering, and Medicine, 2016).

The Canadian Institute for Health Information (CIHI) has produced a framework that mirrors many of the concepts highlighted by the WHO's Commission on Social Determinants of Health. The CIHI framework was introduced in the book's Introduction and will be discussed throughout the remaining chapters. This chapter focuses primarily on explaining the outer circle, as well as the "social determinants of health" section of the CIHI figure, and Part II of this book discusses health system inputs and characteristics, as well as outputs.

> **CRITICAL THINKING QUESTION 1.6:** What determinants of health have been left out of PHAC's 2017 list? And why do you think they are different from Raphael's (2016) list of health determinants?

COMPETENCIES FOR PUBLIC HEALTH

Core public health functions (see Chapter 16) and competencies are critical to guide the behaviour of organizations and individuals involved in public health and assist them in the selection of priority target groups and the development of intervention programs, including workforce considerations. Core competencies transcend the

TABLE 1.4   Landmark Events in Health Promotion Globally from 2000 Onward

Year	Event	Description
2003	WHO Social Determinants of Health: The Solid Facts (Wilkinson & Marmot, 2003)	• Focused on the role that public policy can play in shaping the social environment to improve health • Provided scientific evidence from resource rich countries regarding the social determinants of health • Also acknowledged that as social beings, we need more than good material conditions but also need to feel valued and appreciated.
2005	Bangkok Charter on Health Promotion (WHO, 2005)	• Developed during the 6th Global Conference on Health Promotion in Bangkok, Thailand • Four key commitments included making health promotion: • Central to the global development agenda • A core responsibility for all of government • A key focus for communities and civil society • A requirement for good corporate practice
2008	Commission on Social Determinants of Health releases its final report (Commission on Social Determinants of Health, 2008)	• Final report, titled *Closing the Gap in a Generation: Health Equity through Action on the Social Determinants of Health*, strongly emphasized in a direct and strong way some of the central themes of health promotion, such as: • The notion that inequities are resulting in significant death around the world • Addressing equity is a matter of social justice
2010	Adelaide Statement on Health in All Policies (WHO & Government of South Australia, 2010)	• Was developed at the International Meeting on Health in All Policies • Represented a commitment to focusing on health when building public policies (healthy public policy) and recognizes the contribution of the health sector in actioning difficult societal problems
2011	Rio Political Declaration on the Social Determinants of Health (PHO, 2014b)	• Was developed during the World Conference on Social Determinants of Health. • Reflected a commitment, on a global scale, to action on the social determinants of health to address widespread health inequities
2016	Shanghai Declaration on promoting health in the 2030 Agenda for Sustainable Development (WHO, 2016)	• Was developed during the 9th global conference on Health Promotion • Reflects a global commitment to promote health and well-being in all of the Sustainable Development Goals (SDGs) (global goals that include reducing poverty, food insecurity, inequities, climate change, and so on), as well as enhance funding for and political commitment towards health promotion as a way to accelerate progress on the SDGs

PHO, Public Health Ontario; *WHO*, World Health Organization.

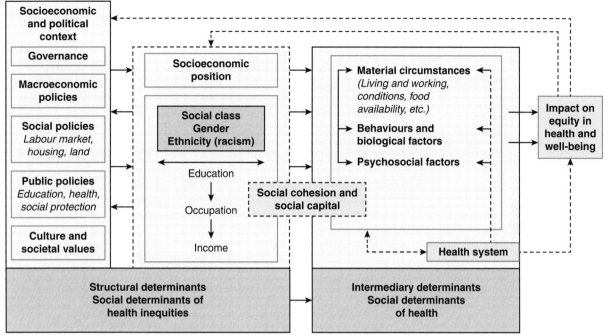

Fig. 1.2 The World Health Organization's Commission on Social Determinants of Health (CSDH) Conceptual Framework. (From Solar, O., & Irwin, A. [2010]. *A conceptual framework for action on the social determinants of health*. Social Determinants of Health Discussion. Paper 2 [Policy and Practice]. Retrieved from https://www.who.int/sdhconference/resources/ConceptualframeworkforactiononSDH_eng.pdf)

boundaries of specific disciplines and are independent of program and topic. They provide a baseline for what is required to fulfill public health system core functions. These include population health assessment, surveillance, disease and injury prevention, health promotion, and health protection. The Public Health Agency of Canada (2017) defines public health competencies as the "essential knowledge, skills and attitudes necessary for the practice of public health" (p. 1). There are 36 public health core competencies (core competencies) that are organized into seven domains:

1. Public Health Sciences (5 competencies)
2. Assessment and Analysis (6 competencies)
3. Policy and Program Planning, Implementation and Evaluation (8 competencies)
4. Partnerships, Collaboration and Advocacy (4 competencies)
5. Diversity and Inclusiveness (3 competencies)
6. Communication (4 competencies)
7. Leadership (6 competencies)

Although these seven domains and their corresponding competencies provide guidance for the practice of public health, Edwards and Davison (2008) argue that social justice should be explicitly included. Edwards and Davison provide examples of how essential attributes of social justice can be integrated within each domain (see Table 1.5).

PUBLIC HEALTH ETHICS

Concern for ethical issues in public health has increased in light of evidence of systematic problems of accountability in Canada's public health system. These concerns relate, for example, to water safety in the aftermath of Walkerton, Ontario, and North Battleford, Saskatchewan, to the importation of serious infectious disease in contaminated food, to access to health information for public health surveillance, to the justification of coercive measures for disease control, and to the communication of environmental risks.

The focus of ethics in public health differs from that of clinical practice in many health professions (Swain, Burns, & Etkind, 2008). In clinical practice, four principles—autonomy (respect for self-determination), beneficence (moral requirement to promote good), nonmalfeasance (do no harm), and justice (fair and

TABLE 1.5   Examples of Potential Social Justice Core Competencies for Public Health

Domain of Core Competencies	Potential Competency Reflecting Social Justice Attributes
Public health sciences	• Describe public health's role in righting social injustices. • Understand relationships between social determinants of health and inequities
Assessment and analysis	• Use data to describe and differentiate *health inequalities* and *health inequities*. • Work with marginalized populations to use quantitative and qualitative data to examine and take action on inequities and inequalities in health status.
Policy and program planning, implementation, and evaluation	• Identify the ways in which each policy option may reduce or increase social and health inequities. • Recognize the potential differential effects of health interventions on populations subgroups.
Partnership, collaboration, and advocacy	• Support governments and community partners to build just institutions. • Solicit input from individuals and organizations to address inequities. • Facilitate dialogue about the fair allocation of resources.
Diversity and inclusiveness	• Understand and apply the Universal Declaration on Human Rights and the Universal Declaration on the Rights of Indigenous Peoples.
Communication	• Develop communication strategies for subpopulations that have been historically oppressed.
Leadership	• Integrate the values of social justice within the mission and strategic plans of an organization. • Identity how the redistribution of public health resources many alter or reinforce inequities.

From Edwards, N., & Davison, C. (2008). Social justice and core competencies for public health: Improving the fit. *Canadian Journal of Public Health, 99*(2), 130–132.

equitable determination distribution of resources and fair treatment for individuals and society)—are well recognized. In public health, the focus is on populations, communities, and the social determinants of health, which are not neatly analogous to a focus on individual patients. There is no set of common principles for public health ethics. The scope of ethical issues in public health is also broader, reflecting the wide range of issues involved (Barrett et al., 2016).The central issues in public health ethics revolve around concerns for weighing individual rights versus community rights. The origins of public health are intimately tied to the application of utilitarian thought (the ethical theory that holds that the criterion for determining the worth or goodness of an action is the maximization of happiness or the greatest good for the greatest number of people). Concerns for equitable distribution of goods and providing for the most vulnerable members of society are also concerns of public health and can be supported by egalitarian concepts of justice.

In most Western countries, legislation supports public health action against individuals. It sets out the justification for communicable disease surveillance, mandatory reporting, detention, and quarantine. The ethical justification rests in the necessity of the community to be able to protect itself from health threats.

A useful framework for analyzing the ethical implications of a public health intervention was proposed by Ross Upshur in 2002 and is still used today. When examining an intervention, Upshur considers the following four principles:

1. **Harm:** Does the intervention protect others from experiencing harm?
2. **Least restrictive means:** Is there another, less coercive or restrictive, intervention that can be implemented that would achieve the same goals?
3. **Reciprocity:** If some people or groups will endure a burden because of the intervention, does the intervention ensure compensation for that hardship?
4. **Transparency:** Was the decision to intervene inclusive and made through a clear and accountable process (Upshur, 2002)?

EXERCISE 1.2: An ongoing and controversial debate exists in Canada with respect to whether men who have sex with men (MSM) should be banned from donating blood because the incidence of HIV is higher in this group. Apply Upshur's framework to tease out arguments for and against this policy.

CRITICAL THINKING QUESTION 1.7: Are the ethical considerations that support and challenge the provision of medical assistance in dying a matter of public health ethics or clinical practice ethics?

CASE STUDY

Medical Assistance in Dying: An Ethical Dilemma?

A growing controversy when it comes to death and dying is the issue of medical assistance in dying (MAiD). With a growing emphasis on quality of life and personal determination around the circumstances of one's death, in June 2016, the government of Canada passed Bill C-14 (Ministry of Health and Long-Term Care, n.d.; Health Canada, 2017), which legalized MAiD. MAiD refers to the administration of a lethal substance by a health care provider (typically a physician or nurse practitioner) to a patient at their request, with the intention of causing death, or the provision by a provider of a lethal substance that the patient then self-administers. Bill C-14 lays out eligibility criteria for patients requesting MAiD, including that the person must be 18 years or older, be capable of making a medical decision, have a grievous and irremediable medical condition, is making a voluntary request, and can provide informed consent.

In October 2017, the second interim report on MAiD was released by the government of Canada. This report showed that from the time the bill passed on June 17, 2016, until the end of 2017, 1982 medically assisted deaths took place across Canada. Although the bill was controversial, a poll commissioned by Dying with Dignity Canada showed that of the 2500 Canadians who were surveyed in February 2016, 85% supported the idea that a person with a serious illness should be able to request MAiD (Dying With Dignity Canada, n.d.).

▋ SUMMARY

This chapter has outlined aspects of population health, the concepts and theories that underlie health and disease, the various conceptualizations of the social determinants of health, health inequalities, inequities, social justice, health promotion, public health competencies, and public health ethics.

Population health is an approach to promoting health. The government of Canada has embraced population health and produced several documents outlining how to take action to improve the health of populations. Health has been defined in various ways. In this book, the WHO's definition is used: *health* is the ability to identify and to realize one's aspirations, to satisfy one's needs, and to change or cope with one's environment Thus, health is a daily resource rather than the objective of living and emphasizes social and personal resources and physical capacities.

There are several views of health. First, the *biomedical model* holds that the body is like a machine that can be corrected by procedures designed to repair damage or restore functioning. The more accepted model,

nowadays, is the socioecological model, which highlights the importance of the political, economic, and psychosocial environment on health.

Impairment is any loss or abnormality of psychosocial, physiological, or anatomical structure or function. *Disability* can be thought of as a broad concept encompassing impairment in addition to participation restriction and activity limitation. A person's environment has an enormous impact on their experience of disability.

The *social determinants of health* are foundational to public health practice and population health and are different than the determinants of health. Often health determinants include an individual's human biology (those aspects of both mental and physical health that arise out of the basic biology of humans or are caused by the individual's organic make-up). However, the social determinants of health include the individual's physical environment (factors include food; drugs; air, water, and soil quality; waste disposal; and animal and insect vectors) and psychosocial environment; lifestyle, behaviour, and modifiable risk factors (aspects of an individual's behaviour and surroundings over which the individual has some control, although they are shaped by the social and economic environmental conditions within which the individual lives); and to some degree the health care organization. The social determinants of health not only influence the state of health of a community or population but also the health inequities within that community. Inequities are underpinned by the values and tenets of social justice, which point to the cause of the inequity as being unfair and unjust.

The Ottawa Charter for Health Promotion (1986), a framework for public health action, was created to address the social inequities in health. Since 2000, a number of landmark global conferences have taken place in the domain of health promotion, which reiterate the foundational principles of health promotion and expand on them.

Public health competencies are critical for the practice of public health. However, social justice being a foundational concept in public health practice must also be made explicit within the competencies if practice is to make a difference addressing health inequities. In recent years, there are increased concerns regarding ethical issues in public health and a demand for more accountability in Canada's public health system. In public health, the ethical focus is on populations, communities, and the social determinants of health, which are not neatly analogous to a focus on individual patients. The scope of ethical issues in public health is broad and reflects a concern for weighing individual rights versus community rights.

KEY WEBSITES

Canadian Hospice Palliative Care Association (CHPCA): http://www.chpca.net
The CHPCA is a national organization that advocates for quality end-of-life care for all Canadians. Its website describes what hospice palliative care is and provides reports and statistics, as well as resources for families, patients, and health care professionals related to palliative care.

National Collaborating Centre for Determinants of Health (NCCDH): http://www.nccdh.ca
One of five Canadian collaborating centres, the NCCDH aims to advance work on equity and social determinants of health. This website profiles their work and provides valuable resources for the public.

National Collaborating Centre for Healthy Public Policy (NCCHPP): http://www.ncchpp.ca/en
One of five collaborating centres, the NCCHPP provides further information, resources, and tools related to healthy public policy like health impact assessment, built environment interventions, and so on.

Nuffield Council on Bioethics: http://nuffieldbioethics.org
The website of the Nuffield Council on Bioethics contains numerous reports that analyze the ethical dimensions of various topics in biology and medicine, including genome editing, research on human embryos, and many other issues.

World Health Organization—Social Determinants of Health: http://www.who.int/social_determinants/en
This website provides more information on the social determinants of health, including descriptions, reports, evidence briefs, and examples of global work.

REFERENCES

Allen, L., Williams, J., Townsend, N., et al. (2017). Socioeconomic status and non-communicable disease behavioural risk factors in low-income and lower-middle-income countries: A systematic review. *The Lancet Global Health, 5*(3), e277–e289. https://doi.org/10.1016/S2214-109X(17)30058-X.

Barrett, D. H., Ortmann, L. H., Dawson, A., et al. (Eds.). (2016). *Public health ethics: Cases spanning the globe* Retrieved from https://www.ncbi.nlm.nih.gov/books/NBK435780/.

Canadian Nurses Association. (2006). *Social justice . . . A means to an end, an end in itself.* Ottawa: Author.

Canadian Public Health Association & World Health Organization. (1986). *Ottawa Charter for Health Promotion.* Ottawa: Health and Welfare Canada.

Canadian Public Health Association. (2017). *Canadian Public Health Association Working Paper: Public health: A conceptual framework.* Retrieved from https://www.cpha.ca/sites/default/files/uploads/policy/ph-framework/phcf_e.pdf.

Commission on Social Determinants of Health. (2008). *Closing the gap in a generation: health equity through action on the social determinants of health. Final Report of the Commission on Social Determinants of Health.* Geneva: World Health Organization. Retrieved from http://www.who.int/social_determinants/thecommission/finalreport/en

Cundiff, J. M., Boylan, J. M., Pardini, D. A., et al. (2017). Moving up matters: Socioeconomic mobility prospectively predicts better physical health. *Health Psychology, 36*(6), 609–617. https://doi.org/10.1037/hea0000473.

Dahlgren, G., & Whitehead, M. (1991). *Policies and strategies to promote social equality in health.* Stockholm: Institute of Future Studies.

Drydakis, N. (2015). The effect of unemployment on self-reported health and mental health in Greece from 2008 to 2013: A longitudinal study before and during the financial crisis. *Social Science & Medicine, 128*, 43–51. https://doi.org/10.1016/j.socscimed.2014.12.025.

Dying With Dignity Canada. (n.d.). *Groundbreaking poll: 8 in 10 Canadians support the right to advance consent for assisted dying.* Retrieved from https://www.dyingwithdignity.ca/advance_consent_assisted_dying_poll.

Edwards, N., & Davison, C. (2008). Social justice and core competencies for public health: Improving the fit. *Canadian Journal of Public Health, 99*(2), 130–132.

Epp, J. (1986). *Achieving health for all: A framework for health promotion.* Ottawa: Health and Welfare Canada.

Evans, R. G., & Stoddart, G. L. (1990). Producing health, consuming health care. *Social Science and Medicine, 31*, 1347–1363.

Fabbris, J. L., Mesquita, A. C., Caldeira, S., et al. (2017). Anxiety and spiritual well-being in nursing students: a cross-sectional study. *Journal of Holistic Nursing, 35*(3), 261–270. https://doi.org/10.1177/0898010116655004.

Frost, D. M., Lehavot, K., & Meyer, I. H. (2015). Minority stress and physical health among sexual minority individuals. *Journal of Behavioral Medicine, 38*(1), 1–8. https://doi.org/10.1007/s10865-013-9523-8.

Government of Canada. (1969). *Task Force reports on the costs of health services in Canada.* Ottawa: Queens Printer.

Government of Canada. (1973). *The community health centre in Canada. (Report of the Community Health Centre project to the Health Ministers).* Ottawa: Information Canada (Hastings Report).

Griep, Y., Kinnunen, U., Nätti, J., et al. (2016). The effects of unemployment and perceived job insecurity: A comparison of their association with psychological and somatic complaints, self-rated health and life satisfaction. *International Archives of Occupational and Environmental Health, 89*(1), 147–162. https://doi.org/10.1007/s00420-015-1059-5.

Hamilton, N., & Bhatti, T. (1996). *Population health promotion: An integrated model of population health and health promotion.* Ottawa: Health Promotion Development Division.

Health Canada. (2017). *2nd interim report on medical assistance in dying in Canada.* Retrieved from https://www.canada.ca/en/health-canada/services/publications/health-system-services/medical-assistance-dying-interim-report-sep-2017.html.

Holt-Lunstad, J., Smith, T. B., Baker, M., et al. (2015). Loneliness and social isolation as risk factors for mortality: A meta-analytic review. *Perspectives on Psychological Science, 10*(2), 227–237. https://doi.org/10.1177/1745691614568352.

Jain, M. M., Khatri, N., & Jamadar, P. (2015). Improved brain function from meditation following an Awareness Training Programme in Spiritual Medicine (ATPiSM).

Journal of Evolution of Medical and Dental Sciences, 4(51), 8881–8893. Retrieved from https://jemds.com/latest-articles.php?at_id=8198.

Kivimäki, M., Virtanen, M., Kawachi, I., et al. (2015). Long working hours, socioeconomic status, and the risk of incident type 2 diabetes: A meta-analysis of published and unpublished data from 222 120 individuals. *The Lancet Diabetes & Endocrinology, 3*(1), 27–34. https://doi.org/10.1016/S2213-8587(14)70178-0.

Labonte, R. (1993). *Health promotion and empowerment: Practice frameworks* (Issues in Health Promotion Series HP-10-0102). Toronto: Centre for Health Promotion.

Labonte, R., & Penfold, S. (1981). Canadian perspectives in health promotion: a critique. *Health Education*, 4–9.

Lago, S., Cantarero, D., Rivera, B., et al. (2017). Socioeconomic status, health inequalities and non-communicable diseases: A systematic review. *Zeitschrift fur Gesundheitswissenschaften (Journal of Public Health), 26*(1), 1–14. https://doi.org/10.1007/s10389-017-0850-z.

Lalonde, M. (1975). *A new perspective on the health of Canadians.* Ottawa: Ministry of Supply and Services.

Lovallo, W. R. (2015). *Stress and health: Biological and psychological interactions.* Thousand Oaks, CA: Sage.

Lynch, J., & Kaplan, G. A. (1997). Understanding how inequality in the distribution of income affects health. *Journal of Health Psychology, 2*, 297–314.

Marinko, J. A., Shi, L., Starfield, B., et al. (2003). Income inequality and health: A critical review of the literature. *Medical Care Research and Reviews, 60*, 407–452.

McGregor, J. (2017). This former surgeon general says there's a "loneliness epidemic" and work is partly to blame. *The Washington Post*, October 4. Retrieved from https://www.washingtonpost.com/news/on-leadership/wp/2017/10/04/this-former-surgeon-general-says-theres-a-loneliness-epidemic-and-work-is-partly-to-blame/.

McPherson, C., Ndumbe-Eyoh, S., Betker, C., et al. (2016). Swimming against the tide: A Canadian qualitative study examining the implementation of a province-wide public health initiative to address health equity. *International Journal for Equity in Health, 15*, 129. https://doi.org/10.1186/s12939-016-0419-4.

Ministry of Health and Long-Term Care. (n.d.). *Medical assistance in dying.* Toronto: Author. Retrieved from http://health.gov.on.ca/en/pro/programs/maid/

National Academies of Sciences, Engineering, and Medicine. (2016). *A framework for educating health professionals to address the social determinants of health.* Washington, DC: National Academies Press. Retrieved from https://www.ncbi.nlm.nih.gov/books/NBK395979/

Navarro, V., & Shi, L. (2001). The political context of social inequalities and health. *Social Science & Medicine, 52,* 481–491.

Nova Scotia. (1972). *Health care in Nova Scotia—a new direction for the seventies.* Halifax: Nova Scotia Council of Health.

Ontario. (1970). *Report of the Committee on the Healing Arts.* Toronto: Queens Printer.

Ontario. (1974). *Report of the Health Planning Task Force* (Mustard Report). Toronto: Ministry of Health.

Park, C. L., Braun, T., & Siegel, T. (2015). Who practices yoga? A systematic review of demographic, health-related, and psychosocial factors associated with yoga practice. *Journal of Behavioral Medicine, 38*(3), 460–471. https://doi.org/10.1007/s10865-015-9618-5.

Peroff-Johnston, N., & Chan, I. (2012). *Evaluation of the social determinants of health nursing initiative among health units in Ontario.* Toronto, ON: Ontario Ministry of Health and Long-Term Care, Public Health Division.

Prüss-Üstün, A., & Neira, M. (2016). *Preventing disease through healthy environments: A global assessment of the burden of disease from environmental risks.* Geneva: World Health Organization.

Public Health Agency of Canada. (2012). *What is the Population Health Approach?* Retrieved from https://www.canada.ca/en/public-health/services/health-promotion/population-health/population-health-approach.html.

Public Health Agency of Canada. (2017). *Core competencies for public health in Canada.* Ottawa: Author. Retrieved from https://www.canada.ca/en/public-health/services/public-health-practice/skills-online/core-competencies-public-health-canada.html

Public Health Agency of Canada. (2018a). *Social determinants of health and health inequalities.* Retrieved from https://www.canada.ca/en/public-health/services/health-promotion/population-health/what-determines-health.html.

Public Health Agency of Canada. (2018b). *Key health inequalities in Canada: A national portrait.* Retrieved from https://www.canada.ca/content/dam/phac-aspc/documents/services/publications/science-research/key-health-inequalities-canada-national-portrait-executive-summary/hir-executive-summary-eng.pdf.

Public Health Agency of Canada. (2018c). *Healthy living.* Retrieved from https://www.canada.ca/en/health-canada/services/healthy-living.html.

Public Health Ontario. (2014a). *Health promotion foundations, Module three: Introduction to models and theories.* [Online Module PowerPoint]. Retrieved from https://www.publichealthontario.ca/en/Learning AndDevelopment/Events/Documents/Webinar2_ Models_and_theories_Apr16_2014.pdf.

Public Health Ontario. (2014b). *Health promotion foundations, Module two: Milestones in the history of health promotion.* [Online Module PowerPoint]. Retrieved from https://www.publichealthontario.ca/en/Learning AndDevelopment/Events/Documents/Webinar1_ History_of_HP_Apr9_2014.pdf.

Puchalski, C. M., Blatt, B., Kogan, M., et al. (2014). Spirituality and health: The development of a field. *Academic Medicine, 89*(1), 10–16. https://doi.org/10.1097/ACM.0000000000 000083.

Quebec. (1970). *Report of the Commission of Inquiry on Health and Social Welfare* (Castonguay—Nepveu Report). Quebec City: Government of Quebec.

Raphael, D. (2008). Getting serious about the social determinants of health: New directions for public health workers. *IUHPE–Promotion and Education, 15*(3), 15–20.

Raphael, D. (Ed.). (2016). *Social determinants of health: Canadian perspectives* (3rd ed.) Toronto: Canadian Scholars' Press.

Raphael, D., & Bryant, T. (2006). Maintaining population health in a period of welfare state decline: Political economy as the missing dimension in health promotion theory and practice. *Promotion & Education, 13*(4), 236–242. https://doi.org/10.1177/17579759061300402.

Sadipun, D. K., Dwidiyanti, M., & Andriany, M. (2018). Effect of spiritual based mindfulness intervention on emotional control in adult patients with pulmonary tuberculosis. *Belitung Nursing Journal, 4*(2), 226–231. Retrieved from http://belitungraya.org/BRP/index.php/bnj/article/view/357/pdf.

Schnall, P. L., Dobson, M., Rosskam, E., et al. (2018). *Unhealthy work: Causes, consequences, cures.* New York: Routledge.

Seeberg, J., & Meinert, L. (2015). Can epidemics be noncommunicable? Reflections on the spread of "noncommunicable" diseases. *Issues, 5,* 2. https://doi.org/10.17157/mat.2.2.171.

Senate Subcommittee on Population Health. (2009). *A healthy, productive Canada: A Determinant of health approach. Final Report of the Subcommittee on Population Health.* Ottawa: The Standing Senate Committee on Social Affairs, Science and Technology.

Shah, C. P. (2003). Places of worship in multicultural settings in Toronto. In *Urban Ethnic Encounters* (pp. 62–76). New York: Routledge.

Swain, G. R., Burns, K. A., & Etkind, P. (2008). Preparedness: Medical ethics versus public health ethics. *Journal of Public Health Management and Practice, 14*(4), 354–357. https://doi.org/10.1097/01.PHH.0000324563.87780.67.

Tan, Ç., Pamuk, M., & Dönder, A. (2013). Loneliness and mobile phone. *Procedia-Social and Behavioral Sciences, 103,* 606–611.

University of Chicago. (2011). *FAIR Toolkit: Strategies, levels, modes*. The University of Chicago and the Robert Wood Johnson Foundation. Retrieved from http://www.solving-disparities.org/sites/default/files/finding_answers_flash-cards2_0.pdf.

Upshur, R. E. (2002). Principles for the justification of public health intervention. *Canadian Journal of Public Health*, 93(2), 101–103.

Virtual Campus for Public Health. (n.d.). *The epidemiological triad*. Retrieved from https://cursos.campusvirtualsp.org/mod/tab/view.php?id=23154.

Wilkinson, R., & Marmot, M. G. (2003). *The solid facts: Social determinants of health*. Geneva: World Health Organization (Regional Office for Europe). Retrieved from http://www.euro.who.int/document/e81384.pdf.

Wilkinson, R., & Pickett, K. (2019). *The inner level: How more equal societies reduce stress, restore sanity and improve everyone's well-being*. London: Penguin Press.

Williams, D. R., Priest, N., & Anderson, N. B. (2016). Understanding associations among race, socioeconomic status, and health: Patterns and prospects. *Health Psychology*, 35(4), 407–411. https://doi.org/10.1037/hea0000242.

World Health Organization. (n.d.-a). *About social determinants of health*. Retrieved from http://www.who.int/social_determinants/sdh_definition/en/.

World Health Organization. (n.d.-b). *Disabilities*. Retrieved from http://www.who.int/topics/disabilities/en/.

World Health Organization. (n.d-c. *WHO definition of palliative care*. Retrieved from http://www.who.int/cancer/palliative/definition/en/.

World Health Organization. (1978). *Alma-Alta Declaration Primary Health Care*. Retrieved from http://www.who.int/publications/almaata_declaration_en.pdf?ua=1.

World Health Organization. (1986). *Ottawa Charter for Health Promotion: First International Conference on Health Promotion, Ottawa, 21 November 1986*. Retrieved from http://www.who.int/healthpromotion/conferences/previous/ottawa/en/index2.html

World Health Organization. (1997). *Jakarta Declaration on Leading Health Promotion into the 21st Century: The Fourth International Conference on Health Promotion: New players for a new era—Leading health promotion into the 21st century, meeting in Jakarta from 21 to 25 July 1997*. Retrieved from http://www.who.int/healthpromotion/conferences/previous/jakarta/declaration/en/index3.html

World Health Organization v. (2005). *The Bangkok Charter for Health Promotion in a Globalized World*. Retrieved from http://www.who.int/healthpromotion/conferences/6gchp/bangkok_charter/en/.

World Health Organization. (2008). *Closing the gap in a generation: Health equity through action on the social determinants of health*. Commission on Social Determinants of Health. Final Report. Executive Summary. Retrieved from http://whqlibdoc.who.int/hq/2008/WHO_IER_CSDH_08.1_eng.pdf.

World Health Organization. (2016). Shanghai declaration on promoting health in the 2030 Agenda for Sustainable Development. *Health Promotion International*, 32(1), 7. Retrieved from http://www.who.int/healthpromotion/conferences/9gchp/shanghai-declaration.pdf?ua=1.

World Health Organization. (2018a). *Disability and health*. Retrieved from http://www.who.int/en/news-room/fact-sheets/detail/disability-and-health.

World Health Organization. (2018b). *Global Action Plan for the Prevention and Control of NCDs 2013–2020*. Retrieved from http://www.who.int/nmh/events/ncd_action_plan/en/.

World Health Organization & the Government of South Australia. (2010). *Adelaide Statement on Health in All Policies: Moving towards a shared governance for health and well-being*. Retrieved from https://www.who.int/social_determinants/hiap_statement_who_sa_final.pdf.

Yeginsu, C. (2018). U.K. appoints a minister for loneliness. *The New York Times* (pp. A7). Retrieved from https://www.nytimes.com/2018/01/17/world/europe/uk-britain-loneliness.html

Zollner, H., & Lessof, S. (1998). *Population health: Putting concepts into action*. Copenhagen, Denmark: World Health Organization, Regional Office for Europe.

2

Methods of Investigation of Population Health Issues

ⓔ Additional resources are available online at http://evolve.elsevier.com/Canada/Shah/publichealth/

LEARNING OBJECTIVES

- Understand ontology, epistemology, and axiology as they relate to the paradigms of positivism, interpretivism, critical approaches, and Indigenous methodologies.
- Define *epidemiology* and describe the various types of epidemiological studies, including their utility, strengths, and limitations.
- Examine the main principles and goals of population-based screening programs.

- Differentiate between different types of qualitative research methodologies.
- Be able to calculate various measures of effect size.
- Define *surveillance* and list the types of data sources available to population health practitioners.
- Understand health informatics and the role it plays in public health.

CHAPTER OUTLINE

KEY TERMS

accuracy
active surveillance
analytic studies
axiology
case-control study
case study
Cochrane Collaboration
confounding
critical research
cross-sectional study

dependent variable
descriptive study
ecological fallacy
ecological studies
epidemic
epidemology
epistemology
ethnography
evidence-informed decision
 making (EIDM)

experimental studies
grounded theory
health informatics
incidence rate
independent variable
Indigenous research paradigm
interpretivism
knowledge translation
lead-time bias
length-time bias

INTRODUCTION

As indicated in Chapter 1, the concepts of health and disease are changing and are multidimensional. A range of tools and methods exist for people working in the health sector to both assess and act to improve health and its determinants. (This chapter is focused specifically on the assessment part.) When it comes to the assessment of complex population health issues, epidemiology is a commonly used tool. Surveillance—one of public health's key functions—is a method used to help understand health and its distribution. Surveillance systems rely on health data sources and health informatics to gather and communicate information.

Before we discuss the various types of epidemiological studies and concepts, it is important to first acknowledge that every investigator has his or her own view of what constitutes truth and knowledge. These views guide our thinking, our beliefs, and our assumptions about society and ourselves, and they frame how we view the world around us and ultimately how we investigate population health issues. These foundational assumptions about the nature of our world (**ontology**) and our knowledge about it (**epistemology**), as well as the role of values in the process of knowledge production (**axiology**) set the foundation for what has been referred to as a **paradigm**. Different paradigms are associated with certain investigative and research methodologies. **Positivism** is a position that holds that the only way to establish truth and objective reality is through the scientific method and that natural science is the only foundation for true knowledge. The belief is that the methods, techniques, and procedures used in natural

science offer the best framework for investigating the social world. The purpose of research in a positivist paradigm is to predict results, test a theory, or find the strength of relationships between variables or a cause-and-effect relationship. Positivist research is related to quantitative methods, wherein questions and hypotheses are posited in advance and are subjected to an empirical test for verification under conditions that are carefully controlled (Guba & Lincoln, 1994). Quantitative researchers begin with ideas, theories, or concepts that are defined as they are used in the study to point to the variables of interest. A majority of this chapter is based on typical methodologies of positivism, including cross-sectional, case control, cohort, observational correlational, and experimental designs. Data-gathering instruments include questionnaires, observations, experiments, and tests.

Interpretivism is another paradigm and differs from positivism in a number of ways. Reality is believed to be socially constructed, and there are as many intangible realities as there are people constructing them. Whereas reality is mind dependent and a personal or social construct, knowledge is subjective. Truth is embedded in human experience—what is true or false is culturally and historically bound and value laden. Understanding people's experiences is the purpose of interpretive methodologies and includes ethnography, phenomenology, case study, and grounded theory. Data-gathering techniques are varied and depend on the choice of design, the population under study, and the research problem. However, typically interviews, observations, photographs, drawings, informal conversations, and artifacts are used.

A third paradigm, **critical research**, includes participatory action research, feminist designs, and research with the aim to transform communities and society. It is this paradigm in which action on the social determinants of health through addressing inequities falls. Social reality is historically bound and is constantly changing, depending on social, political, cultural, and power-based factors. Similarly, with positivism, criticalists believe reality is out there to be discovered but diverge in that they believe the social reality is constantly changing. Knowledge is true when it can be turned into practice that transforms individuals, communities, and society, including the researcher. Knowledge is constructed from the participants' frame of reference. Moral and political activity is the purpose of research in the critical paradigm that requires a value position such as social justice. A range of methods is used, and participants are often involved in all phases of the research process.

Finally, an **Indigenous research paradigm** is a world view that focuses on the shared aspects of ontology, epistemology, axiology, and research methodologies of disempowered or historically oppressed social groups. In his book *Research is Ceremony: Indigenous Research Methods*, Wilson (2008) explains the difference between an Indigenous and a dominant research paradigm:

The major difference between those dominant paradigms and an Indigenous paradigm is that those dominant paradigms build on the fundamental belief that knowledge is an individual entity: the researcher is an individual in search of knowledge, knowledge is something that is gained, and therefore knowledge may be owned by an individual. An indigenous paradigm comes from the fundamental belief that knowledge is relational. Knowledge is shared with all of creation. It is not just interpersonal relationships, or just with the research subjects I may be working with, but it is a relationship with all of creation. It is with the cosmos; it is with the animals, with plants, with the earth that we share this knowledge. It goes beyond the individual's knowledge to the concept of relational knowledge. ... you are answerable to all your relations when you are doing research (Wilson, 2008, p. 56).

Some of the data-gathering techniques from an Indigenous paradigm include methods that are based on oral traditions, talk stories and talking, wisdom circles, and Indigenous knowledge.

Although not all paradigms are discussed here, we have tried to convey a sense of the breadth that can be drawn upon when considering methods of investigation. Dash (2005) provides advice on how to select a research paradigm and corresponding methodology through answering the following questions:

1. What is the nature or essence of the social phenomena being investigated?
2. Is the social phenomenon objective in nature or created by the human mind?
3. What are the bases of knowledge corresponding to the social reality and how can knowledge be acquired and disseminated?
4. What is the relationship of an individual with her environment? Is she conditioned by the environment, or is the environment created by her?

Based on the answers, the researcher can identify whether the research questions pertain to a certain paradigm and choose the appropriate methodology accordingly.

Now that we have covered the basics of paradigms, we will now look at those methods that use more of a positivist or quantitative research paradigm

> **CRTICAL THINKING QUESTION 2.1:** Reflect on the research studies you have read during your training and curriculum. Which paradigm are you most often exposed to, and why do you think that is the case?

EPIDEMIOLOGY

Epidemiology is "the study of the distribution and the determinants of health-related states and events (such as diseases) in specified populations, and the application of this study to the control of health problems" (Last, 1995). The "distribution and the determinants of health-related states" can be thought of in terms of person, place, and time. Person attributes can include innate factors such as age, sex, or factors that determine health (as discussed in Chapter 1), such as socioeconomic status, race, and other factors. Place factors may involve comparisons between urban and rural, between census tracts with high and low income, between north and south, and among different countries. Time factors can include seasonal or diurnal variations in the occurrence of health

BOX 2.1 Social Epidemiology

Over the past 50 years, a new subfield of epidemiology has emerged, called **social epidemiology**. This movement has gained more global momentum in recent years, with an increased focus on the importance of social factors (e.g., housing, income, education) on health (Honjo, 2004).

Social epidemiologists apply epidemiological tools (many of which are explored in this chapter) to investigate the influence of the social determinants of health on well-being and heath equity.

Questions that social epidemiologists might seek to investigate include:

- What is the effect of societal factors such as culture and income security on individual and population health?
- How does the way we have organized society create gaps in health status among various ethnocultural groups?
- How do various healthy public policy solutions influence measures of health equity in the population?

events, differences in the duration of health states, or trends over an extended period of time, for example. Epidemiology seeks to answer questions such as: What are the risk factors for a certain disease state? Do people with disease X have anything in common that may indicate what is causing disease X? How has the rate of disease X changed over time? How is a certain treatment impacting the rate of disease X? What diseases are most common in a population? Are there inequities in the distribution of disease X? (See Box 2.1 for an explanation of social epidemiology, which seeks to answer questions related to health inequities.)

In recent years, the science of epidemiology has been well-recognized for investigating epidemics (**epidemic** is defined as the detection of a higher rate of a health event or disease state in a population over a fixed period of time, compared to a baseline rate) and identifying new health problems in populations. Examples include infectious diseases (e.g., AIDS, Lyme disease, legionnaires disease, toxic shock syndrome), exposure to environmental and occupational hazards (e.g., ozone pollution, pesticides, asbestos), and diseases for which no agent has yet been identified (e.g., Reye's syndrome, Kawasaki disease). Epidemiologists use a range of methodologies to identify and evaluate the causal or

contributing factors to disease, their distribution, and possible means of prevention. The various types of epidemiological studies are described next.

Types of Studies

Descriptive Study

An epidemiological **descriptive study** simply describes a health event, disease state, or other phenomena of interest in terms of person, place, and time. **Prevalence,** which is calculated by dividing the number of individuals who have an attribute or disease at a particular time by the total population at the same point in time, is commonly described in a descriptive study. Prevalence studies can tell us how many people in a specific sociodemographic group, geographic area, or time period have a certain attribute or disease. However, prevalence studies do not go further to look for associations between variables. Thus, one cannot make any causal attribution from descriptive studies; these studies, however, may generate hypotheses that could be further investigated. For example, if a particular report or study finds that the prevalence of food insecurity among people living with diabetes is high, one cannot conclude that food insecurity leads to diabetes. You may hypothesize that there is some connection, but before this can be established, an analytic study needs to be done to actually test this hypothesis and look at whether the rates of food insecurity among people living with diabetes is different than among the general population.

Analytical Studies

In **analytical studies**, a hypothesis is tested to discover if there is an association between a given disease, health state, or other dependent variable (also known as the "outcome" of interest) and possible risk or causative factors (also known as the "exposures" of interest). Analytical studies consist of two types: observational and experimental (refer Fig. 2.1 for a visual depiction of how studies described in this chapter are categorized).

Observational Studies

There are four types of **observational studies**: ecological, cross-sectional, case-control, and cohort studies.

Ecological Studies. **Ecological studies** differ from other observational studies in that the subject of analysis is a an aggregate or group rather than an individual. Usually with other, nonecological observational studies, researchers are assessing both an exposure (e.g., a

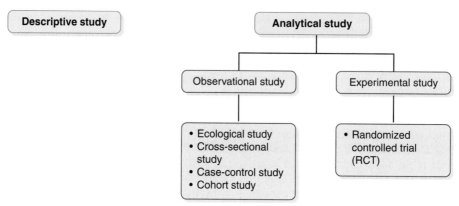

Fig. 2.1 Study types.

risk factor like age) and an outcome (e.g., presence of a certain disease) in each individual person in the study and comparing those exposed to those not exposed or comparing those with the outcome and those without the outcome to find associations (e.g., an association between age and the risk of getting disease X). In ecological studies, however, it is usually geographical areas, such as countries or census tracts, that are used as units of analysis, and differences in exposures and outcomes of interest are compared between the geographical areas as a whole, not between the individual people living in those geographical areas. Ecological studies form a large part of the evidence base that links diet to the risk of developing a number of chronic diseases. For example, researchers who looked at national dietary patterns and rates of chronic diseases across many countries found that countries where people ate a predominantly Mediterranean diet (a diet low in animal fat and high in vegetable consumption) had lower rates of cardiovascular disease (Grant, 2016).

However, one cannot infer from ecological studies alone that a specific type of diet is associated with a disease for an individual person. This pattern might not hold true when you look person to person (versus country to country) because of the differential presence of other associated factors that also influence heart disease (e.g., smoking). Assuming that the country-level trends apply at the individual level is an error known as the **ecological fallacy**—a common downfall of ecological studies. Another way to think about ecological fallacy is inappropriately making inferences about relationships between a risk factor and outcome at the individual level instead of at the level at which the analysis occurred (e.g., country level) (Sedgwick, 2015).

Because they are usually quick and easy to do and make use of readily available data, ecological studies are useful. However, they cannot be used for the direct assessment of causal relationships between risk factors and health outcomes in individuals because the individual is not the unit of analysis. When a variable in question (e.g., income distribution) is either only measurable at the population level or most appropriately measured at this level, then the ecological study may become necessary.

> **EXERCISE 2.1:** What variables can you think of that are best measured at the country level versus person level?

Before we move on to describing other types of descriptive studies, remember the following terms:
1. The **dependent variable**, also known as the outcome, is the particular disease or health state you are trying to investigate.
2. The **independent variable**, also known as the exposure, is the risk or protective factor you are trying to assess against the outcome (i.e., is the factor associated with the outcome or dependent variable).

For example, in a study looking at the association between diet and chronic diseases, diet is the independent variable or exposure, and chronic disease prevalence is the dependent variable or outcome.

Cross-Sectional Study. In a **cross-sectional study**, the investigator measures the outcome and the exposures in the study participants at the same time. Unlike in case-control studies (participants selected based on the outcome status) or cohort studies (participants selected based on the exposure status), the participants in a cross-sectional study are only selected based on the inclusion and exclusion criteria set for the study. In this type of study, the outcome and exposure are examined simultaneously in each person in a defined population at one particular time. The population is divided into those with the disease and those without it, and then various characteristics (or exposures) of the two groups are compared. The total population can also be divided according to different exposure variables such as age or sex, and the disease prevalence rates (outcomes) can be compared among the groups.

Although cross-sectional studies allow for a determination of association between variables, they do not allow for the assessment of the temporal relationship between the variables (e.g., did one variable come before another?). When cross-sectional designs are used to study time-related phenomena, the designs are weaker than longitudinal ones. The advantage of this design is that they are inexpensive and easy to manage.

Drawing on the earlier diet example, a cross-sectional study to investigate the risk of diet on chronic disease prevalence would use the following approach:
- Recruit participants eligible for the study (e.g., adults older than 18 years of age who live in Canada).
- Characterize and record for every participant at a specific time their dietary habits and their chronic disease status.
- For the analysis, group participants into those with a chronic disease (group A) and those without (group B) and then compare the dietary habits between the groups.
- Draw conclusions about whether diet is associated with chronic disease prevalence (e.g., figure out if the dietary patterns of group A differ statistically from the patterns of group B).

Remember that if you do find an association in a cross-sectional study, you cannot simply conclude that it is a causal one (e.g., that an unhealthy diet causes chronic disease). Because you are determining both dietary pattern and chronic disease status in every person at the same point in time, you do not know whether a poor diet preceded the development of the chronic disease or if it was the other way around.

Case-Control Study. A **case-control study** is a type of observational study in which persons with a disease or outcome of interest (cases) are compared with similar persons without the disease (control participants) for exposure to the presumed risk factors. Investigators collect data by examining medical and other relevant records and by interviewing cases and control participants. If a presumed risk factor (exposure, independent variable) is present in cases significantly more often than in control participants, then an association exists between this variable and the disease. This association is expressed by the **odds ratio (OR)**, which is the ratio of the odds of exposure among cases to the odds of exposure among noncases (the next section describes how to calculate the OR). Again, using the diet example, a case-control study would be designed in the following way:
- Recruit participants to the study who have a specific chronic disease (i.e., the case group).
- Recruit other participants to the study (in the same way and drawing from the same or similar general population) who do not have the specific chronic disease (i.e., the control group).
- Interview all participants in both groups and ask them what their dietary habits were in the year before they developed the chronic disease.
- Compare the dietary patterns of the cases with the control participants and see the patterns differ statistically between the two groups.

Case-control studies are less costly and less time-consuming than cohort studies, but they may suffer from **recall bias**; people with a disease may be more prone to recalling, or believing, that they were exposed to a possible causal factor than those who are free of disease because they are often more actively thinking about what they may have been exposed to day to day in their lives to cause a disease they have compared to those without that specific disease. People with a chronic disease may be questioning how they acquired it and so may have a better memory of what they were eating before they developed the disease, compared with those who do not and thus may not remember as well.

Because case-control studies start with an identification of individuals with and without disease, they are good for studying rare disease outcomes. When the disease outcome is rare, the OR is a good estimate of the relative risk (described further later). As with other types of observational studies, case-control studies may also show a spurious association between a factor and a health outcome because of unrecognized confounding. **Confounding** occurs when a variable (known as a confounding variable) is related to the exposure or risk factor in question and is also independently related to the outcome in question but does not lie on the causal pathway between the risk factor and outcome in question (Iles & Barrett, 2011).

If not corrected, a false association between the confounder and the outcome may occur because the confounder is associated with both the outcome and the exposure. For example, a study that sought to investigate the relationship between coffee drinking and heart disease found a strong relationship between increased coffee consumption and heart disease but did not measure cigarette smoking. In this case, it is likely that the association between coffee drinking and heart disease is confounded by cigarette smoking because cigarette smoking is associated with coffee drinking (i.e., those who smoke cigarettes also drink more coffee) and is a known cause of heart disease. Thus, because cigarette smoking was not measured and controlled for, the perceived association between coffee drinking and heart disease may be deceptive, arising from the association between increased cigarette smoking in coffee drinkers and heart disease.

Cohort Study. A cohort is a group of people with a common characteristic, such as year of birth, place of residence, occupation, or exposure to a suspected cause of disease that may be followed forward in time by investigators. Although cohort studies look forward in time (i.e., they focus on exposures that occur before the outcome of interest develops), there are two types: retrospective and prospective. In **retrospective cohort studies**, the whole period of observation is historical; in **prospective cohort studies**, the period of observation starts when the study starts and continues for a period of time into the future. In both types, a cohort that becomes exposed to the hypothesized risk factor (exposure) is chosen from a defined population free of the disease under study, along with a "control cohort" that ideally has the same characteristics except that it is not exposed to this factor. Both groups are followed for

a certain period of time (e.g., 5, 10, or 20 years), and the observed rates of disease or other outcomes in the two cohorts are compared. For example, in a prospective cohort study that is conducted to examine possible association between diet and chronic disease development, a cohort of people that have poor dietary patterns would be chosen, and then a similar group of people with healthier dietary patterns would also be chosen. Both groups would be followed for several years and then compared with respect to how many people in each group developed a chronic disease.

Cohort studies have the great advantage that possible risk factors are identified and recorded before the disease appears, thus reducing the possibility of many sources of **bias** (systematic error in making inferences and recording observations). However, these studies, particularly prospective cohort studies, are expensive, pose great difficulty for studying very rare diseases, and take many years before results can be analyzed. Table 2.1 summarizes the advantages and disadvantages of case-control and cohort studies.

Experimental Studies

Unlike observational studies, **experimental studies** are those in which conditions of the study are under the direct control of the investigator. Observational studies are the best types of studies possible for the study of exposures to risk factors because it would be unethical to expose healthy people intentionally to risk factors. For example, it would be unethical to ask people to follow an unhealthy diet for several years. However, experimental studies are possible when trying to assess the effects of an intervention (which can be thought of as a "positive exposure") to improve health outcomes, either by providing a new treatment to those already ill or by providing an intervention to attempt to prevent a disease. In a **randomized controlled trial (RCT)**, people are randomized into two or more groups (e.g., the group that gets a new medication to treat a chronic disease and the group that gets regular treatment and the usual medications). Usually, as in the example, one group is subjected to the intervention, or positive exposure, being evaluated, usually a new treatment, but all other groups (controls) are given either an inactive treatment (placebo) or current standard treatment. If the health outcomes in the treatment group are statistically significantly better than those in the control group, then the treatment is considered to have been

TABLE 2.1	Comparison of Cohort and Case-Control Studies	
	Cohort Study	**Case-Control Study**
Advantages	Provides incidence rates, relative risk, and attributable risk	Quick to do
	Less bias	Suitable for rare diseases
	Can get natural history of disease	Relatively inexpensive
	Can study many diseases	Can study many factors
Disadvantages	Large number of subjects	Recall bias
	Long follow-up	Provides only odds ratio
	Attrition	Can be challenging to select
	Costly	Does not provide incidence rate
	Changes over time	Locked into disease
	Locked into factor under investigation	

effective in this trial. So, if the chronic disease improves in the group that was given the new medication more so than it does in the group that was given the usual treatment, then the new medication can be considered effective.

The main benefit of an RCT is that you are randomly selecting who gets the intervention being tested and who does not. You are not basing it on anything but a totally random occurrence (e.g., everyone who pulls the number 2 out of the hat receives the treatment). Because of this randomness, you should get two groups that are more or less the same in factors that could be potential confounders (e.g., characteristics of people that influence whether they get the treatment and the outcome). When participants are randomly selected like this, you reduce the chance that all of the people selected for treatment will end up being younger and would therefore be less likely to get the disease anyway, for example.

The Calculation of Relative Risk, Odds Ratio, Attributable Risk, and Attributable Fraction or Population Attributable Risk. Usually, health data take into account the broader population in which certain health events occur. Hence, in most situations, one needs both a numerator, that is, the frequency of occurrence of an event under observation, and a denominator, that is, size of population in which the event occurred to describe trends and statistics in a meaningful way.

Three commonly used measures of data expression are ratio, proportion, and rate. A **ratio** is an expression of the relationship between two items that are usually independent of each other. If there are 6 males and 12 females in a particular situation, then the ratio of males to females in that situation is 1:2. Another public health example is the maternal mortality ratio, which expresses the number of maternal deaths per year relative to the number of live births in that year.

A **proportion** is the relationship of a part to its whole and is generally expressed as a percentage. If there are 25 ill persons of 100 persons, then the proportion of ill persons is 25% or 0.25. This is like prevalence. If there are 25 people with heart disease in a group of 100, then the prevalence of heart disease is 25%, for example.

A **rate** is an expression of the probability of an occurrence of an event in a defined population at risk during a specific time period. For example, if five cases of bladder cancer occur among 500 000 factory workers under study for 1 year, the rate of bladder cancer in this group is 5/500 000 or 1 per 100 000 people over a 1-year period. This latter example is also an incidence rate. The **incidence rate** is the rate at which a new disease or other events in a defined population at risk of having that disease or event occur over a given time. The numerator consists of the number of new events (e.g., new cases of a disease diagnosed or reported) over a given period, and its denominator is the number of people in the defined population who do not have the disease or event at the beginning of the follow-up period. An incidence rate can only be calculated from cohort studies because they follow people in time and thus can track when a new disease or event occurs.

The risk of disease for individuals may be measured by either a relative risk or OR. To calculate these risk measures, you need the number of persons with and without disease, as well as the number of people with

	Disease (cases)	No disease (control)
Positive	a 350	b 220
Negative	c 150	d 280

Exposure

Fig. 2.2 Hypothetical 2 × 2 table.

and without exposure to the suspected causal or risk factor (exposure). These values are often represented using a 2 × 2 table, depicted in Fig. 2.2.

The **relative risk (RR)** is the risk of those exposed developing the disease, compared with the risk of developing the disease in the unexposed, and can be calculated by:

$$\left(\frac{a}{a+b}\right) \div \left(\frac{c}{c+d}\right)$$

In the case of a cohort study, (a/a + b) represents the incidence (i.e., risk of getting the disease) in the exposed, and (c/c + d) represents the incidence in the unexposed.

The OR of a case having been exposed, compared with a control, is (a × d) ÷ (b × c). The OR is essentially the odds that a case was exposed compared with the odds that a control was exposed.

Population attributable risk (PAR), a very commonly used metric in population health, is a measure of the excess incidence of disease associated with an exposure within a population. PAR can be calculated directly from the RR and the prevalence of exposure (Pe) to the risk factor in the population (see Box 2.2 for an example of the PAR calculated for liver cancer and how to interpret it):

$$PAR = Pe \ (RR - 1) \div \{1 + [Pe \ (RR - 1)]\}$$

EXERCISE 2.2:

a. Based on the 2 × 2 table shown in Fig. 2.2, calculate and interpret the relative risk. Assume that this 2 × 2 table was made based on a cohort study looking at the link between smoking (exposure) and cervical cancer (disease).

b. If the prevalence of smoking in the population was 18%, calculate and interpret the population attributable risk.

BOX 2.2   The Population Attributable Risk of Liver Cancer

Population attributable risk (PAR) is often used in health policy and is of particular interest to law makers. It is a simple measure that indicates the proportion of a disease you could eliminate if a risk factor in question (thought to cause that disease) is virtually eliminated.

In the field of environmental health, much attention is paid to biological and chemical agents and their cancer-causing potential. An example of a biological agent that causes hepatocellular carcinoma (a type of liver cancer) is aflatoxin, a substance that is produced by certain fungi found on crops such as corn, peanuts, and others. The most common way people are exposed to aflatoxin is by eating contaminated food products (National Cancer Institute, 2015).

In 2012, researchers aimed to estimate the PAR of aflatoxin by conducting a meta-analysis that pooled summary measures from 17 studies that took place in China, Taiwan, or subSaharan Africa, where exposure to aflatoxin is more common (Liu et al., 2012). The investigators determined that the PAR of aflatoxin is 23%. This means that in these countries, if policy measures were put in place to eliminate exposure to aflatoxin (e.g., testing foods for aflatoxin and removing those testing positive from the shelves, putting into place mandatory practices for those in agriculture to ensure they don't feed livestock contaminated foods), 23% of hepatocellular carcinomas would be prevented.

Systematic Reviews and Meta-Analyses

As the scientific literature grows and numerous studies are published on each health topic, it is increasingly difficult to make sense of the sometimes conflicting results of multiple studies. In recent years, systematic reviews and meta-analyses have become important tools for addressing this issue and are often referred to as one of the most robust tools for assessing a research question within a positivist paradigm. However, it is important to keep in mind that different kinds of reviews offer different kinds of truth: a **systematic review** with meta-analysis deals in probabilistic truth; it is concerned mainly with producing generalizable "facts" to aid prediction. It attempts to overcome biases that might occur through rigorous and systematic methods for searching for papers, retrieving, rating relevance and quality, extracting the data, synthesizing the data, and writing up

---

BOX 2.3 The Cochrane Collaboration

The **Cochrane Collaboration** is a global network of 130 countries, including Canada, that produces systematic reviews independent of commercial funding or influence, for the purpose of advancing evidence-based decision making in the heath care sector. It maintains an accessible database of all evidence related to health care delivery.

Examples of questions that the Cochrane Collaboration has reviewed include the efficacy of various psychological interventions for posttraumatic stress disorder in people with severe mental illness, the impact of community water fluoridation on dental caries, and screening for visual impairment in elderly populations.

The website to access the Cochrane database is listed at the end of this chapter.

---

the review. Criteria for the inclusion of studies, including for rating relevance and quality of the studies, are preset. Often, more than one person independently conducts each stage of the review, compares their results, and discusses the discrepancies. So, for example, if undertaking a systematic review on the effect of vegetable consumption on the incidence of heart disease, an investigator would search for studies undertaken to examine this association, extract the results from each study, analyze how good each study is, give more weight to the results of the studies that were designed better and have less bias, and summarize the findings of the studies as a whole to draw a conclusion.

Meta-analysis takes systematic reviews one step further and quantitatively combines the results of the studies to get an overall summary statistic that represents the combined effect of an intervention across different studies (Moher et al., 2015). If you were undertaking a meta-analysis on the same topic discussed, you would combine, or pool, all the ORs or RRs from each study to look at the association between vegetable consumption and the development of heart disease together into one large summary OR or RR.

The purposes of meta-analyses include increasing statistical power for outcome assessment and subgroup evaluation, resolving uncertainty or conflicting results, improving estimates of effect by increasing sample size, and providing answers to questions not posed by the original trials. See Box 2.3 for an example of a large global network that exists to produce systematic reviews and meta-analyses. Criticism of systematic reviews and meta-analyses have included topic overlap, redundant meta-analyses,

and the same topic meta-analyses, demonstrating they are unnecessary and have been influenced by or produced by industry employees or authors with industry ties that are misleading and conflicted (Ioannidis, 2016).

Although it is always appropriate and desirable to review the literature systematically to answer a question about a health topic, it is not always appropriate to combine the results quantitatively and statistically. Thus, even though a systematic review may be warranted to help answer a particular question, meta-analyses may not be applicable if the independent studies being pooled are too different in their statistical methods.

Narrative Review

A narrative review summarizes different primary studies from which conclusions may be drawn into a holistic interpretation contributed by the reviewers' own experience, existing theories, and models along with critique (Kirkevold, 1997). Results are qualitative rather than quantitative and are conducted using a number of distinctive methodologies. The narrative review, in contrast to a systematic review, deals in plausible truth. Its goal is an argument based on informed wisdom that is convincing to an audience of experts. The author of a narrative review must represent in the written product both the underpinning evidence (including, but not limited to, primary research) and how this evidence has been drawn upon and pulled together to inform the review's conclusions. Narrative reviews not only expand our understanding of the topic in question but also of the reasons why it has been studied in a particular way, the interpretations that have been variously made with respect to what we know about it, and the nature of the knowledge base that informs or might inform clinical practice. An emerging type of narrative review is a **meta-narrative review** that seeks to illustrate a heterogeneous topic area by highlighting the contrasting and complementary ways in which researchers have studied the same or similar topic. A meta-narrative review is a process of sense making of the literature, selecting and combining data from primary sources to produce an account of how a research tradition unfolded and why, and then (in a second phase) comparing and contrasting findings from these different traditions to build a rich picture of the topic area from multiple angles (Wong et al., 2013). Shifting the focus away from comparing findings of studies published at different times, it orients critical reflection to discern how ideas have changed within different scholarly communities at different points in the development of thinking. For an example of a meta-narrative review, see Greenhalgh et al. (2005).

Clinical Epidemiology

An important source of information on the natural history, prognosis, and outcome of disease states comes from the observations and actions of practising health care providers. Clinical epidemiology represents the application, modification, and refinement of epidemiological techniques to individual client care; its purpose is to collect systematic information from clinical practice to increase the accuracy, reliability, validity, and effectiveness of clinical care. Clinicians are often interested in knowing if an intervention works or if it works better than other interventions. There are several types of questions a clinician may ask, such as: How prevalent is a particular condition? Which treatment is the most clinically effective? Which measure of outcome is the most appropriate?

Different types of clinical questions are answered by different types of research studies. PICOT is often used to provide a structure for asking clinical questions (P, population or problem; I, interventions; C, comparison; O, outcomes of interest; and T, time). In all types of health care practice, the concept of **evidence-informed decision making (EIDM)** is being embraced, particularly in nursing practice. EIDM is an ongoing process that incorporates evidence from research findings, clinical expertise, client preferences, and other available resources to inform decisions that health care providers make about clients (Scott & McSherry, 2008). Essentially, it is a move toward using information and all sorts of data to guide clinical decisions.

In line with the EIDM movement, a number of internationally recognized collaboratives regularly publish evidence-based guidelines for the health sector. For example, in England, the National Institute for Health and Care Excellence (NICE) publishes evidence-based guidelines for health and social care. These guidelines, known as the NICE guidelines (see weblink at the end of the chapter), have been developed to assist in decision making in the following sectors: clinical, medical practice, social services, public health, cancer services, and antimicrobial prescribing (NICE, n.d.).

In the Canadian context, the National Collaborating Centre for Methods and Tools (NCCMT), one of six National Collaborating Centres whose aim is to strengthen the Canadian public health system, exists to support EIDM in public health practice. Among other initiatives, the NCCMT has developed a range of methods and tools to support **knowledge translation** (which aims to synthesize, disseminate, exchange, and apply knowledge to practice) (NCCMT, n.d.) and supports Health Evidence, a registry of systematic reviews that evaluate the effectiveness of various public health interventions.

Causal Associations

The types of studies outlined in the previous sections (particularly analytical studies) are frequently undertaken with the overall objective of identifying and establishing associations between exposure to factor(s) and disease.

Although analytical studies are able to draw associations (whether an exposure and outcome are statistically related) between exposures and specific health outcomes, the determination of causation (whether the exposure results in the health outcome) is more challenging. In 1965, Hill published the following criteria for determining whether a causal association exists between an exposure and a disease:

- **Consistency of the association:** Do the findings of studies of the same design, as well as different designs in different populations, demonstrate the same association?
- **Strength of the association:** How large is the RR of the outcome in relation to exposure?
- **Dose response:** Does the severity or the likelihood of the outcome increase as the amount, intensity, or duration of the exposure increases?
- **Temporal relationship:** Did the exposure occur before the onset of the disease?
- **Plausibility:** Is the association possible and does it fit with existing basic science and clinical knowledge about the disease?
- **Coherence:** Does the association make sense in terms of the theory and knowledge about the disease process?
- **Analogy:** Do other established associations provide a model for this type of relationship?
- **Experimental evidence:** Is there experimental or quasi-experimental evidence that removal of the putative causative factor results in reduction of disease incidence?
- **Specificity:** Is the association specific for a particular disease or group of diseases? (In practice, this criterion often is not satisfied, particularly with many chronic diseases that can have multiple causes.)

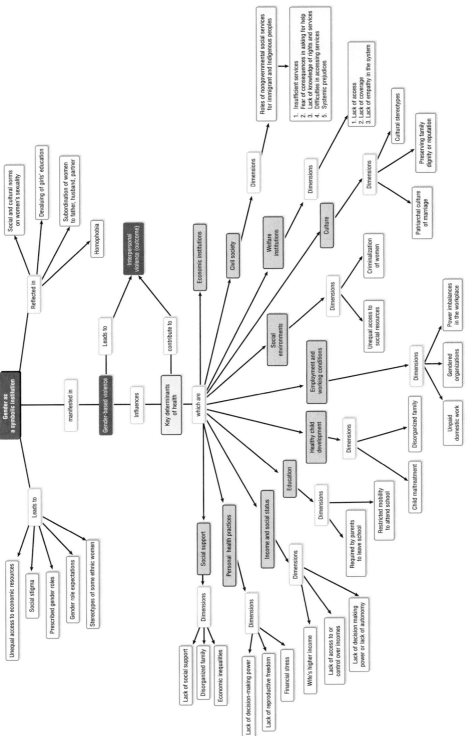

Fig. 2.3 Web of causation for gender-based violence against women. (Montesanti, S. R., & Thurston, W. E. [2015]. Mapping the role of structural and interpersonal violence in the lives of women: implications for public health interventions and policy. *BMC Women's Health*, *15*[1], 100.)

For one to be more confident in the fact that an exposure truly causes a disease, many of these conditions should be met. This criterion may work well when you're thinking about just one risk factor or exposure and one disease (e.g., the link between diet and chronic disease). However, we know that disease states are very complex, and there are multiple determinants of health that go beyond just diet (i.e., socioeconomic status greatly influences diet, so this also needs to be considered).

Causal diagrams, such as the **web of causation**, go beyond the depiction of a single link (e.g., a disease and its proximal causal factor) to focus on a larger causal system showing interrelationships between indirect and direct causes. The web of causation offers a useful way to understand etiology and linking social determinants and social factors and biomedical etiologic factors, which can guide the development of interventions. See Fig. 2.3 for an example in which the web of causation illustrates how structural factors can have negative impacts on the social determinants of health and increase the risk for interpersonal violence among women. This figure, based on the work of Montesanti and Thurston (2015), demonstrates the need to work from a population health perspective to prevent structural violence against women.

In the next section, we move from discussing research in the positivist paradigm to discussing the interpretive and critical paradigms, also known as qualitative research.

Qualitative Research

Many important, complex issues in public health cannot be adequately addressed by quantitative methods. Issues relating to the attitudes and beliefs of community members or health care practitioners may be best explored using qualitative research techniques, which has its origins mostly in the fields of anthropology and sociology. **Qualitative research** uses interpretive and critical approaches and a range of different methodologies and theories to study research questions. Studies are carried out in natural nonexperimental situations. Unlike the quantitative approach, which places a high value on quantitative measurement and analysis, statistical measures, and hypothesis testing, qualitative research focuses on explaining and understanding a particular process and its nuances in depth. More specifically, it aims to explore people's understanding and perceptions of their own lives, the meaning they ascribe to their experiences, and social environments that shape all of this. The goal is usually to explore the *how* and *why* of particular phenomena. Information is usually collected from smaller, nonrandom samples because the goal is not to generalize to entire populations so much so as to enhance the understanding of perceptions of particular groups of people in a specific and given context. Some characteristics of qualitative research include that it is person-centric and exploratory, is based on textual data (e.g., diary entries, case histories from a medical chart, transcripts from interviews) versus numbers, and involves extensive interaction with subjects or research participants, among others (Holloway, 2005; McGill Qualitative Health Research Group, n.d.). Qualitative research methodologies included in this chapter are phenomenology, grounded theory, ethnography, and case study.

Phenomenology is rooted in a philosophical tradition developed by Husserl and Heidegger and is an approach to thinking about people's life experiences and focuses on what all participants have in common while they experience any social phenomenon. A researcher using phenomenology would ask: What is the essence of this phenomenon as experienced by these people, and what does it mean? There is a belief that critical truths about reality are grounded in people's lived experience.

In a phenomenological study, the main data source is in-depth conversations with the participant and the researcher. The researcher helps the participant to describe lived experiences without leading the discussion (see Research Perspective box). Phenomenological studies often involve 10 or fewer participants. Data analysis occurs through a four-step process: bracketing, intuiting, analyzing, and describing. Bracketing involves identifying and holding in abeyance preconceived beliefs and opinions about the phenomenon under study. Intuiting occurs when the researcher remains open to the meanings attributed to the phenomenon by those who have experienced it. Analysis proceeds through extracting significant statements, categorizing, and making sense of the essential meanings of the phenomenon. The descriptive phase occurs when the researcher comes to understand and define the phenomenon.

Understanding Inequalities in Access to Health Care Services for Indigenous People: A Call for Nursing Action

Cameron et al. (2014) reported findings about the experiences of access to health care for Indigenous people seeking emergency care in a large Western Canadian city. An Indigenous-based intervention was implemented to facilitate the access experience of Indigenous people in emergency departments (EDs). This intervention consisted of the placement of two community health representatives in the EDs of one large urban hospital and one rural hospital that served Indigenous communities.

Community health representatives are Indigenous health care workers who are viewed as community health agents in their local communities. An interpretive approach was used through a hermeneutic phenomenological methodology in which context and experience are crucial to knowing and the knower is a large part of what is known. Description and interpretation were the key methodological strategies from hermeneutic phenomenology that were followed. There were 19 participants in the urban study and 35 participants in the rural study, and it used 30-minute interviews focusing on the experience of access to emergency care services, the interaction with health care professionals, the barriers to accessing health services, and the value of having an Indigenous health care worker positioned in the emergency department.

Two stories are presented from the research that report racism, stigmatization, language difficulties, intimidation, harassment, and deep fear. The subjective data demonstrate the need for health care providers to enhance their reflective practice regarding negative behaviours and the health care system itself on others. Recommendations include access to cultural safety workshops for health care providers and to increase the number of Indigenous health care workers in health care settings.

Source: Cameron, B. L., Plazas, M. D. P. C., Salas, A. S., et al. (2014). Understanding inequalities in access to health care services for Aboriginal people. *Advances in Nursing Science, 37*(3), E1–E16.

Grounded theory is a qualitative methodology based on the premise that theory is indispensable for gaining deep knowledge of social phenomena (Glaser & Strauss, 1967). Developed in the 1960s by two sociologists, Barney Glaser and Anselm Strauss, grounded theory is an approach to the study of social processes and social structures. The term "grounded theory" is used to refer to both the process of conducting a study (i.e., the methodology, grounded theory methodology [GTM]) and the product (i.e., the theory produced).

The main reason to use GTM is to create new theories that explain some kind of social phenomena. GTM is particularly useful when there is little pre-existing theory available to explain a certain social process, when theories are underdeveloped for particular populations, or if existing theories are incomplete. A researcher using GTM should "think theoretically" from the start of a study, with the mindset that the goal of the research is to create a grounded theory. It should be clear that initial sampling was dictated by the research question and the goal of developing theory. Data analysis should begin as soon as the first data are collected, and there should be interaction between data analysis and data collection throughout the study. This is referred to as the iterative process of data collection and analysis (Corbin & Strauss, 2015). Theoretical sampling refers to sampling based on the concepts identified during initial data collection and analysis (Strauss & Corbin, 1998).

Coding refers to a range of analytical techniques used to ask questions of data to identify dimensions of concepts and categories (often referred to as themes in other forms of qualitative research) and relationships therein. By coding data, researchers move from interview transcripts (and other raw data) toward interpretation and the production of a grounded theory. Constant comparison involves comparing incident with incident in order to classify data. In the words of Corbin and Strauss, constant comparison is "the analytic process of comparing different pieces of data against each other for similarities and differences" (Corbin & Strauss, 2015, p. 85).

Theoretical saturation is "a matter of reaching the point in the research where collecting new data seems counterproductive; the 'new' that is uncovered does not add that much more to the explanation at this time" (Strauss & Corbin, 1998, p. 136). In other words, with theoretical saturation, there are no more emergent patterns in the theory (i.e., the explanation), as opposed to no new data per se. (See the Research Perspective box on Grounded Theory.)

RESEARCH PERSPECTIVE

A Grounded Theory Model for Reducing Stigma in Health Professionals in Canada

The purpose of the study was to develop a greater theoretical understanding of the process for designing and delivering successful anti-stigma programs for health care providers. The study revolved around the general research question: What is the process for designing and delivering a successful anti-stigma program for health care providers?

The study used a grounded theory methodology, commonly used for building theory from data and for studies of process. Data methods included in-depth interviews with program stakeholders (program leads, facilitators, or instructors; program coordinators; persons with lived experience of mental illness who were involved in program delivery, e.g., as first-voice speakers), direct observation of programs, and review of available program documents.

The data analysis led to the generation of a theoretical model articulating a four-stage process for designing and delivering successful anti-stigma programming for health care providers. The analysis also helped to identify key strategies and activities informing each process stage—from "setting up for success" (preparation and planning), to "building the program using key ingredients," to "making the connection" (program delivery strategies), and to "working toward culture change."

Source: Knaak, S., & Patten, S. (2016). A grounded theory model for reducing stigma in health professionals in Canada. *Acta Psychiatrica Scandinavica, 134,* 53–62.

Ethnography, originating in the field of anthropology, is one of the oldest forms of qualitative research. Ethnography in public health is valuable when considering equity for vulnerable populations (see Research Perspective box). It is a descriptive account of social life and culture in which the researcher investigates the beliefs, ideas, and practices of a particular cultural setting and its influence on people. Rather than studying people, ethnography means learning from people (unlike more positivistic approaches), and knowledge gained from data is intended to inform understanding rather than to control. Examples of a cultural group could include nurses in a certain hospital, female students in a certain department, community members in a certain neighbourhood, and individuals who access short-term shelters in a particular organization.

Researchers who use ethnography may live among the cultural groups to study cultural patterns and their origins to become immersed in a group. Methods for data collection include participant observation (participation in subjects' day-to-day life), making observations, and interviewing participants. Archival research can also be used in an ethnographic study when there is an analysis of existing materials stored for research, service, or other purposes.

According to LeCompte and Schensul (2010), there are seven defining characteristics of ethnography: (1) the study being carried out in a natural setting, not in a laboratory; (2) involving intimate, face-to-face interaction with participants; (3) presenting an accurate reflection of participant perspectives and behaviours; (4) using inductive, interactive, and recursive data collection to build local cultural theories; (5) using both qualitative and quantitative data; (6) framing all human behavior within a sociopolitical and historical context; and (7) using the concept of culture as a lens through which to interpret study results. Ethnography should be used to:

- Define a problem when the problem is not yet clear.
- Identify participants when the participants, population sectors, stakeholders, or the boundaries of the study population are not yet known or identified.
- Clarify the range of settings where a problem or situation currently occurs when not all of the possible settings are fully identified, known, or understood.
- Identify and describe unexpected or unanticipated outcomes.
- Design measures that match the characteristics of the target population, clients, or community participants when existing measures are not a good fit or need to be adapted.
- Answer questions that cannot be addressed with other methods or approaches (LeCompte & Schensul, 2010).

Ethnography can produce vast amounts of data with varied data types and rich interactions that are complex because researchers can spend years in the field. Different types of data analysis can be used depending on the purpose of the study.

An Ethnographic Study to Measure Primary Health Care Indicators Using an Equity Lens

A 4-year ethnographic study by Wong et al. (2011) was conducted at two Primary Health Care (PHC) Centres in Canada that had explicit mandates to provide services to marginalized populations. The aims of the study were to (1) extend an understanding of *how* PHC services are provided to meet the needs of people who have been marginalized by systemic inequities; (2) identify key dimensions of PHC services for marginalized populations; and (3) develop PHC indicators that can account for the quality, process, and outcomes of care when marginalized populations are explicitly targeted.

Observational and interview data were collected at the PHC Centres using in-depth interviews with a total of 114 patients and staff, including (1) individual interviews with 62 patients and three focus groups with 11 patients (*n* = 73 patients) and (2) individual interviews with 33 staff and an additional 8 staff members who participated in focus groups (*n* = 41 staff). An analysis of key organizational documents was also completed to shed light on policy and funding environments. In addition, in-depth interviews were conducted with two decision-makers used by health authorities, within which the PHC Centres were located and funded. Participant observation involved more than 900 hours of intensive immersion, which was essential to developing knowledge about equity-oriented PHC services grounded in the everyday complexities of clinical practice.

An interpretive thematic analysis was conducted using procedures for qualitatively derived data. Through the analysis the investigators identified (1) four key dimensions of equity-oriented PHC services, which are particularly relevant when working with marginalized populations; (2) 10 strategies to guide organizations to enhance their capacity for equity-oriented services; and (3) outcomes related to these dimensions and strategies (Fig. 2.4). Wong et al. (2011) conclude that their data showed that equity-based strategies can result in improved health outcomes and quality of life.

Case study is an approach that uses in-depth investigation of any social phenomenon using various sources of data. Case study can draw upon many disciplines (Yin, 2014) and is conducive to a research approach that is pragmatic. The researcher in a case study becomes a bricoleur; "inventor in the best sense of the word—taking what works from existing methodologies, incorporating what works and is relevant from worldview practices and protocols, and developing a new paradigm to serve the needs of the people" (Denzin & Lincoln, 2005, p. 1061).

Case study research involves the study of an issue explored through one or more cases within a bounded setting (Creswell & Creswell, 2017) and allows researchers to retain the holistic and meaningful characteristics of real-life events (Yin, 2014). There is some discussion regarding whether case study is a research methodology or not (see Stake, 1995; Denzin & Lincoln, 2005; Merriam, 1988; Yin, 2014).

As a methodology, case study research is a qualitative approach in which the investigator explores a bounded system (a case) or multiple bounded systems (cases) over time through detailed, in-depth data collection involving multiple sources of information (e.g., observations, interviews, audiovisual material, and documents and reports) and reports a case description and case-based themes. Types of qualitative case studies are distinguished by the size of the bounded case, such as whether the case involves one individual, several individuals, a group, an entire program (see Research Perspective box), or an activity. They may also be distinguished in terms of the intent of the case analysis.

Mixed methods approaches are also increasingly being used (Tariq & Woodman, 2013). Researchers using mixed methods incorporate methods of collecting or analyzing data from the quantitative and qualitative research approaches in a single research study (Tashakkori & Teddlie, 2003). That is, researchers collect or analyze not only numerical data, which is customary for quantitative research, but also narrative data, which is the norm for qualitative research, to address the research question(s) defined for a particular research study. As an example, to collect a mixture of data, researchers might distribute a survey that contains closed-ended questions to collect the numerical, or quantitative, data and conduct an interview using open-ended questions to collect the narrative, or qualitative, data.

The goal for researchers using the mixed methods approach to research is to draw from the strengths and minimize the weaknesses of the quantitative and qualitative research approaches (Johnson & Onwuegbuzie, 2004). The advantages of a mixed method design that combines data collection or data analysis methods from the quantitative and qualitative research

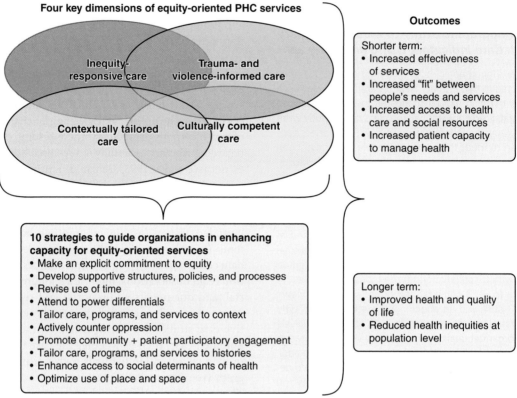

Fig. 2.4 Equity-oriented Primary Health Care services. (From Wong, S. T., Browne, A. J., Varcoe, C., et al. [2011]. Enhancing measurement of primary health care indicators using an equity lens: An ethnographic study. *International Journal for Equity in Health, 10*[1], 38. Retrieved from https://equityhealthj.biomedcentral.com/articles/10.1186/1475-9276-11-59)

approaches are that researchers are now able to test and build theories. Researchers are also able to use deductive and inductive analysis in the same research study.

The mixed methods approach to research provides researchers with the ability to design a single research study that answers questions about both the complex nature of phenomena from the participants' point of view and the relationship between measurable variables. Proponents of the mixed methods approach to research advocate doing "what works" within the precepts of research to investigate, to predict, to explore, to describe, and to understand the phenomenon (Creswell & Creswell, 2017; Tashakkori & Teddlie, 2003). Not only are quantitative and qualitative research approaches compatible, but they are also complementary, which underpins calls for additional research studies that use the mixed methods research approach (Tashakkori & Teddlie, 2003).

INVESTIGATION AND MONITORING OF DISEASE IN POPULATIONS

The preceding section provided an overview of different epidemiological methods for studying health and disease in the population. The following describes several situations in which these methods are applied to monitor or track disease in populations using the spectrum of data available to us in Canada.

Screening

Before the development of symptoms or physical signs, diseases may be present in affected people without their knowledge (i.e., asymptomatic disease). For example, a person can have breast cancer for months before they start to feel a lump or start experiencing any other symptoms, such as pain. The commonly used method for detecting asymptomatic disease in a population is screening. **Screening** is defined as "the presumptive

RESEARCH PERSPECTIVE

The Adoption, Implementation, and Maintenance of a School Food Policy in the Canadian Arctic: A Retrospective Case Study

In Canadian Arctic Indigenous communities, local schools are challenged to support healthy culturally adapted foods. Geography, climate, and changes to cultural traditions have led to a decrease in accessing and consuming traditional foods.

This study took place in a small isolated community in the Canadian Arctic. The goal of this single exploratory case was to gain an understanding of a phenomenon (policy adoption and implementation) experienced by particular individuals (community decision makers, policy champions, and health practitioners) in a particular context (Northern Indigenous community). Therefore, the case is defined as the process of building knowledge and capacity with local decision makers toward policy adoption and implementation of healthy eating and active living policies. The purpose of article was to articulate a policy story retrospectively, exploring the question: What are the stories from decision makers, policy influencers, and health practitioners in the community about their experiences in the policy process related to healthy eating and active living? Data were collected using multiple methods: in-depth interviews, document analysis, and observation at the school and local store. However, because interviews were retrospective, a limitation of the study is that recall about the implementation of the food policy processes may not be as accurate as recall about more recent changes to the policy. The policy processes of a local school food policy to address unhealthy eating were discussed.

The findings indicated that a number of key activities facilitated the successful policy implementation process and the building of a critical mass to support healthy eating and active living in the community. A key contextual factor in school food policies in the Arctic is the influence of traditional (country) foods.

Source: Fournier, B., Illasiak, V., Kushner, K. E., & Raine, K. (2018). The adoption, implementation and maintenance of a school food policy in the Canadian Arctic: A retrospective case study. *Health Promotion International.* https://www.ncbi.nlm.nih.gov/pubmed/31382297 or https://doi.org/10.1093/heapro/day040

EXERCISE 2.3: Determine which of the following research questions may be better suited for quantitative data versus qualitative data:

a. What are working mothers' perceived barriers to good health in the North Kingston community?
b. What are the experiences of emergency nurses and physicians regarding caring for individuals who use drugs and other substances problematically?
c. Is there a significant correlation between annual income and alcohol consumption in the Greater Toronto Area?
d. Does maternal exposure to arsenic in drinking water during pregnancy increase the risk for congenital anomalies in newborns?
e. What are key impressions of needle and syringe use in prisons from the perspective of inmates, law enforcement personnel, and health care providers?
f. Are needle exchange programs effective in preventing hepatitis C infections across 10 provincial prisons?

CRITICAL THINKING QUESTION 2.2: What are some of the challenges with a mixed method design given that both quantitative and qualitative methods are used?

---

identification of unrecognized disease or defect by the application of tests, examinations or other procedures which can be applied rapidly" (Whitby, 1974). Thus, the goal of screening is early detection—identifying which asymptomatic people in the community probably have the disease and which ones probably do not—so that early intervention may be instituted and better health outcomes achieved. Examples of screening procedures include mammography for breast cancer and Papanicolaou (Pap) tests for cervical cancer. Because the goals of public health are to minimize people's interactions with the health care system and keep people healthy, an important public health intervention is screening, which is a form of secondary prevention (described more in Chapters 3 and 8).

CRITICAL THINKING QUESTION 2.3: Can you think of examples of a condition in which a highly sensitive screening test (i.e., a test with a low probability of false negatives) is valued over a specific one (i.e., a test with a low probability of false positives)? What about the other way around?

Types of Screening

Two types of screening can be applied to a community. **Mass screening** is the application of a screening test to an entire population. For example, in Ontario, a universal breast cancer screening program exists that offers free mammograms to all women older than the age of 50 years every 2 years (Government of Ontario, 2015). Another example is the Immigration Medical Examination, which includes screening for tuberculosis in all people older than age 12 years who are relocating to Canada, regardless of their country of origin.

Selective screening is performed on selected subgroups of a population who are increased risk of developing certain diseases. More recently, researchers have called for a more selective tuberculosis (TB) screening program for newcomers to Canada so that only those coming from a country where TB is endemic would be screened (Khan et al., 2015).

Characteristics of Screening

People with positive screening test results do not always have the disease (Fig. 2.5). Screening tests are not diagnostic tests. People with positive or questionable results must be referred for diagnostic evaluation. For screening to be ethical and to fulfill its intended purpose, there should be adequate, effective, and accessible methods of diagnosis and early treatment for those with the disease in question .

Screening tests are evaluated in terms of their accuracy and reliability. **Accuracy** refers to how often the test yields a "true" value, differentiating patients and healthy cases correctly (Baratloo et al., 2015). In other words, accuracy is measured by the frequency with which the result of the test is confirmed by an accurate diagnostic method and is often expressed in terms of its sensitivity and specificity. **Sensitivity** is the proportion (percentage) of those who screened positive who actually have the disease in question. **Specificity** is the proportion (percentage) of those identified by the test as not having the disease in question that truly do not have it (see Fig. 2.5). Both sensitivity and specificity are characteristics of a given test and do not change depending on how common the disease of interest is in a population. Tests with low sensitivity and specificity (i.e., low percentages of correctly identifying those who have and those who do not have the disease) are poor screening tests. To have high sensitivity, screening tests must produce few false-negative results; for high specificity, few false-positive results should arise. A screening test is never 100% sensitive and specific. High sensitivity is gained at the expense of specificity and vice versa. Anything that is done to increase the sensitivity of a test will increase false positives and therefore result in a loss of specificity. Whether sensitivity or specificity is more important will determine which test is test chosen to screen for a particular disease. When there is an important penalty for missing a disease, a highly sensitive test should be chosen. Highly specific tests should be chosen when false-positive results can harm the patient physically, emotionally, or financially (Trevethan, 2017).

The **positive predictive value** is measured as the proportion of true positives in all test positives (i.e., the proportion of cases who truly have the disease among those with positive tests) (Fig. 2.6). The predictive value of a positive test tends to be higher when the disease is more prevalent (see Table 2.2). The **negative predictive value** is the test's ability to identify all those who truly do not have the disease among all those who tested negative. The predictive value of a negative test decreases with increasing disease prevalence.

The **reliability** of a screening test refers to its ability to produce the same or similar results when applied to different populations or even repeatedly to the same individual. It is very closely related to the idea of precision and is often used interchangeably.

> **EXERCISE 2.4:** Based on the values shown in Fig. 2.6, calculate the (1) specificity, (2) positive predictive value, and (3) negative predictive value.

Biases

Two types of biases are particularly important when determining whether screening and early intervention actually lead to improved outcomes (for example, improved survival). **Lead-time bias** refers to the false appearance of a longer survival time or longer time to an outcome of interest with the use of a screening test, occurring because the disease has been detected at an earlier stage in the asymptomatic period but not because of an actual improvement in disease outcome. Essentially, the amount of time with which patients know about and are living with their diagnosis increases even if their chances of survival does not. For example, for diseases in which there is no proven way to intervene early on (such as Huntington's disease, a genetic disorder affecting the nervous system), detecting it earlier not only does not change survival rate but may

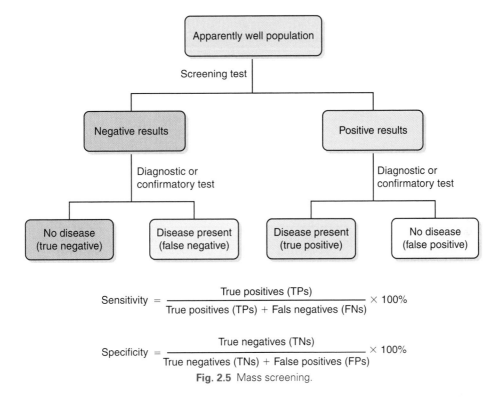

$$\text{Sensitivity} = \frac{\text{True positives (TPs)}}{\text{True positives (TPs)} + \text{Fals negatives (FNs)}} \times 100\%$$

$$\text{Specificity} = \frac{\text{True negatives (TNs)}}{\text{True negatives (TNs)} + \text{False positives (FPs)}} \times 100\%$$

Fig. 2.5 Mass screening.

		Disease present	
		Yes	**No**
Result of test	**Positive**	True positive (TP) 850	False positive (FP) 50
	Negative	False negative (FN) 150	True negative (TN) 950

Fig. 2.6 Result of a hypothetical screening test.

even increase anxiety around diagnosis. For a pictorial representation of lead-time bias, refer to Fig. 2.7. **Length-time bias** is the false appearance of improved disease outcomes as a result of the screening test picking up milder forms of the disease with better prognoses, but diseases with shorter survival outcomes and worse prognoses are less likely to be sampled, causing subjects sampled for the better prognoses to be unrepresentative of the target population (Lee, Ning, & Shen, 2018). Essentially, diseases that have a longer asymptomatic period (making them ideal for screening) tend to be ones that progress more slowly and that are milder. Epidemiologists and statisticians have ways to account for these types of bias to ensure they do not lead to false estimates of survival or other outcomes of interest.

Criteria for a Population-Based Screening Program

As new tests or procedures emerge to screen for a disease, there are pressures on health care professionals and the health care system to adopt and institutionalize them. However, screening of a defined population can only be justified if the following disease, test,

TABLE 2.2 **Predictive Values of a Positive Test with 99% Sensitivity and 95% Specificity at Three Levels of Prevalence**

Item	LEVEL OF PREVALENCE		
	1 percent	10 percent	20 percent
a) Number in population	1 000	1 000	1 000
b) Diseased	10	100	200
c) Not diseased	990	900	800
d) True positive [b × 0.99]	10	99	198
e) False positive [c × (1 − 0.95)]	50	45	40
f) Total positive (d + e)	60	144	238
g) Predictive value of a positive test [d/f]	17%	69%	83%

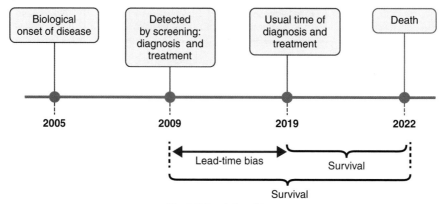

Fig. 2.7 Lead-time bias.

and health system criteria are met (Wilson & Jungner, 1968; Cadman, Chambers, Feldman, et al., 1984):

- Disease
  - The disease must cause significant morbidity or mortality.
  - There is an asymptomatic stage of the disease that is detectable by a test.
  - The natural history of the disease is understood, and early detection and intervention are known to affect health outcomes favourably.
  - Early treatment is effective and acceptable.
  - The disease is not too common and not too rare.
- Test
  - Screening tests should have high sensitivity and specificity; screening must be safe, rapidly and easily applied, relatively inexpensive, and acceptable to health care providers and the screened population (e.g., chest radiographs or a blood test may not bother most individuals, but the discomfort produced by sigmoidoscopy may be unacceptable).

- Ideally, there is randomized control trial evidence of effectiveness.
- Health care system
  - There should be adequate capacity within the health care system for diagnostic follow-up of all those who screen positive and treatment of those diagnosed with disease.
  - Screening and early intervention have been shown to be cost effective.
  - The screening program is sustainable over time.
  - The program will reach those who will benefit from it.
  - Other relevant operational issues have been considered, such as a clear policy on the population to be screened, who is responsible for screening, what constitutes a positive test result, and how findings will become part of the medical record. See the Clinical Example box for a discussion on how these criteria were applied to decide on guidance on prostate cancer screening.

Applying the Criteria to Prostate Cancer Screening

In 2014, the Canadian Task Force on Preventive Health Care (CTFPHC), a federal body that makes evidence-based clinical guidelines to support primary care providers in deciding on preventive clinical interventions such as screening, recommended against the use of a blood test known as the prostate-specific antigen to screen for prostate cancer in adult men (Bell et al., 2014). The rationale for this decision, which spurred quite a bit of controversy, included some of the "disease-specific" criteria discussed above. Essentially, although there is an asymptomatic stage of prostate cancer that is detectable with this blood test, early detection did not seem to affect lifespan (i.e., whether you "catch" the disease early and intervene does not seem to make a difference—the disease it catches is a slow-growing one that would not have caused early death). Additionally, the treatments were not acceptable to many men because of the risk of side effects, such as impotence or problems with urination. Last, the test itself is not great and has a high false-positive rate, which leads to many men unnecessarily having to go through a prostate biopsy to confirm the diagnosis (which itself carries with it the same risks mentioned).

CRITICAL THINKING QUESTION 2.4: Applying the discussed criteria to the question of screening for intimate partner violence, should health care providers working in primary care (e.g., dietitians, nurses, nurse practitioners, physicians) ask their clients questions regarding whether they are currently experiencing intimate partner violence?

SURVEILLANCE AND TRACKING DISEASE USING SOURCES OF HEALTH DATA

There is a large volume of Canadian health data available for interpretation. The abundance of health-related data, from a variety of disparate sources, poses problems for comparability. As well, the need to share information across a variety of jurisdictions creates challenges for developing compatible information systems. These challenges are not merely technical. The advent of powerful computers and algorithms for linking databases has also caused significant ethical and social problems. Consequently, Health Canada

in conjunction with Statistics Canada established the Canadian Institute for Health Information in 1994. The CIHI is a federally chartered, independent, not-for-profit organization (CIHI, 2016). Its primary functions are to collect, process, and maintain a comprehensive number of databases and registries that cover health-related human resources, services, and expenditures and to set national standards for financial, statistical, and clinical data as well as for health information technology.

In this section, the types of data used in the health sector are reviewed.

Census Data

Statistics Canada conducts a national census every 5 years. All citizens across the country are required by law to participate and complete the short census form (Form 2A); a sample of 20% complete a more detailed form (Form 2B, the long form). The census is the major source of information for population and demographic information. Data are collected on many variables, including age, sex, language spoken at home, place of birth, education, and economic status, and are aggregated on a geographical basis according to census tracts.

CRITICAL THINKING QUESTION 2.5: Based on the information discussed, which groups or communities do you think are most likely to be undercounted or are more likely to be missed by the Census?

Canadian Health Surveys

A health survey is either a cross-sectional (administered to respondents once) or longitudinal study (a survey that is repeated to the same respondents over different periods); it is conducted by interview or examination (or both) of a sample of the population. It can also be conducted with a self-administered questionnaire or by telephone, mail, or personal interview. It can be done regularly and repeatedly (to analyze trends) or as needed to investigate a specific problem (e.g., blood lead levels of children living near lead smelters in Toronto). Longitudinal health surveys that are directed at a selected or representative sample of the population follow people over time to examine how health determinants and consequences change among individuals. Most commonly, health surveys are used for surveillance of health behaviour, levels of illness, and health consequences. Because health surveys are often representative samples of entire populations, they can examine many related social factors in people who do not necessarily contact the health care system.

Although simple in theory, surveys pose many methodological problems. Respondents have been shown to forget even major events. If the questionnaire is neither designed properly nor presented conscientiously, it may give ambiguous or misleading results. If interviewers are not adequately trained, they can easily influence the quality of responses. There is also a problem with missing data.

In Canada, there are a few major health-related surveys, conducted by Statistics Canada, that are relied on heavily by health sector decision makers and agencies and that form the basis of a lot of what we know about the health status of Canadians. They will be described below:

1. *Canadian Community Health Survey (CCHS):* The CCHS began in 2000 and is made up of two main surveys: one that is done annually, which typically has more than 100 000 respondents, and a focused survey that is done every 3 years and typically has about 35 000 respondents. The survey questions ask respondents about whether they have certain disease conditions, lifestyle and risk behaviours, use of health care services, and mental health. The CCHS is intended for people 12 years of age and older across Canada. The surveys exclude people living on Indigenous reserves, members of the Canadian Armed Forces, anyone who is living in an institution, and people living in specific regions of Quebec (namely, Région du Nunavik and Région des Terres-Cries-de-la-Baie-James) (Statistics Canada, 2018); however, some of these communities are covered by the First Nations Regional Survey described later.

2. *Canadian Health Measures Survey (CHMS):* The CHMS began in 2007 and collects both self-reported information (i.e., through the administration of a survey, which asks about current health status, lifestyle and physical activity, and medical history, among others) as well as objective health measurements (e.g., measuring height, weight, blood pressure, and physical fitness on every respondent in addition to blood and urine samples to test for chronic diseases, communicable diseases, nutritional status, and environmental exposures). The CHMS is conducted every 2 years, and its target audience is Canadians between 6 and 79 years of age who live in private dwellings

across all provinces and territories. The CHMS typically targets around 5 000 respondents. Those who are excluded from the survey include Indigenous people on reserve or Crown lands, people living in institutions, and members of the Canadian Armed Forces (Statistics Canada, 2007).

3. *First Nations Regional Health Survey (FNRHS):* Initially launched in 2007, the FNRHS is administered by the First Nations Information Governance Centre (FNIGC), a federal, Indigenous, nonprofit organization. It is the only national health survey governed by Indigenous people that incorporates a traditional understanding of well-being into the questions and methodology. To date, there have been three phases of data collection: Phase I in 2003, Phase II in 2008, and Phase III in 2018. Phase III includes three target groups: children (0–11 years), youth (12–17 years), and adults (18–54 years; 55 and older) and includes questions on demographics, physical and mental health, social determinants of health (housing, participation in extracurricular activities, school dropout rates, income, social support, racism, exposure to residential schools, cultural connection), among others (FNIGC, 2018a). The phrase III approach surveyed approximately 24 000 people within 253 communities across Canada, with the goal of understanding health and its determinants among First Nations reserve and Northern communities across the country (FNIGC, 2018b).

4. Other, more focused surveys also exist at the national level (some of which are listed below) as well as at the provincial and territorial levels:
   - Canadian Tobacco, Alcohol, and Drugs Survey
   - The Canadian Health Survey on Children and Youth
   - Canadian Survey on Disability

Administrative Data

Perhaps the most uniformly recorded and reliable health data are administrative (i.e., information that you can obtain from client records such as rates of hospital admission, treatments, and discharge diagnoses). Administrative and professional bodies require this information for planning and evaluating medical care. Administrative data for hospitalization in most provinces are summarized yearly and entered into a central provincial file, such as those maintained by CIHI. One of CIHI's main functions is to prepare easily auditable reports for hospitals to use in quality control and planning, but the data are also suitable for research. Data are also gathered by all provincial health insurance plans, workers' compensation boards, drug utilization plans, and dental health plans. Usually, administrative data are more useful in studying health care rather than the distribution and causes of disease.

Vital Statistics

The record of the basic events of the human life cycle—birth, marriage, and death—is appropriately called vital statistics. Vital statistics are often thought of as being the most reliable because of how consistently they are recorded in the health field.

Birth Certificates

In Canada, parents are responsible for filing a birth certificate with the municipal clerk. It contains relatively limited health information, and there is neither a health history of the mother nor a description of the birth itself. Another form, the Notice of Live Birth or Stillbirth, must be filled out by the attending physician and filed with the provincial registrar. This form provides no information about the father and records the length of the gestation period and the presence of congenital deformities obvious at birth.

Death Certificates

A death certificate must be signed by a licensed physician or nurse practitioner or nurse in remote and isolated communities where they are the primary care provider and includes cause of death, person's name, birth date, sex, and place of residence and death.

The current system for recording cause of death information has been described as unreliable. There are problems with the ambiguity of the instructions and disease definitions set out by World Health Organization for use by the clinician when filling out a death certificate.

Birth and death data usually provide the means to calculate fertility rate, infant mortality rate, crude death rate, life expectancy at birth, potential years of life lost, and all other mortality rates described further in Chapter 4.

Surveillance Systems

Health Surveillance

The Centre for Disease Control (CDC) defines surveillance as the "ongoing, systematic collection, analysis, and interpretation of health-related data essential to planning, implementation, and evaluation of public health practice, closely integrated with the timely dissemination of these data to those responsible for prevention and control" (CDC, 2018).

Thus, it is the continuous, systematic use of routinely collected, nonidentifiable health data used to guide public health action.

Surveillance has the following characteristics:
- It is population based.
- It usually involves the collection of data in a continuous fashion.
- It goes beyond collecting data to produce surveillance products.
- It results in information and analytical products that are made available quickly to public health decision makers for the purposes of public health action (e.g., declaring an outbreak).

Surveillance of a specific disease or risk factor (which can also include an environmental exposure) can be very important in determining how widespread a problem it is, how the problem is changing over time, how effective interventions are in addressing it, detecting new or abhorrent trends in the disease state or risk factor (e.g., identifying an outbreak of a specific communicable disease), and stimulating research (CDC, 2018).

Surveillance is an important function of epidemiological practice, and epidemiologists acquire information used for surveillance through many of the methods, which are described elsewhere in this chapter (i.e., through survey data, administrative data, vital statistics databases, and so on). In some situations, surveillance can be a formal or informal network of medical officers of health, physicians, and other health care professionals who report and share information on unusual occurrences or apparent increases in disease rates to provincial or federal agencies responsible for surveillance. For example, many local public health agencies set up informal networks of partners to conduct surveillance on the opioid crisis in their communities. These informal networks are typically made up of public health, police, fire and rescue, emergency medical services, regional or local coroners, and others with a stake in the opioid crisis. For many communities, this informal way of sharing information is a way to detect any spikes in opioid overdoses and new contaminated drugs products circulating in the community, as well as better understand the response of community members (e.g., to see if emergency departments are being overwhelmed) (Public Health Ontario [PHO], 2016). Just like with informal information sharing, if data sources for a particular disease or risk factor of interest are not available, other means of collecting information can be designed (e.g., requiring by law that physicians report communicable diseases of interest, discussed further below).

There are two main types of surveillance, active and passive, which differ based on the way that information is obtained. With **passive surveillance** (the more common type), information is received by those conducting the surveillance through methods such as mandatory reporting, without their having to initiate or seek out that information.

Many infectious diseases (e.g., measles, chickenpox) and sexually transmitted infections are reportable—that is, the law requires that they be reported to the local health authority. Often, physicians and laboratories must report any positive cases to public health authorities. As such, this type of surveillance is a prime example of passive surveillance because those responsible for surveillance wait for information to be shared with them. In Canada, there are 48 reportable diseases. These include diseases ranging from AIDS to yellow fever.

Active surveillance, on the other hand, requires that those conducting the surveillance actually initiate data collection—by seeking out cases of disease. This typically happens in the setting of an outbreak of a communicable disease at a public health agency. In such cases, the public health staff will initiate contact with members of the community to look for cases that haven't been reported to them or who have not yet seen a clinician for diagnosis (Pan American Health Organization, 2001).

> **EXERCISE 2.5:** List one advantage and one disadvantage of doing active surveillance versus passive surveillance.

Although mandatory reporting often forms the basis of surveillance on communicable diseases, disease registries are important sources of information for surveillance on non-communicable diseases, especially cancer. In all provinces, cancer reports are sent by private practitioners, clinics, and pathology departments, and each patient's name and clinical information are entered in a central registry. The completeness of the registry is checked by searching for notations of cancer on death certificates. If the registry is complete, the name of any person who died of cancer should already be entered in the registry records because cancer is usually detected before death. A 95% agreement between death certificates and registry is the goal in most provinces. Well-kept registries can provide incidence and prevalence data.

The practice for creating disease registries or surveillance systems using health administrative databases or other sources of information not specially designed for surveillance is increasing in Canada.

Health Informatics

With the advent of computers, informatics was born. Good information is critical to providing quality care that is safe to individuals, improving health systems, and reducing health care costs. **Health informatics** is a discipline that focuses on how information is acquired, stored, and used in health care, including technology (Collen & Shortliffe, 2015); it is changing the practice and delivery of health care. Electronic health records, electronic medical records, and telehealth and telemedicine are just a few examples of health informatics that are changing our health care system. The National Institutes of Health Informatics (NIHI) is Canada's first national organization focusing on health informatics innovation, research, and education. NIHI defines the role of health informaticians as managing health information; studying and designing health information flow; developing, deploying, and studying health information systems; analyzing health data; promoting evidence-based health care; and teaching (NIHI, 2018). Many stakeholders are involved in the discipline of health informatics including patients, populations, nurses, doctors, managers, government, and nonprofit organizations such as the Canadian Institute for Health Information (CIHI).

Public health informatics is the application of health informatics methodologies and tools in the public health domain targeting prevention, surveillance, preparedness, and health promotion (Aziz, 2017). As an emerging field, public health informatics focuses on the population's health (and not on individual health), health safety and disease prevention, targets a wide variety of sectors, and creates health information systems to undertake public corrections such as food recalls (Magnuson & O'Carroll, 2014). A noted challenge in public health informatics is the integration of large amounts of data from different sources (El Morr, 2018). Population Data BC supports access to individual-level, de-identified longitudinal data on British Columbia's 4.7 million residents. Data are linkable to each other and to external data sets across sectors, such as health, education, early childhood development, workplace, and the environment to informs health related policy making and investment decisions for healthier communities. Population data science is another emerging field that incorporates health informatics with data science.

The CIHI also deals with health data collection and analysis and works alongside Canada Health Infoway, which was tasked by the federal government in 2002 to implement a pan-Canadian electronic health record system. One of Canada Health Infoway's accomplishments is the creation of "Panorama," a provincial and territorial public health surveillance information system that allows public health professionals to keep track of vaccine inventories, manage immunization programs, investigate and contain the spread of communicable diseases, manage and respond to disease outbreaks, and manage public health workloads (Canada Health Infoway, 2018).

Big data analytics (BDA) is being introduced to the health sector with much promise. However, its capabilities, opportunities, and benefits still need to be tested through clinical and administrative applications. BDA has emerged from two distinct concepts—big data and analytics. It represents a new information management approach that has been designed to derive previously untapped intelligence and insights from data to address many new and important questions.

> **CRITICAL THINKING QUESTION 2.6:** What are some potential ethical issues related to data and specifically to the large amount of data being collected from different data sources?

SUMMARY

This chapter has examined epidemiology, surveillance, screening, data sources, and health informatics.

Health data consist of sets of numerical information about anything related to health and are compiled from many sources. These data must meet three criteria: they must be reliable, be valid, and have sufficient resolution or precision.

Various types of studies are used in the field of epidemiology for data collection and analysis. **Epidemiology** is the study of the distribution (in terms of person, place, and time) of determinants of disease, health-related states, and events in populations. Epidemiology can be applied to control of health problems. The two main types of studies are descriptive and analytic (which include observational and experimental studies), each with their own set of advantages and disadvantages. Systematic and narrative reviews provide evidence from the literature to support population health interventions. Qualitative and mixed method studies are also important in investigating population health issues.

To monitor and track various health states, a number of data sources are used, including census data, survey data, and administrative data, to name a few. **Surveillance** is defined as "the ongoing, systematic collection, analysis, and interpretation of health-related data essential to planning, implementation, and evaluation of public health practice, closely integrated with the timely dissemination of these data to those responsible for prevention and control," and surveillance systems rely heavily on the types of data sources mentioned earlier. The two main types of surveillance are active surveillance (e.g., health practitioners seeking information out) and passive surveillance (e.g., reporting of mandatory reportable diseases by labs and physicians to public health).

Health informatics is a discipline that focuses on how information is acquired, stored, and used in health care, including technology, and is changing the practice and delivery of health care. Public health informatics is the application of health informatics methodologies and tools in the public health domain, targeting prevention, surveillance, preparedness, and health promotion. As an emerging field, public health informatics focuses on the population's health and not on individual health, health safety, and disease prevention; targets a wide variety of sectors; and creates health information systems to undertake public corrections such as food recalls.

KEY WEBSITES

Cochrane Database of Systematic Reviews (CDSR): http://www.cochranelibrary.com/cochrane-database-of-systematic-reviews

The CDSR website is the leading resource for systematic reviews, protocols, and editorials in health care. A wealth of Cochrane Reviews can be explored by topic, Cochrane Review Group, or using the advanced search functions through this site.

Cochrane Canada: http://canada.cochrane.org/about-us

The Cochrane Canada website represents the Canadian arm of the Cochrane collaboration, which is one of 14 worldwide Cochrane Centres. Access the site to learn more about Cochrane Canada's resources, partners, training and events.

Canadian Task Force for Preventive Health Care (CTFPHC): https://canadiantaskforce.ca

The CTFPHC was established by the Public Health Agency of Canada (PHAC). It supports primary care providers to provide preventive care by developing clinical practice guidelines. This website provides access to current and upcoming guidelines, as well as other tools and resources.

National Institute for Health and Care Excellence (NICE): https://www.nice.org.uk/about/what-we-do/our-programmes/nice-guidance

Chartered in the United Kingdom, NICE provides key guidance and advice to improve health and social care. The website provides examples to the NICE frameworks for social value judgements and a variety of guidelines for evidence-based practice.

Health Evidence: https://www.healthevidence.org

Health Evidence aids ongoing knowledge translation for public health decision making by providing more than 5 000 quality-rated systematic reviews that evaluate the effectiveness of public health interventions. Visit the website to access the database, as well as additional information on available tools and consultation services.

National Collaborating Centre for Methods and Tools (NCCMT): https://www.nccmt.ca

The NCCMT collaborates with national and international public health and knowledge-sharing organizations to promote evidence-informed public health practices. The website provides access to the NCCMT's knowledge repositories and a variety of tools.

Canadian Best Practices Portal: http://cbpp-pcpe.phac-aspc.gc.ca/resources

This is a database from PHAC with information and tools for evidence-informed decision making, health indicators, planning public health programs, and developing public health competencies. Visit the website to access detailed resources for those four areas.

Canadian Society for Epidemiology and Biostatistics (CSEB): https://cseb.ca/

The CSEB is a growing network of epidemiologists, biostatisticians, and students. It is a member of the International Joint Policy Committee of the Societies of Epidemiology. The website provides information on webinars, workshops, conferences, and travel grants with the CSEB.

REFERENCES

Aziz, H. A. (2017). A review of the role of public health informatics in healthcare. *Journal of Taibah University Medical Sciences, 12*(1), 78–81.

Baratloo, A., Hosseini, M., Negida, A., et al. (2015). Part 1: Simple definition and calculation of accuracy, sensitivity and specificity. *Emergency, 3*(2), 48–49.

Bell, N., Gorber, S. C., Shane, A., et al. (2014). Recommendations on screening for prostate cancer with the prostate-specific antigen test. *Canadian Medical Association Journal, 186*(16) 1225–123.

Cadman, D., Chambers, L., Feldman, W., et al. (1984). Assessing the effectiveness of community screening programs. *Journal of American Medical Association, 251*(12), 1580–1585.

Canada Health Infoway. (2018). *Public health surveillance.* Retrieved from https://www.infoway-inforoute.ca/en/solutions/digital-health-foundation/electronic-health-records/public-health-surveillance.

Canadian Institute for Health Information. (2016). *CIHI's strategic plan, 2016 to 2021.* Retrieved from https://www.cihi.ca/sites/default/files/document/strategicplan2016-2021-enweb.pdf.

Cameron, B. L., Plazas, M. D. P. C., Salas, A. S., et al. (2014). Understanding inequalities in access to health care services for Aboriginal people. *Advances in Nursing Science, 37*(3), E1–E16.

Centers for Disease Control. (2018). *Introduction to public health surveillance.* Retrieved from https://www.cdc.gov/publichealth101/surveillance.html.

Collen, M. F., & Shortliffe, E. H. (2015). The creation of a new discipline. In *The history of medical informatics in the United States* (pp. 75–120). London: Springer.

Corbin, J., & Strauss, A. L. (2015). *Basics of qualitative research: Techniques and procedures for developing grounded theory* (4th ed.). Thousand Oaks, CA: Sage.

Creswell, J. W., & Creswell, J. D. (2017). *Research design: Qualitative, quantitative, and mixed methods approaches.* Thousand Oaks: Sage Publications.

Dash, N. (2005). *Selection of the research paradigm and methodology*. Manchester: Manchester Metropolitan University. Retrieved from http://www.celt.mmu.ac.uk/researchmethods/Modules/Selection_of_methodology/index.php.

Denzin, N. K., & Lincoln, Y. S. (2005). *The Sage handbook of qualitative research*. Sage.

El Morr, C. (2018). *Introduction to health informatics: A Canadian perspective*. Toronto: Canadian Scholars' Press.

First Nations Information Governance Centre. (2018a). *National Report of The First Nations Regional Health Survey Phase 3* (Vol.1). Retrieved from https://fnigc.ca/sites/default/files/docs/fnigc_rhs_phase_3_national_report_vol_1_en_final_web.pdf.

First Nations Information Governance Centre. (2018b). *New report provides unprecedented look at trends over time in the health and well-being of First Nations communities.* Retrieved from https://fnigc.ca/news/new-report-provides-unprecedented-look-trends-over-time-health-and-well-being-first-nations.

Glaser, B. G., & Strauss, A. L. (1967). *The discovery of grounded theory: Strategies for qualitative research*. Chicago: Aldine Publishing. [seminal].

Government of Ontario. (2015, September 9). *Ontario breast screening program*. Retrieved from https://www.ontario.ca/page/ontario-breast-screening-program.

Grant, W. B. (2016). Using multicountry ecological and observational studies to determine dietary risk factors for Alzheimer's disease. *Journal of the American College of Nutrition, 35*(5), 476–489. https://doi.org/10.1080/07315724.2016.1161566.

Greenhalgh, T., Robert, G., Macfarlane, F., et al. (2005). Storylines of research in diffusion of innovation: A meta-narrative approach to systematic review. *Social Science & Medicine, 61*(2), 417–430.

Guba, E., & Lincoln, Y. (1994). Competing paradigm in qualitative research. In N. Denzin, & Y. Lincoln (Eds.), *Handbook of qualitative research* (pp. 99–136). Sage.

Hill, A. B. (1965). The environment and disease: Association or causation? *Proceedings of Royal Society of Medicine, 58*, 295–300.

Holloway, I. (2005). *Qualitative research in health care*. UK: McGraw-Hill Education.

Honjo, K. (2004). Social epidemiology: Definition, history, and research examples. *Environmental Health and Preventive Medicine, 9*(5), 193–199. https://doi.org/10.1007/BF02898100.

Iles, M. M., & Barrett, J. H. (2011). Single-locus tests of association for population-based studies. In *Analysis of Complex Disease Association Studies* (pp. 109–122). https://doi.org/10.1016/B978-0-12-375142-3.10008-2.

Ioannidis, J. P. (2016). The mass production of redundant, misleading, and conflicted systematic reviews and meta-analyses. *The Milbank Quarterly, 94*(3), 485–514.

Johnson, R. B., & Onwuegbuzie, A. J. (2004). Mixed methods research: A research paradigm whose time has come. *Educational Researcher, 33*(7), 14–26.

Khan, K., Hirji, M. M., Miniota, J., et al. (2015). Domestic impact of tuberculosis screening among new immigrants to Ontario, Canada. *Canadian Medical Association Journal, 187*(16), e473–e481. https://doi.org/10.1503/cmaj.150011.

Kirkevold, M. (1997). Integrative nursing research—an important strategy to further the development of nursing science and nursing practice. *Journal of Advanced Nursing, 25*(5), 977–984.

Last, J. (1995). *A dictionary of epidemiology* (3rd ed.). New York: Oxford University Press.

LeCompte, M. D., & Schensul, J. J. (2010). *Designing and conducting ethnographic research: An introduction* (2nd ed.). Lanham, MD: AltaMira Press, 356.

Lee, C. H., Ning, J., & Shen, Y. (2018). Analysis of restricted mean survival time for length-biased data. *Biometrics, 74*(2), 575–583. https://doi.org/10.1111/biom.12772.

Liu, Y., Chang, C. C. H., Marsh, G. M., et al. (2012). Population attributable risk of aflatoxin-related liver cancer: Systematic review and meta-analysis. *European Journal of Cancer, 48*(14), 2125–2136. https://doi.org/10.1016/j.ejca.2012.02.009.

Magnuson, J. A., & O'Carroll, P. W. (2014). Introduction to public health informatics. In *Public health informatics and information systems* (pp. 3–18). London: Springer.

McGill Qualitative Health Research Group. (n.d.). *Qualitative or quantitative research?* Retrieved from https://www.mcgill.ca/mqhrg/resources/what-difference-between-qualitative-and-quantitative-research.

Merriam, S. (1988). *Case study research in education: A qualitative approach*. San Francisco: Jossey-Bass.

Moher, D., Shamseer, L., Clarke, M., et al. (2015). Preferred reporting items for systematic review and meta-analysis protocols (PRISMA-P) 2015 statement. *Systematic Reviews, 4*(1), 1. https://doi.org/10.1186/2046-4053-4-1.

Montesanti, S. R., & Thurston, W. E. (2015). Mapping the role of structural and interpersonal violence in the lives of women: Implications for public health interventions and policy. *BMC Women's Health, 15*(1), 100.

National Collaborating Centre for Methods and Tools. (n.d.). *About us*. Retrieved from https://www.nccmt.ca.

National Cancer Institute. (2015, March 20). *Aflatoxins*. Retrieved from https://www.cancer.gov/about-cancer/causes-prevention/risk/substances/aflatoxins.

National Institute for Health and Care Excellence. (n.d.). *NICE guidelines*. Retrieved from https://www.nice.org.uk/About/What-we-do/Our-Programmes/NICE-guidance/NICE-guidelines.

National Institutes of Health Informatics. (2018). *About NIHI*. Retrieved from http://www.nihi.ca/index.php?MenuItemID=23.

Pan American Health Organization. (2001). *Virtual course basic epidemiological concepts skills online, passive and active surveillance.* Retrieved from https://cursos.campus-virtualsp.org/mod/tab/view.php?id=23161.

Public Health Ontario (Agency for Health Protection and Promotion), Brecher, R. W., & Copes, R. (2016). *EOH fundamentals: Risk communication.* Toronto: Queen's Printer for Ontario.

Scott, K., & McSherry, R. (2008). Evidence-based nursing: Clarifying the concepts for nurses in practice. *Journal of Clinical Nursing, 18*(8), 1085–1095.

Sedgwick, P. (2015). Understanding the ecological fallacy. *British Medical Journal (Online), 351.* https://doi.org/10.1136/bmj.h4773.

Stake, R. (1995). *The art of case study research.* Thousand Oaks, CA: Sage.

Statistics Canada. (2007). *Canadian Health Measures Survey (CHMS).* Retrieved from http://www23.statcan.gc.ca/imdb/p2SV.pl?Function=getSurvey&Id=10263.

Statistics Canada. (2018). *Canadian Community Health Survey—Annual Component (CCHS).* Retrieved from http://www23.statcan.gc.ca/imdb/p2SV.pl?Function=getSurvey&SDDS=3226.

Strauss, A., & Corbin, J. (1998). *Basics of qualitative research: Grounded theory procedures and techniques* (2nd ed.). Newbury Park, CA: Sage.

Tariq, S., & Woodman, J. (2013). Using mixed methods in health research. *JRSM Short Reports, 4*(6), 2042533313479197. https://doi.org/10.1177/2042533313479197.

Tashakkori, A., & Teddlie, C. (Eds.). (2003). *Handbook of mixed methods in social & behavioral research.* Thousand Oaks, CA: SAGE Publications.

Trevethan, R. (2017). Sensitivity, specificity, and predictive values: Foundations, pliabilities, and pitfalls in research and practice. *Frontiers in Public Health, 5,* 307. https://doi.org/10.3389/fpubh.2017.00307.

Whitby, L. (1974). Screening for disease: Definitions and criteria. *Lancet, 2*(3), 819–821.

Wilson, S. (2008). *Research as ceremony: Indigenous research methods.* Nova Scotia: Fernwood Press.

Wilson, J., & Jungner, F. (1968). *Principles and practice of screening. Public Health Report No. 34.* Geneva: World Health Organization.

Wong, S. T., Browne, A. J., Varcoe, C., et al. (2011). Enhancing measurement of primary health care indicators using an equity lens: An ethnographic study. *International Journal for Equity in Health, 10*(1), 38. Retrieved from https://equityhealthj.biomedcentral.com/articles/10.1186/1475-9276-11-59.

Wong, G., Greenhalgh, T., Westhorp, G., et al. (2013). RAMESES publication standards: Meta-narrative reviews. *BMC Medicine, 11*(1), 20.

Yin, R. K. (2014). *Case study research: Design and methods* (5th ed.). Thousand Oaks, CA: Sage.

Approaches to Achieving Health for All

LEARNING OBJECTIVES

- Define and differentiate between *population health* and *community health*.
- Differentiate among primary, secondary, and tertiary prevention.
- Understand the difference between working downstream, midstream, and upstream.
- Differentiate between population health and community health.
- Define *health communications* and be able to describe its scope and utility in contributing to risk and crisis communication, and media advocacy.

- Define *policy* and be able to understand the complexities of the policy process.
- Examine and analyze various approaches to working midstream and upstream and their underlying theories.
- Describe various approaches to promote community health.
- Examine various approaches to addressing structural determinants and underlying theories, including public health advocacy.

CHAPTER OUTLINE

KEY TERMS

advocacy
asset-based community
   development (ABCD)
community development
community efficacy
community empowerment
community health
community organizing
community resiliency
crisis communication
downstream
health belief model
health communications
health imperialism

health in all policies (HiAP)
health marketing
health promotion
healthy city
healthy public policy
lifestyle drift
media advocacy
midstream
nudge
political economy
population health
public health advocacy
public policy
primary prevention

secondary prevention
self-control
self-efficacy
social enterprise
social entrepreneurship
social innovation
social marketing
social media
stages of change
structural determinants of health
tertiary prevention
theory of social learning
upstream

INTRODUCTION

The key roles of public health for achieving improved health for all include population health assessment, surveillance, health protection, health promotion, and disease and injury prevention. Kickbusch (1995) argues that the aim of public health is to improve the health of communities through advocating for healthy public policies and supportive environments, mediating between different interests in society to benefit health, and enabling communities and individuals to achieve their full potential. The idea of a flexible "continuum of options" that includes both the intermediary and structural determinants of health (see Chapter 1) is required to begin to achieve health for all.

The discussion that follows outlines key concepts as they relate to community and population health, prevention, and the promotion of community and population health. Various frameworks are outlined, with suggestions on how to achieve health for all at the individual, community, and population levels. Traditional models of prevention are discussed, along with health promotion strategies, theories of behaviour change, and finally a political economy approach to addressing the structural determinants of health.

POPULATION HEALTH AND COMMUNITY HEALTH

It is important to begin by defining two key terms that are often used interchangeably but are actually different: *population health* and *community health*. These two concepts have different histories in Canada. As discussed in Chapter 1, **population health** arose from Canadian Institute for Advanced Research (CIAR), a think tank funded by corporate and public sources, within the fields of epidemiology and economics (Poland et al., 1998). The assumption underlying the CIAR model is that change in population health status is brought about by experts, researchers, and governments rather than by social movements or communities. Additionally, the process of how change can occur is absent from the model, ignoring the agency of individuals and communities and disregarding the physical environment. As a result, population health as an approach has been criticized (Raphael & Bryant, 2002; Kindig, 2007; Labonte

et al., 2005) but has been evolving to focus more on inequities and the social determinants of health (SDHs) since the inception of the CIAR model.

Community health, on the other hand, has its roots in community health nursing (CHN), which can be traced back to the early 1700s in Canada (Paul & Ross-Kerr, 2011) and focuses on agency and the process of change. For as long as nursing has existed, CHNs have been focusing on the determinants of health and vulnerable populations. A year after the Ottawa Charter was created, the Community Health Nurses Association of Canada (1987) was formed and later transformed into the Community Health Nurses of Canada (CHNC). Advancing the practice of community health, CHNC developed standards of practice and competencies related to public health and home health nursing (see Chapter 17).

Working in the community, CHNs promote health, prevent illness, partner with community groups to build capacity, and advocate for resources and services that are equitably distributed, focusing on groups and individuals most in need. At the heart of community health are groups of people, whether defined by geography or affinity, who engage in social interaction, build ties, exhibit awareness of identity as a group, and hold direct access to collective decision making. **Community health** is the ability of a community to generate and effectively use assets and resources to support the well-being and quality of life of community members and the community as a whole in the face of challenges and barriers within the context of their environment (Ryan-Nicholls & Racher, 2004).

Community health can be seen as having three dimensions: status, structure, and process (Cottrell, 1976). Status is related to more traditional notions of measurement, such as morbidity, mortality, risk factor profiles, and health indicators for various diseases. Structure includes the services and resources available in the community that reflect health care-to-client ratios, number of hospital beds, and service-use patterns, such as the number of emergency room beds in a specific hospital. The structure of the community is also considered and measured through demographics, such as socioeconomic distributions, age, and educational level. The structure of the community relates directly to the SDHs (conditions where we live, work, learn, and play).

Community health as a process implies action for health promotion. The health and well-being of individuals in a community depends upon how well the community functions, not only in terms of ensuring equitable distribution of the determinants of health but also in terms of the processes of governance in the community, such as the degree of participation, the degree of social cohesion, and civility.

A community health approach is a process of building capacity in a community to implement change by assessing the desire for change and engaging the community in taking action. Participation is an inherent quality of a community, and without participation, there is no community, only the potential for it (Hancock, Labonte, & Edwards, 1999). A key aspect of community health is **community resiliency**, which is the ability of a community to respond to adversity and, in so doing, reach a higher level of functioning, in turn leading to improved health among all individuals in the community (Kulig, 2000).

Several models and theories have been used to improve community health and are discussed later in the chapter. Although CHNs use a population health approach, the relational aspect of community and the process of engaging community members differentiate community health from population health.

Traditional Model of Prevention

A major aspect of community health is the prevention of health problems. Prevention means being proactive and averting problems or identifying them as early as possible to mitigate potential disability or impairment. Traditionally, there have been three approaches to disease prevention: primary, secondary, and tertiary. **Primary prevention** aims at preventing disease before it occurs, thereby reducing the incidence of disease. It includes measures taken to keep illness or injuries from occurring. Examples include immunization programs, dietary recommendations, and the use of seatbelts and other protective devices. **Secondary prevention** involves the early detection of disease and its treatment that may accompany screening. Examples include diabetes, hypertension, and cholesterol screening programs. Mammograms and Pap smears are also examples. Secondary prevention attempts to discover a health problem at an early enough point so that intervening in the health condition may lead to better control and even eradication of the condition. **Tertiary prevention** attempts to reduce death and disease by treatment and rehabilitation of diseased individuals and is carried out by the health care system. Examples of tertiary prevention include

treatment and rehabilitation of individuals after a heart attack or stroke to reduce impairment and restore functioning. For indivdiuals who have an existing illness or disability, its impact on their lives is lessened through tertiary prevention.

Strategies to address the various levels of prevention most often require individuals to change their behaviour. Although primary prevention broadens the strategies to include policy, a scenario referred to as **lifestyle drift** (Whitehead, 2012) can also occur. The drift happens when the design of a policy accepts that improving the health of individuals and communities is about tackling SDHs, only to revert back to addressing lifestyle issues, such as smoking, drinking, and lack of exercise. The policy has the right intention, but reasons for the drift may be more practical in nature (addressing lifestyle issues is easier to visualize and do; there is an existing evidence base weighted towards behavioural interventions) or political in nature (pressure for rapid results or for "doing something"; a growing blame culture, in which the problem lies in the individual rather than acknowledging the causes) (Whitehead, 2012). Nevertheless, policy has been an important strategy for improving the health of populations.

Much work has been done in this area over the past four decades, demonstrating that policies such as vaccinations, seatbelts and child restraints, motorcycle and bicycle helmets, workplace safety monitoring, sanitation requirements, clean indoor air regulations, tobacco control, improvements in food labelling, banning trans fats, and advertisement restrictions, to name a few, have greatly affected disease rates, increased life expectancy, and improved quality of life (Centers for Disease Control and Prevention [CDC], 1999; World Health Organization [WHO] 2018). As a result, there is more emphasis placed on policy change as way to create conditions that support making the healthy choice the easy choice.

> **CRITICAL THINKING QUESTION 3.1:** Is lifestyle drift the same as what is known in health promotion as blaming the victim? How is it or is it not the same?

Medical sociologist Irving Zola's river analogy of 'upstream–downstream' (Fig. 3.1) provides a practical framework for thinking about how we take action to improve health and well-being, which are tied to the three views of health discussed in Chapter 1. Zola

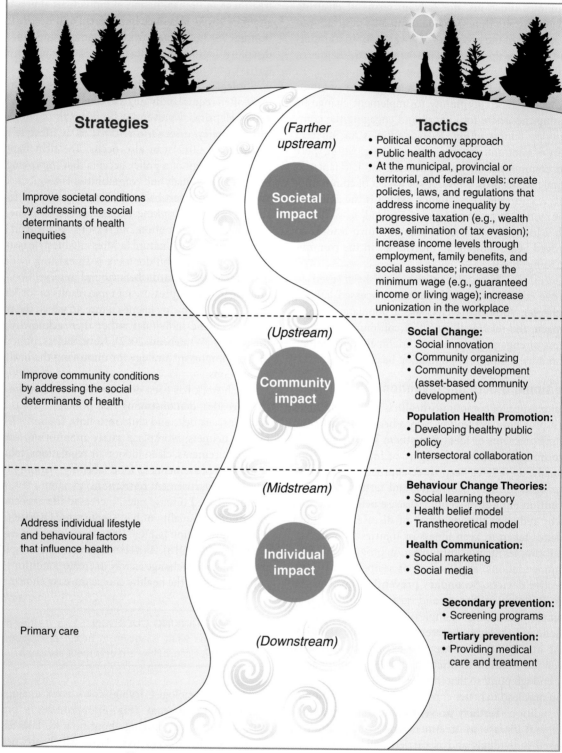

Strategies

Improve societal conditions by addressing the social determinants of health inequities

Improve community conditions by addressing the social determinants of health

Address individual lifestyle and behavioural factors that influence health

Primary care

(Farther upstream)

Societal impact

(Upstream)

Community impact

(Midstream)

Individual impact

(Downstream)

Tactics
- Political economy approach
- Public health advocacy
- At the municipal, provincial or territorial, and federal levels: create policies, laws, and regulations that address income inequality by progressive taxation (e.g., wealth taxes, elimination of tax evasion); increase income levels through employment, family benefits, and social assistance; increase the minimum wage (e.g., guaranteed income or living wage); increase unionization in the workplace

Social Change:
- Social innovation
- Community organizing
- Community development (asset-based community development)

Population Health Promotion:
- Developing healthy public policy
- Intersectoral collaboration

Behaviour Change Theories:
- Social learning theory
- Health belief model
- Transtheoretical model

Health Communication:
- Social marketing
- Social media

Secondary prevention:
- Screening programs

Tertiary prevention:
- Providing medical care and treatment

Fig 3.1 The upstream–downstream approach to community health.

describes modern medical practice as working downstream (biomedical view of health) as follows:

[S}ometimes it feels like this. There I am standing by the shore of a swiftly flowing river and I hear the cry of a drowning man. So I jump into the river, put my arms around him, pull him to the shore and apply artificial respiration. Just when he begins to breathe, there is another cry for help. So I jump into the river, reach him, pull him to shore, apply artificial respiration, and then just as he begins to breathe, another cry for help. So back into the river again, reaching, pulling, applying, breathing and another yell. Again and again, without end, goes the sequence. You know, I am so busy jumping in, pulling them to shore, applying artificial respiration, that I have no time to see who in the hell is upstream pushing them in.

cited in McKinlay, 1979, p.9.

McKinlay also described his frustration with the "**downstream** endeavours," which he characterized as short-term, problem-specific, individual-based interventions, and challenged health professionals to refocus and look **upstream**, where the real problems lie (McKinlay, 1979). "Moving upstream," with a socioenvironmental view of health, focuses on aspects of our social and physical environments that either support or do not support our health. In contrast, downstream activities include biomedical interventions that focus on individual pathology and deal with the diagnosis and treatment of the disease after it has manifested. An "upstream" orientation does not diminish the importance of delivering high-quality, acceptable, affordable, and timely health services downstream or addressing behavioural risks such as smoking and physical inactivity (which are categorized as **midstream** actions by McKinlay & Marceau, 2000). However, remaining "midstream" merely provides people who are more at risk with the knowledge of how to avoid falling into a river and how to save themselves if they do fall in. For example, with regard to cardiovascular disease, this would include preventive messages such as:

1. Control your blood pressure.
2. Keep your cholesterol and triglyceride levels under control.
3. Maintain at a healthy weight.
4. Eat a healthy diet.
5. Get regular exercise.
6. Limit alcohol intake.
7. Don't smoke.
8. Manage stress.
9. Manage diabetes.
10. Get enough sleep.

On the other hand, working upstream to prevent cardiovascular disease requires moving beyond a high-risk approach of population screening (secondary prevention), providing preventive messages as stated earlier, or prescribing medication to reduce blood cholesterol and blood pressure (tertiary prevention). Upstream approaches like, population-wide cardiovascular prevention activities, such as banning dietary artificial trans fats (as was done in Denmark in 2003 and in Canada in 2018) and reducing daily dietary salt intake up to 50% (as was done in Finland in 1970s and the United Kingdom in 2002) translate into substantial reductions in cardiovascular events and deaths (Murray et al., 2003; Federici et al., 2019). Viewing the river in segments such as those outlined earlier—downstream, midstream, and upstream—supports a "way forward" along a flexible continuum of options. As a point of clarification, classifying strategies as either upstream or downstream is an analytical tool to help distinguish between different forms of interventions. However, in recognition of the complexity and the causes of the causes (Rose, 1992), there is a growing body of evidence and models that support working at various levels (individual, organizational, community, policy or municipal, provincial or territorial, federal) using multiple strategies from up-, mid-, and downstream and with multisector partnerships (Edwards, Mill, & Kothari, 2004). Examples of multilevel strategies include the North Karelia Project in Finland, the Stanford Five-City Project, the Minnesota Heart Health Program, and the Community Intervention Trial for Smoking Cessation (COMMIT) (Ferguson, 1998). Initial evidence supporting the effectiveness of multilevel strategies across sectors came from the North Karelia Project in Finland, which showed a reduction in cardiovascular mortality subsequent to a community-wide prevention program (Shea & Basch, 1990a, 1990b).

Despite this evidence, most programs and research still remain focused on individualistic behaviours or lifestyle choices. To support efforts to shift the tide, the remaining sections of this chapter (and this book) focus more on upstream approaches to achieving health for all but also include midstream approaches, with a cautionary note. If any one approach is implemented in isolation, the improvement in health status will be severely reduced. We advocate for multiple interventions to address the SDHs and, in turn, redress health inequities.

EXERCISE 3.1: Identify whether the following examples represent primary prevention, secondary prevention, or tertiary prevention.

1. Recommending to a client that she gets regular Pap tests
2. Writing a prescription for a client to "exercise daily"
3. Implementing a bike-share program in your community
4. Suggesting that a client start on cholesterol-lowering medication after he has had a heart attack
5. Referring a client with severe lung disease to a pulmonary or lung rehabilitation program to improve her exercise tolerance

---

CRITICAL THINKING QUESTIONS 3.2:

1. If you were implementing a program in your community to address the high prevalence of obesity in children younger than 12 years of age, what prevention strategy would you use?
2. Do you need different skills to be working at the individual level versus a community or population level?

STRATEGIES

The strategies discussed in the next section have been organized as midstream and upstream approaches to achieving health for all. However, not all strategies fall into a dichotomous category. Some strategies, for example, social innovation, enterprise, and entrepreneurship for social change, fall more upstream but also use midstream approaches. The categorization of midstream and upstream are used here as a learning strategy to help students to better understand where on the continuum specific strategies may fall. It is important to understand that working upstream has been shown to be more effective in improving population health. Strategies for enhancing community health and addressing the structural determinants are also included in this section and have not been classified as either/or but as separate strategies for achieving health for all.

Midstream Strategies
Behaviour Change Theories
Although the Ottawa Charter emphasizes that health promotion encompasses much more than

building personal skills and focusing on individual level behaviour change, this pillar of the Ottawa Charter remains important and has been embraced by many public health and health care organizations as one important way to improve population health in coordination with other strategies.

Theorists have focused quite a bit on what causes people to continue harmful behaviours and which factors are important for changing people's behaviours into ones that are better for their health. Professionals who work in the area of health promotion should have a good grasp on these theories. The following discussion covers the main aspects of key theories, although it is not comprehensive and is intended only to be introductory overview.

Many behaviour change theorists posit that behaviour is a result of predisposing, reinforcing, and enabling factors. Predisposing factors comprise knowledge (e.g., the health consequences of smoking), attitudes, beliefs, and values. Researchers have found that the intention to change behaviour is also a strong predictor. Reinforcing factors (e.g., those provided by the social context of family, society, or health care professionals) involve reward or feedback for the discontinuation or adoption of behaviour. Enabling factors include skills such as behaviour modification techniques, as well as the availability of relevant supports such as reasonably priced, healthier foods that support dietary change (Center for Community Health and Development, n.d.).

An influential **theory of social learning** has been constructed from a number of related concepts that must be addressed in lifestyle education (Bandura, 1971). There is a strong correlation between social learning principles and some health-related actions. The essential concept is of reciprocal determinism, which is recognition that the social environment influences behaviour, which in turn affects the environment. For example, social norms around behaviours such as smoking are influential in shaping an individual's risk of starting to smoke (i.e., you're less likely to smoke if no one around you smokes and smoking is considered "taboo"), and fewer people smoking over time reinforces not smoking as a norm, like a positive feedback loop.

Apart from components of behavioural capability (the acquisition of skills and knowledge), reinforcements, and supportive social and economic environments (e.g., living in a community that supports not smoking in public spaces), there are other components of social learning theory. These are observation (e.g., having role models who have successfully quit smoking), expectations of positive results from behaviour change, expectancies (e.g., an improved appearance following smoking cessation), perceptions of an individual's situation (e.g., what the consequences of continuing to smoke might be), and emotional factors that may pose barriers to behaviour change (e.g., anxiety associated with the anticipation of giving up a lifestyle habit such as smoking).

Self-efficacy and self-control are components of behaviour change that are increasingly being incorporated into health education for sustained behaviour change. **Self-efficacy** refers to the cognitive state in which a person is confident that they can achieve a behaviour change. This may be reached by the achievement of short-term goals (Hughes, & Naud, 2016). **Self-control** relates to decision-making capacities for healthy choices and self-monitoring, such as those used in guided self-management programs for smoking cessation (Dijkstra, 2017).

An important model, the **health belief model** attempts to explain the factors influencing the uptake of positive health behaviours (Fig. 3.2) (Becker et al., 1977). This model suggests that behaviours undertaken by individuals to remain healthy, including the use of preventive services, are a function of a set of interacting beliefs. To be motivated to take action to avoid illness, an individual must be in a state of readiness to take action and must believe that the action will have positive consequences. To be ready to act, the individual needs to feel susceptible to the disease in question and to believe that it would have a significant impact on his or her life. Beliefs about the benefits of the action in question involve consideration of barriers to action, such as time, cost, and inconvenience.

Current formulations of the health belief model include the role of cues and modifying factors. Cues are specific events that stimulate preventive health behaviours. Modifying factors are sociodemographic variables such as age, sex, and race, sociopsychological variables such as personality and peer group pressure, and other variables such as knowledge of and prior experience with the disease. All these factors influence the individual's perception of susceptibility to disease and seriousness of the disease, as well as perception of the benefits of health-related actions.

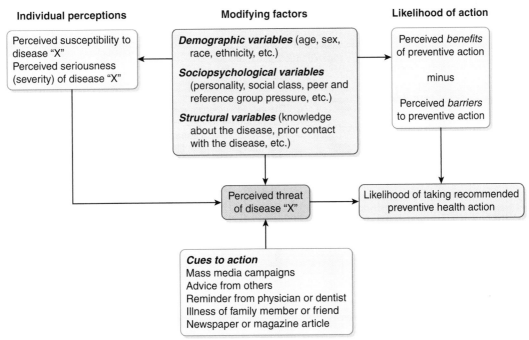

Fig 3.2 Health belief model. (Reproduced with the permission of the publisher, from Becker, M. H., Haefner, D. P., Kasl, S. V., et al. (1977). Selected psychosocial models and correlates of individual health-related behaviours. *Medical Care, 15,* 27–46.)

This model has provided the foundation for many health education and awareness programs. One of its implications is that these programs must be carefully targeted at specific social and cultural groups and must be based on a detailed understanding of their

> **EXERCISE 3.2:** Applying the principles of the health belief model, what key messages might you include in designing a mass health education campaign on the issue of youth who are starting to smoke marijuana?

health beliefs.

Another model based on the **stages of change** has provided a useful framework for understanding how changes of lifestyle behaviour can be facilitated (DiClemente et al., 1991) (Fig. 3.3). In studies of cigarette smokers, four different stages were identified:

the precontemplation stage, when the individual was unaware of a behaviour-related health problem; the contemplation stage, when change was considered; the action stage, when initial attempts at change were made; and maintenance, or long-term change. Individuals may not move through these stages in a linear fashion. There are barriers to change at each stage, as well as facilitative processes.

Health Communications

Health communications is an important tool that is vital to population health activities. The CDC in United States define **health communications** as "the study and use of communication strategies to inform and influence individual decisions that enhance health" (CDC, 2011a). Based on this definition, it is clear that health communications is a broad field and

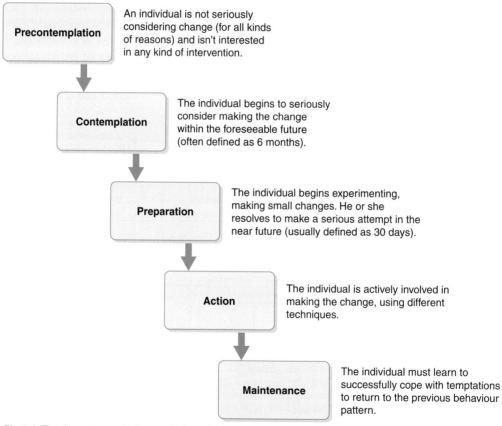

Fig 3.3 The five stages of change. (Adapted from Prochaska, J. O., DiClemente, C. C., & Norcross, J. C. (1992). In search of how people change. Applications to addictive behaviors. *American Psychologist, 47*(9), 1102–1114.)

that decisions that enhance health can include things ranging from following an evacuation order during an emergency to getting immunized during a particularly bad influenza year, choosing healthier meal options, or persuading a policy maker to ban sugar-sweetened beverages in schools. The following section, although not an exhaustive overview of health communications, provides an introduction to the key topics in health communications mentioned earlier.

Risk Communication

Health professionals who are communicating about risk to the public must have a solid understanding of what "risk" entails and the factors that shape how people perceive risk. According to Peter Sandman, a leader in the field of risk communication, risk is the sum of (1) hazard plus (2) outrage (Hooker, Capon, & Leask, 2017). *Hazard* refers to the actual agent and how likely it is to cause harm to the public (e.g., a storm). This is the traditional model of risk—one in which the risk of a hazard is what is considered to be most important when communicating that risk. However, Sandman emphasizes that how people respond to a particular hazard does not have much to do with how likely the hazard is to cause harm or to what extent but actually has much more to do with the perceived concern about a hazard by members of the public (this is known as outrage). Outrage, he argues, is shaped by a complex range of factors, including cultural and economic ones (Hooker et al., 2017). In fact, Sandman has outlined 12 "outrage factors" that interact to influence how a person perceives a specific hazard, and how "outraged" they are by it (Lanard, n.d.). Table 3.1 helps to explain why some hazards such as radon (a colourless, odourless gas that is the second leading cause of lung cancer deaths) go unnoticed by the general public, but others, such as Ebola virus, for example, cause much panic, despite the associated risk of death being relatively low in the Canadian context. Whereas radon is a "natural" hazard that tends to cause disease over a particularly long period of time (i.e., it is "chronic"), Ebola is "exotic" (originating outside of North America), less well known ("unknowable"), and "dreaded" based on how it has been reported in the media, with graphic images and stories of death. Peter Sandman goes on to categorize risks according to hazard and outrage and outlines three main strategies for risk communication based on the level of both hazard and outrage (Fig. 3.4).

EXERCISE 3.3: Use Sandman's 12 outrage factors to explain why eating raw food products (e.g., sushi, beef carpaccio) is a risk that is often underestimated compared with risks related to radiation from cell phone towers, which has caused much outrage in recent years.

As depicted in Fig. 3.4, the three strategies of risk communication are as follows:

1. *Outrage management*, which occurs when outrage is high and the hazard is low. These situations usually call for authorities to calm the public and manage perceived risks, putting them into perspective, increasing understanding, and promoting dialogue. According to some experts, the best way to engage in outrage *management* is to provide clear and evidence-informed information (Ontario Agency for Health Protection and Promotion [OAHPP], 2016).

2. *Precaution advocacy*, which occurs when the hazard is high and outrage is low. In this situation, the goal of health authorities is to increase a risk's profile and encourage people to take a specific risk more seriously. According to Sandman (2007), principles to effectively engage in precaution advocacy include appealing to people's needs and emotions, making messages interesting, and giving people clear actions to take to protect themselves from the specified risk.

TABLE 3.1 Peter Sandman's 12 Outrage Factors

Features of Risks That Produce Low Outrage ("Safe")	Features of Risks That Produce High Outrage ("Risky")
Voluntary	Coerced
Natural	Industrial
Familiar	Exotic
Not memorable	Memorable
Not dreaded	Dreaded
Chronic	Catastrophic
Knowable	Unknowable
Individually controlled	Controlled by others
Fair	Unfair
Morally irrelevant	Morally relevant
Trustworthy sources	Untrustworthy sources
Responsive process	Unresponsive process

From Lanard, J. (n.d.). *A quick introduction to risk perception*. Retrieved from http://www2.wpro.who.int/internet/files/e-ha/toolkit/web/Technical%20References/Risk%20Communication%20and%20Public%20Information/Introduction%20Risk%20Perception.pdf.

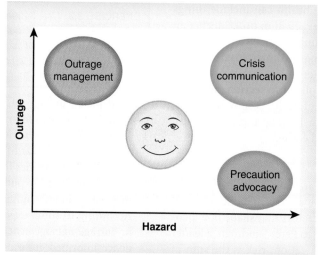

Fig 3.4 Peter Sandman's risk categories. (From Sandman P. [2014]. *Introduction to risk communication and orientation to this Website.* Retrieved from http://psandman.com/index-intro.htm.)

3. *Crisis communication*, which occurs when both the hazard and the outrage are high, and often occurs during an emergency (e.g., pandemic, environmental spill) (Sandman, 2014).

In general, when communicating about risks and specific hazards outside of the context of an emergency, it is important to follow basic principles of risk communication, which include being truthful (e.g., clearly expressing what facts are not known and avoiding unsubstantiated statements), being helpful (e.g., responding directly to the audience without using words that are too technical and that people won't typically understand), being clear (avoiding words that can cause confusion or mean different things to different people), being proactive (e.g., build relationships with communities to establish credibility), and finally, being available (e.g., be responsive to the media and provide information quickly) (OAHPP, 2016).

Social Marketing for Health

Health marketing is an emerging field and represents one of many ways of approaching health education campaigns. **Social marketing** integrates principles from the field of marketing and population health to "create, communicate, and deliver health information and interventions, using customer-centred and science-based strategies to protect and promote the health of diverse populations" (CDC, 2011b). In

this approach, individuals are treated as consumers and campaign designers spend a lot of time trying to understand their audiences and what motivates them, similar to what is done by marketers in the private sector. Central to health marketing is the idea of audience segmentation, which refers to the division of the target audience into "groups who share similar beliefs, attitudes and behavioural patterns" (European Centre for Disease Prevention and Control, 2014). The campaign then is targeted to very specific subgroups and acts on the fundamental reasons for why people behave the way they do.

Social marketing also considers the "competition" or what other factors get in the way of a person adopting healthier behaviours or products (European Centre for Disease Prevention and Control, 2014). In designing social marketing campaigns, the 4 Ps of marketing are applied. The first P stands for *product* and represents the actual good or intervention being promoted. In the case of a traditional marketing campaign, this is often a tangible product like a new soft drink, a new line of clothing, or a specific item such as a computer that companies are trying to sell. In the case of health marketing, examples of products could include on-the-spot HIV test kits or the uptake of a healthier behaviour such as quitting smoking (a less tangible product, which can even be an idea). The second P stands for *price*. In the case of a traditional marketing campaign, the price is how much a good or service costs (in monetary terms). In health marketing, the price can represent monetary costs, practical costs (e.g., the time it takes to get to a health care provider's clinic to obtain smoking cessation aids or HIV tests), social costs (behaving differently than your peers), and emotional costs (the anxiety that can accompany getting an HIV test, for example). *Place* is the third P and represents where a specific product can be accessed (e.g., at a store or a health care provider's office). More emphasis is being placed on bringing key services to the consumer to reduce practical costs, making them more likely to obtain a product or implement behaviour change. Last, *promotion* is the fourth P. Promotion is how a product will be advertised (or how health benefits will be communicated), for example, through posters, on the news, or through bulletins to health care providers (European Centre for Disease Prevention and Control, 2014).

Social Media Communications

The use of social media is gaining much more prominence in the areas of health education, media advocacy, and social marketing, as well as risk communication. One definition of **social media** put forth by Kaplan and Haenlein is "a group of Internet-based applications that allow [for] the creation and exchange of user generated content" (Kaplan & Haenlein, 2010).

One of the unique characteristics of social media applications such as Facebook, Twitter, Instagram, blog sites, and others, is the fact that they allow for two-way communication. Instead of health authorities communicating to users unidirectionally (as is the case with several other strategies described in this section), social media fosters the coming together of peers and collaborations in which content can be generated and shared by users themselves (National Collaborating Centre for Healthy Public Policy, 2015). More recently, population and public health experts have realized the immense potential of reaching large networks of people via social media applications and have begun to draw on them when engaging in messaging and health communications. Social media is being used by health organizations to disseminate health information (e.g., location and hours of specific clinics, information regarding various disease states and action people can take to prevent them) and to complement media advocacy efforts. In the case of **crisis communication**, social media provides an avenue to reach people quickly and in large numbers.

An example of a particularly successful Canadian health care provider who has used social media channels such as YouTube to convey health messaging regarding a variety of topics is Dr. Michael Evans, who has a YouTube channel with more than 3 million views and more than 65 000 subscribers, where he has created a number of short, evidence-based videos related to the importance of physical activity and healthy eating and tips to achieving better productivity and happiness (St. Michael's Hospital, 2019).

Outside of health communications, social media has many uses. For example, it can be used for surveillance activities (discussed earlier) by tracking how many people are experiencing certain symptoms and where they are geographically. This can help identify an emerging disease or outbreak (and is an example of syndromic surveillance). Additionally, social media has many applications in health care, like linking people to health care providers, for example (Newbold, 2015).

Some challenges with the use of social media are also beginning to be articulated. One such challenge is respecting and abiding by privacy laws that protect people's personal health information, making sure it is not shared more widely than necessary or made public. Another challenge pertains to reaching diverse audiences. Some social media channels are more effective than others in reaching specific groups (e.g., youth) and thus, one must always consider the best media for the message and realize that demographic differences exist in the use of various communication mediums. Last, because social media includes content generated by users, this content may not always be verifiable or may take on a shape of its own when generated by people who may not be content experts. For example, many vaccine-hesitant individuals propagate their message using social media channels, and this can generate a large reach and spread information that is not valid. The sheer volume of inaccurate information on social media, as well, contributes to this challenge (Newbold, 2015).

Either way, social media applications are expected to grow, and with more than 80% of Canadians using the Internet, it remains a tool with great potential (Newbold, 2015). The Research Perspective box provides an analysis on the use of social media to further political and policy goals.

Social Media's Influence on Social Movements and Political Protest

In recent years, we have seen a number of influential social media campaigns that have supported and have, in many cases, been critical to movements such as Black Lives Matter, the #Me Too movement, and Idle No More. These campaigns aim to bring awareness and discussion to issues of marginalization and are, fundamentally, a form of social movement and protest against certain inequities and injustices. In many cases, the goal of such movements is to create policy change.

A 2016 article published in the journal *News Media & Society* studied the impact of tweets related to the Black Lives Matter movement over the course of 10 months. The authors of the study found evidence that social media helped the movement attract the media's attention and, in doing so, got political elites to pay attention to the issue of police brutality in the United States (Freelon, McIlwain, & Clark, 2016).

Upstream Strategies

Health Promotion

As discussed in Chapter 1, recognizing and addressing the SDHs has a long history in Canada. The SDHs are the "circumstances in which people are born, grow up, live, work, and age, and the systems put in place to deal with illness" (WHO, 2019, p. 2). Health promotion has become a key cornerstone for taking action on the SDH to address health inequities, decrease the burden of disease, and prevent premature morbidity. **Health promotion** is a multilevel, multisectoral, and multidisciplinary activity. Although the Ottawa Charter for Health Promotion (1986) outlines strategies for improving the health of populations, theories that underpin these strategies have been borrowed from a range of disciplines (e.g., psychology, anthropology, sociology, political science). Strategies and approaches often stop at the individual and focus on behaviour change as a single-level intervention. Individual behaviour change alone is generally not sufficient to produce or sustain widespread improvements in health, let alone sustained behaviour change. Yet despite more than 30 years of health promotion, most activities can be best described as health education or interventions that are aimed at behavioural changes on an individual basis. However, the conceptual framework of health promotion is rooted in the critique of the "downstream" approach of the hegemonic biomedical curative model, with its devotion to "saving drowning swimmers." Health promotion is the development of an alternative "upstream" approach that aims to "tackle the forces that push them into the river" (Canadian Public Health Association & WHO, 1986).

As discussed in Chapter 1, the definition of health expanded from the WHO's 1946 definition to: "a resource for everyday life, not the objective of living. Health is a positive concept emphasizing social and personal resources, as well as physical capacities" (WHO, 1986, p.1). The newer definition conceptualizes health as a resource, as an aspect of a good life but not the ultimate goal of life.

Health promotion approaches in general, as articulated in the Ottawa Charter, involve five key action areas (Fig. 3.5): reorienting health services, enhancing personal skills, strengthening community action, creating supportive environments, and building healthy public policy (see Chapter 1).

Reorienting health services toward prevention of diseases and promotion of health implies the move away from the biomedical approach (see Chapter 1). However, health services continue to remain mostly curative, requiring transformation in the entire health system in Canada to reorient towards health promotion.

Enhancing personal skills is a process of supporting individuals to understand and critically use health information (health literacy). It includes skills in developing the capacity to assess their own health needs and to identify possible changes to their own actions and the wider environment, which has been discussed earlier by providing different frameworks.

Strengthening community action is a process of expanding resources and capacities of communities to make decisions and take collective action to increase their control over the determinants of their health. Actions include community development and advocacy (discussed later).

Creating supportive environments for health means addressing how physical and social environments are organized at the individual, community group, organizational, and government levels. The physical environment includes the natural and built environment, and social environments include the psychosocial, economic, and cultural environments (discussed later).

Building **healthy public policy** means explicitly considering and choosing policies that make positive health

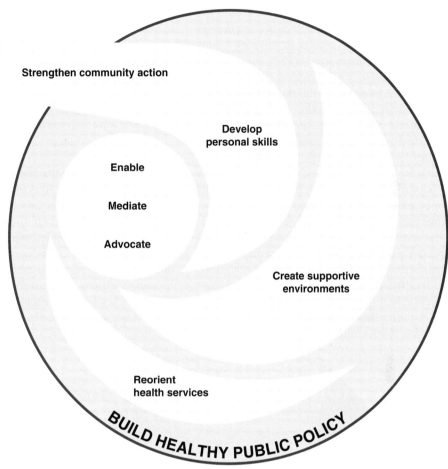

Fig 3.5 The Ottawa Charter for Health Promotion. (From World Health Organization. [1986]. *Ottawa Charter for Health Promotion*. Ottawa: Canadian Public Health Association. Retrieved from https://www.med.uottawa.ca/sim/data/Health_Promotion_e.htm#Ottawa_Charter)

choices easier for people. Advocating for, establishing, and implementing explicit actions by government—including legislation, regulation, and fiscal measures—are specific actions for building healthy public policy. Legislation, regulation, and fiscal measures may affect policy not traditionally under the purview of health (e.g., physical education time in schools, costs associated with eating nutritious foods, incomes associated with the ability to afford nutritious and healthy foods, costs associated with access to recreational spaces). Public and private policies shape how money, power, and material resources flow through society and therefore affect the determinants of health. As a society, creating

healthy public policies is the most important strategy for acting on the determinants of health. A political economy approach (discussed later in the chapter), for example, can support addressing social welfare, universal day care, and securing unemployment insurance, which are important for achieving health for all.

The Ottawa Charter, the Adelaide Recommendations (WHO, 1998), the Jakarta Declaration, and the Helsinki statement on health in all policies call for building healthy public policy: for health care professionals to put health on the agenda of policy makers in all sectors and at all levels, directing them to be aware of the health consequences of their decisions and to accept their responsibilities for health. **Health in all policies** (HiAP) is an intersectoral approach to public policy that systematically takes into account the health consequences of decisions that seek synergies and avoid harmful health impacts to improve population health and health equity (WHO, 2013). However, caution is needed when working across sectors because the perception of **health imperialism**—that is, asserting health above all other important objectives—can thwart efforts. There are several tools that support a HiAP approach to enhance the ability of health issues to be systematically taken into account during decision making. One such tool is the Health Impact Assessment (HIA), which has been repeatedly shown to be effective in influencing decisions in practice (Dannenberg, 2016). HIA is a process that supports health and nonhealth actors to evaluate the potential health-related outcomes of an activity (projects, plans, or policies) before it is built or implemented. Planning, land use, and transportation decisions in a community all have public health consequences. A HIA is helpful to minimize the health risks while enhancing potential health benefits. A streamlined version called the rapid

HIA allows for a summary analysis of either positive or negative effects to be conducted through screening the determinants of health and the various subgroups that may be affected by an activity.

As previously stated, no one strategy is effective on its own; however, used together, they can promote health and prevent disease.

> **CRITICAL THINKING QUESTION 3.3:** What does it mean to work with multisectoral partners or intersectoral partners?

In addition to the Ottawa Charter, the Nuffield Intervention Ladder (Fig. 3.6) is used as a way of categorizing various approaches related to health promotion. The Nuffield Intervention Ladder was first proposed in 2007 by the Nuffield Council on Bioethics (in the United Kingdom), an independent organization that analyzes ethical issues in medicine and biology. This model recognizes that governments can intervene at many levels when influencing the health of a population. At the bottom of the ladder are interventions, such as "provide information" (e.g., health education), which

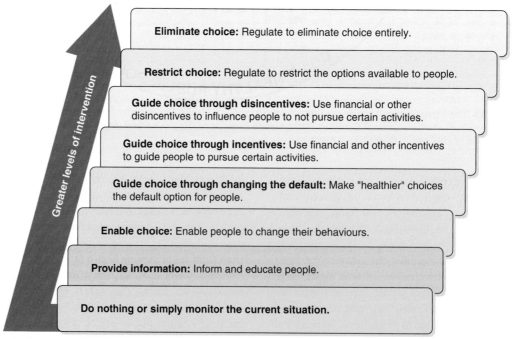

Fig 3.6 The Nuffield Intervention Ladder. (Redrawn from Nuffield Council on Bioethics. [2007]. *Public health: Ethical issues* [p. 42, Box 3.2]. Cambridge: Cambridge Publishers. Retrieved from http://nuffieldbioethics.org/wp-content/uploads/2014/07/Public-health-ethical-issues.pdf)

are nonintrusive and interfere less with people's freedom of choice. However, these nonintrusive interventions are also typically less effective in producing large changes in behaviour at the population level. At the top of the ladder are interventions that governments may take that are seen as being much more intrusive and limiting "free choice" but are also often cited as being much more effective because they result in significant behaviour change, which is again part of creating healthy public policies. For example, when trying to encourage consumption of water instead of sugary drinks, governments may choose among several policy options, such as conducting surveillance of the rates of consumption of sugary drinks in the population, informing the public through health education, limiting the sale of these drinks in public facilities and schools, or banning the sale of sugary drinks by large beverage companies altogether. Health education tends to be a popular intervention among governments, as an option that does not limit "free choice" and can target a range of factors that underlie why someone makes a decision about one behaviour (e.g., drinking a sugary drink) over another (e.g., choosing water). However, many people do not make free choices about, for example, what they eat. Food choices are influenced by habits, food availability,

affordability, and cultural norms (Nuffield Council on Bioethics, 2007). Individuals who experience socioeconomic disadvantage (e.g., those with limited education, low income, or residing in economically deprived areas) may live in neighbourhoods where healthy food is not available, affordable, or acceptable, creating conditions where eating behaviours are not conducive to good health. Health education is not an effective strategy in this instance. An emerging concept, known as "nudges," is being explored more and more; it reflects the idea of "guiding choice through changing the default" (Nuffield Council on Bioethics, 2007) and is explored further in Box 3.1.

EXERCISE 3.4: Using the issue of high levels of unhealthy snack food consumption among school-aged children, apply both the Ottawa Charter for Health Promotion and the Nuffield Intervention Ladder to come up with examples of interventions to address this problem. Is there overlap in the interventions you thought of when using the Ottawa Charter model versus the Nuffield Intervention Ladder model? If so, how? How might you relate or map out what areas of the Nuffield ladder fit within the Ottawa Charter?

BOX 3.1 Behavioural Economics and "Nudges"

Over the years, the value of behavioural economics in shaping public health action has increasingly come to be recognized. Behavioural economics, unlike traditional economics, disagrees that people always act "rationally" and in their own best interests. In fact, it integrates neurology and psychology concepts to highlight that humans can often behave impulsively and in ways that are irrational because of the social and environmental context around them—the same idea that many health promotion practitioners have been supporting for years (Matjasko et al., 2016). Behavioural economists, together with public health practitioners, have written extensively about the idea of a "**nudge**," which can be thought of as an intervention that will predictably change peoples' behaviour without significantly restricting their options or significantly changing their economic incentives (Matjasko, et al., 2016). The idea is that a small "nudge" in the right direction can help a person make a behaviour change. Although new to public health, the food industry has long been nudging the public, often successfully, in the wrong

direction to purchase unhealthy food products through various marketing strategies (e.g., putting snack foods right by the checkout aisle of a grocery store). An example of an intervention that uses nudging for public health to improve the consumption of healthy snacks among youth is changing the names of certain vegetable options to more interesting and appealing names. This small change has been shown to improve the rates of vegetable consumption among youth (Matjasko et al., 2016).

In the Nuffield Intervention Ladder, "nudges" often fall into the category of "making the healthier option the default," or the most convenient option, because people will do what is easiest. However, nudging individuals, for example, to purchase healthier items may be a more effective strategy among individuals with a higher socioeconomic position. Additionally, not all nudges lead to supporting healthier choices; they have shown mixed evidence for their efficacy and should not be used in isolation. See the Research Perspective box for a research example regarding "nudges."

RESEARCH PERSPECTIVE

Choosing Healthier Foods in Recreational Sports Settings

What is the impact of nudging combined with an economic incentive for choosing healthier foods in recreational sports settings?

In Canada, recreational facilities are publicly funded sport complexes providing access to affordable physical activities but are also considered unhealthy food environments. This study used mixed methods to quantify the impact of three environmental interventions on sales of healthy items at an outdoor community pool. An initial pre-intervention control period was followed by three successive interventions, including (1) signage with descriptive menu labels, (2) addition of a taste-testing intervention, and (3) addition of a price-reduction intervention. This study found mixed evidence for the efficacy of three approaches to nudging healthy dietary choices at a population level. Overall, single or multiple nudges or multiple nudges concurrent with price reductions did not influence the sale of healthy items at a community pool. The researchers concluded that given nudging's small and inconsistent impacts to date, it should not replace the use of other proven health promotion strategies but can be used as one more tool that may be helpful in particular contexts.

Source: Olstad, D. L., Goonewardene, L. A., McCargar, L. J., et al. (2014). Choosing healthier foods in recreational sports settings: A mixed methods investigation of the impact of nudging and an economic incentive. *International Journal of Behavioral Nutrition and Physical Activity, 11*(1), 6.

Population Health Promotion

As a response to the CIAR model of population health and absence of health promotion, Hamilton and Bhatti (1996) combined the elements of the two into the framework known now as *Population Health Promotion: An Integrated Model of Population Health and Health Promotion*. This document describes the elements of the population health approach to the broad determinants of health with the strategies and techniques of health promotion as outlined in the Ottawa Charter. Fig. 3.7 shows the interrelationship of the elements of the population health promotion framework. Each element can be extracted so that health promotion strategies can be developed at the social, sectoral (e.g., the agricultural industry), local community, family, or individual level. The framework is also explicit in noting that the choice

depends on values and assumptions about desirable health-related goals that must be mediated through evidence and evaluation. The model provides a synoptic view of the manner by which health promotion strategies can be conceived and implemented. See Box 3.2 to apply the population health promotion model to develop interventions.

EXERCISE 3.5 Developing Interventions by Applying the Population Health Promotion Model: Watch the video *Population Health: The New Agenda* on YouTube (see https://www.youtube.com/watch?v=aJbpRt4r5cE).

Reflect on the following questions:

1. WHAT ("What are the health issues facing this population?"), followed by
2. WHAT ("What are the causes or determinants of these problems?")
3. HOW ("How should we take action?"). Population health then considers the design of interventions using the strategies from the Ottawa Charter.
4. WHO ("With whom should we act?"). Decide at what level you will target your intervention: individual, family, community, sector–organization, or society–policy.

In your class, discuss the stories portrayed in the video as it relates to the population health model.

Decide "WHAT." You may need to do some research on the "WHAT" you have chosen to better understand it. Briefly summarize what the literature says about the health issue and the root causes (socio-environmental view) or determinants of these problems.

Think downstream, midstream, and upstream as you decide the "HOW." You will also need to do a brief search of some promising interventions that are working or best practice interventions. What does the literature say is working really well for the health issue or determinant you have chosen? Base your intervention or "HOW" on best evidence, working midstream and upstream. You can choose more than one intervention if you want to target midstream or upstream.

Then decide at what level you will take action and "WITH WHOM."

Influencing Public Policy

Recognizing that health is determined by more than health services, public policy shifts upstream to focus on the broader structural and SDHs. Understanding how to influence public policy is a necessary skill required by a health care professional to make system change and tackle health inequities. **Public policy** can be defined

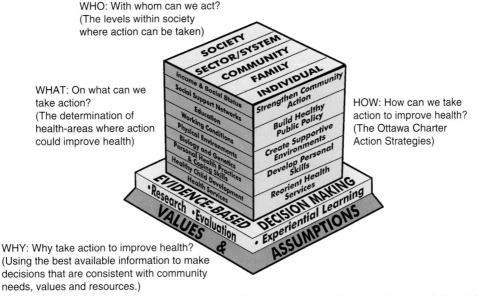

WHO: With whom can we act?
(The levels within society where action can be taken)

WHAT: On what can we take action?
(The determination of health-areas where action could improve health)

HOW: How can we take action to improve health?
(The Ottawa Charter Action Strategies)

WHY: Why take action to improve health?
(Using the best available information to make decisions that are consistent with community needs, values and resources.)

Fig 3.7 An integrated model of population health and health promotion. (From Hamilton, N., & Bhatti, T. [1996]. *Population health promotion: An integrated model of population health and health promotion.* Ottawa: Health Promotion Development Division, Health Canada. Copyright 1996 by Minister of Public Work and Government Services Canada.)

BOX 3.2   Citizens' Jury for Taxing Soft Drinks

A citizens' jury was convened to assess the likely acceptability of taxation to prevent childhood obesity by influencing the purchasing of nutrient-poor food and drinks by parents. The jurors were asked to reach a verdict and make recommendations about taxation as an obesity-prevention strategy based on evidence provided by clinical, policy, and academic expert witnesses from a wide range of perspectives. The jurors were able to "cross-examine" the experts, who provided evidence, and recall "witnesses" to assist them in making their recommendations. The following five questions were developed and put to the jurors for deliberation at the citizens' jury:

1. Is taxation an appropriate strategy for reducing childhood obesity among 0- to 5-year-olds?
2. Is it appropriate to tax sugar-sweetened drinks as a strategy for reducing childhood obesity? (*Sugar-sweetened drinks* refers to all drinks with added sugar, including soft drinks [carbonated drinks], cordials, flavoured milks, fruit juices, fruit drinks, and vitamin waters.)
3. Is it appropriate to tax processed meats as a strategy for reducing childhood obesity? (*Processed meats* refers to meat and meat alternatives that have been processed, including chicken nuggets, sausages, and meats with high fat and sodium content.)
4. Is it appropriate to tax snack foods as a strategy for reducing childhood obesity? (*Snack foods* refers to sweet or savoury snack packs and individually wrapped snacks, including packets of biscuits, potato chips, sweets, muesli bars, small cakes, muffins, and crackers with cheese.)
5. Is it appropriate to tax food eaten away from home as a strategy for reducing childhood obesity? (*Foods eaten outside the home* refers to takeout foods that are purchased or eaten outside the home, including well-known fast food brands and specific items with high fat, sugar, and sodium content.)

Over 2 days, participants were presented with evidence on the topic by experts, were able to question witnesses, and deliberated on the evidence. At the end of their deliberations, jurors unanimously supported taxation on sugar-sweetened drinks but generally did not support taxation on processed meats, snack foods, and foods eaten or purchased outside the home. They also supported taxation on snack foods on the condition that traffic-light labelling was also introduced. Although they were not specifically asked to deliberate strategies outside of taxation, the jurors strongly recommended the inclusion of more nutritional information on all food packaging, using the traffic light and teaspoon labelling systems for sugar, salt, and fat content. It was concluded that these reforms should be considered by government to reduce the future societal costs of obesity.

Source: Moretto, N., Kendall, E., Whitty, J., et al. (2014). Yes, the government should tax soft drinks: Findings from a citizens' jury in Australia. *International Journal of Environmental Research and Public Health, 11*(3), 2456–2471. https://doi.org/10.3390/ijerph110302456

as the decisions, plans, and actions that are undertaken to achieve specific situation within a society (WHO, n.d.). Policies help to support the social rather than the individual good and have the potential to create environments where the healthy choice is the easy choice, thus creating opportunities for everyone, including the most vulnerable, to improve their health (Keen, 2014). Therefore, healthy public policy improves the conditions under which people live, work, learn, and play. Raphael points out that public policy "is primarily concerned with whether a problem is recognized as being a societal rather than an individual problem" (Raphael, 2013, p. 227).

Policy change at any level does not always come about from strong scientific evidence, mobilization of a number of communities, or convincing a few decision makers but rather results from multiple actions in many domains that bring together scientific evidence and political power (Freudenberg & Tsui, 2014). The process of policy change is also not an entirely rational, incremental, or stage-sequential one. Policy making is complex and dynamic and can be described as a cyclical process that involves problem or issue identification; policy formulation, which includes agenda setting and development of legislation; policy implementation, which includes rule making and actual operationalization; and evaluation and modification (Anderson, 2011). An outcome of the dynamic and inherent complexities in policy processes is that health care professionals and other stakeholders often have difficulty determining where and how to engage in the process of supporting policy change (Raine et al., 2014). Even after a policy is developed, policy adoption and implementation remain challenges for many complex and context-specific reasons.

The Alberta Coalition for Chronic Disease Prevention (APCCP) has developed a resource base of policy tools and resources such as the Policy Readiness Tool [PRT] to support healthy public policy change (Nykiforuk et al., 2011). PRT is a self-administered questionnaire that can be used to asses a community's or an organization's readiness for policy change. The tool also provides a series of strategies and resources for working with communities or organizations at different stages of readiness to help encourage the adoption of healthy public policy. PRT has been adapted from the Diffusion of Innovations Theory (Rogers, 1983) and describes policy readiness as a set of behavioural categories: innovator, majority, and late adopter. Readiness is based on the notion of what it means to be an innovator, majority,

or late adopter. The PRT describes innovator communities as adventurous and often serving as role models for other places. Majority communities are described as deliberate because they require time to determine whether to adopt a new initiative. Late-adopter communities are described as being traditional, skeptical of new ideas, and eager to maintain the status quo. The APCCP's website contains many other policy tools and resources that can facilitate policy change (see website address listed at end of the chapter).

Social Innovation, Enterprise, and Entrepreneurship for Social Change

An emerging trend in public health is **social innovation**, which is described as the pursuit of "a novel solution to a social problem that is more effective, efficient, sustainable or just than existing solutions and for which the value created accrues primarily to society as a whole rather than to private individuals" (Cajaiba-Santana, 2014, p. 45). For example, a cell phone isn't a socially innovative product by itself but can be used to diagnose disease. An innovative social service could be a policy change that allows nurses access to student loan deferment or loan forgiveness if they work in communities that are isolated or remote. Providing tandem bicycles and hand cycles to community organizations to enable them to operate para-cycling programs is another example of a social innovation. Ultimately, to truly claim the highest standard of social impact, innovative ideas must be tested. Early evidence suggests that the value of social innovation lies in its capacity to redress system failures at local levels (Mason et al., 2015, p. ii116).

Social enterprise is a business—whether operated for profit or not for profit—that has a double bottom line of maximizing both social and financial return. Although social enterprise may use some philanthropic dollars in the start-up phase or for special projects, it is geared toward the creation of a self-sustaining, market-based business model. The Shelley Gautier Para-Sport Foundation is an example of a social enterprise. This foundation breaks down barriers for people living with disabilities, enabling them to participate in sports activities. An awareness of adaptive sport is created, and the foundation develops resources that encourage inclusive para-cycling programs. Their website can be found at the end of the chapter.

Social entrepreneurship is about mindset. Social entrepreneurs are change agents who are relentless about fashioning bold and creative solutions—through the creation of new organizations or as "intrapreneurs" within existing organizations and communities—to create social change. Intrapreneurs are a catalyst for change to move an organization to pursue social good as a business case. Although they are social entrepreneurs, their organization may or may not be a social enterprise, and their idea may or may not be socially innovative. Purppl (Purposeful People) is a social enterprise accelerator that is focused on building capacity of social entrepreneurs (http://purppl.com). They provide mentorship, training, and tools on sustainable business models to help solve tough community, social, and environmental challenges.

EXERCISE 3.6 Social Procurement: Watch the video *How to Change the World* on YouTube (see https://www.youtube.com/watch?v=pEx-VI1VUj4).

Kevin Vuong is a connector, city builder, and military officer working to build a stronger, resilient, prosperous Canada where no one is left behind. At the Agency for Public & Social Innovation, he is focused on innovating procurement for social impact and improving Ontario's social innovation ecosystem through capital, capacity-building, and scaling services. He sees social entrepreneurship as a vehicle for advancing the sustainable development goals and is playing an active role in its advancement as Canada's Local Pathways Fellow for the United Nations Sustainable Development Solutions Network.

What is social procurement as discussed in the video, and how does it relate to social enterprise?

CRITICAL THINKING QUESTION 3.4: How can you use social enterprise, social innovation, social entrepreneurship, or social procurement to address poverty, a lack of decent work and employment, or some other social determinant of health in your community?

Enhancing Community Health

Many of the strategies discussed in the previous sections can also be used to enhance community health. However, there are specific strategies for community health where the health needs, resources, and capacities are identified by the community members, who then mobilize themselves into collective action. A key concept in all community health work is **community empowerment**, which can be defined as "a social action process

by which individuals, communities and organizations gain mastery over their lives in the context of changing their social and political environment to improve equity and quality of life" (Wallerstein, 2002, p. 73). Importantly, however, Wallerstein stresses that "participation alone is insufficient if strategies do not also build capacity of community organizations and individuals in decision-making and advocacy" (Wallerstein, 2006, p. 4).

Community Development

Public participation was recognized as a right to health in the Alma Ata (see Chapter 1) and is a major strategy in Epp's framework (see Chapter 1). The nature and extent of public participation can be conceptualized along a spectrum of increasing community capacity to respond to issues of community concern. **Community efficacy** represents the state of community confidence necessary to bring about desired social change (Wallerstein, 1992). **Community development** refers to the process of community members identifying issues and problems that affect their community and then developing and acquiring the planning skills and capacity to bring about the implementation of change. Health care providers, such as community health nurses, and health care organizations, such as public health departments, may facilitate this community-initiated and community-directed process. The key to effective facilitation is building relationships within the community and engaging members in a dialogue in the assessment, planning, action, and evaluation of community-based issues.

Asset-Based Community Development. **Asset-based community development (ABCD)** is a positive community engagement approach that aims to facilitate the empowerment of communities to tackle the SDHs by targeting general health and well-being (Kretzmann & McKnight, 1996; Bull, Mittelmark, & Kanyeka, 2013). ABCD is seen as an important innovation in addressing the SDHs as it supports communities to set their own targets in terms of meeting their health and well-being needs (Foot, 2012). Adopting a partnership model, ABCD approaches identify and build on the strengths or "assets" of individuals and communities (Kretzmann & McKnight, 1996), as well as valuing capacity, skills, knowledge, connections, and supportive potential in the community (Foot, 2012). Asset mapping can be used to map the strengths of the community and can be done with community members as a community development strategy.

Citizens' Juries. Citizens' juries (also known as community juries or citizens' assemblies) are an approach to community participation that gives community members a role in democratic decision making around policy questions important to the community. Citizens' juries build on the idea of legal juries, but in the case of health, the jurors are citizens selected to participate in a policy development exercise on behalf of a particular community. Juries usually consist of 12 to 20 randomly selected and demographically representative people. They differ from focus groups in that participants are given reliable information or evidence and time to deliberate, with a verdict delivered by jurors (Street, Duszynski, & Braunack-Mayer, 2014). The issue under discussion should arise from within communities in which there is a high level of commitment to the process and outcomes. The problem or question for consideration and debate is framed and developed collaboratively with the community, and recommendations are context specific and locally developed. The purpose of the recommendations is that they are intended to be acted upon. Thus, the commitment made by ordinary citizens of their time and energy has an outcome. The jury's verdict is not binding, nor does it need to be unanimous. The report of findings must be publicized and the recommendations responded to within a specific timeframe. Explanations must be provided of the decision to follow the recommendations or take another course of action. However, citizen juries can be costly, and the self-selected nature of participation makes participation attractive to those who are more articulate and educated. See Box 3.2 (earlier) for an example of an issue that was tackled by a citizens' jury.

Community Organizing

Community organizing focuses on mobilizing people within a specific neighbourhood or community. Community organizing may be thought of as a way to mobilize small groups of people to accomplish a particular task. Often community organizing uses a problem-oriented approach rather than an asset-based approach. Community residents are mobilized to "solve" a particular problem recognized in their neighbourhood. There are three strategies for mobilizing community members: (1) social planning, which is the rational solution of problems using the existing power structure; (2) community locality development, or the development of a community for an organized approach to a given problem; and (3) social action, which is a shift in power

structures in the community (Rothman, 2001). Social action campaigns are direct actions, like a movement such as Black Lives Matter, that aim to change decisions, societal structures, and cultural beliefs. Social action can be thought of as people with similar self-interests coming together, confronting and making demands on the power structure to create improvements for the community (Alinsky, 1971). Generally, community organizing is better suited than community development for addressing the structural barriers that prevent poor communities from improving their health and well-being.

Community organizing strategies can be integrated into a concept that views an entire community as the focus of health promotion. Within the healthy cities–healthy communities framework, health-enhancing strategies are integrated into urban planning and community design (Kickbusch, 1989). Elements of a **healthy city** include a clean and safe physical environment, a sustainable ecosystem, the meeting of basic human needs, and a strong and supportive community in which decision making is shared by all. The strategy involves including health promotion issues on the political agenda so that key decision makers and the community at large make prevention and health promotion highly visible and community supported. This strategy was emphasized at the WHO's Fifth Global Conference in 2000 on Health Promotion in Mexico and has strengthened the healthy municipalities and communities movement around the world.

ADDRESSING THE STRUCTURAL DETERMINANTS OF HEALTH INEQUALITIES

A Political Economy Approach

Improving health for all through addressing the **structural determinants of health** (the SDH inequalities) (see Chapter 1) directs our attention to a political economy approach (Navarro & Muntaner, 2004; Raphael, 2004). **Political economy** is a broad theoretical framework that emphasizes how the structure of the economy and society affects the lives of individuals. Although other macro-level approaches, such as social ecology (Brofenbrenner, 1979) and complexity science (Byrne, 2002) stress the importance of viewing health and health problems in terms of their relationship to other facets of society and the environment, political economy goes further. The political economy orientation "offers a window into both the micro-level processes by which social structures lead to individual health or illness and the macro-level processes by which power relationships and political ideology shape the quality of these social structures" (Raphael, Bryant, & Rioux, 2006, p. 132).

The assumptions about health made by a political economy approach are as much political as they are social. Health is seen as a reflection of the state of a society's political economy; good health is a state of physical and emotional well-being that includes "access to and control over the basic material and nonmaterial resources that sustain and promote life at a high level of satisfaction" (Baer, Singer, & Johnsen, 1986, p. 95). There are three main areas of social and economic policy that influence health: (1) the industrial relations system, which is how workers are organized and wages set; (2) labour market regulation, which governs hiring and firing; and (3) the welfare state, which is the system for providing benefits (Greer, 2018). Applied to the question of redressing health inequities, a political economy approach highlights the formative role played by power and politics in shaping the social conditions of life and thus the well-being of individuals experiencing inequities and society as a whole. The recommendations in the Commission on Social Determinants of Health report also called for a change in the distribution of power, money, and resources supporting a political economy approach to achieving health for all.

Using a political economy approach to address food insecurity, for example, would focus on structural policies such as fiscal, labour market, or market regulation. Specifically, this would include, but not be limited to, subsidizing the cost of healthy and nutritious foods, progressive tax structures, and increased social assistance rates (Raphael, 2015); reducing poverty through raising minimum wages or social assistance through policies such as universal basic income; and price controls for rent, which can create affordable housing, allowing for more of an individual's budget to go towards necessities such as food. Additionally, this might include strengthening labour markets by centring on unions to protect workers' job security.

The political economy perspective places its focus on how the power and influence of specific groups—primarily the private business and corporate sector—influence public policies that create social inequalities such as food insecurity. Thus, action requires countering and rebalancing the power and influence of these groups

through building political and social movements aimed at the collective empowerment of "whole classes of people," including women, workers, youth, and seniors (Hofrichter, 2003, p. 13). Health care professionals and researchers must advocate for governments to address poverty, unemployment, and housing insecurity along with other key SDHs.

> **CRITICAL THINKING QUESTION 3.5:** Since around 2014, there has been a rise in advocacy (particularly by people in the health care and public health fields) related to a Guaranteed Annual Income, also known as a Basic Income.
>
> Research this policy idea. Do you think it could work? How might it affect health and health equity?

Public Health Advocacy

Advocacy is a core competency of public health practice and is integral to the work of many health care providers in Canada (see the Interprofessional Practice box). Working to achieve health for all requires individuals to be able to "advocate for healthy public policies and services that promote and protect the health and well-being of individuals and communities" (Public Health Agency of Canada, 2008). However, many health care providers and researchers believe that engaging with the political system and advocating for healthy public policy are outside their area of expertise or mandate.

▓▓ INTERPROFESSIONAL PRACTICE
Advocacy As a Competency

Many health professions include advocacy as a core competency for practice:
- Public Health and Home Health Nursing competencies include "Advocate for the reduction of inequities in health through legislative and policy making activities."
- Public Health competencies include "Advocate for healthy public policies and services that promote and protect the health and well-being of individuals and communities."
- Physician competencies include "Advocate for system-level change in a socially accountable manner" (Frank, Snell, & Sherbino, 2015).

Advocacy is a process of influencing outcomes and consists of organized actions to address an issue through speaking, writing, or acting in favour of a particular cause, policy, or group of people. Advocacy can be organized into relationship-based and influenced-based approaches (Vancouver Costal Health, n.d.). Relationship-based approaches include supporting groups and individuals—particularly those who have less social, economic, and political power in society—to express their views and concerns, access information and services, protect their rights and responsibilities, and explore choices and options. Influenced-based approaches include supporting changes to systems and structures (structural determinants of health) and influencing decisions that affect social, economic, and political conditions (political economy).

There are many models to support the "how to" of advocacy work. The National Collaborating Centre for Determinants of Health (2015) has also produced a document to support advocacy work based on the work of Carlisle (2000) and Whitehead (2007) (Fig. 3.8).

The Let's Talk framework helps with choosing a strategy and for considering how each type of advocacy effort

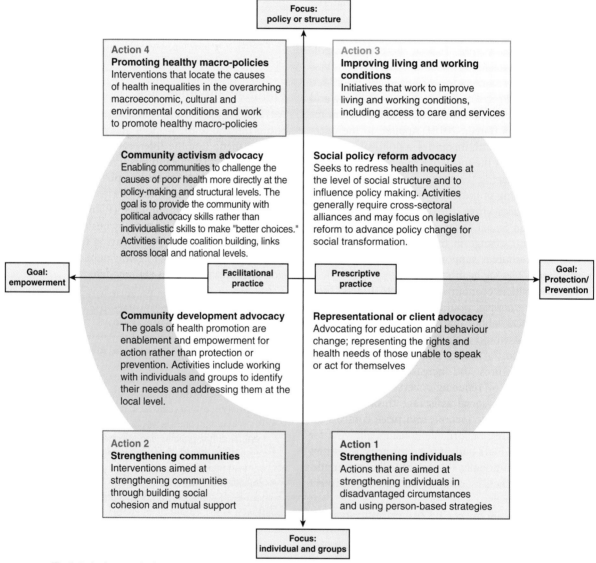

Fig 3.8 Actions and advocacy: categories of action to reduce health inequities and associated types of advocacy. (Adapted from Carlisle, S. Health promotion, advocacy and health inequalities: A conceptual framework. Health Promotion International 2000;15(4):369–376 and Whitehead, M. Glossary: a typology of actions to tackle social inequalities in health. *Journal of Epidemiol Community Health*, 2007;61:473–478. Reproduced with permission of National Collaborating Centre for Determinants of Health.)

aligns with specific actions to reduce health inequities, depending on the goal and focus. The strategies include strengthening individuals, strengthening communities, improving living and working conditions, and promoting healthy macro-policies. Additionally, four different types of advocacy are identified: representational or client advocacy (strengthening individuals), community development advocacy (strengthening communities), social policy reform (improving living and working conditions), and community activism advocacy (promoting healthy macro-policies). The axes of the matrix are best regarded as continua along which practice can be located. The horizontal axes (right-hand half of the matrix) relates to prevention and protection goals and the left-hand side relates to empowerment goals. The vertical axes relate to a focus on either individual or groups or policy or structures. The framework outlined in Fig. 3.8 suggests that both (social) empowerment and (medical) expertise models are needed—"upstream" and "downstream" advocacy for redressing health inequalities.

Media Advocacy

Public health advocacy, particularly through media advocacy, is aimed at promoting public health action targeted at policy makers. As an influenced-based approach, **media advocacy** has evolved as a distinct intervention in the domain of health communications and is defined as "the strategic use of mass media to support community organizing and advance healthy public policy" (Dorfman & Krasnow, 2014, p. 294). See Table 3.2 for a comparison of social marketing, public health, and media advocacy. At the time of its conception, media advocacy was heavily drawn upon to address challenges in the areas of alcohol and tobacco policy and today is being used as a tool to advocate for a variety of other healthy policy interventions, ranging from restricting marketing of junk foods to children to supporting a Basic Income Guarantee for all Canadians. The goal of media advocacy is to shape public opinion around a specific issue and, in doing so, influence people, groups, or organizations with the power to make the desired changes or individuals or groups who can be mobilized to apply pressure on those with the power to make the change. This approach explicitly targets leaders and decision makers for policy change.

The media has a critical role in determining which issues people talk and think about, how they think about various issues, and what sorts of solutions may be plausible when it comes to addressing these issues (Dorfman & Krasnow, 2014). Media advocacy draws heavily on

TABLE 3.2 Comparing Social Marketing, Public Health Advocacy, and Media Advocacy

	Target Audience	Purpose	Tools	Fields
Social marketing	• People who engage in risk behaviours	• To change behaviour (of high-risk people or public)	• Similar • Powerful images	• Marketing
Public health advocacy	• Decision makers • Policy makers, program managers, and those who are in a position to influence actions that affect many people simultaneously	• To effect desired systemic change—a focus on changing upstream factors (e.g., laws, regulations, policies, institutional practices, prices, and product standards)	• Coalitions • News media • Bringing disparate groups together • Gathering and presenting an evidence base for desired changes (e.g., an evidence brief)	• Public health • Politics
Media advocacy	• People, groups, or organizations with the power to make the desired changes. • A secondary target group is composed of individuals or groups who can be mobilized to apply pressure on those with the power to make the change.	• To influence policy makers to support healthy public policy options	• Social math • A relatable and credible spokesperson	• Politics

techniques from political science, communications, and cognitive linguistics to help frame and reframe issues such as the problematic use of substances or eating habits to emphasize the effect the political, social, and economic environment may have on a person's behaviour or "choice" to eat healthy or not smoke.

Experts who engage in media advocacy must be mindful of the speaker, audience, medium, and message. Using the issue of marketing unhealthy foods to children as an example, those who design a media advocacy campaign might wish to specifically target federal Members of Parliament (audience) to pass a bill that bans the advertising of junk food to children younger than 15 years of age. The strategy itself may involve a number of different activities, such as writing opinion pieces in newspapers that politicians read and choosing a prominent spokesperson (speaker) to talk about the issue on the radio as well as on live television and the

news (medium). Those involved in the media advocacy strategy would be drawing on what they know about how people process information and statistics to make sure their messages are relatable, clear, and something people can empathize with. For example, experts who design the campaign would be very careful with how they articulate statistics. Instead of stating what proportion of children consumes more calories than healthy eating guidelines suggest, they might wish instead to use a media advocacy technique called social math to translate that same information into a visual that will be more meaningful to the layperson or provoke an emotional response (e.g., the amount of junk food consumed by children and youth each year is equivalent to five football fields worth of chips and soda) (Dorfman & Krasnow, 2014). Additionally, when thinking through key messages, they must shift public opinion away from the idea that the parent or child is free to choose healthier

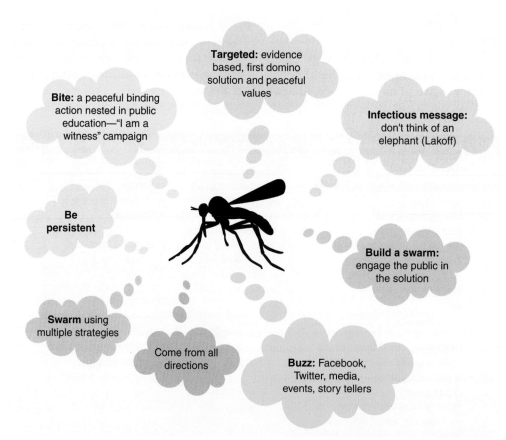

Fig 3.9 Mosquito advocacy. (From Blackstock, C. [2014]. Mosquito advocacy: Change promotion strategies for small groups with big ideas. *Social Issues in Contemporary Native America: Reflections from Turtle Island*, 219.)

options and towards the fact that children's choices are heavily influenced by marketing strategies. Mosquito advocacy was developed by the Caring Society to deal with an urgent need for public policy tools that equip small groups to effectively put pressure on "the big guys" and, in this case, the government to advocate for evidence-based policy in change-resistant environments (Blackstock, 2014, p. 219).

Mosquito advocacy (as depicted in Fig. 3.9) is grounded in having characteristics like a mosquito: (1) being small and agile—quicker than its larger opponent, (2) being goal oriented, (3) being infectious, (4) buzzing, (5) swarming, and (6) biting (using peaceful non-voluntary change techniques). Within this approach, policy

solutions are framed within deeply held public values to optimize their infectious nature and are nested within low-cost public engagement strategies to create a swarm of public dialogue and citizenship (Blackstock, 2014).

EXERCISE 3.7 Public Policy Makes a Difference— Glenda and Jenny's Story: Watch the video *Healthy Living: Public Policy Makes a Difference* on YouTube (see https://www.youtube.com/watch?v=nH-iAXEnb5k).

Use either the mosquito advocacy approach or the National Collaborating Centre for Determinants of Health to build a case to address the structural determinants of health based on the stories shared by Glenda and Jenny.

▌ SUMMARY

Population health can be differentiated from community health by the relationship implied when working in a community and the process of engaging community members in generating and effectively using their assets and resources to support the health of the whole community. Community health as a process implies action for health promotion, and a key aspect is community resiliency. A major aspect of community health is prevention of health problems.

There are three levels of *prevention*: primary, secondary, and tertiary. Primary prevention aims at preventing disease before it occurs. Secondary prevention involves early detection of disease and the treatment that may accompany screening. Tertiary prevention attempts to reduce complications by treatment and rehabilitation. Although primary prevention broadens the strategies to include policy, there can be what is referred to as the lifestyle drift. Lifestyle drift occurs when the design of policy accepts that improving the health of individuals and communities is about tackling SDHs but only to revert back to addressing lifestyle issues, such as smoking, drinking, and lack of exercise (Williams & Fullagar, 2019).

Strategies can be organized into downstream, midstream, and upstream. A number of midstream approaches have been developed or adapted for the promotion of health and include behaviour change, health communications, risk communication, social marketing for health, and social media communications. More upstream strategies have also been developed and include the Ottawa Charter for Health Promotion strategies and the Nuffield Intervention Ladder. The

Population Health Promotion model guides practitioners in thinking about how to develop interventions.

Knowing how to influence public policy is an important skill and can be developed through using the policy readiness toolkit. Social innovation, enterprise, and entrepreneurship for social change is an emerging public health trend that can create solutions for social problems with thinking "outside the box."

Enhancing community health can be done through community empowerment, community development, and community organizing. Focusing on the assets, strengths, and gifts of a community versus the problems can strengthen community action. Citizens' juries are an approach to community participation that gives community members a role in democratic decision-making around policy questions important to the community.

Finally, addressing the structural determinants of health can be done through a political economy approach and public health advocacy. Health is seen as a reflection of the state of a society's political economy; good health is a state of physical and emotional well-being in a political economy approach. Changing the distribution of power, money, and resources are strategies in a political economy approach. **Public health advocacy** is a process of influencing outcomes and taking action to address an issue. Several frameworks have been used to guide public health advocacy, such as the National Collaborating Centre for the Determinants of Health framework and the Mosquito Advocacy framework. Achieving health for all continues, 40 years after the Alma Ata Declaration, we are now only just starting to see the waves upstream.

KEY WEBSITES

POWER UP! Project—Policy Story Topics: http://abpolicy-coalitionforprevention.ca/evidence/stories-of-policy-change/

Part of the Alberta Policy Coalition for Chronic Disease Prevention, the Power Up! Project website showcases case studies and examples of healthy public policies within Canada and around the world.

The Policy Readiness Tool: http://abpolicycoalitionforprevention.ca/portfolio-posts/policy-readiness-tool/

This tool, developed by the Alberta Policy Coalition for Chronic Disease Prevention, is a useful questionnaire to assess readiness for policy change at an organizational level. It not only provides an assessment but also strategies and tools to advance an organizations stage of readiness to adopt policy, specifically healthy public policy.

National Collaborating Centre for Healthy Public Policy (NCCHPP): http://www.ncchpp.ca/en/

One of five collaborating centres, the NCCHPP provides further information, resources, and tools related to healthy public policy, such as health impact assessment and built environment interventions, among others.

Nuffield Council on Bioethics: http://nuffieldbioethics.org/

The Nuffield Council on Bioethics website contains numerous reports that analyze the ethical dimensions of various topics in biology and medicine, including genome editing, research on human embryos, and many other issues.

The Peter Sandman Risk Communication Website: http://www.psandman.com/

This website introduces the topic of risk communication and contains a repository of articles written by the expert in risk communication, Peter Sandman.

The Shelly Gautier Para-Sport Foundation: http://www.sgpsf.ca/index.html

This Foundation breaks down barriers for people living with disabilities, enabling them to participate in sports activities. An awareness of adaptive sport is created, and the foundation develops resources that encourages inclusive para-sport programs.

REFERENCES

Alisnsky, S. D. (1971). *Rules for radicals. A pragmatic primer for realistic radicals*. New York: Random House.

Anderson, J. E. (2011). *Public policy making* (7th ed.). Boston: Wadsworth, Cengage Learnings.

Baer, H., Singer, M., & Johnsen, J. (1986). Toward a critical medical anthropology. *Social Science & Medicine, 34*, 867–884.

Bandura, A. (1971). *Social learning theory*. New York: General Learning Press.

Becker, M. H., Haefner, D. P., Kasl, S. V., et al. (1977). Selected psychosocial models and correlates of individual health-related behaviours. *Medical Care, 15*, 27–46.

Blackstock, C. (2014). Mosquito advocacy: Change promotion strategies for small groups with big ideas. *Social Issues in Contemporary Native America: Reflections from Turtle Island*, 219.

Brofenbrenner, V. (1979). *The ecology of human development*. Cambridge, MA: Harvard University Press.

Bull, T., Mittelmark, M. B., & Kanyeka, N. E. (2013). Assets for well-being for women living in deep poverty: Through a salutogenic looking-glass. *Critical Public Health, 23*, 160–173. https://doi.org/10.1080/09581596.2013.771811.

Byrne, D. (2002). *Complexity theory and the social sciences: An introduction*. New York: Routledge.

Cajaiba-Santana, G. (2014). Social innovation: moving the field forward. A conceptual framework. *Technol Forecast Soc, 82*(0), 42–51.

Canadian Public Health Association & World Health Organization. (1986). *Ottawa Charter for Health Promotion*. Ottawa: Health and Welfare Canada.

Carlisle, S. (2000). Health promotion, advocacy and health inequalities: a conceptual framework. *Health Promotion International, 15*(4), 369–376.

Center for Community Health and Development. (n.d.). Section 2. PRECEDE/PROCEED. Retrieved from https://ctb.ku.edu/en/table-contents/overview/other-models-promoting-community-health-and-development/preceder-proceder/main

Centers for Disease Control and Prevention. (n.d.). Public Health 101 Series: Introduction to public health surveillance. Retrieved from https://www.cdc.gov/publichealth101/documents/introduction-to-surveillance.pdf

Centers for Disease Control and Prevention. (1999). Achievements in public health, 1900–1999: control of infectious diseases. *JAMA, 283*(3), 621–629.

Centers for Disease Control and Prevention. (2011a). What is health communications? Retrieved from https://www.cdc.gov/healthcommunication/healthbasics/WhatIsHC.html.

Centers for Disease Control and Prevention. (2011b). Health marketing. Retrieved from https://www.cdc.gov/health-communication/toolstemplates/Basics.html.

Cottrell, L. S. (1976). The competent community. In B. H. Kaplan, R. N. Wilson, & A. H. Leighton (Eds.), *Further explorations in social psychiatry*. New York: Basic Books.

Dannenberg, A. (2016). Effectiveness of health impact assessment. A synthesis of data of five impact evaluation Reports. *Preventing Chronic Disease, 13*(150559). https://doi.org/10.5888/pcd13.150559.

DiClemente, C., Prochaska, J., Fairhurst, S., et al. (1991). The process of smoking cessation: An analysis of precontemplation, contemplation, and preparation stages of change. *Journal of Consulting and Clinical Psychology, 59*(2), 295–304.

Dijkstra, A. (2017). Self-control in smoking cessation. In *Routledge International handbook of self-control in health and well-being* (pp. 300–313). New York: Routledge. Retrieved from https://www.taylorfrancis.com/books/e/9781317301424/chapters/10.4324%2F9781315648576-24.

Dorfman, L., & Krasnow, I. D. (2014). Public health and media advocacy. *Annual Review of Public Health, 35*(1), 293–306.

Edwards, N., Mill, J., & Kothari, A. R. (2004). Multiple Intervention Research Programs in Community Health. *Canadian Journal of Nursing Research, 36*(1), 40–54.

European Centre for Disease Prevention and Control. (2014). *Social marketing guide for public health managers and practitioners.* Retrieved from https://ecdc.europa.eu/sites/portal/files/media/en/publications/Publications/social-marketing-guide-public-health.pdf.

Federici, C., Detzel, P., Petracca, F., et al. (2019). The impact of food reformulation on nutrient intakes and health, a systematic review of modelling studies. *BMC Nutrition, 5*(1), 9.

Ferguson, J. (1998). Community intervention programs. In R. Wallace (Ed.), *Maxey-Rosenau-Last public health and preventive medicine* (14th ed.). Stamford, CT: Appleton & Lange.

Foot, J. (2012). *What makes us healthy? The asset-based approach in practice: Evidence, action, evaluation.* Retrieved from http://www.assetbasedconsulting.co.uk/uploads/publications/WMUH.pdf.

Frank, J. R., Snell, L., & Sherbino, J. (2015). *CanMeds 2015 physician competency framework.* Ottawa: Royal College of Physicians & Surgeons of Canada.

Freelon, D., McIlwain, C., & Clark, M. (2016). Quantifying the power and consequences of social media protest. *News Media & Society, 20*(3), 990–1011.

Freudenberg, N., & Tsui, E. (2014). Evidence, power, and policy change in community-based participatory research. *American Journal of Public Health, 104*(1), 11–14.

Greer, S. L. (2018). Labour politics as public health: How the politics of industrial relations and workplace regulation affect health. *European Journal of Public Health, 28*(Suppl. 3), 34–37.

Hooker, C., Capon, A., & Leask, J. (2017). Communicating about risk: Strategies for situations where public concern is high but the risk is low. *Public Health Research and Practice, 27*(1), e2711709.

Hancock, T., Labonte, R., & Edwards, R. (1999). Indicators that count! Measuring population health at the community level. *Canadian Journal of Public Health, 90*(1), S22–S26.

Hofrichter, R. (Ed.). (2003). *The politics of health inequities: Contested terrain Health and social justice: a reader on ideology, and inequity in the distribution of disease* (pp. 1–56). San Francisco: Jossey-Bass.

Hughes, J. R., & Naud, S. (2016). Perceived role of motivation and self-efficacy in smoking cessation: A secondary data analysis. *Addictive Behaviors, 61*, 58–61. https://doi.org/10.1016/j.addbeh.2016.05.010.

Kaplan, A. M., & Haenlein, M. (2010). Users of the world, unite! The challenges and opportunities of social media. *Business Horizons, 53*(1), 59–68.

Keen, D. (2014). PanCanadian collaborative approach to improve the health of Canadians. Retrieved from http://www.partnershipagainstcancer.ca/pan-canadian-collaborative-approach-to-improve-the-health-of-canadians/.

Kickbusch, I. (1989). Approaches to an ecological base to public health. *Health Promotion International, 4*, 265–268.

Kickbusch, I. (1995). *Action on health promotion: Approaches to advocacy and implementation.* Copenhagen: WHO.

Kindig, D. A. (2007). Understanding population health terminology. *Milbank Quarterly, 85*(1), 139–161.

Kretzmann, J., & McKnight, J. P. (1996). Assets-based community development. *National Civic Review, 85*(4), 23–29.

Kulig, J. C. (2000). Community resiliency: The potential for community health nursing theory development. *Public Health Nursing, 17*(5), 374–385.

Labonte, R., Polanyi, M., Muhajarine, N., et al. (2005). Beyond the divides: Towards critical population health research. *Critical Public Health, 15*(1), 5–17. https://doi.org/10.1080/09581590500048192.

Lanard, J. (n.d.). A quick introduction to risk perception. Retrieved from http://www2.wpro.who.int/internet/files/eha/toolkit/web/Technical%20References/Risk%20Communication%20and%20Public%20Information/Introduction%20Risk%20Perception.pdf

Mason, C., Barraket, J., Friel, S., et al. (2015). Social innovation for the promotion of health equity. *Health Promotion International, 30*, ii116–ii125.

Matjasko, J. L., Cawley, J. H., Baker-Goering, M. M., et al. (2016). Applying behavioral economics to public health policy: illustrative examples and promising directions. *American Journal of Preventive Medicine, 50*(5), S13–S19. https://doi.org/10.1016/j.amepre.2016.02.007.

McKinlay, J., & Marceau, L. (2000). US public health and the 21st century: diabetes mellitus. *The Lancet, 356*(9231), 757–761.

McKinlay, J. B. (1979). A case for refocusing upstream: The political economy of illness. In E. G. Jaco (Ed.), *Patients, physicians and illness* (pp. 9–25). New York: The Free Press.

Murray, C. J., Lauer, J. A., Hutubessy, R. C., et al. (2003). Effectiveness and costs of interventions to lower systolic blood pressure and cholesterol: A global and regional analysis on reduction of cardiovascular-disease risk. *The Lancet, 361*(9359), 717–725.

National Collaborating Centre for Determinants of Health (2015). *Let's talk…Advocacy for health equity.* Antigonish, NS: National Collaborating Centre for Determinants of Health, St. Francis Xavier University. Retrieved from http://nccdh.ca/images/uploads/comments/Advocacy_EN.pdf

National Collaborating Centre for Healthy Public Policy. (2015). Social media in public health. Retrieved from http://www.ncchpp.ca/docs/2015_TC_KT_SocialMediaPH_en.pdf.

Navarro, V., & Muntaner, C. (Eds.). (2004). *Political and economic determinants of population health and well-being: Controversies and developments.* NY: Baywood: Amityville.

Newbold, B. (2015). *Social media in public health.* Montréal, Québec: National Collaborating Centre for Healthy Public Policy.

Nuffield Council on Bioethics. (2007). *Public health: Ethical issues.* Cambridge, UK: Nuffield Council on Bioethics.

Nykiforuk, C. I. J., Nieuwendyk, L. M., Atkey, K. M., et al. (2011). *Policy readiness tool: Understanding a municipality's readiness for policy change and strategies for taking action.* Edmonton: School of Public Health, University of Alberta.

Ontario Agency for Health Protection and Promotion (Public Health Ontario). (2016). In R. W. Brecher, & R. Copes (Eds.), *EOH fundamentals: Risk communication.* Toronto: Queen's Printer for Ontario.

Paul, P., & Ross-Kerr, J. C. (2011). Nursing in Canada, 1600–present: A brief account. In J. C. Ross-Kerr, & M. J. Wood (Eds.), *Canadian nursing: Issues & perspectives* (5th ed.) (pp. 18–41). Toronto: Elsevier.

Poland, B., Coburn, D., Robertson, A., et al. (1998). Wealth, equity and health care: a critique of a "population health" perspective on the determinants of health. *Social Science & Medicine, 46*(7), 785–798.

Public Health Agency of Canada. (2008). *Core competencies for public health in Canada.* Ottawa: Public Health Agency of Canada. Retrieved from http://www.phac-aspc.gc.ca/php-psp/ccph-cesp/pdfs/cc-manual-eng090407.pdf.

Raine, K. D., Nykiforuk, C. I., Vu–Nguyen, K., et al. (2014). Understanding key influencers' attitudes and beliefs about healthy public policy change for obesity prevention. *Obesity, 22*(11), 2426–2433.

Raphael, D. (2004). *Social determinants of health: Canadian perspectives.* Toronto: Canadian Scholars' Press.

Raphael, D. (2013). Adolescence as a gateway to adult health outcomes. *Maturitas, 75*(2), 137–141.

Raphael, D. (2015). The parameters of children's health: Key concepts from the political economy of health literature. *International Journal of Child Youth and Family Studies, 6*(2), 186–203.

Raphael, D., & Bryant, T. (2002). The limitations of population health as a model for a new public health. *Health Promotion International, 17*(2), 189–199.

Raphael, D., Bryant, T., & Rioux, M. (2006). *Staying alive: Critical perspectives on health, illness, and health care.* Toronto: Canadian Scholars' Press.

Rogers, E. M. (1986). *Diffusion of innovations.* London: Collier Macmillan.

Rose, G. (1992). *Strategy of preventive medicine.* Oxford, UK: Oxford.

Rothman, J. (2001). Approaches to community intervention. In J. Rothman J, L. Erlich, & J. E. Tropman (Eds.), *Strategies of community intervention* (6th ed.) (pp. 27–64). Itasca, IL: F.E. Peacock Publishers.

Ryan-Nicholls, K. D., & Racher, F. E. (2004). Investigating the health of rural communities: Toward framework development. *Rural and Remote Health, 4*(1), 224.

Sandman, P. (2007). "Watch out!"—How to warn apathetic people. Retrieved from http://www.psandman.com/col/watchout.htm.

Sandman, P. (2014). *Introduction to risk communication and orientation to this website.* Retrieved from http://psandman.com/index-intro.htm.

Shea, S., & Basch, C. A. (1990a). Review of five major community-based cardiovascular disease prevention programs. Part 1: Rationale, design, and theoretical framework. *American Journal of Health Promotion, 4*(3), 203–213.

Shea, S., & Basch, C. A. (1990b). Review of five major community-based disease prevention programs. Part 2: Intervention strategies, evaluation methods, and results. *American Journal of Health Promotion, 4*(4), 279–287.

St. Michael's Hospital. (2019). Research: Michael Evans. Retrieved from http://stmichaelshospitalresearch.ca/researchers/michael-evans/.

Street, J., Duszynski, K., & Braunack-Mayer, A. (2014). The use of citizens' juries in health policy decision-making: A systematic review. *Social Science & Medicine, 109*, 1–9. https://doi.org/10.1016/j.socscimed.2014.03.005.

Vancouver Costal Health. (n. d). Vancouver Costal Health Population Health: Advocacy Guideline and Resources. Vancouver: Vancouver Costal Health. Retrieved from http://www.vch.ca/media/PopulationHealth_Advocacy-Guideline-and-Resources.pdf

Wallerstein, N. (1992). Powerlessness, empowerment, and health: Implications for health promotion programs. *American Journal of Health Promotion, 6*(3), 197–205. https://doi.org/10.4278/0890-1171-6.3.197.

Wallerstein, N. (2002). Empowerment to reduce health disparities. *Scandinavian Journal of Public Health, 30,* 72–77. https://doi.org/10.1177/14034948020300031201.

Wallerstein, N. (2006). *What is the evidence on effectiveness of empowerment to improve health?* Copenhagen, Denmark: WHO Europe.

Whitehead, M. (2007). A typology of actions to tackle social inequalities in health. *Journal of Epidemiology & Community Health, 61*(6), 473–478.

Whitehead, M. (2012). Waving or drowning? A view of health equity from Europe. *Australian and New Zealand Journal of Public Health, 36*(6) 523–523.

Williams, O., & Fullagar, S. (2019). Lifestyle drift and the phenomenon of 'citizen shift' in contemporary UK health policy. *Sociology of Health & Illness, 41*(1), 20–35. https://doi.org/10.1111/1467-9566.12783.

World Health Organization. (n.d.). Health policy. Retrieved from http://www.who.int/topics/health_policy/en/

World Health Organization. (1998). *The Adelaide recommendations: Conference statement of the 2nd International Conference on Health Promotion.* Retrieved from www.who.int/hpr/archive/docs/adelaide.html.

World Health Organization. (2013). *Helsinki statement on health in all policies. 8th Global Conference on Health Promotion.* Helsinki, Finland, June 10–14, 2013. Retrieved from http://www.who.int/healthpromotion/conferences/8gchp/8gchp_helsinki_statement.pdf.

World Health Organization. (2018). *Advancing the right to health: The vital role of law.* Geneva: World Health Organization. Retrieved from https://apps.who.int/iris/bitstream/handle/10665/275522/9789241513739-eng.pdf.

World Health Organization. (2019). *Social determinants of health. Backgrounder 3: Key concepts.* Retrieved from https://www.who.int/social_determinants/thecommission/finalreport/key_concepts/en/.

The Health of Canadians

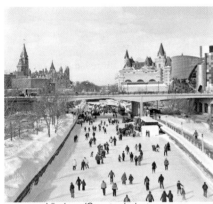

Vladone/Canstockphoto.com

Canadians are shareholders of the public health care system. They own it and are the sole reason the health care system exists. They deserve access to the facts.

Roy J. Romanow, *Building on Values: The Future of Health Care in Canada (2002)*

Evidence and facts are essential for building and developing an effective health care system. Part 2 provides facts about health and the diseases that exist in Canadian society and the factors that influence them. It covers morbidity, mortality, and the economic burden of disease, including communicable and noncommunicable diseases, and it discusses health in relation to the environment and to occupation. Although not exhaustive, this part also considers some population health strategies to prevent disease and, generally, to improve health and its distribution.

4

Health Indicators and the Health Status of Canadians

LEARNING OBJECTIVES

- Define *health indicators* and describe the utility of health indicators, as well as characteristics of good health indicators.
- Be familiar with the various dimensions of the Canadian Institute for Health Information's indicator framework for population health.
- List several indicators that reflect the demographic context of a population, including population growth, net migration, natural increase, and fertility rates.
- List several indicators that describe health status specifically, including those that describe death, health conditions, well-being, and human function.
- Apply the most common community and health status indicators to describe the Canadian population from the perspective of the health system.

CHAPTER OUTLINE

KEY TERMS

age- and sex-specific death rate
case-fatality rate
case-specific death rate
crude birth rate
crude death rate
demography
direct costs
disability-adjusted life years
general fertility rate

health indicators
incidence
indirect costs
infant mortality rate
life expectancy
maternal mortality rate
natural increase
neonatal maternity rate
net migration

perinatal mortality rate
population growth
potential years of life lost
  (PYLLs)
prevalence
proportionate mortality ratio
  (PMR)
quality of life
total fertility rate

INTRODUCTION

The planning and evaluation of services to meet the health needs of a population must be based on the health status of that population. Community health (see Chapter 3) and community health approaches (as described in Chapter 3) are predicated on a deeper understanding of the community where one lives and works. In other words, before one works with the community to mobilize and organize to improve health status, a solid understanding of the community—both its strengths and needs—is required. Often, this means answering questions such as: How healthy is the community as a whole? What are the rates of major chronic diseases? What are the rates of infectious diseases? What are the health perceptions of individuals in the population? How healthy do they consider themselves to be? What are the strengths and enablers to good health in the population of interest? Are there some community groups that have worse health than others and that are being left out of the discussions? As government involvement in the provision of health care has increased, so has interest in the measurement of health and demand for data on the health of the population for which governments are responsible.

The measurement of health dates from the 17th century, when governments first began to collect information on death and its causes. Mortality statistics continue to be a major source of information. However, mortality statistics and associated measures such as life expectancy are no longer adequate indicators of health; they do not take into consideration illness that does not result in death or the often-profound disability and distress, including on a psychosocial level, that may accompany such illness. As seen in Chapter 1, the very concept of health has changed, and a number of other nonmedical determinants have been recognized.

This first half of this chapter describes the various types of health indicators that can be used to describe community health, with examples of specific types of indicators and how they can be useful for understanding health at a population level. The second half of the chapter focuses on how these indicators currently (at the time of writing) reflect the health of the Canadian population for the purpose of getting a better understanding of how healthy Canadians are.

HEALTH INDICATORS

Health indicators are succinct, qualitative, and quantitative statistical measures that summarize information related to the health of a population or the performance of a health system. Broadly speaking, health indicators have three main purposes: (1) to better understand or describe a population or health system, including making comparisons between different communities, regions, systems, or organizations; (2) to monitor progress or performance (in the case of health system indicators) over time; and (3) to help with accountability to the public and funders (Canadian Institute for Health Information [CIHI], n.d.). Refer to the Case Study boxes for a description of how this works in practice in two Canadian provinces.

CASE STUDY

Ontario's Accountability Indicators

In Ontario, the Ministry of Health provides the majority of the funding for its local public health units, which are tasked with protecting and promoting the health of the residents in the health unit's catchment area. For there to be transparency and accountability of these public funds, the Ministry requires that public health units report on various indicators on an annual basis (MOHLTC, 2018). One example of an indicator that is reported on annually is the percentage of school-aged children who have completed immunizations for human papillomavirus (HPV) because one role of local public health agencies is to go into schools and immunize grade 8 students for HPV.

EXERCISE 4.1: What are some advantages and disadvantages of the discussed HPV vaccination indicator (keeping in mind its intent is accountability for public funds)?

CASE STUDY

Saskatchewan's Community Health Indicators Toolkit

Although the Ontario example highlights how indicators can be used to ensure and monitor accountability for public funds, this Saskatchewan example shows how indicators can also be used for the purposes of better understanding the population and monitoring health over time. In 2006, the Saskatchewan Population Health and Evaluation Research Unit at the University of Regina and University of Saskatchewan published the "community health indicators toolkit" for the purpose of helping measure progress on improving community health as part of a First Nations Health Development Project. Recognizing the importance of the social determinants of health, they proposed indicators related to important health determinants, such as economic viability (e.g., unemployment rate), environment (e.g., number of forest fires near the community), identity and culture (e.g., proportion of youth speaking a traditional language), and food security (e.g., cost of food) (Jeffrey et al., 2010). These are all good examples of community health indicators.

It is important to keep in mind that health indicators are intended to be used to describe a population or community (essentially, a group of people) and cannot always be easily applied when trying to ascertain the health status of a single individual. Most indicators have both a numerator and denominator and thus are not applicable to an individual person. For example, mortality rates (i.e., how many deaths occurred in a population over a given period of time) are an indicator of the burden of illness in the population as a whole and rely on knowing how many people are in the population at a given point in time (CIHI, n.d.). Comparing rates between communities can reveal underlying differences between these communities. Mortality rates alone, however, do not suffice to describe the health of a community because they address only one dimension, and as we know, health is a holistic and broad concept.

For an indicator to be useful, it must meet the following criteria:

- Address an important issue
- Be scientifically valid (and, therefore, come from valid data collection methods)
- Be accurate
- Be feasible to collect based on what's available
- Be reliable (i.e., a similar value can be obtained for the indicator on repeat measurements at one point in time)

- Be actionable (Pencheon, 2008).

Ideally, indicators are also collected frequently and are sensitive to changes in the community so that planning and intervention strategies can be promptly implemented when warranted.

The CIHI Health System Performance Measurement Framework (described in this book's Introduction) provides a useful framework for addressing health and its indicators in a broad sense. As a brief recap, this framework highlights how the political, demographic, and economic contexts shape the health system environment. Additionally, health is a product of the social determinants of health (things such as social position, physical environment) as well as both the inputs (leadership, resources) and outputs (effective, high quality, safe services) of the health system, with one of the ultimate goals of the health sector being to improve the health status of Canadians.

This chapter focuses primarily on describing indicators that relate to the demographic context (although this is also touched on again in Chapter 5), as well as those that describe the health status of Canadians. Chapter 5 discusses the social determinants of health, and Part 3 of the book touches on health system inputs, outputs, and outcomes.

Table 4.1 outlines another particularly useful framework, the Health Indicator Framework, developed by both Statistics Canada and CIHI, which focuses specifically on indicators.

The indicators in Table 4.1 are organized into four categories: health status (including health conditions, mortality rates, measures of well-being), nonmedical determinants of health (socioeconomic characteristics and health behaviour), health system performance (measures of accessibility, appropriateness, effectiveness of health care services), and community and health system characteristics (contextual information). The notion of equity spans all dimensions of the framework and can apply equally to any construct or dimension. Therefore, equity is not included as a fifth dimension of the Health Indicators Conceptual framework but is presented as a crosscutting element of the framework that applies to each of the four dimensions. Table 4.2 provides a good overview of examples of health indicators across each category.

The following section focuses on indicators that are related specifically to community characteristics (in particular, the demographic context) and health status.

Before delving into more detail, it is prudent to briefly recap the definitions and key differences between

TABLE 4.1   Health Indicator Framework

HEALTH STATUS					
Health conditions	Human function	Well-being	Deaths	How healthy are Canadians? Health status can be measured in a variety of ways, including well-being, health conditions, disability, or death.	↑ E Q U I T Y ↓
DETERMINANTS OF HEALTH					
Health behaviours	Living and working conditions	Personal resources	Environ-mental factors	These are factors that are known to affect our health and, in some cases, when and how we use health care.	
HEALTH SYSTEM PERFORMANCE					
Acceptability Continuity	Accessibility Effectiveness	Appropriateness Efficiency	Compe-tence Safety	How healthy is the health care system? These indicators measure various aspects of the quality of health care.	
COMMUNITY AND HEALTH SYSTEM CHARACTERISTICS					
Community		Health system	Resources	These measures provide useful contextual information but are not direct measures of health status or the quality of health care.	

Source: Adapted from Canadian Institute for Health Information. (2003). Table 1: Health Indicators Conceptual Framework. *Health indicators conceptual framework: Background paper*, prepared for ISO/TC 215, March 14, 2001. Retrieved from secure.cihi.ca/cihiweb/en/downloads/infostand_ihisd_e_ISO_background.pdf. Reprinted with permission, Canadian Institute for Health Information, Ottawa, Canada.

incidence and *prevalence* (described further in Chapter 2) because these terms will be used throughout this chapter. Both terms can help describe the burden of a health state (e.g., disease) in the population, but whereas **incidence** specifically refers to the number of new cases of this health state or disease over a specified time period (e.g., 12 new cases of diabetes in a community over a year) and more accurately represents the risk or probability that someone may develop a health state, **prevalence** refers to the total number of people affected by a health state or disease in the population, usually at a given point in time (e.g., 12 of the 12000 people in a community are living with diabetes).

Health Status Indicators
Well-Being

When thinking about how to measure and track health status, the various dimensions of health must be kept in mind. According to the World Health Organization (WHO), health has mental, social, and spiritual dimensions, in addition to physical ones. As a result, health status indicators should not only include measures of the prevalence of certain medical conditions or disease states but should also include measures of well-being, functionality, and how well one is able to participate in one's society and in social interactions.

The concept of *quality of life* emerged in the 1960s and has become increasingly popular over time. **Quality of life** (or *health-related quality of life*, as it is sometimes called) has several definitions. It encompasses dimensions such as a person's perceived physical and mental health, perception of and satisfaction with life, satisfaction with level of functioning, and ability to perform everyday activity, among others (Post, 2014).

EXERCISE 4.2:

1. In what situations might it be more useful to gather incidence data versus prevalence data?
2. In what situations might it be more useful to collect prevalence data versus incidence data?
3. Are the following examples of incidence data or prevalence data?
   a. Mortality (e.g., five deaths in the population over a 1-year period)
   b. Lifetime risk (e.g., in community X, there is a 5% risk of getting diabetes over the course of a lifetime)

TABLE 4.2   **Health Indicators**

HEALTH STATUS

Well-Being	Health Conditions	Human Function	Deaths

• Perceived health
• Perceived mental health
• Perceived life stress
	• Adult body mass index
	• Youth body mass index
	• Arthritis
	• Diabetes
	• Asthma
	• High blood pressure
	• Chronic obstructive pulmonary disease (COPD)
	• Pain or discomfort that prevents activities
	• Pain or discomfort by severity
	• Birth-related indicators:
	  • Low birth weight
	  • High birth weight
	  • Small for gestational age
	  • Large for gestational age
	  • Pre-term births
	• Cancer incidence
	• Injury hospitalization
	• Injuries
	• Hospitalized stroke event
	• Hospitalized acute myocardial infarction event
	• Hospitalizations entirely caused by alcohol
		• Functional health
		• Participation and activity limitation
		• Disability-free life expectancy
		• Disability-adjusted life expectancy
		• Health-adjusted life expectancy
			• Infant mortality
			• Perinatal mortality
			• Life expectancy
			• Contribution of selected causes of death to changes (over 1, 5, 10 years) in life expectancy at birth, by sex
			• Contribution of drug poisoning deaths to changes (over 1 and 5 years) in life expectancy at birth, by sex
			• Contribution of age-specific death rates to changes (over 1, 5, 10 years) in life expectancy at birth, by sex
			• Contribution of selected causes of death to differences in life expectancy at birth between males and females
			• Contribution of potentially avoidable causes of death to changes (over 1 and 5 years) in life expectancy at birth, by sex
			• Age-standardized mortality rate (for provincial/territorial level time-series):
			  • Total mortality by selected causes
			  • All diseases of the circulatory system deaths
			  • All malignant neoplasms (cancer) deaths
			  • All disease of the respiratory system deaths
			  • Suicide
			  • Unintentional injury deaths
			  • AIDS deaths
			• Premature mortality
			• Potential years of life lost (PYLL):
			  • for provincial/territorial level time-series
			  • for total mortality
			  • for all cancer deaths
			  • for all circulatory disease deaths
			  • for all respiratory disease deaths
			  • for unintentional injuries
			  • for suicide
			  • for AIDs deaths

continued

NONMEDICAL DETERMINANTS OF HEALTH

Health Behaviours	Living and Working Conditions	Personal Resources	Environmental Factors
• Smoking	• High school graduates	• Sense of community belonging	• Exposure to secondhand smoke at home
• Heavy drinking	• Post-secondary graduates	• Life satisfaction	• Exposure to secondhand smoke in vehicles and public places
• Physical activity during leisure time	• Unemployment rate		• Lead concentration
• Self-reported physical activity, adult (18 years and over0	• Long-term unemployment rate		• Bisphenol A concentration
• Self-reported physical activity, youth (12 to 17 years old)	• Low-income rate		• Mercury concentration
• Breastfeeding practices	• Children in low-income families		
• Fruit and vegetable consumption	• Average personal income		
• Bicycle helmet use	• Median share of income		
	• Government transfer income		
	• Housing affordability		
	• Crime incidents		
	• Adults and youths charge		
	• Household food insecurity		

HEALTH SYSTEM PERFORMANCE

Acceptability	Accessibility	Appropriateness
• Patient satisfaction (and quality rating of services received)	• Influenza immunization	• Caesarean section
	• Mammography	• Patients with repeat hospitalizations for mental illness
	• Pap smear	
	• Colorectal cancer screening	
	• Regular medical doctor	
	• Hip fracture surgery within 48 hours	

Continuity	Effectiveness	Safety
• 30-day readmission for mental illness	• Ambulatory care sensitive conditions	• Hospitalized hip fracture event
	• 30-day AMI in-hospital mortality	
	• 30-day stroke in-hospital mortality	
	• 30-day acute myocardial infarction readmission	
	• 30-day obstetric readmission	
	• 30-day readmission patients aged 19 and younger	
	• 30-day surgical readmission	
	• 30-day medical readmission	
	• Self-injury hospitalization	
	• Potentially avoidable mortality and potential years of life list (PYLL):	
	• Mortality from preventable causes	
	• Mortality from treatable causes	
	• Preventable and treatable mortality, by remoteness geography	

TABLE 4.2   Health Indicators—cont'd

COMMUNITY AND HEALTH SYSTEM CHARACTERISTICS

Community	Health System	Resources
• Population estimates • Population distribution by size and population centre • Population density • Dependency ratio • Indigenous population • Immigrant population • Internal migrant mobility • Metropolitan influenced zones (MIZ) • Lone-parent families • Visible minority population	• Inflow–outflow ratio • Coronary artery bypass graft • Percutaneous coronary intervention • Cardiac revascularization • Hip replacement • Knee replacement • Hysterectomy • Contact with alternative care providers • Contact with medical doctor • Contact with health professionals about mental health • Contact with dental professionals • Mental illness hospitalization rate • Mental illness patient days rate	• Doctors rate

AMI, Acute myocardial infarction

Source: Canadian Institute for Health Information. (2019). *Health Indicators e-publication* (data tables and definitions). Retrieved from http://www
.cihiconferences.ca/indicators/epub/ind_e.html. Reprinted with permission, Canadian Institute for Health Information, Ottawa, Canada.

Indicators of quality of life often include subjective assessments, such as self-rated health, a useful measure by which people gauge their health from their own perspective. Studies have shown that functional status is one of the main criteria used by individuals to rate their health but that self-rated health is also influenced by a person's judgement about the severity of current illness, personal resource to maintain well-being, health behaviour, and family health history (Bonner et al., 2017). Self-rated health is strongly predictive of future health, including the likelihood of dying (Benyamini, 2011).

EXERCISE 4.3: Can you think of some advantages and disadvantages to using self-rated health as an indicator of population health?

Health Conditions

Health conditions include alterations or attributes of the health status of an individual that may lead to distress, interference with daily activities, or contact with health services; such a condition may be a disease (acute or chronic), disorder, injury, or trauma or may reflect other health-related states, such as pregnancy, aging, stress, congenital anomaly, or genetic predisposition (Statistics Canada, 2016a).

Some examples of indicators of health conditions include the following:

- Body mass index (BMI-Canadian standard), which relates weight to height, is a common method of determining if an individual's weight is in a healthy range. BMI is calculated by dividing weight in kilograms by height in metres squared.
- Incidence and prevalence of relevant and common health conditions, such as arthritis, heart disease, diabetes, depression, anxiety, high blood pressure, cancer, and injury
- Pain severity (e.g., on a rated numeric scale, or rated as mild, moderate, or severe) for people who are living with conditions leading to chronic pain

Economic Burden of Disease. The economic burden of disease relates to the use of society's resources towards certain disease states or health conditions. It is one way to capture how much financial stress is placed on the health care system and society at large by various health conditions (e.g., diabetes or heart disease), providing an indication of their importance or impact.

The costs of disease are measured in terms of direct and indirect costs. **Direct costs** measure the expenditure for prevention and treatment of that disease. They include publicly funded health care costs, education, and research, as well as personal health care, which consists of institutional costs, nonhospital medical care costs, and other costs, such as dental care and prescribed drugs. **Indirect costs**, on the other hand, measure the loss of productive services due to being sick or losing one's life. They include financial loss due to premature death or loss of workdays because of temporary or permanent disability. For example, the number of person-years of productive work lost because of automobile collisions is an indirect cost, or indirect burden, of disease.

Human Function

Human function is associated with the ability to function and fulfill your day-to-day roles as a consequence of disease, disorder, injury, or other health conditions. Levels of functionality are considered in terms of impairment (related to function or structure), activity limitations, and ability to participate in day to day endeavours (see Chapter 1) (WHO, 2018; Statistics Canada, 2016b). Information on functionality is often obtained from population surveys, which ask questions such as whether respondents experience certain limitations with respect to specific activities; whether individuals have issues as they related to hearing, seeing, communicating, mobility, and other types of functioning; and to what extent individuals are able to participate in things such as work, leisure activities, or school (Statistics Canada, 2016c).

Death

Death includes a range of age-specific mortality rates (e.g., infant mortality) and condition-specific mortality rates (e.g., AIDS), as well as derived indicators (e.g., life expectancy and **potential years of life lost [PYLLs]**). Box 4.1 presents a description of how these are captured and stored centrally at the global level.

Commonly used health indicators in the category of deaths are listed here, and their derivations are summarized in Table 4.3.

- **Infant mortality rate:** The annual number of deaths in children younger than 1 year of age per 1 000 live births in the same year. The infant mortality rate is commonly used for comparing health among different countries.

The World Health Organization's (WHO's) Global Health Observatory (GHO) provides a repository of country level health-related statistics for all of its 194 member states (WHO, n.d.). The data are publicly accessible and provide for easy comparisons among countries and a way to track progress over time towards the Sustainable Development Goals and other global health targets set out by the WHO.

Included in the GHO are death measures such as life expectancy. According to the GHO, the average life expectancy at birth globally (as of 2016) is 72.0 years. The countries with the highest life expectancies include Monaco (at 89.4 years) and Japan (85.3 years) (Central Intelligence Agency [CIA], 2017). Canada ranks 21st according to some sources, and Canadians have an estimated life expectancy of 82.2 years. The United States has a lower life expectancy than Canada, which is interesting given the fact that it is known to have the largest economy globally and thus has a higher gross domestic product compared with the rest of the world, including Canada. The United States, however, is also known to have poorer access to health care, with a very different health system than Canada (described further in Chapter 13) and greater income inequities (which we know is bad for health, as described further in Chapter 5). See Fig. 4.1 for a visual depiction of life expectancy globally.

The Conference Board of Canada compares life expectancy among various provinces and territories within Canada. Its analysis has revealed that Ontario and British Columbia have the highest life expectancies when looking solely at the provinces, and Manitoba and Saskatchewan are the lower ranking provinces. Life expectancy in British Columbia. is actually about 2.6 years longer than in Saskatchewan. All three territories have life expectancies that are well under the national average. For example, life expectancy in Nunavut is 71.8 years and is closer to that of Ukraine than to other parts of Canada (Conference Board of Canada, 2019).

usually reflects standards of perinatal care, maternal nutrition, and obstetric and pediatric care. Stillbirth is defined as a product of conception of 20 or more weeks' gestation or fetal weight of 500 g or more, which did not breathe or show other signs of life at delivery. Death may occur before or during delivery. At what gestational age a miscarriage becomes a stillbirth depends on the policy or law of each province or country and varies from 20 to 28 weeks.

- **Crude death rate:** The annual number of deaths per 1 000 population.
- **Neonatal mortality rate:** The annual number of deaths in a year of children younger than 28 days of age per 1 000 live births in the same year.
- **Maternal mortality rate:** The annual number of maternal deaths occurring during pregnancy and from puerperal causes (i.e., deaths occurring during delivery; complications of pregnancy, childbirth, and the puerperium) per 1 000 live births in the same year. According to the Public Health Agency of Canada (PHAC), a maternal death is defined by the International Classification of Diseases, Ninth and Tenth Revisions (ICD-9, ICD-10) as the death of a woman while pregnant or within 42 days of termination of pregnancy, irrespective of the duration and the site of pregnancy (e.g., uterine or extrauterine pregnancy), from any cause related to or aggravated by the pregnancy or its management but not from accidental or incidental causes (PHAC, 2013).
- **Age- and sex-specific death rate:** The annual number of deaths in a particular age and gender group per 1 000 population in that subgroup. Suggested:
- **Case-specific death rate:** The annual number of deaths due to a specific cause per 1 000 population
- **PYLLs:** The total years of life lost before age 70 or 75 years for people who become deceased between birth and the 70th or 75th year of life. There is no standard cut-off age. It shows the burden of premature deaths by different causes and the cost in terms of person-years lost to society.
- **Proportionate mortality ratio (PMR):** The ratio of deaths from a specific cause to the total number of deaths in a given period.

- **Perinatal mortality rate:** The annual number of stillbirths (gestation of 20 weeks or more) and early neonatal deaths (within the first 7 days of life) per 1 000 stillbirths and live births. Perinatal mortality

TABLE 4.3   Derivations of Commonly Used Health Status Indicators

$$\text{Incidence rate} = \frac{\text{Number of new cases of disease in a time interval}}{\text{Population at risk}} \times 1\,000$$

$$\text{Prevalence rate} = \frac{\text{Number of existing cases of disease at a point}}{\text{Total population}} \times 1\,000$$

$$\text{Perinatal mortality rate} = \frac{\text{Annual no. of still births + live births dying under 7 days}}{\text{Total births (still and live)}} \times 1\,000$$

$$\text{Neonatal mortality rate} = \frac{\text{Annual no. of deaths of children under 28 days}}{\text{Annual live births}} \times 1\,000$$

$$\text{Maternal mortality rate} = \frac{\text{Annual no. of deaths from puerperal causes per year}}{\text{Annual live births}} = 1\,000$$

$$\text{Infant mortality rate} = \frac{\text{Annual no. of deaths under one year of age}}{\text{Annual live births}} \times 1\,000$$

$$\text{Crude death rate} = \frac{\text{Annual no. of deaths}}{\text{Total population}} \times 1\,000$$

$$\text{Age} - \text{and sex} - \text{specific death rate} = \frac{\text{Annual no. of deaths in a specific subgroup}}{\text{Total population in that subgroup}} \times 1\,000$$

$$\text{Proportionate mortality ratio (PMR)} = \frac{\text{Deaths from a specific cause}}{\text{Total deaths}} \times 100$$

$$\text{Case fatality rate} = \frac{\text{Number of deaths from a specific disease}}{\text{Total no. of cases of that disease}} \times 100$$

- **Case-fatality rate:** The number of deaths from a specific disease per total number of cases of that disease in a given period.

Depending upon the frequency of disease or condition, all the rates and proportion are expressed as per 100 (commonly occurring condition) to per 1 000; per 100 000 or per 1 000 000 (for rare condition) for ease of understanding. The way the rate is expressed is important. For example, 0.65 per 1 000 may be harder to visualize than 65 per 100 000. However, if the rate of 0.65 per 1 000 is meant to be compared with another group-specific rate of 125 per 1 000, then it may be helpful to keep the rate as it is or convert both rates to per 100 000. See Exercise 4.4 for an exercise related to mortality calculations.

Life expectancy is the number of years a person is expected to live, starting from birth (for life expectancy at birth); Organisation for Economic Co-operation and Development [OECD], 2018a or at age 65 years (for life expectancy at age 65 years); OECD, 2018b, if current age-specific death rates continue to apply. See Box 4.1 for more detail on how life expectancy in Canada compares with other countries and how various Canadian provinces and territories fare compared with one another.

EXERCISE 4.4:

1. Can you think of factors that could help to explain why some countries—even those that are relatively similar to each other in terms of their income and resource levels (e.g., the United States and Canada)—may have differing life expectancies?
2. Why might the territories have lower life expectancies compared with provinces such as British Columbia and Ontario?

EXERCISE 4.5 Calculating Mortality Rates:

The table depicts the number of deaths by demographic group from a number of different causes from a hypothetical cohort of 1 500 000 people[a]

| Leading causes of death | AGE AT TIME OF DEATH | | | | | |
	<15 years (n = 200 000)	15–24 years (n = 250 000)	25–44 years (n = 330 000)	45–64 years (n = 450 000)	65+ years (n = 270 000)	Total (n = 1 500 000)
Malignant neoplasms	130	134	1 516	17 381	59 919	79 080
Diabetes mellitus	2	11	130	1 096	5 599	6 838
Alzheimer's disease	0	0	1	73	6 447	6 521
Cardiovascular diseases	22	43	616	6 811	43 892	51 384
Cerebrovascular diseases	4	7	141	1 130	12 268	13 550
Influenza and pneumonia	5	14	100	595	5 491	6 205
Unintentional injuries	146	723	2 281	2 607	6 742	12 499
Intentional self-harm (suicide)	48	487	1 250	1 558	635	3 978
Assault (homicide)	8	87	158	99	44	396
Total	365	1 506	6 193	31 350	141 037	180 451

[a]The information for this exercise is based on selected leading causes of death in 2016 from Statistics Canada, Table 13-10-0394-01, Leading causes of death, total population, by age group.

Questions

1. Calculate the overall condition-specific mortality rate for cardiovascular diseases for this cohort. (NOTE: Typically, with these types of calculations, we only use one or two decimal places because using more may give a false impression of precision—a concept described in Chapter 2.)
2. What is the proportionate mortality ratio (PMR) of cardiovascular diseases for this cohort?
3. Assuming the total number of diagnosed cases of cardiovascular diseases was 220 569 in the year 2016, what is the case-fatality rate of cardiovascular diseases for this cohort?
4. Calculate the age-specific mortality rates for people younger than 15 years old in this cohort.

Summary Measures of Population Health

Summary measures of population health combine measures of death and quality of life into a single measure. A commonly used summary measure is the **disability-adjusted life years (DALY)** (National Collaborating Centre for Infectious Diseases [NCCID], 2015). DALYs build on the mortality indicators of PYLLs and represent the combination of years of life lost due to dying prematurely (PYLLs), as well as years lost because of living with a health condition or disability (also known as *years lived with disability [YLD]*). One DALY can be thought of as 1 year of healthy life lost (either because of death or because of living with the health condition of interest). When you add up all of the DALYs in a particular population, you get a sense of the burden of a specific disease, or how much of a "gap" this disease creates between an ideal health situation in which everyone lives healthily up to an old age and reality (in which people in the population acquire, die from, and live with the consequences of disease X). DALYs can be used to compare the burden of various disease states or chronic conditions. The Case Study box discusses one example of how the WHO has put this into practice.

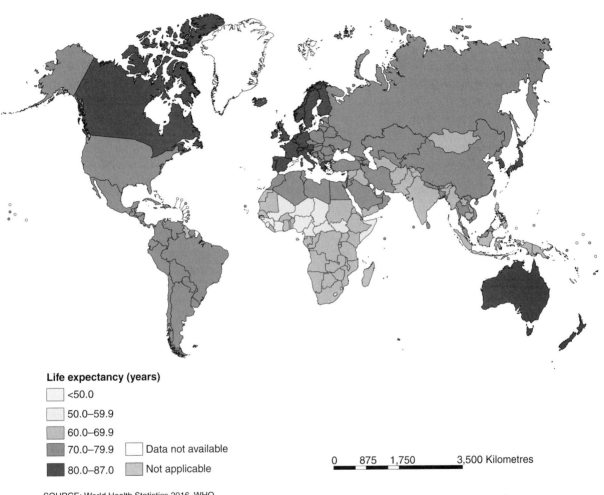

Life expectancy (years)

- ☐ <50.0
- ☐ 50.0–59.9
- ☐ 60.0–69.9
- ☐ 70.0–79.9   ☐ Data not available
- ☐ 80.0–87.0   ☐ Not applicable

0   875   1,750   3,500 Kilometres

SOURCE: World Health Statistics 2016, WHO
NOTE: WHO Member States with a population of less than 90,000 in 2015 were not included in the analysis.
The boundaries and names shown and the designations used on this map do not imply the expression of any
opinion whatsoever on the part of the World Health Organization concerning the legal status of any country,
territory, city or area or of its authorities, or concerning the delimitation of its frontiers or boundaries. Dotted and
dashed lines on maps represent approximate border lines for which there may not yet be full
agreement.

Data Source: World Health Organization Map
Production: Information Evidence and Research (IER)
World Health Organization

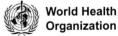

**World Health
Organization**

Fig. 4.1 Life expectancy at birth across the globe (2016 data). (Reprinted from WHO. [2016]. World health
statistics: Life expectancy at birth, both sexes, 2016. Retrieved from http://gamapserver.who.int/mapLibrary/
Files/Maps/Global_LifeExpectancy_bothsexes_2016.png.)

CASE STUDY

The Global Burden of Disease Study

The Global Burden of Disease studies began in 1991 as a collaborative between the World Bank and the World Health Organization, with the goal of quantifying and comparing the magnitude of health lost because of various diseases and risk factors for diseases (Murray & Lopez, 2013, 2017). The idea was to provide policy makers with up-to-date and timely information about what disease states or conditions should be prioritized for intervention.

In 2017, *The Lancet* published a systematic analysis that calculated DALYs for 333 diseases and injuries for 195 countries between 1990 and 2016. From their analysis, they determined that the three leading causes of DALYs (disease states that cause the most burden of disease, both in terms of quality and quantity of life) worldwide are ischemic heart disease, cerebrovascular disease, and lower respiratory infections (Hay et al., 2017).

Nonmedical determinants are discussed in more detail in Chapter 5. Indicators of health system performance are touched on in greater detail in Part 3 of the book. Health system characteristics are also described in Part 3. The discussion in the following section pertains primarily to community characteristics.

Community (Demographic) Characteristics

Indicators that reflect community characteristics, although not indicators of health status or health system performance in themselves, do provide useful contextual information. As can be seen from Table 4.2, many indicators that pertain to the characteristics of a community are demographic in nature. **Demography** is the study of populations, especially with reference to size, density, fertility, mortality, growth, age distribution, migration, geography, and vital statistics. Sociodemographic and socioeconomic indicators represent the interaction of these factors with social and economic conditions and may include things such as percentage of visible minorities, proportion of people living below the poverty line, and so on. Examples of demographic indicators include the age and gender of the population, the population growth rate, ethnicity, language, family size, proportion of single-parent families, and proportion of older adults and Indigenous people (the health of seniors is discussed in Chapter 6 and Indigenous people in Chapter 7).

It is vitally important when reading statistics pertaining to a specific population or community group that the social determinants of health and the wider forces that influence these statistics are kept in mind. For example, one cannot simply read a statistic related to high rates of poverty in a community and take it at face value. One must constantly ask why these rates are so high: Are they high because of government policy, unemployment, racism, discrimination, historical injustice, or some combination of these factors, for example? We know that poverty is borne from other influences, and they must always be considered when reading statistics about a community.

When it comes to demographic indicators specifically, there are a few definitions worth noting.

- **Crude birth rate:** The annual number of live births per 1 000 population.
- **General fertility rate:** The annual number of live births per 1 000 women between ages 15 and 49 years. This is a more refined measure of fertility compared with the crude birth rate because it includes only those likely to give birth.
- **Total fertility rate:** The average number of children who would be born alive to a woman during her lifetime if she were to pass through all her childbearing years conforming to the age-specific fertility rates of a given year.
- **Population growth** represents the sum of natural increase and net migration.
- **Natural increase** is the difference between the number of births and number of deaths.
- **Net migration** is the difference between immigration and emigration.

These demographic characteristics can indicate the "demand" placed on a health system. For example, communities with high fertility rates require perinatal care and services. Communities with a large aging population require more services in the realm of chronic disease and, potentially, long-term care needs.

THE HEALTH STATUS OF CANADIANS

This section applies the indicators discussed earlier to describe the health status of the Canadian population, focusing specifically on demographic indicators and the dimensions of health status, including death, health conditions, human functioning, and well-being. More information relating to demography, social determinants of health, and the health system in the Canadian context are described further in other parts of this book. Equity, as a cross-cutting dimension in CIHI's indicator framework (see Table 4.1), is touched upon throughout the following section and is discussed in more depth in Chapter 6.

Community Characteristics (Demography) of the Canadian Population

In 2018, Canada's estimated population was 36.95 million, of whom 50.37% were male. Of that total, 16%, 67%, and 17% were in the age groups 0 to 14 years, 15 to 64 years, and 65 years and over, respectively. Among those aged 65 years and older, 58.1% of the population was female. The Canadian population is projected to be 51 million people in 2095; 50.05% will be male.

In 2016, the infant mortality rate in Canada established to 4.5 deaths per 1 000 live births, the same value as in 2015. That is the lowest rate on record in Canada. More than half (52%) of the infants (children younger than 1 year old) who died in Canada in 2016 died within 24 hours of birth (Statistics Canada, 2018a).

The distribution of the population by age and sex indicates that the population has more than doubled since 1950, as can be seen in the 1871 and 2016 age pyramid depicted in Fig. 4.2. The ratio of males to females has remained roughly constant, but there has been a definite change in the age distribution. In 1950, there were proportionately more children younger than 14 years of age compared with 2018 because of early age at marriage and large family size. These factors are reflected in the total fertility rate (TFR). Low fertility rates were seen during the Great Depression and World War II; however, the postwar boom increased the number of births and generated more children younger than 14 years of age (Fig. 4.3). In 2011, the TFR was 1.61 children per woman in Canada, which is below the replacement level (2.1) needed for maintaining steady population growth, and it has been this way since 1974 (Statistics Canada, 2017a).

In Canada, fertility rates are falling for a number of reasons, including "postponement transition" (Gietel-Basten, Sobotka, & Zemen, 2017), which is the increasing age at motherhood. In 1965, the mean age was 23.5 years for first birth, and it began increasing steadily to 25.5 years in 1985 and 28.5 years in 2011 (Statistics Canada, 2013a) 28.5 years in 2011 (Statistics Canada, 2013a). Increasing age at motherhood has been attributed to increased educational, employment, and career opportunities for women (Van Bavel, Schwartz, & Esteve, 2018). Other factors that have affected fertility rates include more liberal abortion laws and the availability of contraception. With a decrease in the proportion of young children in the population, the demand for pediatricians and pediatric units in general hospitals has also decreased. A temporary increase in this proportion was predicted to occur when the baby boomers grew up and produced families, but it has not happened.

Geographic distributions also affect the health status of a population, representing an important community indicator. Spread across 10 provinces and three territories, two of three people (66%) are living within 100 km of the southern Canada–United States border, an area that represents about 4% of Canada's territory (Statistics Canada, 2016d). Additionally, approximately 18% of Canada's population lives in rural or remote communities.

As discussed earlier, natural increase (difference in the number of births and deaths) is an important influencer of population growth. In 2016, there were a total of 389 912 births and 267 213 deaths. Thus, the natural increase was 122 699 people. **Net migration** (i.e., the

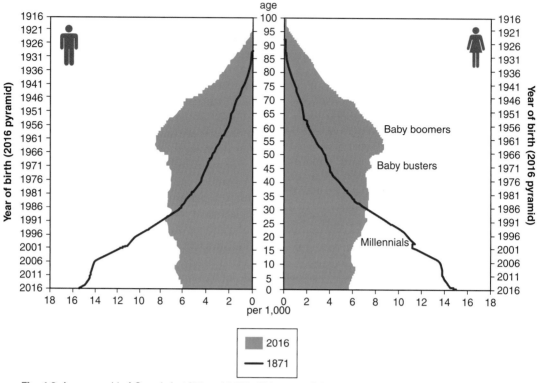

Fig. 4.2 Age pyramid of Canada in 1871 and 2016: 150 years of demographic history. This figure comprises two overlapping pyramids that represent the age–sex structure of the population in 1871 (indicated by *red lines*) and in 2016 (indicated by a *solid blue form*). The 1871 age pyramid has a wide base and a narrow apex, giving it a true pyramid shape. The shape of the 2016 age pyramid is less like a pyramid and more like a mushroom with a narrower base, wider area between the ages of 50 and 70 years, and a pointed apex. The *line* and *horizontal bars* on the y-axis are located in the middle of the chart and divide the pyramids into two. They indicate the ages 0 to 100 years. Men are represented on the left side of the axis and women on the right side. The *horizontal bars* on the x-axis represent the proportion of people for each age per thousand from 0 to 18. They are identical on both the right and left sides of the y-axis. Three areas on the right side of the pyramid represent different generations and where those generations are situated on the 2016 age pyramid. The first area, indicated by a *small peak* in the pyramid, represents individuals who were between 15 and 34 years in 2016, often referred to as millennials. The second area, shown as a *small dip* in the pyramid, represents the smaller generations arising out of the baby bust in the late 1960s and early 1970s. The third area, in the "cap" of the mushroom, represents baby boomers, who were born between 1946 and 1965 and were therefore between the ages of 51 and 70 in 2016. It is much wider than the other areas. (Source: Statistics Canada. [2017]. Age and sex, and type of dwelling data: Key results from the 2016 Census. *The Daily*, May 3, 2017. Retrieved from https://www150.statcan.gc.ca/n1/daily-quotidien/170503/g-a001-eng.htm.)

difference between immigration and emigration) is the other key influencers of population growth. Immigration has always been an important source of population growth in Canada. In 2015, the number of immigrants coming to the country was 259 100, whereas 42 000 people emigrated from Canada. Thus, the net migration was 217 100 persons. In essence, Canada's population increased by 337 800 people in 2015. What may seem like simple calculations, the dynamics behind these numbers are complex. About two thirds of Canada's population growth from 2011 to 2016 was the result of migratory increase. Natural increase accounted for the remaining one third. Migratory increases are playing a larger role in Canada's population growth, unlike in the past when natural increase determined the growth rate. However, with younger immigrants coming to Canada,

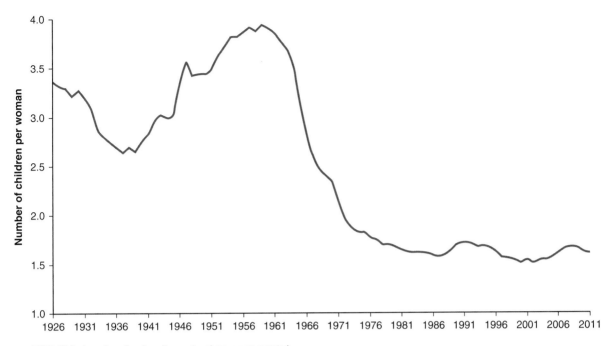

NOTE: Births to mothers for whom the age is unknown were prorated.
SOURCE: Statistics Canada, Demography Division, Population Estimates Program, Canadian Vital Statistics, Births Database, 1926 to 2011, Survey 3231.

Fig. 4.3 Total fertility rate, Canada, 1926 to 2011. (From Statistics Canada. [2018]. Fertility: fewer children, older moms. *The Daily,* May 17, 2018. Retrieved from https://www150.statcan.gc.ca/n1/pub/11-630-x/2014 002/c-g/c-g01-eng.gif.)

fertility rates may also increase over time. Recent migration trends in Canada are reshaping the population and society in ways that may change how we look at the health (Fig. 4.4). Further trends include the baby boomers who will turn 80 years old in 2026, resulting in higher mortality rates in the future.

Health Status

As discussed earlier, when collecting information on the health status of Canadians, indicators pertaining to death, health conditions (including hospitalizations and clinical visits for these health conditions), functional health (disability), and well-being (perceived health) should be taken together. If information on death or health care utilization is presented in isolation, it is easy to forget that for every death, there is a handful of people admitted to hospital, even more that see a health care professional, significantly more that perceive a disability, and quite a large number that perceive that a health problem exists, without ever seeking health care. This must be kept in mind and is best visually depicted by Fig. 4.5 using a theoretical sample of 100 000 Canadians. Conversely, when presented with

self-perceived health, it is important to realize that only a small proportion of people that perceive themselves to have a health problem will seek care, be hospitalized, or die from such a condition.

Death

One of the most common indicators of death, or mortality, is life expectancy. Life expectancy in Canada averages 82.2 years overall (79.8 years for men and 83.9 years for women) (Statistics Canada, 2018b) (refer to Box 4.1 for more details on how life expectancy in Canada compares with other countries and how various provinces and territories compare with one another when it comes to life expectancy). Life expectancy has increased dramatically since the 1920s. For example, in 1920, life expectancy was just 58.8 years (Statistics Canada, 2017b). Health-adjusted life expectancy at birth (i.e., how many years you can expect to live in good health) today is just over 72 years in Canada (PHAC, 2017).

In terms of overall mortality, the crude death rate in Canada in 2016 was 7.4 deaths per 1 000 people (Statistics Canada, 2018c). In general, since the 1920s,

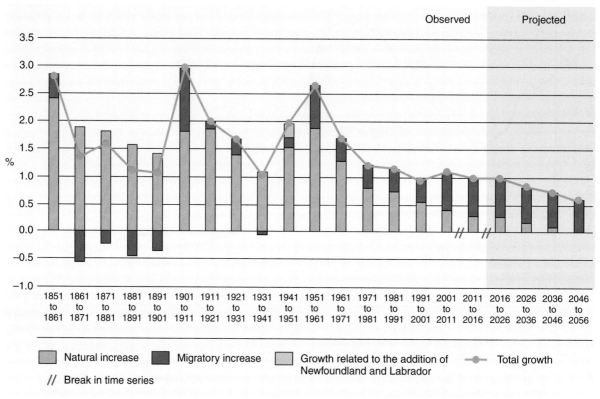

Fig. 4.4 Annual average growth rate, natural increase, and migratory increase per intercensal period, Canada, 1851 to 2056. (From Statistics Canada. [2017]. Population size and growth in Canada: Key results from the 2016 Census.. *The Daily*, February 8, 2017. Retrieved from https://www150.statcan.gc.ca/n1/daily-quotidien/170208/g-a001-eng.htm.)

the crude mortality rate has gone up in Canada. This is largely attributed to an aging population because seniors have a higher mortality rate than the general population (Statistics Canada, 2017b). However, when mortality rates are standardized by age (meaning the influence of having an aging population is accounted for when comparing mortality rates over time), we can see from Fig. 4.6 that standardized mortality rates have actually gone down over time. For example, in 1982, the standardized mortality rate was 16.1 per 1 000, and in 2013, it was 7.2 per 1 000 (Statistics Canada, 2017b). This mirrors the increase in life expectancy we have seen over time.

In the fall of 2018, Canada's chief public health officer warned that the progress we have seen in terms of increasing life expectancy in Canada may be impacted by the opioid crisis. The opioid crisis has its root in a number of different factors (e.g.,

prescriber patterns when it comes to prescription opioids, heavy pharmaceutical marketing of opioids, the prevalence of adverse childhood experiences and mental health issues in society, lack of access to pain treatment), which are described in more detail in Chapter 9. This crisis continues to take an immense toll on populations: in 2017, alone, 4 000 people died of opioid overdoses. The chief public health officer said these types of mortality rates have not been seen since the HIV/AIDS epidemic in the 1980s (Ireland, 2018).

Interestingly, although males typically have a higher death rate than females, over time, death rates between men and women are equalizing—mostly because the lifestyle that men and women lead are converging more now than they ever have before in Canada. For a recently released report on mortality trends in Ontario, see the Research Perspective box.

RESEARCH PERSPECTIVE

Trends in Mortality Across Ontario

In February 2018, the Population Health Analytics Laboratory at the University of Toronto, as part of the Ontario Population Trends in Improved Mortality: Informing Sustainability & Equity of the health care system (OPTIMISE) research program, developed the mortality atlas. This atlas looks at trends in mortality rates across various geographic areas of Ontario. Data analysis revealed that between 1992 and 2015, all-cause mortality declined in Ontario by nearly 40% in males and nearly 30% in females. Mirroring Canadian trends, cardiovascular disease and cancers accounted for two thirds of all deaths during this time period. Additionally, after analyzing the data by socioeconomic status, a clear trend was observed: premature mortality rates were correlated with socioeconomic status across the province, in both men and women. Unfortunately, inequities in death rates according to socioeconomic status have actually widened since 1992.

Source: Buajitti, E., Chiodo, S., Watson, T., et al. (2018). *Ontario atlas of adult mortality, 1992-2015, Version 2.0: Trends in Public Health Units.* Toronto, ON: Population Health Analytics Lab. Retrieved from https://pophealthanalytics.com/wp-content/uploads/2018/09/OntarioAtlasOfAdultMortality_12Sept2018.pdf

As indicated at the beginning of this chapter, infant mortality is often used to compare health status among countries because it tends to be an accurate indicator of overall health and reflects important determinants of health like poverty and availability of health services (Centers for Disease Control and Prevention, 2018). In 2016, Canada's infant mortality rate was 4.5 per 1 000 people (Statistics Canada, 2018b). Although infant mortality has fallen over time in Canada, a 2013 report by UNICEF highlighted that Canada ranked 22 of 29 high-income countries when it came to infant mortality specifically (UNICEF Office of Research, 2013).

Most experts agree that this is due in large part to the higher rates of infant mortality among Indigenous people in Canada (discussed further in Chapter 7). Infant mortality rates are higher in some Indigenous communities because of the influence that the social determinants have on health and health inequities.

Infant mortality may be influenced by poorer access to health care in rural and remote areas, lower incomes, unemployment or precarious employment, unsafe housing conditions, differential access to affordable nutritious foods, among others. It is critical remember, however, that these inequities in social determinants of health are not the result of chance. Rather, they are a result of historical government policy and colonialism, which caused widespread inequities relating to employment, housing, income, and so on for Indigenous people across the country (discussed further in Chapter 7) and which continues to cause inequities today.

The leading causes of death in Canada vary based on age group. As described further in Chapter 8, the top leading causes of death among the general population are cancers, cardiovascular disease, cerebrovascular disease, unintentional injuries, and chronic lower respiratory diseases (Statistics Canada, 2018d). Among children aged 1 to 14 years, however, the leading causes of death include unintentional injuries, cancers, intentional self-harm (i.e., suicide), and influenza and pneumonia (Statistics Canada, 2018e). Table 4.4 provides a breakdown of the leading causes of death by age group in Canada. Overall, mortality rates from the leading causes of deaths caused by the four common noncommunicable diseases (NCDs) (e.g., heart disease, lung disease, cancer, and diabetes) have gone down by almost one third over an 18-year period, as has the probability of dying from one of these major NCDs prematurely (i.e., between the ages of 30 and 69 years) (Public Health Agency of Canada, 2018c).

Health Conditions

Noncommunicable diseases (discussed in Chapter 8) are the leading cause of disability and poor health in Canada, with one in three Canadians living with at least one major chronic or NCD (Roberts et al., 2015). In fact, a 2018 study showed that increasingly more Canadians are living with multiple chronic diseases. Nearly 13% of Canadians report living with two chronic diseases, and 4% report living with three or more chronic diseases. However, although the actual number of Canadians living with NCDs has increased over time—largely because of an aging population and availability of better treatments enabling people to live longer with their disease—the actual incidence

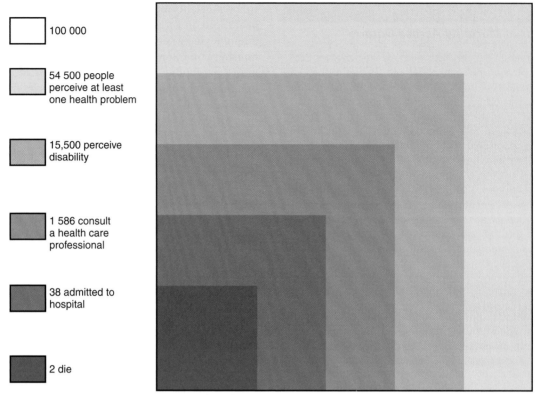

100 000

54 500 people perceive at least one health problem

15,500 perceive disability

1 586 consult a health care professional

38 admitted to hospital

2 die

Fig. 4.5 Health of a population sample of 100 000 Canadians on an average day. (Adapted from Kohn, R. [1967]. Royal Commission on Health Services: The health of the Canadian people. Ottawa: Queen's Printer. © All rights reserved. Organization of Health Canada: Branches and Agencies. Health Canada, 2017. Adapted and reproduced with permission from the Minister of Health, 2019

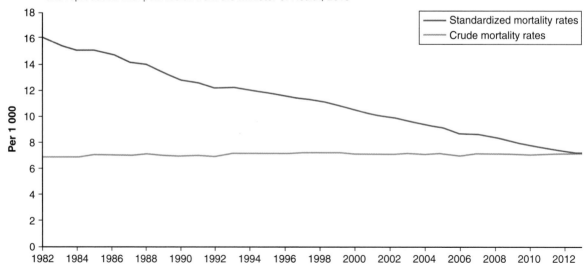

NOTE: Deaths for which the age of death is unknown were prorated using the observed distribution.
SOURCES: Statistics Canada, Canadian Vital Statistics, Deaths Database, 1982 to 2013, Survey 3233 and Demography Division, Population Estimates Program (PEP).

Fig. 4.6 Crude and standardized mortality trends in Canada, 1982 to 2013. (Statistics Canada. (2017) Lebel, A., & Hallman, S. *Report on the Demographic Situation in Canada. Mortality Overview: 2012 and 2013* (Figure 4). Retrieved from https://www150.statcan.gc.ca/n1/pub/91-209-x/2017001/article/14793-eng.htm)

(number of new cases of specific illnesses) is slowly decreasing for many NCDs (PHAC, 2018c).

Similar to causes of death, the leading conditions causing the most suffering to Canadians depend on age and how one measures suffering or burden of disease. In the first half of this chapter, several indicators reflecting morbidity were described, including health conditions and their respective rates. One can use an indicator such as hospitalization rate or years lived with disability to reflect what health conditions cause the most impact to Canadians.

The leading diseases contributing to hospitalizations in Canada among children and youth include respiratory system diseases, infectious diseases, unintentional injuries, congenital anomalies, digestive system diseases, and mental health disorders (discussed further in Chapter 9). Among adults older than 55 years, however, leading conditions resulting in hospitalization include heart disease, lung disease, cancer, digestive system diseases, and unintentional injuries (PHAC, 2016a).

In Manitoba, data are analyzed to determine the most common reasons for a visit to a primary care provider. The three most common disease specific reasons for a visit include visits related to heart disease (making up 10% of all visits to a primary care provider), lung disease (accounting for 9.5% of all visits), and mental health disorders (accounting for 9.4% of all visits) (Manitoba Health, 2017).

In 2016, the Institute for Health Metrics and Evaluation reported that the top causes of years lived with disability among the general Canadian population included low back and neck pain, sense organ diseases, skin diseases, migraines, depression, anxiety, and diabetes (refer to Chapter 8 for more detail) (Institute for Health Metrics and Evaluation, n.d.).

A 2017 report published by the Public Health Agency of Canada pointed to the importance of some of the health conditions mentioned. For example, the prevalence of both heart and lung disease have increased since the year 2000, and it is now estimated that one in five Canadian adults lives with one of either heart disease, lung disease, cancer, or diabetes (PHAC, 2017). The high prevalence of mental health issues is also a growing concern in Canada and is covered in more depth in Chapter 9.

A 2018 report released by the Canada's Chief Public Health Officer highlights that nearly one in three Canadians is affected by a mental illness at some point in their lifetimes, and one in five is affected by a substance use disorder, with alcohol use disorder being most common (PHAC, 2018a).

When considering the impact of various health conditions, the direct and indirect costs associated with them must be factored in. In 2017, the Public Health Agency of Canada published a report called the *Economic Burden of Illness*, in which the direct and indirect costs of major health conditions were summarized. The diseases with the highest total costs (including both direct and indirect) included digestive system diseases (accounting for nearly 14.9% of costs associated with all major health conditions), injuries (accounting for 14.2% of all costs), circulatory system diseases (10.4% of all costs), and mental health disorders (8.9% of all costs) (PHAC, 2018b).

Interestingly, not all diseases that resulted in high direct costs had high indirect costs. Musculoskeletal disorders, for example, resulted in high indirect costs but low direct costs, implying the cost that actually goes into treatment isn't as high as the cost associated from loss of productivity, or days of work lost as a result of having this type of a health condition. On the other hand, digestive system diseases result in a high level of direct costs (because often treatment may require expensive surgical procedures) but low levels of indirect costs.

Functional Health

Both health conditions and functional health reflect morbidity or levels of disease in the population. Indicators of functional health (as described above) often include disability days, disability-free life expectancy (i.e., the number of years a person is expected to live without disability at a given age), years lost because of disability, and prevalence of people reporting disabilities limiting functioning, among others.

Nearly 14% of the Canadian population older than 15 years of age reports having a disability that limits their functioning. The rates of Canadians reporting living with a disability that impairs function increases with

TABLE 4.4   Top Five Leading Causes of Death By Age Group (2016)

		AGE CATEGORY							
Rank	1–14	15–24	25–34	35–44	45–54	55–64	65–74	75–84	85+
1	Unintentional injuries	Unintentional injuries	Unintentional injuries	Cancer	Cancer	Cancer	Cancer	Cancer	Diseases of the heart
2	Cancer	Suicide	Suicide	Unintentional injuries	Diseases of the heart	Diseases of the heart	Diseases of the heart	Diseases of the heart	Cancer
3	Suicide	Cancer	Cancer	Suicide	Unintentional injuries	Unintentional injuries	Chronic lower respiratory diseases	Chronic lower respiratory diseases	Cerebro-vascular disease
4	Influenza or pneumonia	Homicide	Diseases of the heart	Diseases of the heart	Suicide	Chronic liver disease	Cerebro-vascular disease	Cerebro-vascular disease	Alzheimer's disease
5	Diseases of the heart	Diseases of the heart	Homicide	Chronic liver disease	Chronic liver disease	Chronic lower respiratory diseases	Diabetes	Diabetes	Chronic lower respiratory diseases

From Public Health Agency of Canada. (2018). *Canadian chronic disease indicators, Quick stats* (2018 Edition). Ottawa: Public Health Agency of Canada.

age from 4% among people age 15 to 24 years to just over 40% in people 75 years or older (Statistics Canada, 2017c).

A 2014 study looked at trends in disability-free life expectancy over time and found that years spent with a disability increased in both men and women. The authors highlighted that gains in life expectancy that have been seen in Canada are not matched by gains in disability-free life expectancy and that the proportion of Canadians that are limited in their functioning (and need assistance to carry out activities of daily living) is actually increasing countrywide (Mandich & Margolis, 2014).

A particularly interesting indicator that can also reflect functional health (and that is being reported more and more in institutional settings) is that of absenteeism, or habitual and unscheduled days of work or school lost due to personal reasons, which include illness (Statistics Canada, 2015). The assumption in using an indicator such as absenteeism to reflect functional health is that a person that is ill from a disease state (whether acute or chronic) is not able to function well enough in a work environment, to the point where they need to stay home. Statistics Canada's Labour Force Survey captures the number of days lost because of illness and has found that since the early 2000s, the number of days lost has increased across the country but has levelled off since the later 2000s. In 2011, 6% of full-time employees missed some work each week (which amounted to nearly 7.7 workdays lost because of illness or disability over the course of that year (Statistics Canada, 2015)).

Well-Being

As discussed in Part 1, self-perceived health is a reliable health status indicator; thus, agencies spend time collecting this information across Canada. When asked to rate their health according to the descriptors excellent, very good, good, fair, or poor, approximately 60% of Canadians older than 12 years of age say their health is "very good" or "excellent" (PHAC, 2016b). Over time, the proportion of Canadians

responding in this way has not changed significantly. In fact, in 2003, 58% of Canadians rated their health as "very good" or "excellent" compared with nearly 60% in 2014 (PHAC, 2016b). Equal proportions of men and women rank their perceived health highly; however, as with other indicators of health status, inequities among certain groups do exist. For example, Indigenous communities (including First Nations on reserve a well as First Nations off reserve, Inuit, and Métis people) are less likely to report that their health is "very good" or "excellent" (PHAC, 2016b). Additionally, people who live in households with lower income levels do not tend to rate their health as highly as those living in households with higher income levels. The proportion of people who rated their health as "very good" or "excellent" among the lowest decile of income was only about 40% in 2014. In comparison, the proportion of people living in the highest income decile that rated their health as "very good" or "excellent" was nearly 70% (PHAC, 2016b).

Interestingly, when comparing across other G7 countries, Canada is at the top in terms of its populations perceived health—on par with the United States and higher than countries such as the United Kingdom, France, Italy, Germany, and Japan (PHAC, 2016b).

CRITICAL THINKING QUESTION 4.2: As described earlier, the opioid crisis may be having an impact on the Canadian life expectancy. Research the health effects of opioids, and then, using the Indicator Framework that was presented in Table 4.1, describe how the opioid crisis might change the current health status of Canadians (including health conditions, human function, and well-being).

Based on your predictions, how might you most effectively communicate or "warn" the public of this information for the purposes of mobilizing people, including decision makers, to take action? Who on your interdisciplinary team might you involve to support these communication efforts?

SUMMARY

This chapter has discussed health indicators, which are qualitative and quantitative measures that indicate the health of a population and are examined on four dimensions, namely health status, nonmedical determinants of health, health system performance, and community and health system characteristics. The chapter focused specifically on indicators that reflect health status and community (demographic) characteristics. Health status indicators include indicators of well-being, health conditions of human function, and deaths. All of these must be considered together to paint an accurate picture of health in a community. Using indicators related solely to death, for example, does not adequately capture important aspects of health, such as quality of life, participation in society, and perceived health and well-being. Although each of these indicators has its limitations, together they can be used to depict health in a more comprehensive and holistic way. As will be emphasized in later chapters, indicators related to health equity are also important as a way of highlighting the spread of ill health in a population because often, health does not improve over time equally for all groups. Indicators, however, do not tell the full story, so although they are necessary to describe and monitor population health, on their own, they are not sufficient and may be complemented with narrative stories, lived experience, and observation.

Characteristics of the community can be most often thought of as those that reflect demography (e.g., the age and sex of the population and population growth rate, as well as fertility rates). They are important for the health system because they can represent changing "demand" on health services. For example, an aging population can mean things such as increasing client complexity and a growing cohort of people having multiple chronic conditions. Similarly, declining fertility has implications for the number and mix of reproductive health services needed.

Community and health indicators were used to describe the Canadian population. From a demographic standpoint, the age distribution of Canadians has seen a change over the past several decades towards an aging population. Fertility rates have been declining as well, for a number of reasons (e.g., policy changes and delayed age at which women are having children). Population growth is continuing but is mostly driven by immigration.

When it comes to health status (which is described according to morbidity, mortality, well-being, and functionality), overall, Canadians are healthy compared to people from other countries and, specifically, have very high rates of self-perceived health. Although mortality rates are decreasing over time, years lived with disability and in particular, with one or more NCDs are increasing as the population continues to age and treatments for NCDs improve. Last, significant challenges remain when it comes to achieving equitable health for all groups; groups with less access to important social determinants of health (e.g., income) are at a disadvantage. This is examined extensively in Chapter 5, "Determinants of Health and Disease," and Chapter 6, "Inequities in Health."

KEY WEBSITES

Canadian Institute for Health Information (CIHI): https://www.cihi.ca/en

CIHI provides information about Canadian health care and health systems, contributing to improvements in health care, health system performance, and population health in Canada. This independent and not-for-profit organization provides a wide variety of databases and measurements to aid evidence-informed decision making.

Canadian Socioeconomic Information Management (CANSIM) Database: https://www.statcan.gc.ca/eng/developers/concordance

CANSIM is a part of Statistics Canada and provides socioeconomic data that may not be found in the Census of Canada. Specific data can be searched by topic on the StatsCan website and can be provided by CANSIM table numbers. Access the site for a list of all CANSIM tables or search for tables by topic.

Global Burden of Disease (GBD) by the Institute for Health Metrics and Evaluation (IHME): http://www.healthdata.org/gbd

As an initiative from the IHME at the University of Washington, the GBD is an online resource providing quantified information about health loss, injuries, and risk factors to help inform policy makers and researchers about health statuses across countries, time, age, and sex. The site provides access to data, data visualization tools, training and workshop opportunities, and publications.

Global Health Observatory (GHO): http://www.who.int/gho/en/

The GHO is a World Health Organization database with more than 1 000 health-related indicators for the WHO's 194 member states. The indicators help monitor progress of health-related targets as part of the WHO's Sustainable Development Goals.

Population Health Analytics Laboratory: https://pophealthanalytics.com/

The team at the Population Health Analytics Laboratory works to gain a comprehensive perspective on population health from demographic, clinical, behavioural, social, and health outcome data. Visit the link to learn check out projects like the Local Health Integration Networks Mortality Atlas that the team developed with the Ontario Population Trends in Improved Mortality: Informing Sustainability & Equity of the health care system (OPTIMISE) research program.

Statistics Canada (StatCan): https://www.statcan.gc.ca/eng/start

The StatsCan mission is "serving Canada with high-quality statistical information that matters." Fulfilling an important federal responsibility, StatsCan provides quality, objective statistical information to help elected representatives, businesses, unions, health care providers, individual Canadians, and other organizations make informed decisions. Explore the link to learn more about what StatsCan does and access datasets including the 2016 Canadian Census Profile.

The World Factbook: Central Intelligence Agency (CIA): https://www.cia.gov/library/publications/the-world-factbook

This massive database from the CIA contains information about 267 world entities and links to maps, photos, and information about the geography, history, government, economy, transnational issues, and more.

REFERENCES

Benyamini, Y. (2011). Why does self-rated health predict mortality? An update on current knowledge and a research agenda for psychologists. *Psychology & Health*, *26*(11), 1407–1413. https://doi.org/10.1080/08870446.2011.621703.

Bonner, W. I. A., Weiler, R., Orisatoki, R., et al. (2017). Determinants of self-perceived health for Canadians aged 40 and older and policy implications. *International Journal for Equity in Health*, *16*, 94. https://doi.org/10.1186/s12939-017-0595-x.

Canadian Institute for Health Information. (n.d.). Health indicators. Retrieved from https://www.cihi.ca/en/health-indicators

Centers for Disease Control and Prevention. (2018). *Infant mortality*. Retrieved from https://www.cdc.gov/reproductivehealth/MaternalInfantHealth/InfantMortality.htm.

Central Intelligence Agency. (2017). *Country comparison: Life expectancy at birth*. Retrieved from https://www.cia.gov/library/publications/the-world-factbook/rankorder/2102rank.html.

Conference Board of Canada. (2019). *Provincial and territorial ranking: Life expectancy*. Retrieved from https://www.conferenceboard.ca/hcp/provincial/health/life.aspx?AspxAutoDetectCookieSupport=1.

Gietel-Basten, S., Sobotka, T., & Zeman, K. (2017). Future fertility in low fertility countries. In W. Lutz, W. Butz, & S. KC (Eds.), *World population & human capital in the twenty-first century: An overview*. Oxford, UK: Oxford University Press.

Hay, S. I., Abajobir, A. A., Abate, K. H., et al. (2017). Global, regional, and national disability-adjusted life-years (DALYs) for 333 diseases and injuries and healthy life expectancy (HALE) for 195 countries and territories, 1990–2016: A systematic analysis for the Global Burden of Disease Study 2016. *The Lancet*, *390*(10100), 1260–1344. https://doi.org/10.1016/S0140-6736(17)32130-X.

Ireland, N. (2018). *Life expectancy in Canada may be decreasing as opioid crisis rages on*. CBC News. Retrieved from https://www.cbc.ca/news/health/life-expectancy-canada-decrease-opioid-crisis-1.4874651.

Jeffrey, B., Abonyi, S., Hamilton, C., et al. (2010). *Community health indicators toolkit* (2nd ed.). University of Regina and University of Saskatchewan: Saskatchewan Population Health and Evaluation Research Unit (SPHERU). Retrieved from. http://www.spheru.ca/publications/files/Tools-1-community-health-indictors-toolkit-2nd-edition-2010-rev-1-Apr-2016.pdf.

Mandich, S., & Margolis, R. (2014). Changes in disability-free life expectancy in Canada between 1994 and 2007. *Canadian Studies in Population*, *411*(1–2), 192–208.

Manitoba Health. (2017). *Seniors and active living information management and analytics. Annual Statistics 2016–2017*. Retrieved from https://www.gov.mb.ca/health/annstats/as1617.pdf.

Ministry of Health and Long-Term Care. (2018). *Ontario Public Health Standards: Requirements for programs, services, and accountability*. Retrieved from http://www.health.gov.on.ca/en/pro/programs/publichealth/oph_standards/docs/protocols_guidelines/Ontario_Public_Health_Standards_2018_en.pdf.

Murray, C. J., & Lopez, A. D. (2013). Measuring the global burden of disease. *New England Journal of Medicine, 369*(5), 448–457. https://doi.org/10.1056/NEJMra1201534.

Murray, C. J., & Lopez, A. D. (2017). Measuring global health: motivation and evolution of the Global Burden of Disease Study. *The Lancet, 390*(10100), 1460–1464. https://doi.org/10.1016/S0140-6736(17)32367-X.

National Collaborating Centre for Infectious Diseases. (2015). *Understanding summary measures used to estimate the burden of disease: All about HALYs, DALYs and QALYs.* Retrieved from https://nccid.ca/publications/understanding-summary-measures-used-to-estimate-the-burden-of-disease/.

Organisation for Economic Co-operation and Development. (2018a). *Life expectancy at birth (indicator).* https://doi.org/10.1787/27e0fc9d-en.

Organisation for Economic Co-operation and Development. (2018b). *Life expectancy at 65 (indicator).* https://doi.org/10.1787/0e9a3f00-en.

Pencheon, D. (2008). *The good indicators guide: Understanding how to use and choose indicators [PDF].* Coventry, UK: NHS Institute for Innovation and Improvement. Retrieved from https://fingertips.phe.org.uk/documents/The%20Good%20Indicators%20Guide.pdf.

Post, M. W. M. (2014). Definitions of quality of life: What has happened and how to move on. *Topics in Spinal Cord Injury Rehabilitation, 20*(3), 167–180. https://doi.org/10.1310/sci2003-167.

Public Health Agency of Canada. (2013). *Maternal mortality in Canada.* Retrieved from https://sogc.org/wp-content/uploads/2014/05/REVISEDMortality-EN-Final-PDF.pdf.

Public Health Agency of Canada. (2016a). *Leading causes of hospitalizations, Canada, 2009/10, males and females combined, counts (age-specific hospitalization rate per 100,000).* Retrieved from https://www.canada.ca/en/public-health/services/reports-publications/leading-causes-death-hospitalization-canada/2009-10-males-females-combined-counts-specific-hospitalization-rate.html.

Public Health Agency of Canada. (2016b). *Health status of Canadians, 2016.* Retrieved from http://healthycanadians.gc.ca/publications/department-ministere/state-public-health-status-2016-etat-sante-publique-statut/alt/pdf-eng.pdf.

Public Health Agency of Canada. (2017). *How Healthy are Canadians? A trend analysis of the health of Canadians from a healthy living and chronic disease perspective.* Retrieved from https://www.canada.ca/en/public-health/services/publications/healthy-living/how-healthy-canadians.html#s3-5-4.

Public Health Agency of Canada. (2018a). *The Chief Public Health Officer's report on the state of public health in Canada 2018: Preventing problematic substance use in youth.* Retrieved from https://www.canada.ca/en/public-health/corporate/publications/chief-public-health-officer-reports-state-public-health-canada/2018-preventing-problematic-substance-use-youth.html.

Public Health Agency of Canada. (2018b). *Economic burden of illness in Canada, 2010, Table 8.* Retrieved from https://www.canada.ca/en/public-health/services/publications/science-research-data/economic-burden-illness-canada-2010.html#tb8.

Public Health Agency of Canada. (2018c). *Canadian chronic disease indicators: Quick stats* (2018 ed.). Ottawa: Author.

Roberts, K. C., Rao, D. P., Bennett, T. L., et al. (2015). Prevalence and patterns of chronic disease multimorbidity and associated determinants in Canada. *Health Promotion and Chronic Disease Prevention in Canada: Research, Policy and Practice, 35*(6), 87–94. Retrieved from https://www.ncbi.nlm.nih.gov/pmc/articles/PMC4910465/.

Statistics Canada. (2013a). *Health fact sheets: The 10 leading causes of death, 2013.* Retrieved from https://www150.statcan.gc.ca/n1/pub/82-625-x/2017001/article/14776-eng.htm.

Statistics Canada. (2015). *Analysis, work absences in 2011.* Retrieved from https://www150.statcan.gc.ca/n1/pub/71-211-x/2012000/part-partie1-eng.htm.

Statistics Canada. (2016a). Health status. Retrieved from https://www150.statcan.gc.ca/n1/pub/82-229-x/2009001/status/int4-eng.htm.

Statistics Canada. (2016b). Health indicators framework. Retrieved from https://www150.statcan.gc.ca/n1/pub/82-221-x/2013001/hifw-eng.htm.

Statistics Canada. (2016c). *Participation and activity limitation.* Retrieved from https://www150.statcan.gc.ca/n1/pub/82-229-x/2009001/status/pal-eng.htm.

Statistics Canada. (2016d). *Population size and growth in Canada: Key results from the 2016 Census.* Retrieved from https://www150.statcan.gc.ca/n1/daily-quotidien/170208/dq170208a-eng.htm.

Statistics Canada. (2017a). *Fertility: Fewer children, older moms.* Retrieved from https://www.statcan.gc.ca/pub/11-630-x/11-630-x2014002-eng.htm.

Statistics Canada. (2017b). *Report on the demographic situation in Canada, mortality: Overview, 2012 and 2013.* Retrieved from https://www150.statcan.gc.ca/n1/pub/91-209-x/2017001/article/14793-eng.htm.

Statistics Canada. (2017c). *A profile of persons with disabilities among Canadians aged 15 years or older, 2012.* Retrieved from https://www150.statcan.gc.ca/n1/pub/89-654-x/89-654-x2015001-eng.htm.

Statistics Canada. (2018a). *Mortality: Overview, 2014-2016.* Retrieved from: https://www150.statcan.gc.ca/n1/pub/91-209-x/2018001/article/54957-eng.htm.

Statistics Canada. (2018b). *Health reports: Health-adjusted life expectancy in Canada.* Retrieved from https://www150.statcan.gc.ca/n1/pub/82-003-x/2018004/article/54950-eng.htm.

Statistics Canada. (2018c). *Table 13-10-0710-01 Deaths and mortality rates, by age group.* Retrieved from https://www150.statcan.gc.ca/t1/tbl1/en/tv.action?pid=1310071001.

Statistics Canada. (2018d). *Table 13-10-0394-01 Leading causes of death, total population, by age group.* Retrieved from https://www150.statcan.gc.ca/t1/tbl1/en/tv.action?pid=1310039401.

Statistics Canada. (2018e). *Table 13-10-0394-01 Leading causes of death, total population, by age group.* Retrieved from https://www150.statcan.gc.ca/t1/tbl1/en/tv.action?pid=1310039401&pickMembers%5B0%5D=2.21&pickMembers%5B1%5D=3.1.

UNICEF Office of Research. (2013). *Child Well-being in Rich Countries: A comparative overview. Innocenti Report Card 11, Figure 2.1a.* Retrieved from https://www.unicef.no/sites/default/files/child_well-being_in_rich_countries.pdf.

Van Bavel, J., Schwartz, C., & Esteve, A. (2018). The reversal of the gender gap in education and its consequences for family life. *Annual Review of Sociology, 44,* 341–360. https://doi.org/10.1146/annurev-soc-073117-041215.

World Health Organization. (2018). *International classification of functioning, disability and health.* Retrieved from http://www.who.int/classifications/icf/en/.

World Health Organization. (n.d.). About the GHO. Global Health Observatory (GHO) data. Retrieved from http://www.who.int/gho/about/en/.

5

Determinants of Health and Disease

ⓔ Additional resources are available online at http://evolve.elsevier.com/Canada/Shah/publichealth/

LEARNING OBJECTIVES

- Describe the distribution of various determinants of health that influence health status and health inequities in Canada, particularly biology and genetics, sociodemographics, socioeconomic factors, the physical environment, lifestyle and behaviour, and health care access.
- Explain the possible mechanisms by which various determinants influence health status.

- Analyze how the ultimate drivers of health status (i.e., politics, policy environment) shape other determinants of health such as income, employment, and health behaviours.
- Explore various community health issues through a social determinants of health lens.

CHAPTER OUTLINE

KEY TERMS

alternative medicine
at risk of homelessness
body mass index (BMI)
complementary medicine
couch surfing
chronic stress
demography
distracted driving
emergency sheltered
epigenetics
food environments

food insecure
health literacy
low income cut-off (LICO)
nutrition transition
obese
overweight
physical literacy
protective devices
provisionally accommodated
unsheltered

INTRODUCTION

The determinants of health, often broadly referred to as any nonmedical factors that influence health, have a profound direct and indirect effect on the health of populations. What makes us sick are the factors that influence where we work, live, play, learn, grow, and age, contributing 50% to our health, with biology or genetics and the environment contributing 25%, and health care the remaining 25%. (See Fig. 1.2 in Chapter 1 for the World Health Organization's [WHO's] framework on the social determinants of health [SDHs].)

Before we start, it is important to briefly recap some of the key concepts that were described in Chapter 1 as they relate to health determinants. The SDHs, or "the conditions in which people are born, grow, live, work and age" (listed in Box 5.1) are all ultimately shaped by how we've chosen to structure our societies—that is, how we distribute power, money, and resources and the political and policy environments in which we exist. SDHs not only shape health at an individual level but also at a population level—they are the reason why some groups in our society are healthier than others (WHO, 2019a). It is vital for health sector trainees to be aware of the determinants of health and how they manifest in Canadian society.

As such, this chapter is dedicated to discussing various different determinants in a Canadian context. The chapter highlights some examples of community-based and policy interventions to address the SDHs, but its main focus is "describing the problem" (as in Chapter 3, as well as Chapters 6 through 12) and describing action that can be taken at a community level.

Last, it is clear that most of what determines whether we are healthy or sick lies outside the health sector and, as such, health sector students must become skilled at working in a multidisciplinary interprofessional environment with experts from various fields, including education, law, finance, transport, and others, to best implement community health approaches (defined and described in Chapter 3). Approaches described in future chapters will highlight interdisciplinary and cross-sector collaboration.

CRITICAL THINKING QUESTION 5.1: Reflect on how the determinants of health are framed. Consider whether it is "gender," "race," or "Indigenous status" that shapes health or whether it is more sexism, racism, colonialism, and so on that have a larger influence on the health of these groups.

If you were creating a SDHs framework, how might you characterize the fact that while "race" and "gender" have some bearing on health, in many cases, inequities suffered by groups that are in the nondominant category (e.g., females, visible minorities) are due mainly to their experiences in society that have nothing to do with genetic make-up (e.g., having a Y chromosome or darker skin tone)?

BIOLOGY AND GENETIC ENDOWMENT

An individual's genetic make-up affects that person's health in complex ways, many of which are poorly understood. In general, genes are thought to predispose an individual to certain health conditions, which may manifest themselves when the individual is exposed to certain socioeconomic or environmental factors. Within specific populations in Canada, the clustering of certain gene mutations can lead to an increased incidence of specific genetic disorders. For example, among Canadian (Old Colony) Mennonites, because of familial aggregations of autosomal recessive and dominant conditions, diseases that occur more frequently are insulin-dependent diabetes mellitus, autoimmune diseases, Tourette's syndrome,

---

BOX 5.1 The Social Determinants of Health

- Income and income distribution
- Education
- Unemployment and job security
- Employment and working conditions
- Early childhood development
- Food insecurity
- Housing
- Social exclusion
- Social safety net
- Health services
- Indigenous status
- Gender
- Race
- Disability

Source: Raphael, D. (2009). *Social determinants of health: Canadian perspectives* (2nd ed.). Toronto: Canadian Scholars' Press.

some malformations, inborn errors of metabolism, and other inherited disorders (Baird & Scriver, 1998). Similarly, Nova Scotia has an indigenous black population that is genetically predisposed to carrying or expressing the gene for sickle-cell anemia. The genes for sickle-cell anemia are thought to be more prevalent in certain populations because of the protective advantage they may confer under certain environmental conditions. For example, in carriers, the sickle-cell mutation may protect against malaria (Goheen, Campino, & Cerami, 2017).

Within the area of genetics, epigenetics is emerging to the forefront, demonstrating that genes alone may not be sufficient to determine health status. In many cases, social environments play important roles in shaping and reshaping the genetic endowment of individuals (Landecker & Panofsky, 2013). **Epigenetics** is the study of heritable changes in gene expression (phenotype) that do not involve changes to the underlying DNA sequence, which in turn affect how cells read the genes (Schierding et al., 2017). Epigenetics is concerned with the interaction between genes, the environment (social, physical), and inheritance (Loi, Del Savio, & Stupka, 2013). A particularly interesting area of research that has implications for community health is that of epigenetics and early childhood experiences (see the Research Perspective box).

⟨⟩ RESEARCH PERSPECTIVE

Epigenetics and Early Childhood

It is now well known that the quality of one's early childhood experiences (e.g., whether one received emotional warmth, high-quality interactions with one's caregiver or parent, sensory stimulation) has a lasting impact on a person's physical and mental health in later life. Some researchers are focusing on why this is the case and point to the role that epigenetics plays in linking positive early childhood experiences with good mental health later in life. Emerging evidence points to the fact that the quality of a parent–offspring relationship results in epigenetic changes in the brain (changes to how specific brain genes are expressed) that then affects how a person responds to and copes with stress later in life—which we know is a strong predictor of mental health (Kundakovik & Champage, 2015).

Exercise

Using a community health approach, what programs or policies at a community level do you think may help foster good quality relationships between a parent and her or his offspring soon after birth?

THE DEMOGRAPHY OF THE CANADIAN POPULATION

Demography is the study of populations, especially with reference to size, density, fertility, mortality, growth, age distribution, migration, geography, and vital statistics, all of which can influence health at the population level. A summary of the demography of the Canadian population (when it comes to population size, growth and migration, age structure, and fertility) is presented in Chapter 4. Here we highlight relevant sociodemographic and socioeconomic demographic factors, specifically, that have a bearing on health and its distribution.

Sociodemographic Indicators
Aging

One important demographic change with far-reaching implications, is the rise in the proportion of the population older than 65 years of age. According to new population projections, Canada's population will continue growing in the next quarter century but will age considerably, and the proportion of young people will shrink significantly (Statistics Canada, 2013a). An enormous increase in the number of seniors, attributable to the aging of the baby boomers, combined with continuing low fertility levels and increasing longevity, will age the population rapidly.

The baby boomers—those born in the two decades after World War II—will have the most profound impact on the nation's demographics over the next 25 years. By 2026, one in every five people will be a senior. In 2016, Canada had more seniors than children aged 14 years and younger (Fig. 5.1), a phenomenon never before recorded and a trajectory that is predicted to continue for the next 15 years unless radical changes occur in migration or fertility rates. Because older Canadians are far more likely than younger Canadians to have physical health problems, seniors have been found to account for a disproportionately larger percentage of patient days spent in general hospitals, allied special hospitals, and even mental health hospitals (Canadian Medical Association, 2016). Thus, the growing proportion of seniors in our population will have significant implications for the planning of health care services because our health care system was not built to meet the challenges of our aging population. The health of seniors is discussed in more detail in Chapter 6.

For the first time, the number of persons aged 65 years and older exceed the number of children aged 0 to 14 years

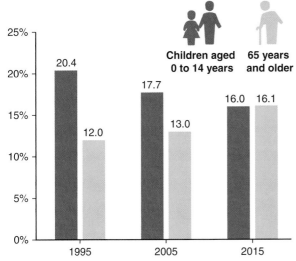

Children aged 0 to 14 years   65 years and older

Fig 5.1 Number of Canadians aged 65 years and older compared to children aged 0 to 14 years. (From Statistics Canada. [2018]. Population estimates, Canada, 2015. Retrieved from https://www150.statcan.gc.ca/n1/pub/11-627-m/11-627-m2015003-eng.htm)

Immigrant Population

The composition of the Canadian population is changing in relation to ethnicity and is expected to continue to change as immigrants migrate into Canada from diverse areas of the world. The impact of immigration policies has offset the decreasing Canadian fertility rate. The number of immigrants coming into Canada has been in the range of 200 000 to 300 000 over the past decade (Statistics Canada, 2016b). (See Chapter 6 for a more detailed discussion regarding the impact of immigration on health and the health status of immigrant communities.)

The 2016 census showed that 7.5 million foreign-born people came to Canada through the immigration process, representing more than one in five persons in Canada (Fig. 5.2). There has been an almost 16% increase since 2016 (Statistics Canada, 2016c). Canada has the highest proportion of foreign-born citizens in the industrialized democracies.

The sources of immigration to Canada have also changed greatly. Asia—including the Middle East—provides the majority of new Canadians: about 60% of all immigrants. The Philippines was the top source country, providing about 16% of all newcomers in 2016. China

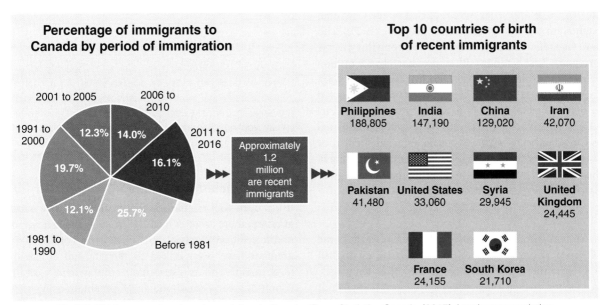

Fig 5.2 2016 census: immigrant population in Canada. (From Statistics Canada. [2017]. Immigrant population in Canada, 2016 Census of population. Retrieved from https://www150.statcan.gc.ca/n1/pub/11-627-m/11-627-m2017028-eng.htm)

and India were third and fourth. More people from Africa are now immigrating to Canada. The number of African immigrants rose from 10% in 2011 to 13.4%, in 2016, with most new Canadians coming from Nigeria, Algeria, Egypt, Morocco, and Cameroon (Statistics Canada, 2017c). Many new immigrants are settling in the Prairie Provinces. Alberta saw a rise from 6.9% in 2001 to 17.1% in 2016, Saskatchewan saw a rise from 1.0% in 2001 to 4.0% in 2016, and Manitoba a rise from 1.8% to 5.2% during the same period. These increases are attributed to government programs and employment availability.

The impact of recent immigration is most clearly seen in big cities. In 2016, immigrants represented 46.1% of Toronto's population, 40.8% of Vancouver's, and 23.4% of Montréal's (Statistics Canada, 2016c).

Ethnicity

Ethnic origin, as defined in the Canadian Census, refers to the ethnic or cultural group(s) to which the respondent's ancestors belong. An ancestor is someone from whom a person is descended and is usually more distant than a grandparent. Ethnic origin pertains to the ancestral roots or background of the population and should not be confused with citizenship or nationality (Statistics Canada, 2015a). In 2016, more than 250 ethnic origins or ancestries were reported by the Canadian population, including 2.1 million people, or 6.2%, who have Canadian Indigenous ancestry. Among this diverse group are First Nations with approximately 1.5 million people, including Cree (356 660), Mi'kmaq (168 480), and Ojibway (125 725). Métis ancestry was reported by 600 000 people, and Inuit ancestry was reported by 79 125 (Statistics Canada, 2017c). Most people listed as Canadian were born in Canada and had English or French as their first language. This suggests that many of these respondents come from families that have been in Canada for several generations.

Language

Canadians who reported speaking only English at home fell from 58.0% in 2011 to 56.8% in 2016, as English is spoken more and more alongside other languages. In Quebec, two in three people who spoke English at home also spoke another language. Outside Quebec, the proportion of the population who reported speaking English at home remained stable at 91.2%. There has been a decline in French as a mother tongue and

a language spoken at home in Canada. In 2016, close to 8.2 million Canadians, or 23.4% of the population, reported speaking French at home, down from 23.8% in 2011. In Quebec, the number of people with French as their first official language spoken (FOLS) rose from 7.7 million in 2011 to 7.9 million in 2016.

Given the recent immigration trends in Canada, it is not surprising that in 2016, 7.6 million persons (21% of the population) reported a first language other than French or English, an increase of almost 1 million (+14.5%) people since 2011. Moreover, the proportion of the Canadian population who speak more than one language at home rose from 17.5% in 2011 to 19.4% in 2016 (Statistics Canada, 2017b). The most common non-official languages spoken in 2016 were Mandarin (641 100 people), Cantonese (594 705 people), Punjabi (568 375 people), Spanish (553 495 people), Tagalog (Filipino; 525 375 people), and Arabic (514 200 people). Proportionally speaking, the number of people who speak each of these languages individually represents between 1.4% and 1.9% of the Canadian population.

EXERCISE 5.1: What are some ways that old age, immigrant status, and speaking a language other than English or French can affect health?

CRITICAL THINKING QUESTION 5.2: Canada's population is changing in many diverse ways. As a health care professional, how do you anticipate your work will change in the next decade, and what new knowledge may you need to learn to better serve these populations?

Socioeconomic Indicators

It has been well established that health follows a social gradient: there is better health with increasing socioeconomic position (Raphael, 2016). The causes of this social gradient have been linked to literacy and education level, income and its distribution, employment, working conditions, early childhood development, housing quality, access to health care, and others as listed in Box 5.1 (Marmot et al., 2008). This section describes how some of these SDHs are distributed within the Canadian population.

Literacy and Educational Attainment

Educational attainment is positively associated with health through a number of factors, such as higher income and better health literacy (Raphael, 2016). From 1990 to 2014, the levels of schooling continued to increase for all population groups in Canada. Education levels reported here are for ages 25 to 64 years (i.e., the working-age population)—people who are old enough to have completed their education but still young enough to work. In 2016, more than half (54.0%) of Canadians had either college or university qualifications, up from 48.3% in 2006 (Fig. 5.3).

Each year the Organisation for Economic Cooperation and Development (OECD) conducts an international comparison of education levels in the working-age population of 30 countries. In 2016, Canada ranked fourth among OECD countries, with 20% of its population aged 25 to 64 years having a university education. The proportion of Canadians aged 25 to 64 years who had completed a high school diploma or equivalency certificate was 91%. The Czech Republic (94%) and Poland (92%) had higher proportions, and the United States was comparable with Canada at 90% (Statistics Canada, 2016d).

The proportions of Canadians aged 25 years and older who had a university education were 31% for women and 26% for men; college education was 25% for women and 19% for men; apprenticeship trades education was 2% women and 8% for men; and nonapprenticeship trades education was 5% for women and 7% for men (Statistics Canada, 2016e).

In 2016, 8.5% of men and 5.4% of women aged 25 to 34 years had less than a high school diploma, representing about 340 000 young Canadians. The level of education attained at the college level increased for both the Métis (from 23% to 26%) and Inuit (from 16% to 19%) from 2011 to 2016. The high school level of education attained among First Nations, Métis, and Inuit aged 25 to 64 years also rose from 71% in 2011 to 74% in 2016 (Statistics Canada, 2016h). Although educational levels are somewhat lower among First Nations, Inuit, and Métis than for the rest of the population, there has been considerable improvement over the previous decades. Additionally, the driving forces behind why some Indigenous communities have lower educational attainment than others in Canada must be considered. As discussed in further detail in Chapter 7, colonialism

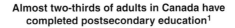

Almost two-thirds of adults in Canada have completed postsecondary education[1]

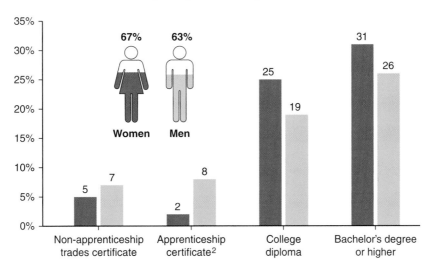

1. The precentages do not add up to the total due to rounding and the exclusion of university qualifications below the bachelor's level.
2. Including journeyperson

Fig 5.3 Postsecondary education in Canada. (From Statistics Canada. [2017]. Canada's educational portrait, 2016 Census of population [Cat. No. 11-627-M]. Retrieved from https://www150.statcan.gc.ca/n1/pub/11-627-m/11-627-m2017036-eng.htm)

and the inequitable funding of education for Indigenous people versus non-Indigenous people have significantly impacted education rates among Indigenous groups. In addition, trauma, the residential school system, and the terms of the *Indian Act* have also affected the gap we see in high school completion rates between the general Canadian population and some Indigenous groups.

Literacy is also an important factor that influences health. Four out of ten Canadian adults have low literacy levels (Statistics Canada, 2012). The ability to access information for the purposes of maintaining or improving health has been termed **health literacy**. Access to and use of information communication technology may have an impact on health literacy (Mackert et al., 2016). According to the Canadian Internet Use Survey (Statistics Canada, 2011), Internet access in Canada has been on an upward trend from 51% of the population in 2000 to 80% in 2009 and 90% in 2018, with education, geography (northern Canada), and income being significant predictors of Internet access (Van Deursen & van Dijk, 2014).

CRITICAL THINKING QUESTION 5.3: Health agencies that do health promotion and health education can improve significantly in terms of making their materials more accessible to people with low levels of literacy. Look at a health promotion campaign (e.g., website, poster, brochure) from your local area or nearest public institution, whether it is a hospital or public heath agency. How does this health promotion material fare in terms of being accessible to people with low levels of literacy? How might you redesign it or communicate the same message in a way that is more accessible?

Income

Income is another major socioeconomic indicator. According to the 2016 Census, the average total income of Canadian households rose from $63 457 in 2005 to $70 336 in 2015, a 10.8% increase. (Statistics Canada, 2016f). Same-sex couples have a higher average income than opposite-sex couples. This may be because a greater proportion of same-sex couples are in their prime working years. Female same-sex couples had a median total income of $92 857 in 2015, while male same-sex couples had a median income of $100 707—the highest among all couple types. Higher education was associated with higher income. Recent immigrants earn substantially less than their Canadian-born counterparts, even after

10 years in the country. This is true for immigrants with low levels of education, as well as for those with a university degree.

To determine whether a person (or family) has low income, Statistics Canada uses **low-income cut-off (LICO)** points (Statistics Canada 2015a), which are based on a survey of family expenditures. The appropriate LICO (given the family size and community size) is compared with the income of the person's economic family. A family that spends more than 54.7% of its income on the basic needs of accommodation, food, and clothing is considered to live under strained circumstances and thus falls below the LICO. Because there is no accepted definition of poverty, the LICO is used by many to study the characteristics of relatively deprived groups in Canada.

In 2015, there were 1.2 million Canadian children (younger than 18 years) living in poverty in Canada (Statistics Canada, 2017d). Certain groups of children are more affected by poverty than others: children in lone-parent families, particularly those headed by a female; Indigenous children; visible minority children; and children of immigrants and refugees. The rate of children living in low-income households varies across the country, with Quebec having the second-lowest rate after Alberta. The reasons may be attributed to Quebec having lower childcare costs and higher child benefits per family than any other province. Quebec is also the only province where children were less likely to live in low-income households than adults (14.3% of children compared with 14.7% of adults) (Statistics Canada, 2017d). The Quebec statistics highlight how important politics and the policy environment are for shaping the SDHs. Policies such as providing tax benefits and subsidizing childcare can reduce rates of childhood poverty, both improving health status for children and reducing the gap that exists between the health of children in low- and high-income households.

Welfare recipients are those who cannot adequately meet their own needs or the needs of their dependents because of their inability to find work, the loss of a spouse who was the main financial support for the family, illness, disability, or other reasons. Welfare payments typically fall substantially below the previously described LICOs set by Statistics Canada. In 2017, 1.1 million people received social assistance in Canada; these included adults who were actual recipients and children living in their households (Maytree, 2019).

BOX 5.2 The Influence of Income and Dental Insurance on Dental Care Utilization

Income and dental insurance are the two most important determinants of dental care utilization. With each step up the income ladder, Canadians were more likely to have visited a dentist. Low-income populations receive oral health care services less frequently than the general population and more so for emergency situations when in pain rather than for preventive care (Canadian Dental Association, 2017).

Low-income Canadians are more likely to die earlier and suffer more illnesses than Canadians with higher incomes, regardless of age, sex, race, and place of residence (see Box 5.2 for an example of how income correlates with dental care utilization). At each rung going up the income ladder, Canadians have less sickness, longer life expectancies, and improved health (Raphael, 2011). Likely, this is because income influences the ability to obtain things one needs for good health (e.g., services, safe housing, nutritious foods) is correlated with education level (which we know is a determinant of health) and can impact things such as stress, quality of the neighbourhood in which you live, exposure to crime, and so on. Income and all that it impacts must be considered when designing programs to improve health (refer to Box 5.3).

Employment and Working Conditions

Improved employment prospects are generally linked to higher education attainment. In 2016, the Canadian employment rate for adults aged 25 to 64 years who had not completed high school (upper secondary education) was 55%, below the OECD average of 58%. By comparison, the employment rate among individuals of the same age group was highest for those who had a community college or university credential at 82%. This was still slightly below the OECD average of 84%.

The working environment includes many factors that affect an individual's health. Safety in the work environment is a key factor and is illustrated by the fact that there are hundreds of work-related fatalities every year in Canada. The Association of Workers' Compensation Boards of Canada (AWCBC, 2002) reported 905 fatalities in 2016. The number and characteristics of work-related health problems are changing as working environments

---

BOX 5.3 The Importance of Considering Income when Planning Community Health Services

The barriers people face when living on a low income must be considered when planning or implementing community health programming, including health promotion. For example, program planners must factor the cost of transportation that people and families have to bear when travelling to and from community health care spaces. Transportation is not cheap and can represent a significant barrier to accessing supports. Many low-income earners do not own cars and need to find other modes of transportation in order to access services. Thus, locating care close to where people are, or even within home settings, can be beneficial and can improve access for those who may need care the most. In some rural and remote communities, where places are quite spread out, this can be a significant challenge.

Second, health promotion messaging must be viewed through a social determinants of health lens. Often public health messaging advises peoples to eat healthier or be more active. However, health sector care providers must consider that in some cases people do not have ready access to affordable fresh and healthy foods, nor do they have the time or money to participate in leisure time activities. Approaches and health promotion messaging must consider the very real barriers that some people face with incorporating healthy eating and active living into day-to-day living.

---

change. Since World War II, the labour force has shifted gradually from goods-producing jobs in manufacturing, construction, and primary industries to less physically hazardous service-producing jobs, for example, in the financial, technology, and business services. Thus, the nature of the hazards has changed from those that are physical to those that are psychosocial. The increased participation of women in the workforce, generally in the service sector, has led to new concerns regarding safety of the working environment for pregnant mothers and their fetuses. The effect of the physical working environment on health is described in Chapter 12.

Labour markets have also changed dramatically in the past decade due in part to a response to globalization, trade competition, and technological innovation. Many workers in advanced economies now face limited employment prospects and poor working conditions (Sweet & Meiksins, 2015). Adverse labour conditions are related to either the availability of work (e.g., unemployment, job insecurity, and overwork) or to the nature of work (e.g., increasing job demands, low job position within a firm, and contingent employment). Overall, unemployment rates in Canada have decreased since the 1990s from 11.0% to 5.8% in 2018. Employment has grown by 1.5% from 2017 to 2018 and can be attributable to gains in full-time work, while part-time employment remained unchanged. Over the same period, hours worked rose by 3.2%. There has recently been a shift to longer standard working hours in some provinces, including Ontario. Globally, there has been a move toward lean production models (input of fewer resources to do the same job), leading to job strain (Landsbergis et al., 2017).

All these changes can have profound health consequences. For example, unemployed adults have been found to have gains of over 10% in body mass index (BMI), earlier deaths, and other health problems compared to employed adults (Hughes et al., 2017; Monsivais et al., 2015). This, in turn, can result in the use of extra health services by unemployed persons, costing millions of dollars to the health care system (Canadian Public Health Association, 1996).

Having a sick or aging relative often imposes additional, unpaid, work, especially for women. For caregivers who are also employed, it can increase work stress and harm their job security because of absences to care for the relative. The resulting reduced income affects the whole family. See Box 5.4 for an intervention that helps with those caring for others.

EXERCISE 5.2: How might unemployment affect health?

Homelessness

Homelessness describes the situation of an individual, family, or community without stable, safe, permanent, appropriate housing, or the immediate prospect, means and ability of acquiring it (Gaetz et al., 2012).

BOX 5.5   Social Determinants of Homelessness

A social determinants of health perspective helps us to focus on the causes or determinants of homelessness and explains how homelessness can contribute to a range of health challenges. For example, a number of social determinants can influence the health status of an individual who is experiencing homelessness: income, housing, level of education, ability access to health services, ethnicity, social exclusion, federal, provincial, and local policies can all interact together to negatively impact the experience of homelessness, and will influence how being homeless can negatively impact health.

Group Exercise

1. What are some challenges of providing preventive and curative services to someone who is homeless in an urban centre versus in a rural community?
2. What are the major health risks that are associated with homelessness?

The causes of homelessness are complex. They include poverty, changes in the housing market, reductions in social assistance, family violence, substance abuse, and changing mental health services (Box 5.5). As a result, the composition of this group now includes (1) **unsheltered**, or absolutely homeless and living on the streets or in places not intended for human habitation; (2) **emergency sheltered**, including those staying in overnight shelters for people who are homeless, as well as shelters for those impacted by family violence; (3) **provisionally accommodated**, referring to those whose accommodation is temporary or lacks security of tenure, often referred to as **couch surfing**, hidden homelessness describes people who are staying with relatives, friends, neighbours, or strangers because they have no other option; and finally, 4) **at risk of homelessness**, referring to people who are not homeless but whose current economic or housing situation is precarious or does not meet public health and safety standards. It should be noted that for many people, homelessness is a fluid experience, in which one's shelter circumstances and options may shift and change quite dramatically and with frequency.

Homelessness is associated with increased health risks (see the In the News box for an example of how homelessness contributes to injury and mortality).

Cardiovascular disease is a leading cause of death among homeless people and particularly among men (Gozdzik et al., 2015). There is also evidence that homelessness may add to poor health by posing barriers to the management of health conditions such as diabetes (White, Logan, & Magwood, 2016). Additionally, many homeless persons are ex-clients (former clients) of mental health institutions, runaway teenagers, women and children escaping from domestic violence, seniors, and Indigenous people. In 2016, the first nationally coordinated point-in-time homeless count was conducted with 32 communities and, in 2018, with more than 60 communities across Canada. Estimates for the number of homeless vary because it is difficult to count them; however, the various estimates suggest that each year, approximately 235 000 Canadians experience homelessness (Homeless Hub, 2018a).

In 2017, the Canadian National Housing Strategy (NHS) was released with a $40 billion commitment over 10 years (2018–2028), of which approximately $11 billion is new funding; the rest is reallocated from existing ongoing programs (Government of Canada, 2017).

Community health providers, recognizing the effect of homelessness on multiple aspects of health, have developed targeted services for people who experience homelessness that are multidisciplinary in nature. One example of an organization like this is the Inner City Health Associates (ICHA) in Toronto, which provides primary care, mental health, and palliative care services to people experiencing homelessness in shelters and drop-in centres across the city. To address the multidimensional nature of the challenges encountered by people experiencing homelessness or at risk of homelessness, ICHA employs a range of professionals, including registered nurses, nurse practitioners, social workers, psychiatrists, family doctors, and outreach coordinators (ICHA, n.d.). Social workers are instrumental to this team because they can provide counselling services, as well as link people with much-needed income support programs (including social assistance and unemployment benefits, as appropriate) and connect people to the services they need to obtain social or subsidized housing or emergency shelter. For an innovative example of multidisciplinary care serving the justice needs of people at risk of or experiencing homelessness, refer to the Interprofessional Practice box.

IN THE NEWS

Risks of Being Homeless

In 2015, a man who was believed to have been homeless was found dead inside a makeshift shelter in Toronto that had burned down because of a fire. The hypothesis at the time was that the man may have started the fire to keep himself warm in the wake of freezing temperatures. This incident followed the deaths of three homeless people in Toronto the previous week. All three were believed to have died as a result of freezing temperatures. The issue of fatal accidents and injuries, resulting from living in harsh environmental conditions, continues to be a major concern regarding individuals who are homeless.

Source: Mangione, K. (2015). Homeless man's body found in burned makeshift shelter in Toronto. *CTV News*, January 14. Retrieved from https://www.ctvnews.ca/canada/homeless-man-s-body-found-in-burned-makeshift-shelter-in-toronto-1.2187847.

INTERPROFESSIONAL PRACTICE

The Health Justice Program at St. Michael's Hospital

The housing and legal sectors often overlap. For example, having a criminal record can predispose someone to homelessness (because it affects a person's opportunities to access employment and housing, and people with criminal records often face overt discrimination in these two areas), people who are homeless or at risk of homelessness may be victims of criminal activity (e.g., domestic violence, unfair evictions), and being homeless may put people at risk for being incarcerated because seeking shelter in certain places may be criminalized. As such, people at risk of or experiencing homelessness often have the need for a range of legal services, including support for issues like evictions, tenant–landlord disputes, employee rights, family law, child custody, denied benefits, and so on (Homeless Hub, 2018b).

The Health Justice Program at St. Michaels Hospital (a hospital in downtown Toronto that serves inner-city populations) recognized this need and brought together health and legal partners who don't often come together under one roof. As a result, social workers, primary care nurse practitioners, and others working in health settings that serve homeless communities can work together and learn from legal professionals, as well as refer their clients for consultation with lawyers who offer

🏛 INTERPROFESSIONAL PRACTICE

The Health Justice Program at St. Michael's Hospital

free legal education, brief services, and connection to longer term legal services (St. Michael's Hospital, 2019). This unique interprofessional partnership means that people working in the legal sector can learn more about the health challenges that their clients face, and those working in the health sector can learn more about the influence of the justice sector (another important determinant of health) on the well-being of their clients.

Stress

Chronic stress has a significant impact on the health of Canadians, and how it affects health is described in Chapters 1, 8, and 9. **Chronic stress** can occur in response to everyday stressors that are ignored or poorly managed, as well as to exposure to traumatic events (American Psychological Association, n.d.). In 2016, one in four (23%) Canadians reported experiencing high chronic stress. Women are more likely than men to report stress (29% vs 25% respectively, age 35–49 years old) (Statistics Canada, 2016g). People in these age groups are most likely to be managing multiple responsibilities with their careers and families. In contrast, 10.0% of men and 12.3% of women aged 65 years of age or older were least likely to find their days stressful. The least educated group is more than twice as likely as university graduates to report high stress.

> **EXERCISE 5.3:** What are some reasons why people with lower levels of educational attainment may experience high levels of stress?

Research published in the past decade or so has highlighted the issue of chronic stress among Indigenous women in particular. Faced with a range of stressors as a direct result of the historical impact of colonialism and residential schools on generations of Indigenous people (including separation from family and friends, loss of languages and cultures, forced assimilation, violence, trauma, and racism, to name a few), Indigenous women have demonstrated very high levels of perceived stress (see Chapter 7). This is an important issue, given the impact that chronic stress has on the development of cardiovascular disease and mental health issues (Benoit et al., 2016). It is important, therefore, to focus on not only finding ways to enhance community resiliency and coping but also to also shift the underlying conditions that result in chronic stress, such as exposure to violence, homelessness, poverty, and others.

> **CRITICAL THINKING QUESTION 5.4:** Think about the last time you offered healthy living advice to a client in a health care setting. Were these recommendations easy to follow for your client? Might your client have experienced any barriers related to the SDHs when it came to consistently following your advice? How could you have shifted your approach, and what else can you do to be an advocate for your clients who face barriers such as low income?

THE PHYSICAL ENVIRONMENT

The physical environment includes physical, biological, chemical, and radiological factors found in food, water, soil, indoor and outdoor air, the built environment, and animal and insect vectors. Public interest in environmental issues has generally increased over the past 50 years, and concomitantly, so has public support for more extensive and strict control of environmental agents.

Although the negative impact of the environment on health has been widely publicized, the positive impact of the environment must not be forgotten; being immersed in nature and the outdoor environment can be a source of calm and healing, with positive mental health impacts, and substances such as fluoride in the water can be of great benefit when it comes to protecting against dental cavities. Information on specific physical environmental contaminants is presented in Chapter 11, which deals with environmental health.

Agricultural Exposure

The agricultural sector continues to be important sector across Canada. However, there are concerns about health and safety issues in modern, competitive agriculture, which depends heavily on mechanization and the use of pesticides, herbicides, fertilizers, fungicides, and efficient feeding techniques to achieve economies of scale. Recent widely publicized concerns include the use of genetic technology to produce genetically modified food crops, the widespread use of antibiotics as growth factors in animal agriculture, the suspected relationship of a new variant of Creutzfeldt-Jacob disease in humans to bovine spongiform encephalopathy in beef-industry cows fed animal-containing products, the fecal contamination of drinking water supplies by run-offs from nearby farms, and the adequacy of drinking water regulations and legislation in safeguarding the drinking water supply.

Occupational hazards also exist for those working within agricultural industries. Grain workers and swine and poultry producers are at significant risk for respiratory disorders as a result of intensive feeding techniques and of confinement of poultry. Disabling injuries from accidents also occur.

Outdoor Air Quality

Air quality affects human health and well-being, ecosystems, and climate change. Health effects related to air pollution include impacts on pulmonary, cardiac, vascular, and neurologic systems. In Canada, it is estimated that there are 14 400 deaths attributable to air pollution each year (Statistics Canada, 2017e).

Over the past 30 years, Canada has made significant gains in improving outdoor air quality. There has been a decline in the concentration of hazardous air pollutants such as sulphur dioxide, nitrogen dioxide, lead, dust, and smoke. Ground-level ozone (ozone within 11 km of the Earth's surface) creates smog and is one of the most serious air pollution problems in Canadian cities, with significant associations to both respiratory hospital admissions and respiratory mortality. However, the ozone layer (located 11 to 47 km above the Earth's surface in the stratosphere) acts as a barrier to ultraviolet B radiation. The discovery of the depletion of this ozone layer has led to concerns about the increased risks of skin cancer. There has also been concern about global warming, a phenomenon of rising temperatures on Earth that are thought to result from increases in the concentrations of certain greenhouse gases (described in detail in Chapter 11).

CRITICAL THINKING QUESTION 5.5: Climate change is one of the pressing issues of our time. How might climate change affect health status? How do you think climate change might affect health equity?

LIFESTYLE AND BEHAVIOURAL RISK FACTORS

The Lalonde report (see Chapter 1) placed great emphasis on lifestyle elements and the personal behaviour of Canadians as major factors in determining their health. Emphasis continues to be placed on modifying these risk factors (e.g., improving healthy eating, reducing alcohol and tobacco intake) in disease prevention and health promotion, although there is increasing recognition that the social and economic environment in which individuals live and work also affects their ability and motivation to change their behaviour and lifestyle. As mentioned earlier, people living with low incomes or in precarious employment may face significant challenges when it comes to accessing affordable healthy and fresh foods and may not have leisure time in which to engage in structured physical activity. Thus, factors such as the policy environment, income, employment, and built environment have a very large influence on people's lifestyle and behaviours, including taking up health care interventions that are preventive in nature (e.g., immunization, screening, and preventive sexual practices such as using a condom).

Preventive Health Practices
Immunization

The routine use of vaccines has led to significant reductions in vaccine-preventable diseases. Vaccination programs are considered to be the most cost-beneficial health intervention, leading to far more dollar benefits than costs. Routine immunization programs for children are among the most cost-effective interventions. Vaccines are discussed in more detail in Chapter 10.

Because of the success of vaccination programs, the mortality and morbidity previously associated with many vaccine-preventable diseases have been forgotten. Although this is a good thing, it has also contributed to the rise in vaccine hesitancy, which the WHO named in 2019 as one of top 10 threats to global public health (see Chapter 10 for more detail on this growing problem) (WHO, 2019b).

The Childhood National Immunization Coverage Survey (cNICS) is conducted approximately every 2 years to estimate national uptake for all routine childhood immunizations recommended by the National Advisory Committee on Immunization (NACI). It is a representation of how many people in our nation get vaccinated. Overall, the results demonstrated that Canadians are not meeting the national targets set by the NACI (Health Canada, 2018). The survey also asked parents questions regarding their knowledge, attitudes, and beliefs regarding vaccines. The majority of respondents strongly agreed or somewhat agreed that childhood vaccines are safe (95%), effective (97%), and important for children's health (97%). On the other hand, respondents strongly agreed (34%) or somewhat agreed (36%) that they were concerned about potential side effects from vaccines. Thus, vaccine hesitancy remains an issue in the Canadian context.

Preventive Sexual Health Practices

In addition to unplanned pregnancies, unsafe sexual behaviour can lead to serious conditions such as sexually transmitted infections (STIs), infertility, HIV, and other infections. In a recent study, Canadians aged 40 to 59 years were less likely to use condoms than their younger counterparts. The online survey found that 65% of men in that age bracket reported not using a condom the last time they had sex; the number jumped to 72% for women (McKay, Quinn-Nilas, & Milhausen, 2017). Respondents had a surprisingly cavalier attitude towards STIs, with 58% saying they were either not very or not at all concerned about contracting an STI.

The Health Behaviour in School-Aged Children study (HBSC)—a WHO collaborative cross-national study focusing on relationships—evaluated health outcomes, attitudes, and behaviours during the 2013 to 2014 academic year. Overall, the majority of Canadian 15-year-olds had not had sexual intercourse; they appeared to be waiting longer to have sexual intercourse than in previous years (Statistics Canada, 2016i). The majority of sexually experienced students used a condom the last time they had sexual intercourse, and more than 80% used some form of contraception. Higher family, school, and community support were found to be related to lower likelihood of having had sexual intercourse.

> **CRITICAL THINKING QUESTION 5.6:** What individual level factors may help to explain why a person might not use a condom or might be cavalier about contracting an STI? How might the various SDHs described in Box 5.1 influence the factors you have described?

Injury Prevention Practices

Use of Protective Devices. Seatbelts and bicycle helmets are examples of **protective devices.** Although vital for preventing morbidity and mortality, the use of protective devices exemplifies how preventive health practices are not always universally adopted.

Motor vehicle collisions are a leading cause of death and injury in Canada, especially in young adults. The established role of seatbelts in reducing fatalities has been well publicized. Seatbelts save about 1 000 lives a year in Canada, yet Transport Canada reports that although 93% of Canadians buckle up, the 7% who don't account for almost 40% of fatalities in vehicle collisions. Data released by the Ontario Provincial Police in 2018 indicated that six of seven people killed in motor vehicle collisions between September 7 and 13 of that year were not wearing seatbelts (Canadian Safety Council, 2013).

Similarly, helmet use is known to be protective for head injuries, but helmets are still inconsistently used. In 2013 and 2014, of the estimated 12 million cyclists aged 12 years or older, 5 million (42%) reported "always" wearing a helmet (users); the remaining 7 million did so "most of the time," "rarely" or "never." However, the number of cyclists wearing helmets is up significantly from 25 years ago, when helmet use was much less common. In 1994, only 19% of those who had cycled in the past 3 months "always" wore a helmet, compared with 45% in 2013 and 2014. The increase among 12- to 14-year-olds was almost threefold—from 18% to 50%—which may reflect, at least in part, introduction of bicycle helmet legislation.

Although females were less likely than males to cycle, they were more likely to wear a helmet—46% compared with 39%. Higher helmet use (47%) in the early teen years coincided with the ages when cycling prevalence was highest. These are also the years when parents and caregivers may find it easier to enforce helmet use, which is legislated in several provinces, territories, and cities. However, in the later teen (15–17) and early adult (18–24) years, helmet use dropped to 28% and 25%, respectively. At older ages, the percentage rose again—49% of cyclists aged 50 years or older "always" wore a helmet.

Distracted Driving. Distracted driving is a national safety issue. The Canadian Council of Motor Transport Administrators' Distracted Driving Subcommittee defines **distracted driving** as "the diversion of attention from driving, as a result of the driver focusing on a non-driving object, activity, event, or person. This diversion reduces awareness, decision making, or performance leading to increased risk of driver error, near-crashes, or crashes. The diversion of attention is not attributable to a medical condition, alcohol/drug use and/or fatigue" (Canadian Council of Motor Transport Administrators, 2018, p. 4).

There are numerous possible driver distractions, including:

- Use of electronic devices, such as global positioning systems (GPS), CD and DVD players, radios, cell phones, laptops, personal digital assistants (PDAs) and MP3 players
- Reading maps, directions or other material
- Grooming (e.g. combing hair, putting on make-up or shaving)
- Eating or drinking
- Talking with passengers or tending to children or pets
- Visual distractions outside the vehicle, such as collisions, police activity, or looking at street signs or billboards

The availability of cells phones offers some benefit to drivers, such as allowing them to make emergency calls quickly. However, cellphone use during driving appears to increase the risk of a motor vehicle collision. In a study of 700 drivers who had cellular telephones and were involved in motor vehicle collisions resulting in substantial property damage but no personal injury, the risk of a collision when using a cellular telephone was four times higher than the risk when a cellular telephone was not used (Redelmeier & Tibshirani, 1997). This relative risk is similar to the hazard associated with driving with a blood alcohol level at the legal limit. Hands-free devices offered no safety advantage over handheld units. Thus, these vehicle collisions may have been the result of a decrease in the driver's attention rather than dexterity.

Driving Under the Influence of Marijuana. In Canada, cannabis became legalized in 2018, although before legalization, it was still a very commonly consumed substance (see Chapter 9 for more detail on cannabis and cannabis legalization). A 2018 survey undertaken by Statistics Canada found that around 19% of men and 11% of women reported using cannabis in the past 3 months (Statistics Canada, 2019). Perhaps more surprisingly, the survey found that around one in seven people who consumed cannabis regularly reported driving a vehicle within 2 hours of using cannabis over the previous three months (Tasker, 2018).

Cannabis affects our ability to drive because it can impact attention, vigilance, perception of time and speed, and the use of knowledge. Drivers under the effects of cannabis tend to have slower reaction times, drive more slowly, and keep a larger distance from the car ahead. The brain effects of cannabis also vary with how the drug is absorbed—via the lungs, digestive tract, or the skin. The current recommendations from the evidence-based publication, *Canada's Lower-Risk Cannabis Use Guidelines*, endorse not driving for at least 6 hours after using cannabis (Fischer et al., 2017). However, the wait time can be longer, depending on the user and the properties of the specific cannabis product used. Using new simulation technology, the iDAPT Driver Lab (see http://www.idapt.org/index-.php/labs-services/research-labs/ceal-labs/driverlab) is testing various conditions that affect driving performance, including cannabis use for both for medical and recreational purposes.

The Importance of the Policy Environment for Injury Prevention Practices

Although education efforts can support the uptake of injury prevention practices (e.g., use of helmets or seatbelts, not engaging in distracted driving or consuming cannabis before driving), often the policy environment can have a much more major effect. Policy interventions such as legislation to mandate the use of seatbelts is correlated to these preventive practices and as such, when thinking through why the uptake of such practices might be low one must be very mindful and consider the policy environment.

For example, one of the main reasons traffic fatalities decreased by just over 50% between 1975 and 2003 is because of seatbelt laws across the country (Government of Canada, 2008). Following the very tragic accident killing 16 young hockey players in a bus crash in Humboldt, Saskatchewan, which devastated the community and drew widespread national attention, new legislation regarding seatbelt use on buses will come into effect by 2020. Transport Canada is making seatbelts mandatory on newly built medium and large highway buses. As a result of these changes, all highway buses built on September 1, 2020, or later will require seatbelts (Transport Canada, 2018), which will undoubtedly influence seatbelt use on buses.

Similar to seatbelt laws, a variety of laws exist in Canada around mandating the use of helmets, which also impacts people's behaviours. For example, in Saskatchewan, no laws exist mandating the use of bike helmets, whereas in Manitoba, minors must wear bike helmets (Cycle Helmets, n.d.).

When it comes to legislation related to distracted driving, in December 2002, Newfoundland and Labrador was the first Canadian province to pass legislation banning cellular phones while driving. Currently, all 10 provinces in Canada have some form of cell phone or distracted driving legislation in place. However, although legislation that bans cell phone use or bans eating or drinking in vehicles helps with some types of distraction, it does not cover all forms of distracted driving. It is harder to pass laws that address distracted driving as a result of talking to another passenger or even being distracted by thoughts or problems, for example. Enforcing these types of bans would be nearly impossible and public acceptance would be low and, as such, distracted driving remains a policy challenge.

Last as a result of the legalization of cannabis, new laws have been put into place regarding driving under the influence. For example, Bill C-46s create new provisions in the Criminal Code of Canada for drug-impaired driving, with penalties ranging from fines to prison time.

EXERCISE 5.4: Look up Bill C-46 and the new laws and penalties that accompany drug-impaired driving.

What are some of the health equity implications of such a law?

Diet and Nutrition

Good nutrition is vital to maintaining good health, preventing disease, and reducing the severity of disease all throughout the life cycle. (The impact of nutrition on health is discussed in Chapter 8.) Overall, dietary habits have changed quite a bit over the past 50 to 100 years and are significantly influenced by income and education levels, pointing to the importance of the policy and upstream determinants of health on lifestyle and behaviours. According to the Canadian Community Health Survey, for example, 10% of the population consume most of their calories from snacks (which tend to be high in unhealthy ingredients such as salt, sugar, and fat). Additionally, on any given day, about 20 to 30% of the population ate food prepared at a fast food outlet.

It is also reported that most Canadians consume more than the recommended amount of saturated fat (fat found in baked goods that is particularly bad for health) (Nishi, Jessri, & L'Abbé, 2018). In terms of fruit and vegetable consumption (important sources of fibre and other nutrients), only 30% of Canadians aged 12 years and older reported consuming fruits and vegetables five or more times per day. Interestingly, both education and income are correlated with fruit and vegetable intake. In families in which the highest level of education is below a postsecondary degree, 24% consumed fruits and vegetables five or more times a day. However, in families in which the highest level of education is postsecondary or above, nearly 32% of people consumed fruits and vegetables five or more times a day. Similarly, families that fall into the highest income quintile consume more fruits and vegetables per day than families that are in the lowest quintile group (Statistics Canada, 2017g).

Food Environments

As mentioned earlier, food environments greatly influence the availability, affordability, and social acceptability of food and nutrition "choices." **Food environments** include the physical, social, economic, cultural, and political factors within a community or region (Rideout, Mah, & Minaker, 2015). There is an association between food environments and diet-related outcomes. People who are socioeconomically disadvantaged tend to have decreased access to grocery stores where healthy foods are available and affordable. They have increased access to fast food outlets, where unhealthy foods tend to be more available (Luan, Minaker, & Law, 2016).

Food Insecurity

Being food insecure means you have limited or unsustainable access to nutritionally adequate, safe foods, or the inability to acquire personally acceptable foods in socially acceptable ways (Food and Agriculture Organization, 2001). The Household Food Security Survey Module (HFSSM) in the CCHS measured food insecurity; however, not all provinces and territories participated. Combining the results of Alberta, Saskatchewan, Ontario, Quebec, New Brunswick, Nova Scotia, Prince Edward Island, the Northwest Territories, and Nunavut, 12% of households experienced some level of food insecurity during the previous 12 months in 2014. This represents 1.3 million households, or 3.2 million individuals, including nearly 1 million children younger

BOX 5.6 Food Access in Nunavut

Nunavut is Canada's geographically largest and least-populated territory. It is home to about 32 000 people in 25 fly-in-only communities. There are very high rates of food insecurity among the Inuit, with 70% of Inuit preschoolers living in food-insecure households. The reasons for this are complex and multifold and include things such as the high cost of transporting food in rural areas, colonialism and the loss of traditional ways of being (such as hunting and sourcing food locally), and poverty and unemployment caused by historical legacies such as colonialism and the *Indian Act* (Arriagada, 2017). As a result, a number of community initiatives have been developed to help support food-insecure households, including food banks, community kitchens, community freezer programs, and greenhouses (Feeding Nunavut, n.d.).

Often, however, these programs provide an abundance of nonperishable food items, but what people really want is a return to traditional country foods, including foods such as caribou or maktaaq. A community organization known as Feeding Nunavut is helping to solve this challenge by helping to support hunters. The organization is starting a pilot program to cover the costs of gas and ammunition so that hunters can hunt traditional foods and return some of their catch back to soup kitchens, food banks, and other programs to support food-insecure families (Murray, 2016). This helps to promote the consumption of traditional country foods (which tend to be healthier), support the traditional practice of hunting, and reduce rates of food insecurity in the population.

income was social assistance, 61% were food insecure, as were 35.6% of those reliant on employment insurance or workers' compensation. However, the majority of food-insecure households (62.2%) were reliant on wages or salaries from employment. Other household characteristics associated with a higher likelihood of food insecurity included having an income below the Low Income Measure (29.2%), being Indigenous (25.7%), being Black (29.4%), and renting rather than owning one's home (24.5%). The lowest rate of food insecurity was in Quebec City, where 1 in 14 households were food insecure.

Food insecurity has been identified as a significant social and health problem in Canada. Limited budgets for those in food-insecure households result in purchasing cheaper, nutrient-poor foods that are high in fat, sugar, and salt, which can contribute to weight gain and an increased risk of many chronic diseases, including type 2 diabetes. The lack of access to nutritious foods is not only a risk factor for developing chronic illness but also compromises the ability to manage health conditions that involve specific dietary regimens.

In 1981, Canadian charities began setting up food banks as a temporary measure to help people deal with food-insecure emergencies. The pressure on food banks to deliver other kinds of social services has also increased well beyond their capacity to deal with them. Other services, run mainly by civil society organizations, occasionally with support from provincial/territorial or municipal governments, include community kitchens and gardens, food-buying clubs, and school-based breakfast and lunch programs. There is a current need for interventions to target economic factors at the root of food insecurity and the broader systemic factors that shape food environments, production, and distribution (Tait et al., 2018). Most provinces and territories in Canada have initiated poverty reduction strategies; however, they have not prioritized reducing food insecurity as part of the strategy.

than the age of 18 years. More than 1 in 6 children younger than the age of 18 years lived in households that experienced food insecurity. Food insecurity was most prevalent in Canada's North (especially Nunavut; see Box 5.6) and the Maritimes in 2014. In Nunavut and the Northwest Territories, the prevalence rose to the highest levels observed since monitoring began in 2005, 46.8%, and 24.1%, respectively.

Some groups of people may be more at risk to food insecurity than others, as shown in a number of studies on food bank use, poverty, and dietary intake. Poverty is one of several factors that impede access to sufficient, safe, and nutritious foods. There are vulnerable people with low incomes who cannot meet their food requirements without compromising other basic needs, such as shelter. Among households whose major source of

---

EXERCISE 5.5: Research the Nutrition North Program. Keeping in mind the principles of community health—including empowerment, sustainability, and fostering self-determination—what are some of the concerns you might have about this program? Suggest ways to improve the program while at the same time improving self-determination and community empowerment.

Physical Activity and Literacy

Physical activity is important for health and well-being. Physical activity with health benefits includes moderate to vigorous physical activity, causing children to sweat, breathe harder, or be out of breath. Only one third of kids are meeting the physical activity recommendation (Colley et al., 2017). Research has shown that 82% of adults in Canada do not attain the recommended minimum of 150 minutes of moderate to vigorous physical activity per week (Statistics Canada, 2013b). It is estimated that physical inactivity is responsible for 6% of coronary heart disease, 7% of type 2 diabetes, 10% of breast cancer, 10% of colon cancer, and 9% of premature mortality worldwide (Ding et al., 2016). Being physically active is strongly linked to healthy aging; reduced risk for premature death; reduced risk of diseases and conditions such as obesity, heart disease, some types of cancer, diabetes, dementia, osteoporosis, and cardiovascular issues; and better health in people who are living with various diseases and conditions (e.g., cancer, diabetes, mood disorders). In general, males are more likely than females to engage in vigorous activity.

The top eight leisure-time physical activities for the Canadian population aged 12 years and older are walking, gardening, home exercises, swimming, cycling, jogging, dancing, and weight training (Gilmour, 2007). Leisure-time physical activity is less prevalent among people in lower income groups, compared with the highest income group, even when sociodemographic characteristics, non–leisure-time activity, and activity restrictions are taken into account. Immigrants, regardless of how long they had been in Canada, were less likely to be moderately active in their leisure time than Canadians overall, even when adjustments were made to account for the different age distributions of the two groups (Mahmood et al., 2018). Off-reserve Indigenous people were more likely to be at least moderately active than were Canadians overall (Findlay, 2015). Canadians are more likely to be active if their neighborhoods have places to walk to (e.g., stores), free or low-cost recreational facilities, areas specifically for cycling, good sidewalks, interesting features, and higher levels of safety.

The concept of physical literacy has gained prominence in recent years. Educational organizations and researchers have argued that physical literacy should be given the same educational value as literacy and numeracy. **Physical literacy** is defined as the motivation, confidence, physical competence, knowledge, and understanding to value and take responsibility for engagement in physical activities for life (ParticipACTION, 2018). Physical literacy is an antecedent of physical activity, while also being developed through physical activity. The promotion of physical literacy is a key opportunity to generate significant health benefits in both children and adults.

> **EXERCISE 5.6:** What are some reasons that might explain why leisure-time physical activity is less prevalent among people in lower income groups?

Body Mass Index and Obesity

The **body mass index (BMI)** is commonly used to determine if an individual is in a healthy weight range. BMI is calculated by dividing a person's weight in kilograms by their height in metres squared. However, BMI does not consider lifestyle behaviours like dietary quality and physical activity, which are, in fact, stronger determinants of death and disease. A BMI of 30 kg/m² or higher is considered obese for adults aged 18 years and older. A BMI between 25 and 30 kg/m² is considered overweight. In 2014, 20.2% of Canadians aged 18 years and older, roughly 5.3 million adults, reported height and weight that classified them as **obese** (Statistics Canada 2015c). The rate of obesity among men increased to 21.8% in 2014 from 20.1% in 2013 and is the highest obesity rate for men reported since 2003 (in 2003, 16.0% of men were obese). Among women, the rate of obesity in 2014 (18.7%) was an increase over 2013 and was also up significantly from 2003, when it was 14.5%. The rates of adults who reported height and weight that classified them as **overweight** in 2014 were 40.0% for men and 27.5% for women. The percentage of men who were overweight was about the same as 2012 but was a decrease from 41.9% in 2013. The rate among women has been stable since 2003 (Statistics Canada, 2015b). Individuals with lower income, those with lower educational attainment or working in lower grade occupation, are more likely to have higher BMIs than individuals in higher-income groups (Lebel et al., 2018), and this may be a result of a number of factors, such as access to healthy built environments, adequate food environments, and leisure time. Obesity is a risk factor for multiple health problems, including type 2 diabetes, cardiovascular diseases, and certain types of cancers. Common risk factors for many of these conditions include unhealthy eating, physical inactivity, harmful use of alcohol, and tobacco use. Obesity is often considered both a health problem and a risk condition associated with other diseases.

The rise in obesity and overweight has been linked to what some call the **nutrition transition**, a shift in diet, food practices, and food supply chains towards greater quantity and variety of foods, accompanied by an increase in consumption of meats, fats, and processed foods (Drewnowski, 2017; Popkin, 2015).

It is important to keep in mind, however, that both the issue of obesity and physical inactivity are strongly linked to the policy and food environments. As described earlier, the more access people have to affordable healthy food outlets and built environments that foster walking and other forms of active transport, the better everyone's health can be, and as such, policy approaches must be considered when thinking through how to address these complex issues.

CRITICAL THINKING QUESTIONS 5.7: Thinking about the community in which you live, ask yourself the following:

1. What are the food environments like around the schools?
2. How do you think the food environment around schools influences what students eat before, during, and after school?
3. What are some solutions that could positively influence the neighbourhoods where schools are located?

THE USE OF HEALTH CARE SERVICES

Health care organization (also discussed in Part 3 of this book) is also a major determinant of health. The major feature is the availability of universal health insurance for all Canadians, which has significantly contributed to reducing the inequities in access to health care within the population.

Contact with Health Care Professionals

In 2014, 14.9% of Canadians aged 12 years and older, roughly 4.5 million people, reported that they did not have a regular medical doctor. Men were more likely than women to report being without a regular doctor in

all age groups from 20 to 64 years of age. Canadians visit the emergency department (ED) more than other countries—and we wait longer, too: It takes about 4 hours of waiting to see a doctor when you're in the emergency department. More than 40% of Canadians said the last time they went to the ED, it was to treat something their family doctor could have helped with if they were available. These issues ranged from throat inflammation, ear infections, to needing antibiotics. Canadians also report the longest wait times for specialists, with more than half (56%) waiting longer than 4 weeks to see a specialist, compared with the international average of 36% (Canadian Institute for Health Information, 2016) (Fig. 5.4). Wait times are discussed in Part 3 of this book.

Complementary and Alternative Medicine

Complementary medicine refers to a range of services offered outside of the traditional health care system that is used alongside conventional medical treatments, whereas **alternative medicine** is generally used instead of conventional medical treatment. Examples include traditional Chinese medicine, homeopathy, naturopathy, acupuncture, massage therapy, tai chi, herbs, dietary supplements, and probiotics. (For the purposes of this discussion, chiropractors are included among alternative health care providers.)

A survey conducted by the Fraser Institute revealed that more than three quarters of Canadians (79%) had used at least one complementary or alternative therapy sometime in their lives in 2016. This compares with 74% in 2006 and 73% in 1997. Among the provinces in 2016, British Columbians were most likely to have used an alternative therapy during their lifetime (89%) followed by Albertans (84%) and Ontarians (81%). Conversely, those in Quebec (69%) were least likely to have done so. In this survey, massage was the most common therapy used: 44% tried it, followed by chiropractic care (42%), yoga (27%), relaxation techniques (25%), and acupuncture (22%). In 2016, the most likely users of complementary and alternative therapies were between the ages of 35 to 44 years old (61%). The use of complementary and alternative medicines and treatments diminished with age and generally rose with both income and education (Fraser Institute, 2016).

The following Case Study brings together all the learning from this chapter about the determinants of health.

EXERCISE 5.7: How might the use of complementary therapies impact health (both positively and negatively)?

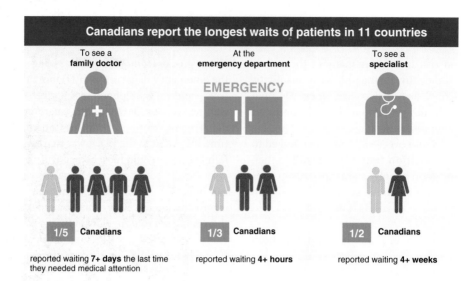

Canadians report the longest waits of patients in 11 countries

To see a
family doctor

At the
emergency department

EMERGENCY

To see a
specialist

1/5 Canadians

1/3 Canadians

1/2 Canadians

reported waiting **7+ days** the last time
they needed medical attention

reported waiting **4+ hours**

reported waiting **4+ weeks**

Fig 5.4 Canadian emergency department wait times. (From Canadian Institute of Health Information [CIHI]. [2017]. Commonwealth Fund Survey 2016: Infographic. Retrieved from https://www.cihi.ca/en/commonwealth-fund-survey-2016-infographic)

CASE STUDY

Determinants of Health

Jimmy was terribly sick, but Nurse J. could tell from the faint smile he formed as she entered the room that he was very happy to see her familiar face. Young Jimmy Brown, 9 years old, was no stranger to her care. This was his third visit to the ED since the fall. She clutched his hand and said, "Everything will be all right now, Jimmy. We'll look after you."

Jimmy Brown has chronic asthma, and his condition had deteriorated since his last visit. This time, Nurse J. was very worried, from the signs she saw. They would look after him and give him the best care possible, and probably he would get better. But everything wouldn't be all right. In a week or so, if everything went well, he would go home, but that wouldn't make everything all right. Far from it. That was where the cycle would begin again.

Since his father had abandoned him and his mother 2 years ago, Jimmy had lived in a dilapidated old house on the outskirts of town. And in that house, which others might call a shack, was a wood stove that served as the only source of heat. Jimmy's mother knew that the fumes from the smoke aggravated his asthma, but there was nothing she could do. She didn't have the money to buy a furnace or to move into a better place. And the welfare system wouldn't cover the purchase of a furnace. Nurse J. and the social worker had tried their best to intervene on the Browns' behalf, but to no avail.

Nurse J. felt frustrated and angry. The system could not or would not do anything to remedy the problem causing Jimmy's sickness, but whenever he got really sick, the system would go into high gear and spend many times more money than the cost of a furnace to fix him up. And the cycle would begin again.

It didn't make sense: not for Jimmy, not for his mother, and not for society. They wouldn't look after him, not really. It wouldn't be all right. It was only February, and there were more cold months ahead.

Questions

1. What are the determinants of health (according to Box 5.1) in this case study that are influencing Jimmy's health?
2. Which determinant is most prominent and how would you address Jimmy's situation from a health promotion perspective, keeping in mind the influence of the policy environment on health?
3. *Ethical question:* In some cases, the costs of treating someone who is sick and in need are very great, and the anticipated benefit is uncertain and slight at best. In other cases, however, tremendous benefits can be had for very little cost. If you had to choose between producing a very slight benefit for one very sick person and a greater benefit for 10 people who were less sick, which would you choose and why?

> **CRITICAL THINKING QUESTION 5.8:** In your mind, reflecting on your own community, of all the determinants of health mentioned in Box 5.1 and discussed in this chapter, which determinants of health do you believe are most important in shaping health and its distribution? Why?

▌ SUMMARY

This chapter has dealt with the determinants of health in the Canadian population. The determinants of health are many and include genetics and human biology, demography, socioeconomics, physical environment, lifestyle and behavioural and risk factors, and health care organizations (which are discussed elsewhere in this book). Politics and the policy environment have the potential to shape all of these determinants and thus represent an important place for health sector workers to intervene.

Sociodemographic indicators affect health and include aging, immigration, language, and family environments. An important demographic change is the rise in the proportion of the population older than age 65 years. The composition of the Canadian population is also changing in relation to ethnicity and is expected to continue changing as more immigrants from non-European countries are migrating to Canada.

The composition of the population in terms of literacy, education, income, and employment influences health. It does so directly because of access to things needed for good health (e.g., housing, nutritious foods, health literacy), as well as indirectly because it can be correlated with things like living in unsafe neighbourhoods and experiencing poor working conditions.

Inadequate housing and homelessness are associated with many health risks. The composition of this group now includes increasing numbers of women and children and other groups in special circumstances, such as adolescents, persons with mental illness, and Indigenous people.

Chronic stress has a significant impact on Canadians. Longitudinal data show that feeling personal stress was predictive of developing chronic conditions.

The physical environment includes physical, biological, chemical, and radiologic factors found in food, water, soil, indoor and outdoor air, the built environment, and animal and insect vectors. Public interest and knowledge in environmental issues have increased over the past 50 years and concomitantly so has public support for more extensive and strict control of environmental agents.

The lifestyle of Canadians is also a major factor in determining their health. The most common causes of mortality, potential years of life lost, hospitalizations, and disability are cardiovascular diseases, cancer, diabetes, and injuries. Key to preventing such noncommunicable diseases are activities such as eating healthy, exercising, undertaking preventive health practices, and practices related to injury prevention.

Finally, health care organization is also a determinant of health. The major feature is the availability of universal health insurance for all Canadians, which has significantly contributed to reducing the inequities in access to health care within the population.

KEY WEBSITES

Homeless Hub: http://homelesshub.ca

The Homeless Hub, hosted by the Canadian Observatory on Homelessness (a research institute focused on homelessness research) houses a number of great resources related to the topic. Resources include those related to the causes of homelessness and interventions and community solutions to address this complex issue.

World Health Organization—Social Determinants of Health: https://www.who.int/social_determinants/en/

This landing page includes global resources about the social determinants of health, including evidence about various determinants, calls to action, and policy solutions such as health in all policies approaches.

Food Secure Canada: https://foodsecurecanada.org

Food Secure Canada is an alliance of people and organizations formed in 2001 dedicated to ending hunger, ensuring healthy and safe food across the country and creating sustainable food systems.

National Collaborating Centre for Determinants of Health (NCCDH): http://www.nccdh.ca

The NCCDH is one of six collaborating centres funded by the Public Health Agency of Canada. As an organization focused on knowledge translation efforts, NCCDH helps provide the health and public health sector with information and resources to help it take action social determinants of health to improve health equity.

REFERENCES

American Psychological Association (n.d.). Understanding chronic stress. Retrieved from http://www.apa.org/helpcenter/understanding-chronic-stress.aspx

Arriagada, P. (2017). *Insights on Canadian Society: Food insecurity among Inuit living in Inuit Nunangat. Ottawa: Statistics Canada.* Retrieved from https://www150.statcan.gc.ca/n1/pub/75-006-x/2017001/article/14774-eng.htm.

Association of Workers' Compensation Boards of Canada. (2002). *Lost time claims in Canada.* Retrieved from http://awcbc.org/?page_id=14#fatalities.

Baird, P., & Scriver, C. (1998). Genetics and the public health. In R. Wallace (Ed.), *Maxey-Rosenau-Last public health and preventive medicine* (14th ed.). Stamford, CT: Appleton & Lange. [seminal reference].

Benoit, A. C., Cotnam, J., Raboud, J., et al. (2016). Experiences of chronic stress and mental health concerns among urban Indigenous women. *Archives of Women's Mental Health, 19*(5), 809–823.

Canadian Council of Motor Transport Administrators. (2018). *Distracted driving white paper.* Ottawa: Author. Retrieved from https://www.ccmta.ca/images/publications/pdf//CCMTA_Distracting_Driving_White_Paper_-_Revised_December_2018.pdf.

Canadian Dental Association. (2017). *The state of oral health in Canada.* Retrieved from https://www.cda-adc.ca/stateoforalhealth/_files/TheStateofOralHealthinCanada.pdf.

Canadian Institute for Health Information. (2016). *Results from The Commonwealth Fund's 2016 International health policy survey of adults in 11 countries.* Retrieved from https://www.cihi.ca/sites/default/files/document/text-alternative-version-2016-cmwf-en-web.pdf.

Canadian Medical Association. (2016). *The state of seniors' health care in Canada.* Retrieved from https://www.cma.ca/En/Lists/Medias/the-state-of-seniors-health-care-in-canada-september-2016.pdf.

Canadian Public Health Association. (1996). *Discussion paper on the health impact of unemployment.* Retrieved from https://www.cpha.ca/sites/default/files/assets/resolutions/1996-dp1_e.pdf.

Canadian Safety Council. (2013). *Safety on the road ahead.* Retrieved from https://canadasafetycouncil.org/safety-on-the-road-ahead/.

Colley, R. C., Carson, V., Garriguet, D., et al. (2017). Physical activity of Canadian children and youth, 2007 to 2015. *Health Reports, 28*(10), 8–16.

Cycle Helmets. (n.d.). Mandatory bicycle helmet laws in Canada. Retrieved from http://www.cycle-helmets.com/canada_helmets.html

Ding, D., Lawson, K. D., Kolbe-Alexander, & Lancet Physical Activity Series 2 Executive Committee., et al. (2016). The economic burden of physical inactivity: A global analysis of major non-communicable diseases. *The Lancet, 388*(10051), 1311–1324.

Drewnowski, A. (2017). Nutrient density: Addressing the challenge of obesity. *British Journal of Nutrition, 120*(s1), S8–S14. https://doi.org/10.1017/S0007114517002240.

Feeding Nunavut. (n.d.). Inuit community-based food initiatives. Retrieved from https://www.feedingnunavut.com/inuit-community-based-food-initiatives/

Findlay, L. (2015). Physical activity among First Nations people off reserve, Métis and Inuit. *Health Reports, 22*(1). (Cat. No. 82-003-x.) Retrieved from https://www150.statcan.gc.ca/n1/pub/82-003-x/2011001/article/11403-eng.htm.

Fischer, B., Russell, C., Sabioni, P., et al. (2017). Lower-risk cannabis use guidelines: a comprehensive update of evidence and recommendations. *American Journal of Public Health, 107*(8), e1–e12.

Food and Agricultural Organization. (2001). *Food insecurity.* Retrieved from http://www.fao.org/3/a-y1500e.pdf.

Fraser Institute. (2016). *Complementary and Alternative Medicine: Use and Public Attitudes 1997, 2006, and 2016.* Retrieved from https://www.fraserinstitute.org/studies/complementary-and-alternative-medicine-use-and-public-attitudes-1997-2006-and-2016.

Gaetz, S., Barr, C., Friesen, A., et al. (2012). *Canadian definition of homelessness.* Toronto: Canadian Observatory on Homelessness Press.

Gilmour, H. (2007). Physically active Canadians. *Health Reports, 18*(3), 45–66 Statistics Canada, Catalogue 82-003.

Goheen, M. M., Campino, S., & Cerami, C. (2017). The role of the red blood cell in host defence against falciparum malaria: an expanding repertoire of evolutionary alterations. *British Journal of Haematology, 179*(4), 543–556. https://doi.org/10.1111/bjh.14886.

Government of Canada. (2017). *National Housing Strategy: A Place to Call Home.* Retrieved from https://www.placetocallhome.ca/.

Government of Canada. (2008). *Chapter 2: The Chief Public Health Officer's report on the state of public health in Canada 2008—Canada's public health history.* Retrieved from https://www.canada.ca/en/public-health/corporate/publications/chief-public-health-officer-reports-state-public-health-canada/report-on-state-public-health-canada-2008/chapter-2b.html.

Gozdzik, A., Salehi, R., O'Campo, P., et al. (2015). Cardiovascular risk factors and 30-year cardiovascular risk in homeless adults with mental illness. *BMC Public Health, 15*(1), 165. https://doi.org/10.1186/s12889-015-1472-4.

Health Canada. (2018). *Vaccine uptake in Canadian children: Highlights from childhood National Immunization Coverage Survey.* Retrieved from https://www.canada.ca/en/public-health/services/publications/healthy-living/2015-vaccine-uptake-canadian-children-survey.html.

Homeless Hub. (2018a). How many people are homeless in Canada? Retrieved from https://www.homelesshub.ca/about-homelessness/homelessness-101/how-many-people-are-homeless-canada.

Homeless Hub. (2018b). *Legal & justice issues*. Retrieved from https://www.homelesshub.ca/about-homelessness/topics/legal-justice-issues.

Hughes, A., Kumari, M., McMunn, A., et al. (2017). Unemployment and inflammatory markers in England, Wales and Scotland, 1998–2012: Meta-analysis of results from 12 studies. *Brain Behavior and Immunity*, 64, 91–102. https://doi.org/10.1016/j.bbi.2017.03.012.

Inner City Health Associates. (n.d.). *About us*. Retrieved from http://www.icha-toronto.ca/about-us

Kundakovic, M., & Champagne, F. (2015). Early-life experience, epigenetics, and the developing brain. *Neuropsychopharmacology*, 40, 141–153.

Landecker, H., & Panofsky, A. (2013). From social structure to gene regulation, and back: a critical introduction to environmental epigenetics for sociology. *Annual Review Sociology*, 39, 333–357. https://doi.org/10.1146/annurev-soc-071312-145707.

Landsbergis, P. A., Dobson, M., LaMontagne, A. D., et al. (2017). Occupational stress. In B. S. Levy, D. H. Wegman, S. L. Baron, & R. K Sokas (Eds.), *Occupational and environmental health* (pp. 325–344). Oxford UK: Oxford University Press.

Lebel, A., Subramanian, S. V., Hamel, D., et al. (2018). Population-level trends in the distribution of body mass index in Canada, 2000–2014. *Canadian Journal of Public Health*, 1–10. https://doi.org/10.17269/s41997-018-0060-7.

Loi, M., Del Savio, L., & Stupka, E. (2013). Social epigenetics and equality of opportunity. *Public Health Ethics*, 6(2), 142–153. https://doi.org/10.1093/phe/pht019.

Luan, H., Minaker, L. M., & Law, J. (2016). Do marginalized neighbourhoods have less healthy retail food environments? An analysis using Bayesian spatial latent factor and hurdle models. *International Journal of Health Geographics*, 15(1), 29. https://doi.org/10.1186/s12942-016-0060-x.

Mackert, M., Mabry-Flynn, A., Champlin, S., et al. (2016). Health literacy and health information technology adoption: The potential for a new digital divide (G. Eysenbach, Ed.). *Journal of Medical Internet Research*, 18(10), e264. https://doi.org/10.2196/jmir.6349.

Mahmood, B., Bhatti, J. A., Leon, A., et al. (2018). Leisure time physical activity levels in immigrants by ethnicity and time since immigration to Canada: Findings from the 2011–2012 Canadian Community Health Survey. *Journal of Immigrant and Minority Health (online)*, 1–10.

Marmot, M., Friel, S., Bell, R., & Commission on Social Determinants of Health., et al. (2008). Closing the gap in a generation: Health equity through action on the social determinants of health. *The Lancet*, 372(9650), 1661–1669.

Maytree. (2019). *Social Assistance Summaries*. Retrieved from https://maytree.com/social-assistance-summaries/.

McKay, A., Quinn-Nilas, C., & Milhausen, R. (2017). Prevalence and correlates of condom use among single midlife Canadian women and men aged 40 to 59. *The Canadian Journal of Human Sexuality*, 26(1), 38–47. https://doi.org/10.3138/cjhs.261-A6.

Monsivais, P., Martin, A., Suhrcke, M., et al. (2015). Job-loss and weight gain in British adults: Evidence from two longitudinal studies. *Social Science & Medicine*, 143, 223–231. https://doi.org/10.1016/j.socscimed.2015.08.052.

Murray, N. (2016). *Non-profit funds Nunavut hunters to supply country food to the needy*. CBC News, June 16. Retrieved from https://www.cbc.ca/news/canada/north/feeding-nunavut-traditional-food-pilot-project-1.3637841.

Nishi, S. K., Jessri, M., & L'Abbé, M. (2018). Assessing the dietary habits of Canadians by eating location and occasion: Findings from the Canadian Community Health Survey, Cycle 2.2. *Nutrients*, 10(6), 682.

ParticipACTION. (2018). *Physical literacy*. Retrieved from https://www.participaction.com/en-ca/thought-leadership/physical-literacy.

Popkin, B. M. (2015). Nutrition transition and the global diabetes epidemic. *Current Diabetes Reports*, 15(9), 64. https://doi.org/10.1007/s11892-015-0631-4.

Raphael, D. (2011). *Poverty in Canada: Implications for health and quality of life*. Toronto: Canadian Scholars' Press.

Raphael, D. (2016). Social structure, living conditions, and health. *Social determinants of health: Canadian perspectives* (3rd ed.) (pp. 32 -56). Toronto: Canadian Scholars' Press.

Redelmeier, D., & Tibshirani, R. (1997). Association between cellular-telephone calls and motor vehicle collisions. *New England Journal of Medicine*, 336(7), 453–458 [seminal].

Rideout, K., Mah, C. L., & Minaker, L. (2015). *Food environments: An introduction for public health practice*. Vancouver: National Collaborating Centre for Environmental Health. Retrieved from http://www.ncceh.ca/sites/default/files/Food_Environments_Public_Health_Practice_Dec_2015.pdf.

Schierding, W., Vickers, M. H., O'Sullivan, J. M., et al. (2017). *Epigenetics. Fetal and neonatal physiology* (5th ed.). London: Elsevier, 89–100. https://doi.org/10.1016/B978-0-323-35214-7.00009-3.

Statistics Canada. (2011). *Canadian Internet Use Survey (CIUS): Detailed information for 2010*. Ottawa: Author. Retrieved from http://www23.statcan.gc.ca/imdb/p2SV.pl?Function=getSurvey&Id=66116.

Statistics Canada. (2012). *Problem-solving skills and labour market outcomes*. Retrieved from http://www.statcan.gc.ca/pub/81-004-x/2012001/article/11651-eng.htm.

Statistics Canada. (2013a). *Population projections for Canada (2013 to 2063)*. Retrieved from https://www.statcan.gc.ca/pub/91-520-x/91-520-x2014001-eng.htm.

Statistics Canada. (2013b). *Table 13-10-0337-01: Household population meeting/not meeting the Canadian physical activity guidelines*. Retrieved from https://www150.statcan.gc.ca/n1/pub/82-625-x/2015001/article/14135-eng.htm.

Statistics Canada. (2015a). *Low income cut-offs*. Retrieved from https://www150.statcan.gc.ca/n1/pub/75f0002m/2009002/s2-eng.htm#n7.

Statistics Canada. (2015b). *Ethnic origin of person*. Retrieved from http://www23.statcan.gc.ca/imdb/p3Var.pl?Function=DEC&Id=103475.

Statistics Canada. (2015c). *Overweight and obese adults (self-reported), 2014*. Retrieved from https://www150.statcan.gc.ca/n1/pub/82-625-x/2015001/article/14185-eng.htm.

Statistics Canada. (2016b). *2016 Census topic: Immigration and ethnocultural diversity*. Retrieved https://www12.statcan.gc.ca/census-recensement/2016/rt-td/imm-eng.cfm.

Statistics Canada. (2016c). *Immigration and ethnocultural diversity: Key results from the 2016 Census*. Retrieved from https://www.statcan.gc.ca/daily-quotidien/171025/d-q171025b-eng.htm.

Statistics Canada. (2016d). *Education indicators in Canada: An international perspective, 2017*. Retrieved from https://www150.statcan.gc.ca/n1/daily-quotidien/171212/dq171212a-eng.htm.

Statistics Canada. (2016e). *Education indicators in Canada, biannual*. Retrieved from http://www.statcan.gc.ca/daily-quotidien/180321/dq180321f-eng.htm.

Statistics Canada. (2016f). *Household income in Canada: Key results from the 2016 Census*. Retrieved from https://www150.statcan.gc.ca/n1/daily-quotidien/170913/d-q170913a-eng.htm.

Statistics Canada. (2016g). *Perceived life stress, by age group*. Retrieved from https://www150.statcan.gc.ca/t1/tbl1/en/tv.action?pid=1310009604&pickMembers%5B0%5D=1.1&pickMembers%5B1%5D=3.2&pickMembers%5B2%5D=4.5.

Statistics Canada. (2016h). *Farm and farm operator data*. Retrieved from https://www150.statcan.gc.ca/n1/pub/95-640-x/95-640-x2016001-eng.htm.

Statistics Canada. (2016i). *Health behaviour in school-aged children in Canada: Focus on relationships*. Retrieved from http://healthycanadians.gc.ca/publications/science-research-sciences-recherches/health-behaviour-children-canada-2015-comportements-sante-jeunes/index-eng.php?_ga=2.256199755.1562579534.1531680887-1406384625.1530393908#c14a3.

Statistics Canada. (2017b). *An increasingly diverse linguistic profile: Corrected data from the 2016 Census*. Retrieved from https://www150.statcan.gc.ca/n1/daily-quotidien/170817/dq170817a-eng.htm.

Statistics Canada. (2017c). *Ethnic and cultural origins of Canadians: Portrait of a rich heritage*. Retrieved from https://www12.statcan.gc.ca/census-recensement/2016/as-sa/98-200-x/2016016/98-200-x2016016-eng.cfm.

Statistics Canada. (2017d). *Children living in low-income households*. Retrieved from https://www12.statcan.gc.ca/census-recensement/2016/as-sa/98-200-x/2016012/98-200-x2016012-eng.cfm#n4.

Statistics Canada. (2017e). *Health impacts from air pollution in Canada*. Retrieved from http://publications.gc.ca/collections/collection_2018/sc-hc/H144-51-2017-eng.pdf.

Statistics Canada. (2017g). *Fruit and vegetable consumption, 2016*. Retrieved from https://www150.statcan.gc.ca/n1/pub/82-625-x/2017001/article/54860-eng.htm.

Statistics Canada. (2019). *Cannabis Stats Hub*. Retrieved from https://www150.statcan.gc.ca/n1/pub/13-610-x/cannabis-eng.htm.

Michael's Hospital, St. (2019). *Department of Family and Community Medicine and St. Michael's Academic Family Health Team—Health Justice Program*. Retrieved from http://www.stmichaelshospital.com/programs/familypractice/health-justice-program.php.

Sweet, S., & Meiksins, P. (2015). *Changing contours of work: Jobs and opportunities in the new economy*. Thousand Oaks, CA: Sage Publications.

Tait, C. A., L'Abbé, M. R., Smith, P. M., et al. (2018). The association between food insecurity and incident type 2 diabetes in Canada: A population-based cohort study. *PloS One, 13*(5), e0195962.

Tasker, J. P. (2018). *Many Canadians driving after consuming cannabis, according to new StatsCan data*. CBC News. Retrieved from https://www.cbc.ca/news/politics/statcan-cannabis-driving-high-1.4779004.

Transport Canada. (2018). *Transport Canada to make seat belts mandatory on highway buses*. Retrieved from https://www.canada.ca/en/transport-canada/news/2018/07/transport-canada-to-make-seat-belts-mandatory-on-highway-buses.html.

Van Deursen, A. J., & van Dijk, J. A. (2014). *Digital skills: Unlocking the information society*. New York: Springer.

White, B. M., Logan, A., & Magwood, G. S. (2016). Access to diabetes care for populations experiencing homelessness: An integrated review. *Current Diabetes Reports, 16*(11), 112.

World Health Organization. (2019a). *About social determinants of health*. Retrieved from https://www.who.int/social_determinants/sdh_definition/en/.

World Health Organization. (2019b). *Ten threats to global health in 2019*. Retrieved from https://www.who.int/emergencies/ten-threats-to-global-health-in-2019.

6

Groups Experiencing Health Inequities

ⓔ Additional resources are available online at http://evolve.elsevier.com/Canada/Shah/publichealth/

LEARNING OBJECTIVES

- Be familiar with key principles and terms related to exploring health inequities among specific groups in Canadian society.
- Describe the demography, health gap, and determinants of the health gap of key populations, including racialized Canadians, people with disabilities, seniors, homeless people, LGBT2SQIA+, and rural populations.

- Use the social determinants of health to analyze health inequities facing other groups in Canadian society.
- List strategies at the individual, institutional, and societal levels to remedy inequities faced by certain populations.

CHAPTER OUTLINE

KEY TERMS

acculturation	family-class immigrants	proportionate universalism
centenarians	frailty	race
cultural awareness	gender identity	racialized persons
cultural competence	healthy immigrant effect	refugees
cultural humility	heterogeneity	rural
cultural safety	high-risk populations	sexual orientation
cultural sensitivity	interpersonal racism	social isolation
economic-class immigrants	intersectionality	structural racism
ethnicity	loneliness	visible minority
equity-seeking groups	marginalized populations	vulnerable populations

INTRODUCTION

In earlier chapters, we have discussed the determinants of health, health status, consequences in the Canadian population as a whole and strategies for achieving health for all. This chapter examines inequities in health that are faced by certain groups in Canada.

Not all groups enjoy equal opportunities for health—significant inequities continue to exist because of societal factors that influence health and its distribution, as well as characteristics of our health system. This topic is a complex one, and not all populations that experience inequities will be covered comprehensively. Additionally, **intersectionality** (the interconnectedness of different systems of oppression such as racism and sexism that make it hard to tease out the influence of one versus another) and **heterogeneity** (the idea that not all racism is experienced the same way and that many differences exist between members of a particular group or community) complicate matters. The health of groups that face inequities reflects the influence of the determinants of health. For the purposes of brevity, we will focus on a few groups that either highlight key social determinants of health (SDHs) or represent a large or rapidly growing segment of the Canadian population and introduce some key principles that can be applied in examining the health of any group that may be experiencing health inequities.

Key Terminology and Principles

Often, the terms *vulnerable, disadvantaged, hard-to-reach, marginalized,* and *priority groups* are used interchangeably to describe people facing inequities; however, there are actually nuanced differences in the meanings of these terms. As well, the language we use to describe groups of people must be thoughtful and intentional and must not further stigmatize them. In general, as terminology continues to evolve, we must be mindful of any connotations—negative or positive—that may be associated with certain terminology.

Putting the preface "people" before describing a behaviour of some groups is generally preferred. For example, instead of using the term "injection drug users" as was often done in the recent past, it is now preferable to say "people who inject drugs" to recognize that, above all, people are people. The idea behind using this kind of "people-first" terminology is that people's identity is much more than a behaviour they engage in or a condition or illness they may have. By saying "people" first, their humanity is emphasized above their behaviour or illness, and they are less medicalized. Emphasizing behaviours or conditions can actually be quite dehumanizing and possibly pave the way for notions that the people they describe are inferior, wrong, or deviant.

Another good rule of thumb, especially for front-line workers, is to ask people how they want to be referred to. It is fundamental to avoid assumptions regarding gender, race, or ethnicity, and when in doubt, asking a client you are serving is the most ideal way to ensure respect and prevent further stigmatization.

High-risk populations is the term used in the Lalonde Report (see Chapter 1) to describe groups that engage in risk behaviours such as smoking, substance use, physical inactivity, and others. However, this term has largely fallen out of favour because it does not capture any of the SDHs that account for people's "choice" to engage in risk behaviors. **Vulnerable populations** is a term that is also used quite commonly. It most often refers to "groups that have increased susceptibility to adverse health outcomes as a result of inequitable access to the resources needed to address risks to health" (National Collaborating Centre for Determinants of Health [NCCDH], 2013). In its most basic sense, the word *vulnerable* actually refers to a susceptibility to be harmed (i.e., the Latin term *vulnerare* for vulnerable means "to wound"; Vamanu, Gheorghe, & Katina, 2016). In a somewhat similar light, the term **marginalized populations** is also used to refer to "groups denied opportunities to meaningfully participate in society due to their lack of economic resources, knowledge about political rights, recognition, and other forms of oppression." The terms *vulnerable* and *marginalized* have been criticized for being disempowering and for suggesting that these individuals or groups are lacking agency (i.e., the perceived ability to change or control their own circumstances; Bentley-Edwards, 2016). The term **equity-seeking groups** is being used in some places to refer to socially and economically disadvantaged groups that are "taking an active role in altering processes and structures that influence health" (NCCDH, 2013). However, this term implies that all groups that are experiencing inequities have agency, which also isn't necessarily true. For the purposes of our discussion, we will use the phrase "groups experiencing health inequities" to reflect the context of groups and populations discussed. Specific details on the context and diversity among groups of people will be expanded upon in this chapter.

For a list of additional key principles to consider regarding health inequities (in addition to being purposeful about language) that will be applied throughout this chapter, see Box 6.1.

Chapter Overview

Each group that is discussed in this chapter will be described in terms of their prevalence and mix in the Canadian population (*demography*), the health inequities experienced by this group (*health gap*), and an exploration of the key determinants that influence the inequitable distribution of health in the group when compared with the general population (*understanding the health gap*). Although not every group that experiences inequities in Canada will be discussed in this chapter, this way of approaching the examination of certain groups (demography, health gap, understanding

> **BOX 6.1 Key Principles for Understanding Health Inequities**
>
> In addition to being intentional about the terminology used, a few other key principles must be kept in mind as you read this chapter:
> 1. **Strengths-based approach:** When studying the health of specific groups, a strengths-based approach must be used. It is important to examine an issue not only from a health inequity and gap perspective but also to consider the resources, capacities, and abilities of a person or community that are protective. In this chapter, we discuss the health gap and focus on factors to explain this gap, for the sake of brevity and to highlight differences in health status between Canadian groups. However, as you read, be mindful of the *resources, capacities,* and *abilities* of the populations discussed as well.
> 2. **Nuanced discussions:** Nothing is black and white, and discussions regarding health inequities should remain nuanced. For example, much diversity and heterogeneity exist within groups that experience health inequities. People experience disadvantage on multiple and intersecting levels. For example, a person can experience racism and sexism at the same time, and these experiences may be difficult to tease apart, but this same person may also experience some advantages over others if they are also high on the social hierarchy due to their income or occupation. Essentially, no two experiences are alike.
> 3. **Reflexivity:** Practitioners must be aware of their own biases, work to improve their knowledge and understanding of diverse groups, and ensure that their practice does not further stigmatize but instead reduces power imbalances that exist in society.

the health gap) can be applied to any population. Key determinants of inequities in health that will be specifically highlighted in the discussions that follow are listed in Table 6.1, with a brief explanation of how each determinant may influence health outcomes in a particular group. A more comprehensive discussion of health determinants and determinants of equity can be found in Chapters 1 and 5.

> **CRITICAL THINKING QUESTION 6.1:** What is the term you have been using to date to refer to individuals who experience health inequities? What are some of the advantages and drawbacks of using that terminology?

TABLE 6.1   Key Determinants of Health and Equity and the Mechanisms by Which They Affect Health and Equity

Determinant of Health	Effects on Health and Equity
Income	Affects access to resources for health (e.g., transportation to and from appointments, healthy foods, healthy recreational activities, medications, adequate housing)
	Lack of income and financial hardship can cause significant stress on individuals and families
Social support network	Allows for mental and material support in times of need and crisis
	Lack of social supports causes isolation, loneliness
Housing	Provides shelter from harsh environmental conditions, stability, and safety
	Lack of housing or unsafe housing causes exposures that affect health (e.g., mold, stress)
Employment and working conditions	Provides meaning and purpose to many
	Provides families with income and other benefits and resources for health (e.g., drug coverage)
	Lack of secure and safe employment causes injuries, lack of income, significant stress
Health services	Provides access to preventive, curative, diagnostic, rehabilitation, and palliative care
Racism and discrimination	Results in discrimination when it comes to services, access to employment, and other resources
	Results in stress, feelings of exclusion, and marginalization
Early childhood development	Positive interactions and attachment foster positive mental and physical health later in life
	Adverse childhood experiences (e.g., neglect, abuse, trauma) result in stress, substance use, chronic disease, and altered brain development

THE HEALTH OF RACIALIZED CANADIANS

In keeping with the introductory discussion about use of language, it is also important to distinguish between the terms *race* and *ethnicity*. Whereas **ethnicity** often refers to a self-chosen category that encompasses dimensions of culture, religion, language, and geographic location (e.g., Greek, Arab), **race** is a political and social construct that classifies people into categories based on skin colour (e.g., black, white) and other phenotypes (and assumes that human value is linked to these categories; Nestel, 2012). These categories are not scientific in nature (i.e., there are no genetic differences between the various racial categories), and they were created to legitimize power and privilege of white people over others (Barndt, 2007, p. 72). Just like racial diversity exists among different ethnicities, ethnic diversity also exists among racial groups (Nestel, 2012).

The federal government and its organizations, such as Statistics Canada, often use the term **visible minority**, which refers to "persons, other than Aboriginal peoples, who are non-Caucasian in race or non-white in colour" (Statistics Canada, 2017a). Examples of visible minorities in Canada include South Asian, Chinese, Black, Filipino, Latin American, and Arab people, among others (see Chapter 4 for statistics).

The preferred term, which we will adopt in our discussions (except when referring to Statistics Canada data), is **racialized persons** or groups because this term more explicitly recognizes the fact that race is socially constructed (i.e., created by society with no biological basis; Ontario Human Rights Commission, n.d.). Racialized groups, unlike visible minorities, encompass Indigenous people.

According to Statistics Canada, just over one fifth of Canadians are considered to be visible minorities (the term adopted by Statistics Canada to refer to non-Indigenous racialized groups). By 2036, it is expected that visible minorities will make up about one third of the Canadian population. In Canada, the most populous visible minority groups include South Asians, Chinese, and Black Canadians (Catalyst, 2018). Foreign-born Canadians also make up about one fifth of the Canadian population, many of whom are visible minorities. The top 10 countries of origin for foreign-born Canadians are listed in Box 6.2. Additionally, Toronto is one of the world's most diverse cities in the world (see In the News box).

🌐 IN THE NEWS

Toronto Named Most Diverse City in the World

Toronto's population is made up of 51% of residents born outside of Canada, is home to 230 different nationalities, and is growing by 100 000 people annually. According to BBC Radio, Toronto is the most diverse city in the world.

Source: From Flack, D. (2016). Toronto named the most diverse city in the world. *BlogTO*, May 15. Retrieved from https://www.blogto.com/city/2016/05/toronto_named_most_diverse_city_in_the_world/

BOX 6.2 Top 10 Countries of Origin for Foreign-Born Canadians

Philippines
India
China
Iran
Pakistan
United States
Syria
United Kingdom
France
South Korea

Data from Statistics Canada. (2017). *Immigrant population in Canada, 2016 Census of Population*. Retrieved from https://www150.statcan.gc.ca/n1/pub/11-627-m/11-627-m2017028-eng.htm

---

Because racialized and foreign-born Canadians make up a significant proportion of the population and to highlight the importance of racialization as a determinant of health and equity, the health of two specific groups that experience inequities in Canada—Black Canadians and new Canadians—will be highlighted next.

Black Canadians

The term "Black Canadians" requires closer investigation and thought. As discussed earlier, race is a social construct (with no basis in biology or genetics). As a result, calling a group of individuals "Black" or "White" is arbitrary. *Black Canadians* describes a category of people who are diverse and represent individuals from a number of different backgrounds, including those who originate from Africa and the Caribbean. Thus, although this term is commonly used and will be used in this chapter (because racism is an important determinant of health), the implications of using this term and the ideas that it propagates should be reflected upon.

Demography

According to the 2016 Census, there were just over 1 million Black Canadians across the country, making up around 16% of the visible minority population (Statistics Canada, 2017c) and just around 3% of the Canadian population in total (Veenstra & Patterson, 2016).

The first documented person of African ancestry to come to Canada came in the early 1600s. Between 1749 and 1782, significant numbers of Africans came to Nova Scotia as runaway slaves. Because slavery had not yet been abolished in the United States, it is estimated that around 30 000 Africans escaped to Canada between 1800 and 1865 via the Underground Railway. Black communities settled across the country. It wasn't until 1833, however, that slavery was completely abolished in Canada and other British colonies (Canadian Heritage, 2018). For a more detailed history of slavery in Canada, see Box 6.3.

The Health Gap

Unfortunately, the existence of data and research on racial health inequities in Canada is limited, in large part because most health databases and health care encounters do not tend to track race.

However, some health inequities experienced by Black Canadians have been well described, both in terms of communicable and noncommunicable diseases (NCDs). With respect to communicable diseases, Black Canadians are reported to have a higher prevalence of HIV compared with the general Canadian population. For example, in 2009, Black Canadians accounted for around 9% of all HIV cases in the country (Nestel, 2012). In terms of NCDs and their risk factors, a recent analysis examining Black–White inequities in Canada found that when controlling for factors such as education, income, smoking, body mass index (BMI), and physical activity, Black Canadians were more likely to report having diabetes and hypertension (Veenstra & Patterson, 2016). Other studies have shown that Black Canadians are more likely to experience risk factors that promote the development of NCDs, such as smoking and having a high BMI (Siddiqi et al., 2017).

BOX 6.3 Slavery in Canada

Just like the United States, Canada participated in the transatlantic slave trade for nearly two centuries. Although Canada represented a safe haven for some time since slavery was abolished nation wide in Canada before it was in the United States, Canada too has its own long history of enslavement, dating back to the early 1600s. Owning Black and Indigenous slaves was a common practice across this country during its early history, and many slaves worked as domestic servants, sailors, hunters, and agricultural workers without any rights or freedoms. At the peak of slavery in Canada, there were just over 4 000 slaves. Many were subjected to harsh and cruel treatment.

In the late 1700s, several American states (including Vermont and New York) banned slavery, and a number of Canadians escaped there over time. The abolitionist movements eventually began to spread in Canada, too, and by the early 1800s, New Brunswick, Nova Scotia, and Upper Canada had all attempted to pass laws to end slavery but were unsuccessful (Henry, 2018).

Many legal cases also set precedents for abolishing slavery, until finally, in 1793, the *Act to Limit Slavery* was passed, which prevented the introduction of new slaves in Upper Canada and set forth a provision that any child born to an enslaved woman would be freed at age 25 years. In 1825, Prince Edward Island took this restriction a step further and went so far as to ban the practice of slavery completely (McRae, 2014). After this, the *Slavery Abolition Act* came into effect in 1834 and officially made slavery illegal across Canada and all other British colonies.

In terms of rates of injury, interestingly, research in both the United States and Canada has shown that mortality associated with drowning is higher among people of African descent, as well as among new Canadians, compared with those of European descent (Gallinger, Fralick, & Hwang, 2015). The most common explanation for this finding is that people from these groups are less likely to have engaged in swimming lessons because of a variety of different factors (e.g., cost, proximity to pools).

EXERCISE 6.1 If you were the Health Minister of a province or territory, would you insist on tracking race when it comes to health system encounters? Why or why not?

Understanding the Health Gap

The determinants of health inequities were introduced and described in Chapter 1 and Chapter 5. Here we will draw on that concept to explore why inequities in health continue to exist between certain groups. In the case of Black Canadians, an important reason frequently cited as a core or root cause of inequities is that of racism. Racism is generally categorized in two different forms: *structural racism* and *interpersonal racism*. **Structural racism** refers to the impact of factors related to how we have organized society (i.e., politics, policies) and how they affect access to opportunity for some groups over others. For example, slavery (as mentioned earlier) has had a massive impact on opportunities for good health and access to SDHs (e.g., safe housing, income, employment) for Black people compared with White people. Additionally, a few studies have reported on the discrimination that Black people face in the labour market compared with their White counterparts. A 2011 study found that Canadian-born racialized men earned, on average, 18% less than Canadian-born White men. Racial inequities also continue to exist in the educational system and justice system, with much media attention being paid in recent years to the disproportional rate of arrests and incarceration of Black Canadians (Nestel, 2012).

Interpersonal racism is the more direct and visible form of racism, which usually involves treating a person differently (whether consciously or unconsciously) based on their race because of negatively held views about non-White people (Siddiqi et al., 2017). Although this form of racism is thought to be less prevalent, it does still exist, particularly in the health care sector. A range of qualitative studies have examined client perceptions of racism during health system encounters. One such study, which took place in Toronto, examined the perceptions of racialized women and found that one in five of them encountered racism in the Canadian health system, in the form of name calling, cultural insensitivity, and poorer quality care (Nestel, 2012).

Both types of racism can produce and perpetuate health inequities because both limit access to key resources needed for health and also result in stress, which influences the adoption of risk behaviours.

Immigrants and Refugees

Demography

In 2016, new Canadians (i.e., those who had settled in Canada during the previous 5 years) made up around 3.5% of Canada's population (Statistics Canada, 2017c). Of these new Canadians, 60% were **economic-class immigrants** (meaning they are selected on the basis of the skills they can contribute to the Canadian economy), 27% were **family-class immigrants** (meaning their Canadian family members have sponsored them to settle in Canada), and 12% were **refugees** (defined as a person who came to Canada because they were forced to flee from persecution). These numbers are quite different from the 1980s, when about 40% of immigrants were economic-class immigrants, 30% were family-class immigrants, and just over 20% were refugees. Today, most newcomers to Canada are from Asia. In terms of geographic dispersion, nearly half of all newcomers to Canada settle in Toronto, Montreal, or Vancouver. In Toronto, for example, immigrants represent about 46% of the population. However, as per the most recent Statistics Canada data, more immigrants are beginning to settle in the Prairies and Atlantic provinces (Statistics Canada, 2017c).

The Health Gap

Much has been written about a phenomenon known as the **healthy immigrant effect**. The healthy immigrant effect reflects the fact that recent newcomers often experience better health compared with their Canadian-born counterparts. However, researchers have discovered that with more time spent in Canada, the health experience of these immigrants declines. For example, on the whole, recent immigrants tend to have lower rates of cancer, heart disease, and diabetes, as well as age-standardized death rates initially, but after 20 to 25 years of living in Canada, their rates of NCDs, in particular, mirror those of Canadian-born individuals.

This phenomenon, however, does not apply equally to all new Canadians. Refugees, for example, often arrive having poorer health than the average Canadian-born citizen, and non-European immigrants' health often declines more rapidly than that of European immigrants (Lane et al., 2018).

In terms of specific health outcomes of new immigrant and refugee populations, a recent meta-analysis has shown that first-generation Canadian children experience less psychological distress than Canadian-born youth. First-generation Canadian youth also experienced lower rates of alcohol consumption compared with second- or third-generation Canadian youth. Studies analyzing adult health have reported that immigrants who have been in Canada for less than 10 years reported lower rates of depression and anxiety. It is hypothesized, however, that this advantage decreases over a period of time living in Canada. This same trend is said to hold true for a number of other chronic conditions, including asthma, cancer, and cardiovascular disease. Compared with Canadian-born women, however, immigrant women are more likely to have small-for-gestational-age babies, as well as deliver preterm babies. Recent immigrant women, in particular, are more likely to report postpartum depression than Canadian-born mothers. With respect to communicable diseases, immigrant women are more likely to die from HIV/AIDS than Canadian-born women (Vang et al., 2017). As discussed in Chapter 10, 70% of new cases of active tuberculosis (TB) in Canada occur among foreign-born individuals (Public Health Agency of Canada [PHAC], 2018), mostly because TB is more common in their countries of origin compared with Canada.

Understanding the Health Gap

Reasons to explain the healthy immigrant effect are plentiful. One explanation is that immigrants tend to be people in their country of origin who are the most well-off and are able to leave in search of a different life experience. Additionally, immigration policies tend to select the best-off migrants for the contributions they are expected to make to the economy. Increasingly more often, Canada is selecting immigrants with higher levels of education, work experience, and those who are fluent in either French or English. Probably the most commonly cited reason for why the health of new Canadians tends to decline over time spent in Canada is the notion of **acculturation**—when new Canadians adopt lifestyle and risk behaviours similar to Canadians, for example, tobacco smoking, physical inactivity, and a fast-food diet (Vang et al., 2017).

It is also important to keep in mind differential access to the SDHs. Social disadvantage is another reason to explain why some immigrants and refugees experience rapid declines in health after settling in Canada. Factors such as labour market discrimination, barriers to social integration, and poverty and poorer access to health care services also influence the health of some new Canadians. It has been documented that immigrants coming to Canada after the 1970s were more likely to be socially disadvantaged (which we know impacts health) than immigrants who arrived in Canada before the 1970s (Vang et al., 2017).

THE HEALTH OF SENIORS

This section identifies some characteristics relevant to the health of seniors, often defined as people older than 65 years of age. Seniors are a heterogeneous group, each generation having a different social history. The number of seniors and their proportion in the population of Canada continues to grow and, thus, this group has been chosen as one to highlight.

Aging is a lifelong process, encompassing a series of transitions from birth to death. Reaching the age of 65 years does not therefore herald old age. Even though functional impairment increases with age, aging and poor health are not synonymous. It is not clear how much functional disability is intrinsic to the aging process or whether death is always the result of a disease process, which is the prevalent biomedical model. The degree of limitations experienced by seniors also depends on society's response. Successful aging has been defined in terms of retaining the ability to function independently, remaining mobile, and undertaking all the activities of daily living (e.g., dressing, bathing, using stairs, getting in and out of bed, eating).

Demography

According to the 2016 Canadian Census, seniors make up close to 17% of the Canadian population, and this proportion now exceeds the percentage of Canadians younger than 15 years of age (see Fig 4.2 in Chapter 4) (Statistics Canada, 2017g). According to demographers, it is expected that by 2031, nearly one in four Canadians will be over the age of 65 years. People over age 85 years make up 2.2% of the Canadian population and represent the fastest growing age group in the country. Interestingly, according to the most recent Census, there were 8230 **centenarians** (people older than 100 years of age) living in Canada, and the proportion of centenarians increased by over 40% between 2011 and 2016 (Statistics Canada, 2017d). This increase is attributed to an increase in average life expectancy, the aging of the baby boomers, and the projected decline in fertility (Statistics Canada, 2015b).

Another striking trend is the expanding population of senior women, particularly among those aged 85 years and older. As a result of the increased life expectancy of women compared with men, for every man age 85 years and older, there are two women of that age. When looking at centenarians, for every one man older than the age of 100 years, there are five women older than 100 years of age (Statistics Canada, 2017d).

The Health Gap

Although the health of seniors has improved over the past 100 years, between 75% to 80% of seniors report having one or more chronic health condition (Canadian Medical Association, 2016). In terms of life satisfaction, seniors tend to be more satisfied with their lives compared with people aged 20 to 64 years. However, when asked about health, which is correlated with life satisfaction, nearly one in five Canadian seniors reported having "fair" or "poor" health, and 6% stated that their mental health was either "fair" or "poor" (Uppal & Barayandema, 2018).

Frailty is a commonly used term to describe seniors with a complex mix of health conditions that results in a state of vulnerability and reduced likelihood of adapting or recovering from an acute injury or illness. Frailty is correlated with the risk of death, hospitalization, and institutionalization (Hoover et al., 2015). Recent estimates produced by Statistics Canada show that nearly one quarter of community dwelling seniors are considered to be "frail." In general, frailty increases with age, and more women than men are considered frail (Hoover et al., 2015).

With age, people tend to use more health care system services. A recent study examining a large cohort of community-dwelling seniors found that about one quarter of the cohort required hospital services at least once during the study duration (which ranged between 2 and 3 years) (Ramage-Morin, Gilmour, & Rotermann, 2017). Nearly 7% of the senior population resides in special care facilities (e.g., nursing homes), and this proportion increases to almost 30% among people aged 85 years or older (Statistics Canada, 2018a).

Understanding the Health Gap

As mentioned earlier, seniors are a very heterogenous group, and their health is heavily influenced by a number of SDHs. Some of the most influential factors affecting the health of seniors specifically will be discussed here, including marital status, social isolation, income, and elder abuse.

Among seniors, marital status is a known determinant of well-being, with seniors who are married reporting higher levels of well-being than those who are widowed, divorced, separated, or never married. In Canada, approximately one fifth of seniors are widowed—7% of men and 30% of women, and 2% of Canadian seniors are separated (Uppal & Barayandema, 2018). In addition to providing physical and practical assistance, spouses are also an important source of social interaction for seniors, and this may be one mechanism by which spousal status affects well-being. **Social isolation** (defined as a lack of quantity and quality of human connection) is an emerging issue among seniors in Canada. It is closely tied to the concept of **loneliness**, which is the perception of social isolation. Both social isolation and loneliness are important determinants of physical and mental health (as discussed in both Chapters 1 and 5). In fact, loneliness is associated with disrupted sleep, increased risk of heart disease, suicide, falls, and worse cognition (National Seniors Council, 2017). In Canada, nearly a quarter of seniors report wanting to participate more in social activities, and about one in five seniors reports feeling a lack of companionship (National Seniors Council, 2016).

Income is a strong determinant of health for all age groups. When it comes to poverty among seniors, Canada ranks third best regarding poverty rates for seniors compared with other OECD countries, largely because of the presence of its publicly supported retirement security system (described further later). In general, the rate of poverty among seniors has decreased from the 1970s. More specifically, between 1976 to the mid-1990s, the number of seniors living in poverty decreased from around 30% to about 5% (Conference Board of Canada, 2013). Alarmingly, however, since the mid-1990s, the rates are beginning to rise again, with most recent estimates showing that just over 12% of Canadian seniors are living in poverty (Statistics Canada, 2018b). Women and seniors who live alone are more likely to have low income compared with other seniors (Conference Board of Canada, 2013).

An increasingly recognized determinant of poor physical and mental health among seniors is elder abuse, defined as mistreatment towards seniors that can include neglect and abandonment, in addition to financial, physical, psychological or sexual abuse (Royal Canadian Mounted Police, 2018). A recent study that examined a large cohort of adults older than the age of 55 years in Canada in an attempt to determine the prevalence of mistreatment among seniors found that, overall, 8% of community-dwelling older adults were mistreated. More specifically, 2.2% of people older than the age of 55 years were physically abused, 1.6% were sexually abused, 2.7% were emotionally abused, and 2.6% were financially abused. The most common perpetrators of abuse included spouses, children or grandchildren, friends, and service providers. Interestingly, both social isolation and depression were correlated with mistreatment, although it's difficult to tease out whether isolation or depression leads to abuse or whether it is the other way around (McDonald, 2018).

> **EXERCISE 6.2:** List four risk factors for social isolation among seniors.

THE HEALTH OF PEOPLE LIVING WITH DISABILITIES

People who live with disabilities face many challenges in both their daily activities and their meaningful participation in society; physical and social environment influences a great deal in their functioning. Given that this group makes up a significant portion of the Canadian population and is anticipated to grow as the number of seniors grows, it has been chosen as a focal point for discussions on inequities.

Demography

According to recent estimates, 3.8 million Canadians over age 15 (which represents 14% of the population of Canada) live with some form of disability (Statistics Canada, 2017e). Although the causes and range of disability are quite broad, it is estimated that about 32% of Canadians living with a disability have a "mild" disability, 20% have a "moderate" disability, 23% have a "severe" disability, and nearly 26% have a "very severe" disability. The most common types of disability reported in Canada are disabilities related to pain, flexibility, mobility, mental health, dexterity, and hearing (Statistics Canada, 2017e).

The proportion of people reporting a disability that interferes with their daily activities rises with age, with 43% of people over age 75 years reporting a disability. Women are more likely than men, on average, to report a disability.

The Health Gap

Disability status is a known determinant of health because people who live with a disability are more likely to experience ill health in terms of morbidity, mortality, and quality of life (Frier et al., 2018). For example, just over three quarters of people over the age of 15 years living with disabilities take a prescription medication at least once a week (Statistics Canada, 2017e). Additionally, among a subgroup of working women living with disabilities, satisfaction with their health was rated as being only 5.5 out of 10 on average (Crompton, 2010).

Understanding the Health Gap

For people living with disabilities, the key drivers of health inequities according to recent research include social support (as discussed previously in the section on seniors); transport-related barriers; and employment status, which affects income (Frier et al., 2018).

Access to affordable transportation is important when it comes to attending work and social activities and participating in everyday activities (e.g., grocery shopping and going to health appointments), all of which can affect health either directly or indirectly. People who live with disabilities face some barriers when it comes to transport, including requiring modifications when it comes to driving; reduced capacity to drive an automobile independently; and an increased reliance on the assistance of friends, family, and public transport to get around (Frier et al., 2018). Furthermore, when it comes to accessing public or specialized transit services, 26% of people with disabilities experienced "some" or "a lot" of difficulty using these services. Common challenges were overcrowding, issues getting in and out of a vehicle and getting to and from bus stops (Statistics Canada, 2017e).

Perhaps one of the most written about SDHs for people living with disabilities is employment status. The employment rate for people living with disabilities is significantly lower than for people without disabilities. For example, the employment rate among 15- to 64-year-olds living with a disability was 47% compared to a rate of 74% among those without disabilities (Statistics Canada, 2017e). Some people have attributed this low rate to the fact that people with disabilities tend to be older and are less likely to hold a university degree. However,

a recent report by Statistics Canada has found that even after accounting for these factors, on the whole, people with disabilities in Canada are still less likely than people without disabilities to be employed. Thus, discrimination in the labour market also accounts for some of these differences. Around 12% of people living with a disability in Canada reported being denied a job because of their disability (Turcotte, 2015).

The relationship between labour market inequities and disability status is complex, however. For example, a promising trend is that among people in professional occupations, the employment rate for people with mild to moderate disabilities is similar to that for people without any disability (Turcotte, 2015).

Even when employed, people with disabilities may face inequities in terms of type of employment, retention, and promotion and may experience job-related discrimination. For example, just over 40% of workers with a disability considered themselves to be at a disadvantage in their career because of their disability (Statistics Canada, 2017e). On the whole, the median income of people with disabilities in Canada is about $10000 less than those without disabilities. Although this is attributed in part to differences in unemployment rates, even when employed, differences exist with respect to income. For example, the median employment income among men with a university degree who have a disability is about $69 200, quite a bit lower than the employment income for men without a disability who hold a university degree (which is $92 700) (Turcotte, 2015).

THE HEALTH OF LGBT2SQIA + CANADIANS

The acronym LGBT2SQIA+ is used for the discussion below to represent a very broad and diverse group of people who identify as lesbian, gay, bisexual, transgender, two-spirit, queer, questioning, intersex, and asexual. The plus indicates that there may be other identities not fully represented by the categories in the acronym. It is important to keep in mind that although this group of categories is aggregated together, many of the categories represent different concepts altogether. For example, although terms such as *lesbian* and *gay* often denote **sexual orientation** (i.e., attraction to others), terms such as *transgender* represent gender identity (i.e., how one perceives oneself in terms of a gender continuum), which is independent of sexual orientation. For example, a transgender male may be attracted to either men or women (Positive Space Campaign, n.d.).

This diverse population has been chosen for inclusion in this chapter because it represents a growing community, with increased rates of acceptance across our country.

Demography

As with other groups discussed in this chapter, LGBT2SQIA+ people in Canada represent a very diverse range of individuals, and the full extent of this diversity is difficult to capture through tools such as data collection and statistics. In fact, before 2014, no data were collected by Statistics Canada on sexual orientation. Cycle 2.1 of the Canadian Community Health Survey (CCHS) (described in Chapter 2) was the first Statistics Canada survey to include a question on sexual orientation (Statistics Canada, 2015a). After the legalization of same-sex marriages in 2005, the Census began to capture data on same-sex couples who are married or common law (only one subset of some LGBT2SQIA+ individuals) (Statistics Canada, 2017f).

According to 2016 census data, 1% of all married or common law couples in Canada are same-sex couples. Between 2006 and 2016, the number of same-sex couples enumerated on the Census grew by 60%, perhaps in part because of increased social and legal acceptability of being married or in a common-law same-sex relationship.

The proportion of same-sex couples that are males (51.9%) is roughly the same as females (48.1%). Nearly one third of same-sex couples who were enumerated by Statistics Canada are married. Notably, nearly 50% of married or common law same-sex couples live in Toronto, Montréal, Vancouver, and Ottawa–Gatineau. The proportion of same-sex couples with children is 12% (compared with ~50% for couples that are not same sex) (Statistics Canada, 2017f).

According to the CCHS data that specifically asked people about whether they consider themselves to be heterosexual, homosexual, or bisexual, approximately 1.7% of respondents aged 18 to 59 years reported that they consider themselves to be homosexual, and 1.3% of respondents considered themselves to be bisexual (Statistics Canada, 2015a).

EXERCISE 6.3: In terms of data validity, what are some advantages and disadvantages to asking questions about sexual orientation in the following way: "Do you consider yourself to be heterosexual, homosexual, or bisexual?"

Is there a better way that you can think of to capture this same information by using a different question?

The Health Gap

Several studies have outlined some of the differences in health outcomes and their risk factors that are more prevalent among LGBT2SQIA+ Canadians. For example, in the domain of sexual health, LGBT2SQIA+ populations tend to have higher rates of HIV, gonorrhea, and syphilis infections. Additionally, rates of smoking tend to be higher in this group compared with the general Canadian population, which puts this population at undue risk for a number of chronic conditions associated with smoking (including cancer and heart disease). Mental health outcomes, including higher rates of depression and suicidal ideation, have also been well studied in this population (Gahagan & Colpitts, 2017). In fact, according to the most recent CCHS data, the population of homosexual and bisexual individuals captured in the data was more likely than the general population to have had a consultation with a psychologist over the past 12 months (Statistics Canada, 2015a). Lifetime risk of a mood disorder diagnosis is around 25% for bisexual women and 11% in lesbian women compared with only 8% in heterosexual women (Steele et al., 2017). Broader North American data have also found that this population is less likely to engage in screening behaviours (e.g., Pap tests) (Cahill, 2017). Rates of stress (which may explain some of the inequities in health status) are also different between LGBT2SQIA+ people and the general Canadian cohort. According to the CCHS data, just over one third of people identifying as homosexual or bisexual reported that their days were either "quite a bit or extremely stressful," compared with 27% of the general population (Statistics Canada, 2015a). Finally, data on LGBT2SQIA+ youth have found higher rates of unwanted pregnancies, intravenous drug use, and sexual abuse in this population (Knight et al., 2014). For a discussion specifically on the health and determinants of health of transgendered Canadians, see Box 6.4.

Understanding the Health Gap

Differences in health status and adoption of risk behaviours can partially be explained through the increased rates of stress faced by LGBT2SQIA+ people (as discussed earlier) because stress is known to affect the adoption of risk behaviours, as well as influence physical and mental health.

Access to health care services and discrimination faced in the health sector is another important determinant of health inequities in this population.

BOX 6.4   The Health of Transgendered People in Canada

Transgendered people are individuals who "experience a different gender identity from their sex at birth" (Bauer et al., 2014). In Canada, transgendered people face disproportionately high rates of disease, even compared with the general LGBT2SQIA+ population. More specifically, rates of mental health issues and suicide are quite a bit higher in this population than in the general Canadian population. A sample of Ontario transgendered people, for example, revealed that more than 50% of respondents had symptoms consistent with depression, and 43% had a history of attempting suicide (Bauer & Scheim, 2016).

The inequities faced by transgendered Canadians are partially due to the discrimination they face in accessing health services. A recent study from Ontario found that of 400 transgendered respondents, one in five actually avoided going to the emergency department because of fear of discrimination, and one in two reported a negative encounter related to their gender identity when accessing emergency care (Bauer et al., 2014). In terms of social determinants of health beyond the health sector, trans people in Canada are also known to face higher rates of unemployment, food insecurity, and social ex-

clusion, as well as lower rates of postsecondary education completion—all of which are known to affect health (Giblon, 2016). Among a sample of transgendered Ontarians, 13% reported being fired because they were trans. Transphobia, significant discrimination, and even violence have been reported by a shockingly large proportion of transgendered individuals. In the same Ontario sample described, nearly 20% of transgendered people reported being physically or sexually assaulted, and just over one in three reported being verbally abused because of being transgendered (Bauer & Scheim, 2016).

These experiences have a huge impact on social participation and inclusion, and many trans people avoid public spaces (e.g., washrooms, libraries, gyms, malls, restaurants) because of fear of discrimination or embarrassment. Some are even forced to move from their home communities and places of origin because of either discrimination or a lack of availability of trans-specific services (Bauer & Scheim, 2016). Thus, although racism and discrimination are important determinants of health, so is violence against a group or a community.

According to recent CCHS data, for example, people who identified as being homosexual or bisexual were less likely to have a regular medical doctor, compared with those who identified as heterosexual. Additionally, more people who identified as homosexual or bisexual reported having unmet health care needs (i.e., needing medical care but not receiving it over the past 12 months) (Statistics Canada, 2015a). Reasons to explain this are plentiful. Health care trainees, for example, are not well-trained in the area of LGBT2SQIA+ health and often approach their work using a heterosexual lens (Gahagan & Subirana-Malaret, 2018). Research that examined clinician experiences has found that many health care professionals feel "uncomfortable and underprepared" when providing care to LGBT2SQIA+ youth (Knight et al., 2014). This may cause problems when it comes to asking questions or giving advice about LGBT2SQIA+ health and may lead people belonging to these groups to feel uncomfortable, not heard, or worse—further stigmatized. LGBT2SQIA+ groups also often actively avoid health care services because of fear of stigma or discrimination—a very real and often-described phenomenon in the Canadian

health care system (Gahagan & Subirana-Malaret, 2018). A recent study conducted in Nova Scotia found that a large proportion of LGBT2SQIA+ participants in a qualitative study described experiencing negative interactions with health system services (Colpitts & Gahagan, 2016).

It is important to keep in mind that, until recently, homosexuality was considered to be a pathological psychiatric condition requiring "treatment". As well, our health care institutions can be very heteronormative, without doing so consciously. For example, when filling out demographic information about patients, many hospitals only have categories for "man" or "woman" and, often, bathrooms are designed for the either/or category.

Lastly, as with many other groups, social support has been found to be a critical determinant of health for LGBT2SQIA+ people (Colpitts & Gahagan, 2016). With many groups feeling disconnected or even unaccepted by their communities or families because of their gender identity or sexual orientation, support from families, friends, and other members of the LGBT2SQIA+ community can be very protective for health (Colpitts & Gahagan, 2016).

EXERCISE 6.4: Imagine that you are a nurse practitioner working at a sexual health clinic. When gathering clinical information regarding behaviour and sexual practices, what questions might you ask, and how might you frame these questions so that they are neutral, sensitive, and nonjudgemental? Provide examples.

EXERCISE 6.5: In addition to social supports and social connectedness, what other protective factors might groups that experience inequities possess that would help to mitigate the health risks of being marginalized or oppressed?

CRITICAL THINKING QUESTION 6.2: Think of an institution you are affiliated with (e.g., a clinic, hospital, university). In what ways does this institution perpetuate a heteronormative approach to dealing with individuals?

THE HEALTH OF PEOPLE WHO EXPERIENCE HOMELESSNESS

Demography

As discussed in Chapter 5, defining and counting homelessness is a complex task and underreporting is a significant problem, especially because of the challenges involved with identifying people who are considered to be "the hidden homeless" or people who are temporarily living with friends or family. Nevertheless, recent statistics indicate that over the course of 12 months, between 150 000 and 300 000 Canadians will experience homelessness (Piat et al., 2015). In terms of youth homelessness, it is estimated that over the course of a year, between 25 000 and 35 000 Canadian youth experience homelessness (Kidd, Gaetz, & O'Grady, 2017).

Homeless Canadians are highlighted in this chapter to emphasize the importance of housing as a determinant of health and to demonstrate the interplay between housing and other determinants of health, such as adverse childhood experiences and poverty.

The Health Gap

Perhaps most striking are the inequities in mortality experienced by homeless Canadians compared with the general population. One study found that homeless youth in Canada die at rates 11 to 40 times higher than the general adolescent population, mostly as a result of drug overdose and suicide (Kidd et al., 2017). A landmark study conducted in 2009 found a significant association between the risk of death and living in shelters, rooming houses, or hotels. Alarmingly, this study found that among Canadians who were experiencing homelessness, the probability of surviving to age 75 years was only 32% (Hwang et al., 2009).

Much has been written about the correlation between homelessness and poor mental health. For example, up to one third of people who experience homelessness have a serious mental illness (which includes schizophrenia and bipolar disorder), and up to one half suffer from substance misuse (Piat et al., 2015). The relationship between poor mental health and homelessness is, of course, complex, with evidence showing both that homelessness is a risk factor for poor mental health and that poor mental health can be a risk factor for homelessness (Piat et al., 2015).

In addition to poor mental health, homeless Canadians also have higher rates of physical health issues. Homeless individuals tend to have disproportionately higher rates of certain NCDs (e.g., cardiovascular disease, high blood pressure [Baggett, Liauw, & Hwang, 2018], lung disease), injuries—both intentional (e.g., suicide) and unintentional, as well as higher rates of communicable diseases (including HIV, hepatitis, and TB). They also tend to have an earlier onset of NCDs compared with the general population (Smith et al., 2017). Additionally, when it comes to health care utilization, homeless Canadians have higher rates of hospitalizations and longer durations of admission compared with the general population (Smith et al., 2017).

Understanding the Health Gap

Housing is a critical determinant of health, and there are a number of pathways by which people who are homeless or living in places such as shelters or rooming houses are at risk of poor health. For example, people without shelter are at a greater risk of assault and victimization (and this is worse for youth or women who experience homelessness), as well as the effects of things such as heat and cold. Overcrowding and poor sanitation in shelters also put one at risk of certain health conditions, such as TB. Trauma and stress experienced as a result of not having a stable home are ways in which homeless Canadians are at higher risk of poor health. Additionally, not having a stable place to live presents many barriers to be able to access health care consistently, engage in preventive health practices, take medications, and follow up for treatment services.

When explaining the inequities in health between people who experience homelessness and other Canadians, however, we must go beyond considering housing as a key determinant of health and also consider how some of the factors that put people at risk of homelessness to begin with influence their health and development. For example, people who are experiencing or have experienced homelessness are much more likely to report a history of physical or sexual violence in their younger years, poverty, and family conflict and violence—all of which we know significantly influence health, particularly when experienced in the early years of life (Piat et al., 2015). Expanding on this, homeless Canadians are more likely to have experienced extremely stressful life events such as placement in foster care, incarceration, major financial disruptions, death, or the loss of important relationships (including parental abandonment) (Piat et al., 2015).

Last, it is very important to consider social and political factors when it comes to explaining health inequities. Rising costs of shelter coupled with a lack of adequate financial supports for people living in poverty and a lack of affordable housing options increases the risk of homelessness and its ill health effects (Piat et al., 2015). Social and political factors such as political will, social policies (e.g income and housing policy) are key to understanding the health gaps of many groups and must change in order to achieve health for all.

EXERCISE 6.6: Apply the determinants of health and equity listed in Table 6.1 to analyze the determinants of health and mechanisms by which another group in Canadian society experiences inequities—people who are incarcerated. Which determinants of health are likely to influence health inequities and poor health status among the prison population, and how?

THE HEALTH OF RURAL AND REMOTE POPULATIONS IN CANADA

According to Statistics Canada's Population Centre and Rural Area Classification, there are 918 small population centres (with a population between 1 000 and 29 999) in Canada. Additionally, all areas outside of population centres (which have a population of at least 1 000 people) are classified as rural areas. (Statistics Canada, 2016). However, it is important to keep in mind that the language used to describe rural communities matters. The classifications impact the perception of the community and those who live there, as well as acting as factors of inclusion or exclusion for various programs and funding opportunities, which can impact health equity. Definitions of **rural** emphasize different criteria and ask

different questions: number of residents, population size, and geographic distances are measured in diverse ways. As a result, definitions generate varied information about being rural that makes it difficult to capture accurate data on health status; Canadians who live in rural communities; and the human health workforce, including the number of physicians and nurses, who practise in rural communities. Much of the data that are being captured relate specifically to facility utilization. Consequently, measuring and responding to rural population outcomes as they relate to the specifics of individual community services (e.g., prevention of diabetic complications) is challenging (Grzybowski & Kornelsen, 2013).

Demography

As discussed in the book's Introduction, Rural Canada constitutes 95% of the country's land mass, with approximately 18% of Canada's population living in rural and remote communities (Statistics Canada, 2017h). Commonly in rural communities, there are fewer immigrant and visible minority populations (with some exceptions—see Box 6.5, regarding Brooks, Alberta), higher proportions of Indigenous peoples, and unique religious groups (i.e., Amish, Hutterites, and Mennonites). The diversity of populations in rural and remote areas poses significant challenges to the health care systems in these regions. These demographic characteristics play a large role in the comparative vulnerability that rural Canadians experience across a number of determinants of health determinants.

BOX 6.5   The Changing Landscape of Brooks, Alberta

In the mid-1990s, the town of Brooks, Alberta, had a population of approximately 10 000 people, with the number of visible minorities sitting at approximately 315 (Broadway, 2007). Since then, the population of Brooks has grown considerably. Sometimes called *The City of 100 Hellos*, more than 100 languages are now spoken in Brooks (City of Brooks, n.d., p. 8). Demographic data shows a substantial increase in the immigrant population between 1996 and 2012. The percentage of the population consisting of immigrant and nonpermanent residents increased from 6.7% in 1996 to 23.9% in 2011. The largest number of newcomers arrived between 2006 and 2011, with 1 245 newcomers arriving in Brooks in that period, resulting in a total immigrant population of 2 680 immigrants, or 19.5 % of the total population (Statistics Canada, 2013).

EXERCISE 6.7:
1. What happened in Brooks, Alberta, between 1996 and 2012 that created an influx of immigrants to this town?
2. What services were impacted and created to address the needs of this new population?

The Health Gap

As mentioned earlier, data tend to be quite dated regarding rural health outcomes, however, there is evidence that rural Canadians do not enjoy the same health status as individuals living in more urban settings. In general, rural Canadians tend to be older in age, experience worse health outcomes, and have a lower income compared with their urban counterparts. Increased urbanization and centralization of medical services has further stressed this situation. Inequities in Indigenous health and access to care for Indigenous people in rural Canada are also evident (see Chapter 7). Rural Canadians generally have a lower socioeconomic position because of higher unemployment rates and lower education levels than do their urban Canadian counterparts (Kirby & LeBreton, 2002).

Rural residents have a shorter life expectancy and higher mortality and infant mortality rates than the Canadian average (Canadian Institute for Health Information [CIHI], 2013). In contrast to urban residents, rural residents show higher levels of high blood pressure and obesity, higher levels of arthritis or rheumatism and depression, and lower levels of self-reported functional health, self-assessed health status, and health-promoting behaviours (CIHI, 2006). Furthermore, Canadians who live in rural areas tend to have higher rates of injury and premature death than their urban counterparts and have higher rates of cardiovascular disease and respiratory illness (CIHI, 2006). Rural residents' health indicators such as lifestyle-related illnesses, injuries, and poisoning are inferior to those of their urban counterparts (Hay, Varga-Toth, & Hines, 2006). Among women living in rural Canada, screening rates for breast cancer are lower than in urban areas (Roberts & Falk, 2002).

Understanding the Health Gap

Factors such as gender, age, occupation, environment, and geography must be considered as determinants of rural health. Rural women are disproportionately affected by social factors such as poverty and violence and are negatively impacted by "the urban bias of specialized services for family violence, combined with the centralization of more generalized services such as Social Services, Legal Aid … creates a serious issue of accessibility for rural women and their families" (Martz & Saraurer, 2000, p. ii). Women who live in rural areas are also disadvantaged by the lack of subsidized daycare, inadequate employment opportunities, and lack of access to affordable housing.

Young children, adolescents, and seniors are often over-represented in rural regions. These age groups present unique challenges to the health care systems of rural areas. Health promotion and education for children and adolescents tend to be underdeveloped in many rural communities. Rural youth benefit from early exposure to information on matters such as healthy diets and fitness; healthy sexuality; and the dangers of smoking, alcohol, and drug abuse.

Many rural and remote communities are reliant on natural resources and have chronic high unemployment, and the vulnerability of single-industry towns can pose significant economic challenges to many communities. Occupations in rural areas, such as forestry, fishing, mining, farming, and the meatpacking industry, face important health concerns. High accident rates and high incidence of occupational diseases such as lung cancer; obstructive pulmonary diseases; and cancers of the bowel, stomach, bone, bladder, and pancreas can be found among many miners.

Economic growth of rural communities can become a threat to a region's water supply, air and soil quality, and overall health of residents. For example, in areas where there are livestock operations, gastrointestinal illnesses can occur with the danger of manure—and the bacteria, parasites, and phosphorus it contains—getting into local lakes, rivers, and underground aquifers when it is not properly contained, which becomes a serious health concern. Recent water-contamination tragedies in North Battleford, Saskatchewan, and in Walkerton, Ontario, demonstrate that these threats are very real (see Chapter 11).

Geography is a critical determinant of health for rural Canadians. Challenges include distance to clinics, not having enough family practitioners or specialists, the cost of disseminating information (as well as goods and services), and young people who move away to attend school and find work who do not often return, creating a much older demographic. There are often large distances between farms and reasonably sized towns or major urban centres where health services may be available, and with harsh Canadian winters, travelling to health care facilities is also risky and hazardous. These geographic realities directly impact the ease of access to and utilization of health services, as well as other health promoting goods and resources. They also decrease

TABLE 6.2   Individual-Level, Institution-Level, and Society-Level Interventions to Improve Health Equity

Level Of Intervention	Actual Intervention	Social Determinant Of Health
Individual level	Practice cultural humility	(racism and discrimination, health services)
	File and pay income tax	(income)
	Advocate for healthy public policies at the institutional and societal levels	(all)
	Practice equitable employment practices	(employment, income, discrimination)
Institutional level	Cultural humility training	(racism and discrimination)
	Clubs and associations	(social support)
	Mentoring programs	(social support)
	Pay employees a living wage	(income)
	Offer benefits like ancillary health services to employees	(health services)
Societal level	Guaranteed income	(income)
	Minimum wage	(income)
	Living wage	(income)
	Universal day care	(early childhood development)
	Employment equity laws	(employment, discrimination)
	Affordable housing units	(housing)
	Accessible parenting programs	(early childhood development)
	Home visitation programs	(early childhood development)
	Social assistance for people living in poverty, or with disabilities	(income)
	Design inclusive communities	(social isolation, employment, income)
	Housing first	(housing)

the response capability and timeliness of emergency health responders to rural residents when the need may arise.

INTERVENTIONS TO ADDRESS INEQUITIES AMONG VARIOUS GROUPS IN CANADA

Inequities in the Canadian population are avoidable and preventable. Action on key SDHs (as listed in Table 6.2) can help reduce the health gap that is seen in certain segments of the population. As discussed in Chapter 3, various strategies can be leveraged to redress inequities among various groups in Canada. In general, strategies to reduce inequities among various groups can be divided into three levels: (1) strategies at the individual or provider level, (2) strategies at the institutional level, and (3) strategies at the societal level. Health care providers can engage in many of these strategies, either directly as they care for members of groups experiencing inequities, design health

promotion or other programs for and with these groups, or act as leaders of institutions and become social entrepreneurs (see Chapter 3) or indirectly, via advocacy to their institutions or governments (see Chapter 3).

Individual-Level Strategies to Reduce Inequities

When engaging clients who are members of groups that experience inequities, providers must ensure that they treat these clients in appropriate and safe ways. A common framework that is used in many practice disciplines is the continuum of cultural awareness, sensitivity, competence, and safety. **Cultural awareness** simply means being conscious of the differences among various cultural groups. **Cultural sensitivity** takes cultural awareness a step further and refers to a deeper understanding of how culture shapes health and being mindful of your own culture and cultural biases. **Cultural competence** refers to the skill and ability of practitioners to provide effective care to people of different cultures. **Cultural safety** is a step beyond cultural competence that encompasses self-reflection (i.e., being mindful of your biases and your own culture and how it influences the care you provide to others) as well as working to reduce power imbalances (through advocacy, for example) (University of Ottawa, 2017).

Although cultural awareness, sensitivity, and competence do not require explicit reflection on or action towards reducing power imbalances, cultural safety and humility do. The notion of **cultural humility,** a somewhat newer concept that is emerging in the literature, was initially defined as "a lifelong commitment to self-evaluation and critique, to redressing the power imbalances in the [health care provider]-patient dynamic, and to developing mutually beneficial and non-paternalistic partnerships with communities on behalf of individuals and defined populations" (Foronda et al., 2016). Key principles underlying the idea of cultural humility are:
- Open-mindedness
- Self-awareness and self-reflection
- Critique
- Supportive interactions (Foronda, et al., 2016)

Institution-Level Strategies to Reduce Inequities

According to the NCCDH, health agencies can work on inequities through assessing and reporting on them (e.g., reporting on health care–associated infections by race or income to uncover inequities and an institution's role in those inequities), as well as designing and reorienting existing programs and interventions to meet the needs of groups facing inequities (NCCDH, 2010). A concept that is receiving international attention is called **proportionate universalism**. First outlined in 2010 in the *Strategic Review of Health Inequalities in England*, this concept refers to interventions that are universal (not targeted to specific groups) but designed in such a way that their scale and intensity matches the level of disadvantage faced by the beneficiaries of such an intervention (Carey, Crammond, & De Leeuw, 2015). For example, if one is designing a public health communication campaign for smoking cessation, although everyone is targeted, the messages for lower income parents may be more prominent or frequent (because low income is associated with higher smoking rates) or may be written in a way that respects differing literacy levels. Other institutional-level practices that can help to better serve groups facing inequities include training and development for staff to teach principles of cultural humility, ensuring safe and inclusive

spaces (e.g., many hospitals now contain nondenominational religious spaces to allow groups to practice their faith), and taking steps internally to ensure equity when it comes to hiring, retention, and promotion of staff.

Societal-Level Strategies to Reduce Inequities

Perhaps the most impactful of interventions include those at the societal level, for example, public policies and legislation that are health and equity promoting (also known as "healthy public policies," which are described in Chapter 3).

Internationally, several declarations exist that respect equity among all people. The United Nations Declaration of Human Rights, for example, was proclaimed in Paris in 1948 and represents a standard that all states should work towards. A few significant statements made in the proclamation are as follows:
- "All human beings are born free and equal in dignity and rights."
- "Everyone has the right to life, liberty and security of person."
- "Everyone has the right to recognition everywhere as a person before the law."
- "Everyone is entitled to all the rights and freedoms set forth in this Declaration, without distinction of any kind, such as race, colour, sex, language, religion, political or other opinion, national or social origin, property, birth or other status" (United Nations, 1948).

Often inspired by international declarations and conventions or treaties, countries, provinces, and territories develop their own human rights laws, which can be enforced at the appropriate level. In Ontario, for example, the *Ontario Human Rights Code* was enacted in 1962 and represented Canada's first such code. Under this law, every person is protected against discrimination when it comes to things like obtaining jobs, housing, and other services. Under the Code, there are 17 grounds for protection, including race, sex, disability, and age. Box 6.6 presents a full list of the protected grounds covered under the *Ontario Human Rights Code.*

The United Nations has also set forth various conventions (or treaties) respecting the rights of specific groups facing inequities. In 2006, for example, the United Nations Convention on the Rights of Persons with Disabilities was adopted in New York and signed by 82 countries around the world. The convention emphasizes the fundamental rights and freedoms of people living with all types of disabilities globally (United Nations, 2006).

A number of other societal-level strategies implemented at the municipal level exist, as well, to ensure the inclusion and success of groups facing health inequities. The age-friendly cities project, for example, was developed in 2006 by the World Health Organization to support municipalities in becoming more age friendly. Four Canadian cities participated, and the government has been supporting more Canadian communities to become age friendly. As part of this strategy, age-friendly communities focus on the following areas: improving outdoor spaces and buildings (e.g., ensuring wide sidewalks, adequate lighting), transportation (ensuring affordable and accessible transport options), housing (making sure houses are affordable and safe for seniors), social participation (making sure there are enough opportunities for seniors to volunteer and become active participating members of society), respect and social inclusion, civic participation and employment (addressing agism in employment), communication and information, and community support and health services (ensuring access to primary care providers for example) (PHAC, 2016). Another example of a municipally based program to address SDHs (particularly housing) is discussed in the Case Study box.

Similar to the general human rights laws, many provinces and territories have also followed suit and transformed these declarations into local, enforceable laws. Many provinces and territories have passed laws that require agencies to be accessible to people living with disabilities, for example. Other laws that help remedy social inequities include social policies related to income (e.g., minimum wage laws, welfare policies), housing (e.g., ensuring affordable housing), and employment (e.g., making hiring discrimination illegal). These can be enacted either provincially and territorially or federally.

One of the most successful Canadian interventions has been the implementation of a Guaranteed Annual Income program for seniors, known as Old Age Security (OAS). Through this program, all Canadians over the age of 65 years who have lived in Canada for 10 years or more after the age of 18 years receive a public pension. Seniors who are richer get less of this benefit compared with those who have lower total incomes. Additionally, low-income seniors below a certain threshold are entitled to receive a Guaranteed Income Supplement (GIS) to "top them up" to a livable amount. This program has resulted in low rates of poverty and food insecurity among seniors in Canada and is thought to have a beneficial impact on mental health, self-reported health, and functionality (McIntyre et al., 2016).

CASE STUDY

"Housing First" Strategy to Address Homelessness

In 2008, the federal government gave the Mental Health Commission of Canada more than $100 million to research a strategy known as Housing First. The idea behind Housing First is that to work on health issues, people first and foremost need a safe and secure place to live.

Housing is seen as a critical determinant of health and one of the most significant barriers to success in other programming efforts. So, in Housing First programs, the emphasis is on housing people who experience homelessness (in addition to providing them with other support services), as opposed to providing them with supports as a prerequisite to obtaining housing (Mental Health Commission of Canada, n.d.). The At Home study, which randomized participants to either a Housing First approach or usual supports, took place in five cities across Canada—Toronto, Vancouver, Montreal, Winnipeg and Moncton—and followed nearly 2 000 people over the course of 2 years. The results were significant. A housing first program resulted in lower rates of homelessness, significant cost savings, improved quality of life, and improved community functioning (Goering et al., 2014).

SUMMARY

This chapter examined key terms and principles to keep in mind when examining the health of certain groups facing health inequities in Canada. Terms such as *vulnerable, marginalized, high risk,* and *equity seeking* have their advantages and disadvantages. The language used to describe groups must be intentional and not contribute further to stigma. Additionally, we must recognize that groups facing inequities are extremely heterogenous and that much intersectionality exists among various dimensions of disadvantage.

The health of Canadian populations that experience inequities was described, including racialized Canadians (with a focus on new Canadians and Black Canadians), people living with disabilities, seniors, people experiencing homelessness, LGBT2SQIA+ populations, and individuals living in rural communities. These groups were focused on because of their prevalence or growth in the population over the years or because they highlight unique determinants of health and equity. However, when discussing any group that experiences inequities, analyses of these inequities should include a focus on key determinants of health (e.g., income, employment, social support, housing, health services, early childhood experiences, safe working conditions, racism, and discrimination).

Strategies to alleviate inequities are multifactorial and can be thought of as being categorized into various levels—those that occur at the individual level, the institutional level, and the societal level. Individual-level strategies can include advocacy in addition to practising principles of cultural humility. Institutional-level policies may include fair hiring and employment policies, providing employees with a decent wage and benefits, ensuring a safe and welcoming space for clients with differing backgrounds, and instituting training for staff on things like cultural humility and safety. Last, societal-level policies can exist at the international, national, provincial or territorial, and municipal levels and may include things such guaranteed income, Housing First initiatives, and laws banning discrimination in housing or employment based on certain grounds, to name a few.

KEY WEBSITES

Canadian Civil Liberties Association (CCLA): https://ccla.org
The CCLA has been involved in a variety of civil liberties movements throughout history in Canada. This independent nongovernmental organization partakes in legal, legislative, educational, and public advocacy efforts to protect constitutional rights and freedoms of Canadians. Visit the website to learn more.

Canadian Network for the Prevention of Elder Abuse (CNPEA): https://cnpea.ca/en
The CNPEA works at the local, regional, provincial or territorial, and national levels on programs and policy development to prevent elder abuse. This website provides information on the knowledge exchange tools and resources facilitated by CNPEA and ways of getting involved.

CARP: http://www.carp.ca
CARP was formerly known as the Canadian Association for Retired Persons. Currently, it is the largest nonpartisan association advocating for the health care, financial security, and freedom from discrimination for all older Canadians. Follow the link to find out about CARP chapters, membership, and work in the media.

National Collaborating Centre for Determinants of Health, National Collaborating Centre for Determinants of Health: *Let's Talk Racism and Health Equity* Resource: http://nccdh.ca/images/uploads/comments/Lets_Talk_Racism_and_health_equity_EN_web.pdf
This document is designed to encourage public health to act on racism as a key structural determinant of health inequities.

Ontario Human Rights Commission (OHRC): http://www.ohrc.on.ca/en
Since 1961, the OHRC has been working to prevent discriminate and promote as well as advance human rights for peoples in Ontario. Visit the link to learn about rights in Ontario, education and outreach resources, and works by the OHRC.

Trans PULSE: http://transpulseproject.ca/about-us
This community-based research project aims to understand how social exclusion, cisnormativity, and transphobia impact access to health and social services for trans people. Access the weblink to learn about the project history, Trans PULSE resource guide, research, and study results.

REFERENCES

Auger, N., Authier, M. A., Martinez, J., et al. (2009). The association between rural–urban continuum, maternal education and adverse birth outcomes in Quebec, Canada. *The Journal of Rural Health*, 25(4), 342–351.

Baggett, T. P., Liauw, S. S., & Hwang, S. W. (2018). Cardiovascular disease and homelessness. *Journal of the American College of Cardiology*, 71(22), 2585–2597. https://doi.org/10.1016/j.jacc.2018.02.077.

Barndt, J. R. (2007). *Understanding and dismantling racism*. Minneapolis: Fortress Press.

Bauer, G. R., Scheim, A. I., Deutsch, M. B., et al. (2014). Reported emergency department avoidance, use, and experiences of transgender persons in Ontario, Canada: Results from a respondent-driven sampling survey. *Annals of Emergency Medicine*, 63(6), 713–720. https://doi.org/10.1016/j.annemergmed.2013.09.027.

Bauer, G., & Scheim, A. (2016). *Transgender people in Ontario, Canada: Statistics from the Trans PULSE Project to inform human rights policy*. University of Western Ontario. Retrieved from https://www.rainbowhealthontario.ca/wp-content/uploads/woocommerce_uploads/2015/09/Trans-PULSE-Statistics-Relevant-for-Human-Rights-Policy-June-2015.pdf.

Bentley-Edwards, K. L. (2016). Hope, agency, or disconnect: Scale construction for measures of Black racial cohesion and dissonance. *Journal of Black Psychology*, 42(1), 73–99. https://doi.org/10.1177/0095798414557670.

Broadway, M. (2007). Meatpacking and the transformation of rural communities: A comparison of Brooks, Alberta and Garden City, Kansas. *Rural Sociology*, 72(4), 560–582.

Cahill, S. (2017). LGBT experiences with health care. *Health Affairs*, 36(4), 773–774. https://doi.org/10.1377/hlthaff.2017.0277.

Canadian, Heritage (2018). *Historic Black Canadian communities*. Ottawa: Government of Canada. Retrieved from https://www.canada.ca/en/canadian-heritage/campaigns/black-history-month/historic-black-communities.html.

Canadian Institute for Health Information. (2006). *How healthy are rural Canadians? An assessment of their health status and health determinants*. Ottawa: Author. Retrieved from https://secure.cihi.ca/free_products/rural_canadians_2006_report_e.pdf.

Canadian Institute for Health Information). (2013). *Hospital births in Canada: A focus on women living in rural and remote areas*. Ottawa: Author. Retrieved from https://secure.cihi.ca/free_products/Hospital%20Births%20in%20Canada.pdf.

Canadian Medical Association. (2016). *The state of seniors health care in Canada*. Retrieved from https://www.cma.ca/En/Lists/Medias/the-state-of-seniors-health-care-in-canada-september-2016.pdf.

Carey, G., Crammond, B., & De Leeuw, E. (2015). Towards health equity: A framework for the application of proportionate universalism. *International Journal for Equity in Health*, 14(1), 81. https://doi.org/10.1186/s12939-015-0207-6.

Catalyst. (2018). Quick take: Visible minorities in Canada. Retrieved from https://www.catalyst.org/knowledge/visible-minorities-canada.

City of Brooks. (n.d.). Community profile. Retrieved from http://www.brooks.ca/DocumentCenter/Home/View/255

Colpitts, E., & Gahagan, J. (2016). "I feel like I am surviving the health care system": Understanding LGBTQ health in Nova Scotia, Canada. *BMC Public Health*, 16(1), 1005. https://doi.org/10.1186/s12889-016-3675-8.

Conference Board of Canada. (2013). Elderly poverty. Retrieved from https://www.conferenceboard.ca/hcp/Details/society/elderly-poverty.aspx.

Crompton, S. (2010). *Living with disability series: Life satisfaction of working-age women with disabilities*. Ottawa: Statistics Canada. Retrieved from https://www150.statcan.gc.ca/n1/pub/11-008-x/2010001/article/11124-eng.htm.

Foronda, C., Baptiste, D. L., Reinholdt, M. M., et al. (2016). Cultural humility: A concept analysis. *Journal of Transcultural Nursing*, 27(3), 210–217. https://doi.org/10.1177/1043659615592677.

Frier, A., Barnett, F., Devine, S., et al. (2018). Understanding disability and the "social determinants of health": How does disability affect peoples' social determinants of health? *Disability and Rehabilitation*, 40(5), 538–547. https://doi.org/10.1080/09638288.2016.1258090.

Gahagan, J., & Colpitts, E. (2017). Understanding and measuring LGBTQ pathways to health: A scoping review of strengths-based health promotion approaches in LGBTQ health research. *Journal of Homosexuality*, 64(1), 95–121. https://doi.org/10.1080/00918369.2016.1172893.

Gahagan, J., & Subirana-Malaret, M. (2018). Improving pathways to primary health care among LGBTQ populations and health care providers: Key findings from Nova Scotia, Canada. *International Journal for Equity in Health*, 17(1), 76. https://doi.org/10.1186/s12939-018-0786-0.

Gallinger, Z. R., Fralick, M., & Hwang, S. W. (2015). Ethnic differences in drowning rates in Ontario, Canada. *Journal of Immigrant and Minority Health*, 17(5), 1436–1443. https://doi.org/10.1007/s10903-014-0095-7.

Giblon, R. E. (2016). *Inequalities in social determinants of health in the Ontario transgender population*. Retrieved from https://ir.lib.uwo.ca/etd/3875.

Goering, P., Veldhuizen, S., Watson, A., et al. (2014). *National at home/chez soi final report*. Ottawa: Mental Health Commission of Canada. Retrieved from https://www.mentalhealthcommission.ca/sites/default/files/mhcc_at_home_report_national_cross-site_eng_2_0.pdf.

Grzybowski, S., & Kornelsen, J. (2013). Rural health services: Finding the light at the end of the tunnel. *Healthcare Policy Politiques de sante*, 8(3), 10–16.

Hay, D., Varga-Toth, J., & Hines, E. (2006). *Frontline health care in Canada: Innovations in delivering services to vulnerable populations*. Ottawa (Canada): Canadian Policy Research Networks. Retrieved from http://www.cprn.org/doc.cfm?doc=1554&l=en.

Henry, N. (2018). Black enslavement in Canada. *The Canadian Encyclopedia*. Retrieved from https://www.thecanadianen-cyclopedia.ca/en/article/black-enslavement.

Hoover, M., Rotermann, M., Sanmartin, C., et al. (2015). *Validation of an index to estimate the prevalence of frailty among community-dwelling seniors*. Ottawa: Statistics Canada. Retrieved from https://www150.statcan.gc.ca/n1/pub/82-003-x/2013009/article/11864-eng.htm.

Hwang, S. W., Wilkins, R., Tjepkema, M., et al. (2009). Mortality among residents of shelters, rooming houses, and hotels in Canada: 11 year follow-up study. *British Medical Journal, 339*, b4036. https://doi.org/10.1136/bmj.b4036.

Kidd, S. A., Gaetz, S., & O'Grady, B. (2017). The 2015 National Canadian Homeless Youth Survey: Mental health and addiction findings. *Canadian Journal of Psychiatry, 62*(7), 493–500. https://doi.org/10.1177/0706743717702076.

Kirby, M., & LeBreton (2002). *The Health of Canadians: The Federal Role Volume 2: Recommendations for Reform*. Ottawa: Standing Senate Committee on Social Affairs.

Knight, R. E., Shoveller, J. A., Carson, A. M., et al. (2014). Examining clinicians' experiences providing sexual health services for LGBTQ youth: Considering social and structural determinants of health in clinical practice. *Health Education Research, 29*(4), 662–670. https://doi.org/10.1093/her/cyt116.

Lane, G., Farag, M., White, J., et al. (2018). Chronic health disparities among refugee and immigrant children in Canada. *Applied Physiology Nutrition and Metabolism, 43*(10), 1043–1058. https://doi.org/10.1139/apnm-2017-0407.

Martz, D., & Sarurer, D. (2000). *Domestic violence and the experiences of rural women in east central Saskatchewan (p. ii), Muenster, SK: Prairie Women's Health Centre of Excellence*. Retrieved from http://www.pwhce.ca/pdf/do-mestic-viol.pdf.

McDonald, L. (2018). The mistreatment of older Canadians: Findings from the 2015 national prevalence study. *Journal of Elder Abuse & Neglect, 30*(3), 176–208. https://doi.org/10.1080/08946566.2018.1452657.

McIntyre, L., Kwok, C., Emery, J. H., et al. (2016). Impact of a guaranteed annual income program on Canadian seniors' physical, mental and functional health. *Canadian Journal of Public Health, 107*(2), 176–182. https://doi.org/10.17269/CJPH.107.5372.

McRae, M. (2014). *It happened here, too: The story of slavery in Canada*. Retrieved from https://humanrights.ca/blog/it-happened-here-too-story-slavery-canada.

Mental Health Commission of Canada. (n.d.). **What is Housing First?** Retrieved from https://www.mentalhealthcom-mission.ca/sites/default/files/Housing_Housing_First_Summary_0_1.pdf

National Collaborating Centre for Determinants of Health. (2010). *Integrating social determinants of health and health equity into Canadian public health practice: Environmental Scan 2010. Antigonish, NS: National Collaborating Centre for Determinants of Health*. St: Francis Xavier University. Retrieved from http://nccdh.ca/images/uploads/Envi-ron_Report_EN.pdf.

National Collaborating Centre for Determinants of Health. (2013). *Let's talk: Populations and the power of language*. Antigonish, NS: National Collaborating Centre for Determinants of Health. St: Francis Xavier University. Retrieved from http://nccdh.ca/images/uploads/Population_EN_web2.pdf.

National Seniors Council. (2016). *Report on the social isolation of seniors*. Retrieved from https://www.canada.ca/en/national-seniors-council/programs/publications-reports/2014/social-isolation-seniors/page03.html.

National Seniors Council. (2017). *Who's at risk and what can be done about it? A review of the literature on the social isolation of different groups of seniors*. Retrieved from https://www.canada.ca/en/national-seniors-council/pro-grams/publications-reports/2017/review-social-isolation-seniors.html.

Nestel, S. (2012). *Colour-coded health care: The impact of race and racism on Canadians' health*. Toronto: Wellesley Institute. Retrieved from http://www.wellesleyinsti-tute.com/wp-content/uploads/2012/02/Colour-Cod-ed-Health-Care-Sheryl-Nestel.pdf.

Ontario Human Rights Commission. (n.d). *(Racial discrimination, race and racism (fact sheet)*. Retrieved from http://www.ohrc.on.ca/en/racial-discrimina-tion-race-and-racism-fact-sheet.

Piat, M., Polvere, L., Kirst, M., et al. (2015). Pathways into homelessness: Understanding how both individual and structural factors contribute to and sustain homelessness in Canada. *Urban Studies, 52*(13), 2366–2382. https://doi.org/10.1177/0042098014548138.

Positive Space Campaign. (n.d.). *Terminology: What do all the LGBT2SQIA+ terms mean?* University of British Columbia. Retrieved from http://positivespace.ubc.ca/terminology/

Public Health Agency of Canada. (2016). *Age-friendly communities*. Retrieved from https://www.canada.ca/en/public-health/services/health-promotion/aging-seniors/friendly-communities.html.

Public Health Agency of Canada. (2018). *Surveillance of tuberculosis (TB)*. Retrieved from https://www.canada.ca/en/public-health/services/diseases/tuberculosis-tb/sur-veillance-tuberculosis-tb.html.

Ramage-Morin, P. L., Gilmour, H., & Rotermann, M. (2017). *Health reports: Nutritional risk, hospitalization and mortality among community-dwelling Canadians aged 65 or older*. Ottawa: Statistics Canada. Retrieved from https://www150.stat-can.gc.ca/n1/pub/82-003-x/2017009/article/54856-eng.htm.

Roberts, J., & Falk, M. (2002). *Women and health: Experiences in a rural regional health authority*. Winnipeg, MB: Prairie Women's Health Centre of Excellence. Retrieved from http://www.pwhce.ca/pdf/rha.pdf.

Royal Canadian Mounted Police. (2018). *Elder abuse*. Retrieved from http://www.rcmp-grc.gc.ca/ccaps-spcca/elder-aine-eng.htm.

Siddiqi, A., Shahidi, F. V., Ramraj, C., et al. (2017). Associations between race, discrimination and risk for chronic disease in a population-based sample from Canada. *Social Science & Medicine, 194*, 135–141. https://doi.org/10.1016/j.socscimed.2017.10.009.

Smith, O. M., Chant, C., Burns, K. E., et al. (2017). Characteristics, clinical course, and outcomes of homeless and non-homeless patients admitted to ICU: A retrospective cohort study. *PloS One, 12*(6), e0179207. https://doi.org/10.1371/journal.pone.0179207.

Statistics Canada. (2013). *Brooks, CY, Alberta (Code 4802034) (table). National Household Survey (NHS) Profile. 2011 National Household Survey. Statistics Canada Catalogue no. 99-004-XWE*. Ottawa. Retrieved from http://www12.statcan.gc.ca/nhs-enm/2011/dp-pd/prof/index.cfm?Lang=E.

Statistics Canada. (2015a). *Same-sex couples and sexual orientation ... by the numbers*. Retrieved from https://www.statcan.gc.ca/eng/dai/smr08/2015/smr08_203_2015.

Statistics Canada. (2015b). *Section 3: Analysis of the results of the long-term projections*. Retrieved from https://www150.statcan.gc.ca/n1/pub/91-520-x/2010001/part-partie3-eng.htm.

Statistics Canada. (2016). *Population centre and rural area classification 2016*. Retrieved from https://www.statcan.gc.ca/eng/subjects/standard/pcrac/2016/introduction.

Statistics Canada. (2017a). *Visible minority and population group reference guide, Census of Population, 2016*. Retrieved from https://www12.statcan.gc.ca/census-recensement/2016/ref/guides/006/98-500-x2016006-eng.cfm.

Statistics Canada. (2017b). *Immigrant population in Canada, 2016 Census of Population*. Retrieved from https://www150.statcan.gc.ca/n1/pub/11-627-m/11-627-m2017028-eng.htm.

Statistics Canada. (2017c). *Immigration and ethnocultural diversity: Key results from the 2016 Census*. Retrieved from https://www150.statcan.gc.ca/n1/en/daily-quotidien/171025/dq171025b-eng.pdf?st=Piyme-Gs.

Statistics Canada. (2017d). *A portrait of the population aged 85 and older in 2016 in Canada*. Retrieved from https://www12.statcan.gc.ca/census-recensement/2016/as-sa/98-200-x/2016004/98-200-x2016004-eng.cfm.

Statistics Canada. (2017e). *A profile of persons with disabilities among Canadians aged 15 years or older, 2012*. Retrieved from https://www150.statcan.gc.ca/n1/pub/89-654-x/89-654-x2015001-eng.htm.

Statistics Canada. (2017f). *Census in brief: Same-sex couples in Canada in 2016*. Retrieved from https://www12.statcan.gc.ca/census-recensement/2016/as-sa/98-200-x/2016007/98-200-x2016007-eng.cfm.

Statistics Canada. (2017g). *Age and sex, and type of dwelling data: Key results from the 2016 Census*. Retrieved from https://www150.statcan.gc.ca/n1/daily-quotidien/170503/dq170503a-eng.htm.

Statistics Canada. (2017h). *Population size and growth in Canada: Key results from the 2016 Census*. Retrieved from https://www150.statcan.gc.ca/n1/daily-quotiden/170208/dq170208a-eng.htm.

Statistics Canada. (2018a). *Living arrangements of seniors*. Retrieved from https://www12.statcan.gc.ca/census-recensement/2011/as-sa/98-312-x/98-312-x2011003_4-eng.cfm.

Statistics Canada. (2018b). *Seniors' income from 1976 to 2014: Four decades, two stories*. Retrieved from https://www150.statcan.gc.ca/n1/pub/11-630-x/11-630-x2016008-eng.htm.

Steele, L. S., Daley, A., Curling, D., et al. (2017). LGBT identity, untreated depression, and unmet need for mental health services by sexual minority women and trans-identified people. *Journal of Women's Health, 26*(2), 116–127. https://doi.org/10.1089/jwh.2015.5677.

Turcotte, M. (2015). *Persons with disabilities and employment*. Ottawa: Statistics Canada. Retrieved from https://www150.statcan.gc.ca/n1/pub/75-006-x/2014001/article/14115-eng.htm.

United Nations. (1948). *The Universal Declaration of Human Rights*. Paris: Author. Retrieved from http://www.un-.org/en/universal-declaration-human-rights/.

United Nations. (2006). *Convention on the Rights of Persons with Disabilities (CRPD)*. Retrieved from https://www.un.org/development/desa/disabilities/convention-on-the-rights-of-persons-with-disabilities.html.

University of Ottawa. (2017). *From cultural awareness to cultural competency*. Ottawa: Author. Retrieved from https://www.med.uottawa.ca/sim/data/Serv_Culture_e.htm.

Uppal, S., & Barayandema, A. (2018). *Insights on Canadian society: Life satisfaction among Canadian seniors*. Ottawa: Statistics Canada. Retrieved from https://www150.statcan.gc.ca/n1/pub/75-006-x/2018001/article/54977-eng.htm.

Vamanu, B. I., Gheorghe, A. V., & Katina, P. F. (2016). The vulnerability issue. In *Critical infrastructures: Risk and vulnerability assessment in transportation of dangerous goods* (pp. 91–105). New York: Springer.

Vang, Z. M., Sigouin, J., Flenon, A., et al. (2017). Are immigrants healthier than native-born Canadians? A systematic review of the healthy immigrant effect in Canada. *Ethnicity & Health, 22*(3), 209–241. https://doi.org/10.1080/13557858.2016.1246518.

Veenstra, G., & Patterson, A. C. (2016). Black–white health inequalities in Canada. *Journal of Immigrant and Minority Health, 18*(1), 51–57. https://doi.org/10.1007/s10903-014-0140-6.

7

Indigenous Health

Ⓔ Additional resources are available online at http://evolve.elsevier.com/Canada/Shah/publichealth/

LEARNING OBJECTIVES

- Differentiate among the terms Aboriginal, Indigenous, First Nations, Métis, and Inuit.
- Describe, in general and at a high level, the demographic makeup of Indigenous people in Canada.
- Understand the effects of racism, colonialism, and self-determination on the health of Indigenous people, as well as the impact of decolonization.
- Summarize the health gaps that exist between Indigenous and non-Indigenous Canadians in the areas of morbidity, mortality, self-perceived health, and health care utilization.
- Describe Indigenous views on health.
- List challenges in health care provision and access to Indigenous communities, on and off reserve.
- Be familiar with strategies that the health sector can take to reduce health inequities facing Indigenous people.
- Define the terms *ally* and *accomplice* and reflect on how one can be an aspiring ally of Indigenous people.

CHAPTER OUTLINE

KEY TERMS

Aboriginal
accomplice
ally
colonialism
colonization
cultural appropriation
cultural hegemony
decolonization
ethnocentrism
First Nations

Indian Act
Indigenous
intergenerational trauma
Inuit
Jordan's Principle
medicine wheel
Métis
Non-Insured Health Benefits Program (NIHB)
residential schools

resiliency
Royal Commission on Aboriginal People (RCAP)
Royal Proclamation
self-determination
Sixties Scoop
Truth and Reconciliation Commission (TRC)

INTRODUCTION

Before embarking on an exploration of Indigenous health issues, it is important to keep in mind that although this chapter has been extensively researched and reviewed with support and in consultation with Indigenous partners, its primary authors are settlers of this land. Thus, this chapter is being written from the perspective of settlers aspiring to be allies—people who are committed to the rights of nondominant groups and the elimination of social inequities and who establish meaningful relationships with communities to support and show accountability to those communities (refer to Box 7.1 for a more detailed understanding of what it means to be an *ally* and an *accomplice*) (Smith, Puckett, & Simon, 2015). As with any piece of published work, it is important that readers keep in mind the perspective (with all its strengths and limitations) from which it is written.

When thinking through issues of inequity and groups experiencing inequities, one must be mindful of the distinct but interrelated concepts of cultural hegemony and ethnocentricity. **Cultural hegemony** occurs when the dominant (or ruling) class maintains its dominance through cultural or ideological means—meaning through the perpetuation of self-serving norms, ideas, values, and worldviews (Cole, 2019). **Ethnocentrism** can be thought of as the tendency that people have to view or evaluate other societal groups according to the values and standards of their own group (which they often perceive as being superior to others) (Cambridge Dictionary, 2019). For example, in science and health care, we often have established "ways of knowing"—that is, methods and tools that we feel are reliable and credible places from which to obtain knowledge from. These include things such as randomized controlled trials, program evaluations, written reports reflecting indicators, and the like. Underlying this are the assumptions that some studies are rigorous and objective, that quantitative information is the most reliable kind of information, and that information and data should be written down. However, many non–North American and European

---

BOX 7.1   What It Means To Be an Ally and an Accomplice

Aspiring to be an **ally** (because it is a process, not a designation) means constantly engaging in a process of self-reflection, thinking about how one chooses to live and how one's actions and behaviours affect (either directly or indirectly) nondominant groups. As alluded to earlier, being an Indigenous ally goes beyond understanding history or displaying minimal prejudice towards Indigenous peoples. It means actually supporting (not leading) and working alongside Indigenous peoples to promote rights and change the political and social structures that contribute to health inequities (Smith et al., 2015).

The term **accomplice** is increasingly being used by social justice advocates to refer to people who move beyond working with and standing by individuals or communities to explicitly focus on dismantling oppressive structures. The focus of being an accomplice then is on social structures and addressing root cause of inequities (Clemens, 2017).

A common example to highlight the differences between the two terms is that whereas an Indigenous ally might read about Indigenous history, reflect on their own behaviours (e.g., being affiliated with an institution that may have in the past contributed to the process of colonialization), and attend marches and demonstrations organized by the community to show support, an accomplice might work specifically for an organization that aims to support the process of self-determination and creation of systems whereby Indigenous people self-govern in the areas education, health, and other social systems (Clemens, 2017). The two concepts, of course, overlap, and it is essential to keep in mind that one cannot self-identify as an ally or accomplice but might be considered a person who is aspiring to be one or both from the perspective of the nondominant community itself (Smith et al., 2015).

Exercise

Being an aspiring ally involves reflecting on your own privilege and position in society. For the categories listed below, identify who the "dominant group" is considered to be within that category and whether your own identity is aligned with that dominant group or not. (For example, for the "gender" category, the dominant group is male. Nondominant groups you may otherwise identify with could be female, transgender, other.):

- Gender
- Age
- Sexual orientation
- Language
- Ability
- Body type
- Geographic region
- Social class

cultures and traditions value other ways of knowing or understanding complex phenomena, with very different underlying values and assumptions. Indigenous ways of knowing, for example, are predicated on the fact that knowledge is primarily experiential and personal. Knowledge is often orally transmitted through story and narrative, and the process of knowing something can be as valuable as the knowledge itself. Because this way of knowing differs from Western tradition, for many generations, Indigenous knowledge has been discredited because Westerners approached it from an ethnocentric perspective. Many Western institutions, including schools, universities, and colleges, advance the assumptions discussed (i.e., that quantitative, written-down information is the most valuable), further contributing to this problem (University of Toronto Ontario Institute for Studies in Education [OISE], n.d.). Another example of ethnocentrism (from health care) is the common dominant Western societal value that when it comes to health decision making, individuals have the right to make their own informed choices without undue influence; anything contrary to this may be framed as being inferior, a "challenge or issue" or the "wrong way to do things." However, in many other ethnocultural groups, family-based decision making is valued. Overall, although everyone approaches issues with their own conscious or unconscious biases (framed by their worldview and culture), the goal for learners reading this chapter is simply to be aware of the dominant worldview and how that may get perpetuated when speaking about nondominant groups. Being reflective of your own values, beliefs, and assumptions will also frame how you read and interpret learning material.

The area of Indigenous health is one of great complexity. It is vital that trainees and practitioners in various health disciplines have a solid understanding of Indigenous health matters. The Truth and Reconciliation Commission (TRC) (described in detail later in the chapter) calls for all nursing and medical students and, really, all health care providers across disciplines, to have an understanding of the history of Indigenous people, of how their history shapes health and its distribution, and how practitioners can ensure they are practising in culturally safe and competent ways (concepts related to cultural safety and competency are covered in Chapter 6). Across Canada, many faculties, schools, and departments are taking up the calls of the TRC by teaching required courses in Indigenous peoples' history

and health. The pedagogical approaches are more in line with Indigenous ways of knowing, bringing students on the land in their local communities to learn from Elders and community members about their language, history, and traditional medicine. Because we are all treaty people (discussed later), it is incumbent on all of us, including those who work in the health sector, to further the TRC's calls to action.

This chapter will, as a result, attempt to educate about and address various nuances related to the area of Indigenous health, but it does not represent a comprehensive or exhaustive exploration of all issues. Its goal is to introduce learners to the topic and present an overview of key areas relating to Indigenous health and their determinants. The main purpose of this chapter is to apply the concepts discussed in Chapter 6 to Indigenous people of Canada—a heterogenous group of people with a long history in North America (referred to by Indigenous people as Turtle Island). Similar to the discussions of other Canadian population groups in this book, the principles of using a strength-based approach, considering intersectionality, and engaging in reflexive practice must be kept in mind. Resources that provide more in-depth education and training are included in the Key Websites section at the end of this chapter, for those seeking further knowledge.

Two related concepts will be supported, applied, and discussed throughout this chapter: decolonization and self-determination. Whereas **decolonization** is defined as the "revalorization, recognition, and re-establishment of Indigenous cultures, traditions, and values within the institutions, rules, and arrangements that govern society" (Rice, 2016), **self-determination** refers to the individual and collective right to have control over health, education, and economic systems (i.e., self-government) (Auger, Howell, & Gomes, 2016). Both concepts aim to reverse the effects of colonialization (discussed further later) and put Indigenous people and their respective values and traditions at the centre of any change process or organization. This shifts the focus away from Indigenous people needing to be "helped" by broader societal efforts and towards community-led change processes and an infusion of Indigenous cultures, values, and traditions within society's institutions and processes.

The chapter presents an overview of the demographics of Indigenous people in Canada at this point in history, discusses health status and health determinants relating to Indigenous communities (recognizing the diversity and heterogeneity that exists between Indigenous groups), and touches on how health care and preventive health services are organized for Indigenous Canadians.

A Note about Terminology

Aboriginal is a term used in the Canadian Constitution of 1982 and thus has a very specific legal meaning. It is a broader term referring to the three major Indigenous groups in Canada—the First Nations, Inuit, and Métis people. Many members of these communities, however, may prefer to be identified not as Aboriginal or First Nations, Inuit, or Métis but as people of a specific local nation (e.g., Mohawk, Cree, Ojibwe) (Smith et al., 2015). The term **Indigenous** (i.e., people who inhabited a place before there was any colonial contact) is also commonly used, especially internationally and by many countries other than Canada that also have Indigenous communities (Smith et al., 2015). Use of the term *Indigenous* is often preferred to *Aboriginal* because it is not associated with federal law and better highlights the relationship between Indigenous people and land (Smylie & Firestone, 2016). Box 7.2 describes how the international community is supporting the advancement of Indigenous people around the world.

First Nations

The term **First Nations** became popular in the 1970s and replaced the term *Indian*, which increasingly was being recognized as offensive and often confused with people immigrating from India. The federal government classifies First Nations people based on whether they are registered under the *Indian Act* (i.e., Status First Nations) and thus are eligible to receive certain rights, or not (i.e., nonstatus First Nations) (Smylie & Firestone, 2016). This classification and Act remains problematic, and is discussed later in the Chapter

First Nations people are very diverse in their traditions and languages, with more than 50 cultural groups living in more than 1000 communities across the country (Smith et al., 2015).

Inuit

The **Inuit** in Canada have historical links to the Inuit in Greenland, Alaska, and Russia and have traditional homelands in four Canadian regions—Nunavut, Northern Québec (Nunavik), Labrador (Nunatsiavut), and Northwest Territories (Inuvialuit region) (McGhee, 2013) (Fig. 7.1). *Inuk* is the term used to refer to a person who identifies as Inuit (Smylie & Firestone, 2016).

> ### BOX 7.2   The United Nations Declaration on the Rights of Indigenous Peoples
>
> In September 2007, the United Nations (UN) General Assembly adopted the UN Declaration on the Rights of Indigenous Peoples, which outlines the minimum standards for assuring the rights, dignity, and well-being of the world's Indigenous communities (United Nations, 2008). Interestingly, Canada was one of four countries (along with the United States, Australia, and New Zealand) that initially voted against adopting this declaration but later reversed its decision (UNDESA, n.d.).
>
> Some of the articles included in the declaration state that Indigenous people:
> - Are free and equal to all other peoples
> - Have the right to self-determination
> - Have the right to all rights and freedoms contained in the Universal Declaration of Human Rights
> - Have the right to a nationality
> - Have the right not to be subjected to forced assimilation or destruction of their culture
> - Shall not be forcibly removed from their lands or territories
> - Have the right to practise and revitalize their cultural traditions and customs
> - Have the right to participate in decision making in matters which would affect their rights. (UN, 2008)
>
> The impetus for this global declaration was the growing recognition that around the world, not only in Canada, Indigenous peoples face varying levels of discrimination, oppression, and marginalization, leading to health inequities (UNDESA, n.d.).

Métis

Métis people include individuals who historically emerged from the mixing and intermarriage of First Nations and European people dating back to the 17th century and developed a distinct culture and language (Smylie & Firestone, 2016).

> **CRITICAL THINKING QUESTION 7.1:** Review the Indigenous Ally Toolkit developed by the Montreal Urban Aboriginal Community Strategy Network: https://exchange.youthrex.com/toolkit/indigenous-ally-toolkit.
>
> Reflect on your own interest in being an aspiring ally. Discuss the questions asked in the toolkit: Where does this interest stem from? What steps can you take personally to support the voices of marginalized groups, and what do you have that can be leveraged?

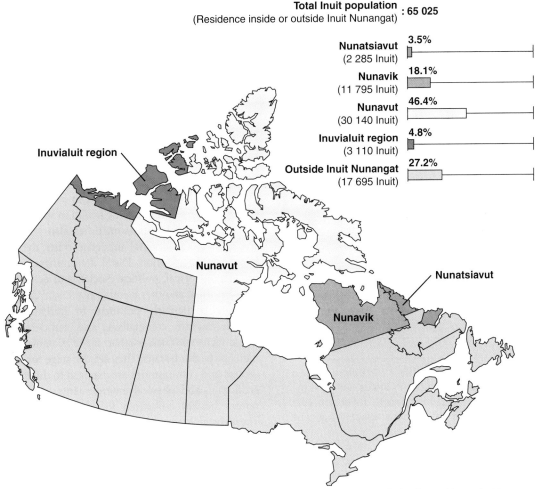

Fig. 7.1 Inuit Territories in Canada. (From Statistics Canada. [2016]. Inuit population by residence inside or outside Inuit Nunangat, 2016. *Census of Population 2016*. Retrieved from https://www150.statcan.gc.ca/n1/daily-quotidien/171025/mc-a001-eng.htm.)

DEMOGRAPHY

In Canada, there are more than 1.6 million Indigenous people, making up 4.9% of the population. Indigenous people are a fast-growing subset of the population. For comparison, in 1996, Indigenous people in Canada made up only about 2.8% of the population. Indigenous communities have grown at a rate almost four times that of non-Indigenous populations in the country and are expected to exceed 2.5 million people by 2036. Part of this increase is thought to be caused by more people identifying as Indigenous on the Census, and part by actual population growth (Statistics Canada, 2017a).

The Indigenous population is, on average, younger than the general Canadian population. The average age of Indigenous people in Canada is 32.1 years compared with 40.9 years for non-Indigenous Canadians (Statistics Canada, 2017a).

The majority of Indigenous people in Canada are First Nations, and they make up approximately 60% of Indigenous people in the country. In Canada, there are more than 600 First Nations bands. In contrast, Métis people represent about 35% of Indigenous people in Canada, and Inuit make up approximately 4% (Statistics Canada, 2017a).

In recent years, there has been an increase in the proportion of Indigenous people who live in cities and large metropolitan areas. In 2016, it was estimated that just over half of Indigenous people lived in a metropolitan area with a population of at least 30 000 people. In terms of geographic spread, Indigenous people live across the country. Of note, almost three of four Inuit people live in Inuit Nunangat—a region which includes the Northern coast of Labrador, Norther Quebec, Nunavur, and Northwest Territories; Ontario has the largest Métis population in Canada; and over half of the First Nations population lives in the Western provinces (Statistics Canada, 2017a).

In terms of the diversity of Canada's Indigenous population, the 2016 census estimated that there are more than 70 Indigenous languages (Statistics Canada, 2017a).

EXERCISE 7.1: It is important to note that most of our modern-day data collection tools, including the Census, may undercount Indigenous people. What are some reasons for this?

CRITICAL THINKING QUESTION 7.2: Before reading the next section about the health status and determinants of health of Indigenous people, reflect on your own perceptions and assumptions about Indigenous health.

What specific health issues come to mind when you think of the health of Indigenous people, and why? Are the issues that are top of mind informed by media coverage, your own experiences, research studies, or something else?

Similarly, reflect on the factors that you believe are most important for shaping the health of Indigenous people across the country. Make note, as you read through these next sections, about which of your notions of health status and determinants hold true and which ones do not hold true.

FACTORS INFLUENCING THE HEALTH OF INDIGENOUS PEOPLE IN CANADA

Before discussing the health of Indigenous peoples, it is important to discuss the factors that are critical in shaping Indigenous health, specifically. In previous sections of this book, we have made mention of a range of health determinants, including things such as education, access to health care, income level, housing conditions, and so on. These factors all intersect to influence health and its distribution

for Indigenous people; however, some other factors also need to explicitly be considered when thinking through the health inequities faced by Indigenous peoples, including racism, colonialism, and self-determination. We will highlight how these are all interconnected.

As discussed in Chapter 5, the many listed determinants of health can be categorized in different ways. For example, some determinants of health are more proximal (i.e., they affect health more directly). Examples of proximal determinants are things such as the physical or social environment (e.g., exposure to asbestos or loneliness) and health behaviours (e.g., fruit and vegetable consumption)—things that you can point to and more clearly identify as influencing health in some way.

Distal determinants (sometimes also referred to as structural determinants) influence other determinants in a cascading fashion. Distal determinants reflect the broader historical, political, social, and economic contexts in which all other factors exist. Distal determinants that are particularly pertinent to Indigenous health include racism, colonialism, and self-determination. These factors influence other, more proximal, determinants of health because they set the stage for why some groups and communities are exposed to different social, economic, and physical environments (and thus have poorer health) compared to others (Reading, 2015). These distal factors are discussed later and should always be kept in mind when statistics are presented that reflect inequities in health. For example, if you are reading a statistic stating that rates of social cohesion are higher in some Indigenous communities compared with the non-Indigenous Canadian population, you must always ask why and try to make the link between how things such as colonialism, racism, and self-determination play a role in explaining the statistic (Reading & Wien, 2009).

Racism

The issue of racism (both interpersonal and structural racism) has been defined and explored in Chapter 6. This section explores racism as it relates specifically to Indigenous communities.

Racism against Indigenous people in Canada is widespread. According to the Regional Health Survey, nearly 40% of First Nations surveyed had experienced overt forms of interpersonal racism in the past 12 months, and nearly two thirds of those reporting the experience stated that it negatively affected their self-esteem (Loppie, Reading, & de Leeuw, 2014). A range of negative stereotypes exist about Indigenous people, and at times these notions can be internalized by the very people who are being stereotyped. The media and popular culture may also reinforce these stereotypes, even simply by reporting on the gaps that exist in areas such as health, education, and employment—highlighting the need to take a strengths-based approach when communicating about issues related to Indigenous health.

Structural racism affecting Indigenous people is also prominent, even today. An example of this is lower rates of investment in Indigenous education systems, housing, and water treatment systems compared with those serving non-Indigenous people. Structural racism as it pertains to the justice system is also evident in this country. Not only are Indigenous people overrepresented in the prison system, but Indigenous offenders are also more likely to be imprisoned when convicted of a crime (Loppie et al., 2014). Indigenous victims of crime are also treated differently than non-Indigenous people, as evidenced by the inquiry into Missing and Murdered Indigenous Women (see Case Study box).

CASE STUDY

Missing and Murdered Indigenous Women and Girls in Canada

In recent years, the rate of violence, including violent deaths, among Indigenous women and girls has received greater recognition, largely because of the advocacy efforts of many Indigenous groups and leaders. Landmark reports have highlighted how Indigenous women are 12 times more likely to be murdered or missing than other Canadian women, 7 times more likely to be murdered by serial killers, and 3 times more likely to be assaulted or robbed.

These worrying statistics and calls to action by Indigenous leaders and human rights and community groups led to the Canadian government launching an independent inquiry into the Missing and Murdered Indigenous Women and Girls in 2016. The goal of this inquiry was to report on the root causes of all forms of violence (including sexual violence) against Indigenous women and girls. In its interim reports, the inquiry pointed to racism, colonialism, and a lack of self-determination as key underlying factors that influence the high rates of violence among Indigenous women and girls. Other more proximal reasons to explain the issue (which actually stem from the above mentioned factors) include an overrepresentation of Indigenous people in child welfare services, poverty, homelessness, the failure of police and child welfare systems in addressing the higher rates of violence, and intergenerational trauma (National Inquiry into Missing and Murdered Indigenous Women and Girls, 2017).

Racism is experienced by Indigenous people in nearly all sectors of society, and the health care sector is no exception. In 2015, the Wellesley Institute published a report titled *First Peoples, Second Class Treatment*, that highlighted the impact of racism on health and well-being and called attention to the explicit racism faced by Indigenous people in the health care sector. According to the Wellesley Institute, the very system of health care delivery to Indigenous people is flawed and may result in inequities between Indigenous people and non Indigenous Canadians (Allan & Smylie, 2015).

As will be discussed later in the chapter, only Status First Nations and Inuit people (as defined by the federal government) are entitled to specific health benefits under the Non-Insured Health Benefits (NIHB) program; Métis people and non-Status First Nations are not. The Wellesley report also presented some disturbing findings about how many Indigenous people may avoid health care or strategize around how to mitigate negative responses from health care providers who perceive them to be less credible or provide them with poorer quality care. One particular case that received much media attention was that of Mr. Brian Sinclair, a 45-year-old Indigenous man who waited more than 30 hours in a Winnipeg emergency department (ED) without being treated. He died of a bladder infection in the ED waiting room (Allan & Smylie, 2015).

Finally, as will be discussed more in the next section, federal laws such as the *Indian Act*, as well as the residential school system, are clear examples of structural racism that continue to affect health inequities for Indigenous people to this day.

Colonialism

Colonialism is defined as the imposition of systems (including policies, laws, cultures, and so on) by settlers on Indigenous people, resulting in thought patterns that support and perpetuate the occupation and subjugation of Indigenous people. Cultural hegemony—the imposition of thought patterns, ideas, and culture (as discussed in the introduction)—is one way of achieving colonialism. Colonialism is different from **colonization** (which is the process by which settlers occupied Indigenous lands) but is related to it in the sense that colonialism is the underlying ideology that allows for colonization to take place (National Inquiry into Missing and Murdered Indigenous Women and Girls, 2017).

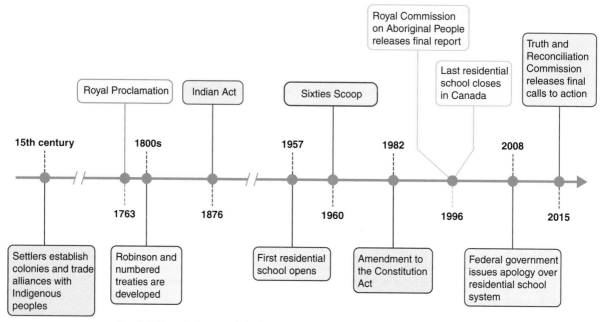

Fig. 7.2 Historical events in Indigenous history from European contact onwards.

As noted earlier, racism and colonialism are interrelated, with colonialism resulting in racist thoughts and practices and in racism being used as a justification for colonialism (Allan & Smylie, 2015).

To understand the extent of colonialism and its influence on the health of Indigenous people in Canada, a brief history of Indigenous contact with settlers and resulting government policies and systems must be recounted. This history is summarized in a timeline format in Fig. 7.2.

The first European explorers came to North America in the 11th century. For thousands of years before this, however, Indigenous people occupied land across the continent, developing rich traditions and systems of transportation, trade, and social life. In the 15th century, Europeans (predominantly French and British settlers and fisherman) began establishing colonies and trade alliances with Indigenous people (Government of Canada, 2017a). However, as more and more settlements occurred, there was increasing conflict between the British and French, and both sides also established military alliances with Indigenous peoples. Conflict also occurred between the settlers and Indigenous communities, particularly

around issues related to land. In 1763, France gave up its colonial territories, and the British became the primary European power in what is now Canada. To secure their position of power, the British decided that they required the support and cooperation of Canada's Indigenous people. As such, they drafted what is known as the **Royal Proclamation** in 1763—a landmark document that promised a specific area of land to Indigenous people, where no settlements or trade could occur without their explicit permission. In this proclamation, it was decided that only the crown could purchase land from an Indigenous person; the Indian Department was the liaison between Indigenous communities and the settler colonies. Over time, however, more and more European settlers arrived in Canada, and the agreement to not impede on Indigenous peoples' land was starting to be seen as a hindrance to growth for Europeans. The power balance began to shift towards British settlers. In the 1800s, the Robinson treaties and the numbered treaties were developed with the purpose of ensuring that Indigenous people gave up their share of the land. These treaties resulted in much of the land being given up by Indigenous communities in exchange for annuities (money, schools) and the promise of what turned out to be much smaller areas of protected reserve land where they could fish and hunt (Hall, 2017).

It is important to keep in mind that upon arrival of European settlers, the Indigenous population was reduced significantly in size—some estimate that the population was reduced by nearly 90% (Boksa, Joober, & Kirmayer, 2015). The Europeans exposed Indigenous communities to new diseases to which they had little or no immunity, including measles, smallpox, tuberculosis, and influenza (Smylie & Firestone, 2016), as well as violence and displacement (Boksa et al., 2015). These harsh conditions often meant that in the negotiation of these land treaties, Indigenous communities did not have much negotiating power (Smylie & Firestone, 2016).

In 1876, a major piece of legislation known as the *Indian Act* was passed, which continues to have long lasting effects on communities to this day. The *Indian Act*, although amended many times over history, still exists as a federal law. Under the *Indian Act* of 1876, much power was given to the Department of Indian Affairs. The Department was given the ability to intervene in Indigenous issues, manage reserve lands and resources, and actually determine who was classified as an "Indian" and who was not (Government of Canada, 2017a). Under the *Indian Act*, if a First Nations person did not wish to register their status, they were no longer considered a First Nations person. Additionally, if a First Nations woman married a man who was not considered First Nations under the act, she would lose her status. The *Indian Act* also banned various traditional ceremonies and was clearly based on a goal of "assimilating" and "civilizing" Indigenous people. Interestingly, provisions were also included so that any First Nations person who obtained a university degree would lose their status, showing the direct relationship between the *Indian Act* and a critical determinant of health—education (Smylie & Firestone, 2016; Government of Canada, 2017a).

Perhaps one of the most traumatizing and harmful policies implemented by the Canadian government was that of the residential school system—which was made mandatory under the *Indian Act* (Smylie & Firestone, 2016). Across Canada, nearly 132 **residential schools** were established by the federal government, sometimes in partnership with various church organizations, to support this process of "civilization" and "assimilation." The schools forced children out of their homes and away from their family supports and traditional lands. The schools did not allow, and actually punished, speaking in traditional languages or practising any type of cultural traditions. It is estimated that more than 150 000 children attended these schools between 1957 and 1996 (Government of Canada, 2017a). Unfortunately, many children suffered abuse (physical, emotional, and sexual) and starvation and died from infectious and other diseases. This had an immense impact on First Nations and Métis people across the country. The trauma; isolation; and loss of culture, tradition, and spirituality have had long-lasting effects on health, including mental health (Smylie & Firestone, 2016). In 2008, the federal government issued an apology for its role in the residential school system. This, along with several other initiatives (described later), has brought much-needed attention to the suffering Indigenous people faced at the hands of the government during this time (Government of Canada, 2017a).

In the 1960s, a set of amendments to the *Indian Act* gave provinces and territories control over child welfare systems related to Indigenous children. This resulted in a country-wide phenomenon, known as the **Sixties Scoop**, which, similar to residential schools, perpetuated trauma, isolation, and loss of culture. The Sixties Scoop resulted in a mass apprehension of Indigenous children by child welfare agencies without consent from their own parents or band councils. Children were adopted primarily into non-Indigenous homes and separated from their family supports. It is estimated that in the 1960s, after this change in policy, Indigenous children made up about 30% of children involved with child protective services—a significant increase from 1950 when Indigenous children made up just about 1% of children in protective service agencies. Just over 20 000 First Nations, Inuit, and Métis children were apprehended, and many were sent overseas. Although the laws moved towards giving local bands control over child protective services, Indigenous children today are still overrepresented in the child welfare system (Niigaanwewidam & Dainard, 2017).

CRITICAL THINKING QUESTION 7.3: before the Euro-peans' arrival, the Indigenous people spread across Turtle Island had rich traditions, languages, and distinct and diverse cultures. Do some research about the first peo-ple who lived in the city or region where you practice or train (i.e., find out what traditional territory you currently reside in).

Which Indigenous groups existed there before Euro-pean settlers arrived? What languages were spoken? How easy or difficult was it to find this information? Are your peers or institution(s) aware of the history of the land they currently occupy?

Intergenerational Trauma

Trauma resulting from exposure to residential schools and removal from family and community has over time been further exacerbated by subsequent high rates of poverty, sometimes complicated by illness and addiction within surviving communities. The idea of intergenera-tional trauma (also known as historical trauma) is one that needs to be considered when exploring the health status of Indigenous people in Canada. **Intergenerational trauma** can be defined as "collective complex trauma inflicted on a group of people who share a specific group identity or affiliation—ethnicity, nationality, and religious affiliation. It is the legacy of numerous traumatic events a com-munity experiences over generations and encompasses the psychological and social responses to such events"

(University of Calgary, 2012). Essentially, it represents the idea that trauma can be "passed on" from generation to generation, and even people in more recent generations who have themselves not been directly exposed to resi-dential schools can still suffer the consequences. This occurs for many reasons: children of residential school survivors are still subject to racism and oppression, and many may be parented by individuals who suffered immensely from these experiences. In some situations, trauma and its effects are actually amplified in subsequent generations. Although it may not initially seem intuitive, this type of collective or shared trauma has been linked to many health issues, including post-traumatic stress disor-der, depression, and chronic communicable diseases such as HIV and hepatitis C (University of Calgary, 2012). See Fig. 7.3 for a pictorial representation of how colonial pol-icies result in trauma and related health effects. Health care providers must be very aware and sensitive to this in their interactions with clients, and there is a need for trauma-informed approaches and training in the health sector (as discussed further in Chapter 9).

Promising Developments

It is encouraging that in recent decades, a number of positive developments have not only increased aware-ness of these issues among the Canadian population but have also tried to reduce and help rectify the impact of colonialism of Indigenous people.

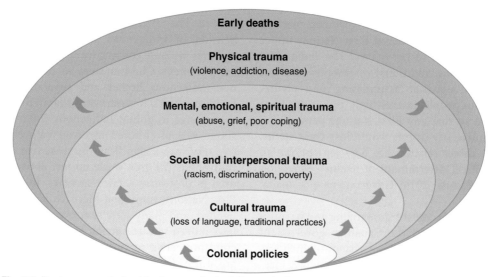

Fig. 7.3 Root cause analysis of the impact of colonialism on indigenous health: delayed tsunami effect. (From Shah, C. P., Klair, R., & Reeves, A. [2014]. Early deaths among members of Toronto Aboriginal community. Retrieved from https://www.toronto.ca/legdocs/mmis/2013/hl/bgrd/backgroundfile-64668.pdf.)

BOX 7.3 Truth and Reconciliation Calls to Action Specific to the Health Sector

We call upon the federal, provincial, territorial, and Aboriginal governments to acknowledge that the current state of Aboriginal health in Canada is a direct result of previous Canadian government policies, including residential schools, and to recognize and implement the health-care rights of Aboriginal people as identified in international law, constitutional law, and under the Treaties.

We call upon the federal government, in consultation with Aboriginal peoples, to establish measurable goals to identify and close the gaps in health outcomes between Aboriginal and non-Aboriginal communities, and to publish annual progress reports and assess longterm trends. Such efforts would focus on indicators such as: infant mortality, maternal health, suicide, mental health, addictions, life expectancy, birth rates, infant and child health issues, chronic diseases, illness and injury incidence, and the availability of appropriate health services

In order to address the jurisdictional disputes concerning Aboriginal people who do not reside on reserves, we call upon the federal government to recognize, respect, and address the distinct health needs of the Métis, Inuit, and off-reserve Aboriginal peoples.

We call upon the federal government to provide sustainable funding for existing and new Aboriginal healing centres to address the physical, mental, emotional, and spiritual harms caused by residential schools, and to ensure that the funding of healing centres in Nunavut and the Northwest Territories is a priority.

We call upon those who can effect change within the Canadian health-care system to recognize the value of Aboriginal healing practices and use them in the treatment of Aboriginal patients in collaboration with Aboriginal healers and Elders, where requested by Aboriginal patients.

We call upon all levels of government to: i. Increase the number of Aboriginal professionals working in the health-care field. ii. Ensure the retention of Aboriginal health-care providers in Aboriginal communities. iii. Provide cultural competency training for all healthcare professionals.

We call upon medical and nursing schools in Canada to require all students to take a course dealing with Aboriginal health issues, including the history and legacy of residential schools, the United Nations Declaration on the Rights of Indigenous Peoples, Treaties and Aboriginal rights, and Indigenous teachings and practices. This will require skills-based training in intercultural competency, conflict resolution, human rights, and anti-racism.

Source: The Truth and Reconciliation Commission of Canada. (2015). *Honouring the truth, reconciling for the future: Summary of the Final Report of the Truth and Reconciliation Commission of Canada.* Retrieved from http://www.trc.ca/websites/trcinstitution/File/2015/Honouring_the_Truth_Reconciling_for_the_Future_July_23_2015.pdf

Amendment to the Constitution and the Indian Act. In the 1982, the Constitution was amended, and Section 35 of our current constitution now explicitly recognizes Indigenous treaty rights. The constitution was also adjusted to include in the definition of Aboriginal, all three major Indigenous groups: First Nations, Inuit, and Métis (Government of Canada, 2017a).

In 1985, the *Indian Act* was amended. Many of the negative provisions mentioned earlier were removed, and Indigenous people were given more control over defining who is considered a status First Nations. Through this process, nearly 60 000 people regained their status (Government of Canada, 2017a).

Royal Commission on Aboriginal People. In 1991, the federal government established the **Royal Commission on Aboriginal People (RCAP),** which published its 20-year plan to improve the relationship between Indigenous people and the government of Canada in 1996. The commission recommended that the government invest significantly in healing, economic development, human resource development and the building of Indigenous institutions. RCAP also emphasized the need for self-determination (discussed further later), giving Indigenous people control over their welfare (Government of Canada, 2016).

The Truth and Reconciliation Commission. Indigenous organizations supported survivors of residential schools to launch the largest class action lawsuit in Canadian history against the federal government and the churches. The lawsuit resulted in the Indian Residential Schools Settlement Agreement, in which it was specified that a commission should be established to document what occurred in the residential school system and recommend ways to move forward. In 2015, the **Truth and Reconciliation Commission (TRC)** published 94 calls to action, focused in the areas of child welfare, education, health, language and culture, and justice. Box 7.3 lists the calls to action in the area of health (TRC, 2015). Part of the spirit of the TRC involves increasing awareness and educating all Canadians about the history of Indigenous people. This awareness and education lay the foundation upon which further calls to action can be implemented. The Case Study box presents an example of a successful advocacy campaign aimed at enhancing awareness of Indigenous history among new Canadians.

CASE STUDY

An Ally at Work: Lobbying for the Inclusion of Indigenous History in Canada's Citizenship Guide

Dr. Chandrakant Shah (the originator of this textbook), a prominent physician and Indigenous ally, was able to make great strides in changing Canada's Citizenship Guide and Examination to include more Indigenous content. Recognizing that the Citizenship Guide provided only a cursory mention of Indigenous history and lacked key details relating to the treaties that were signed, the impact of the *Indian Act*, the residential school system, the Sixties Scoop, and other historical facts, Dr. Shah set out on a letter-writing campaign in 1991. For nearly 3 years, he wrote letters to various levels of government, social organizations, and churches pointing out the need for change. He urged them to include more historical content in their programs so that new Canadians could have a deeper understanding of the complex history between Canada and Indigenous people. Finally, in 1994, materials in the *Canadian Citizenship Guide and Examination* were updated to include much more information about Indigenous people and the importance of their history for Canada. As a result, more than 4 million new Canadians now have a greater understanding of Indigenous people and their history—a great step towards helping realize the TRC's calls to action (Canadian Race Relations Foundation, 2019).

EXERCISE 7.2: The following is a TRC call to action: We call upon all levels of government to:
i) Increase the number of Aboriginal professionals working in the health-care field.
ii) Ensure the retention of Aboriginal health-care providers in Aboriginal communities.
iii) Provide cultural competency training for all health-care professionals. (TRC, 2015)
What sorts of policies might you advocate for locally, provincially, or federally to help further goals i and ii?

Self-Determination

As the United Nations (UN) Declaration on the Rights of Indigenous People, the Truth and Reconciliation Commission, and the Royal Commission on Aboriginal People all point out, all people in Canada should enable and support the move towards self-determination (e.g., the right for Indigenous people to have control over their own political, cultural, and social institutions) (National Inquiry into Missing and Murdered Indigenous Women and Girls, 2017). Self-determination is a recognized determinant of Indigenous health and, through its promotion, can help in addressing some of the health inequities we see between Indigenous people and the general Canadian population (Auger et al., 2016). As mentioned in the chapter introduction, self-determination and decolonization are related concepts. Self-determination is a way to counter the effects of colonialism: instead of focusing on Indigenous people as a "problem in need of change" through societal efforts, self-determination allows for a thoughtful, purposeful, and meaningful infusion of Indigenous culture, values, and traditions into the processes and institutions of society trying to move towards change (Rice, 2016).

The phrase "We are all treaty people" is particularly relevant in this context and supports reconciliation between Indigenous and non-Indigenous peoples. Some people consider treaty rights to be unique or special rights that Indigenous people hold, when in fact, all people living in an area (whether they are new to the area, Indigenous, or settlers who have been there for generations) are influenced by treaties. Treaties are agreements that were negotiated between Indigenous people and the Crown for the benefit of all people living in specific geographic areas of Canada. This means each and every person living on Turtle Island has a responsibility to uphold treaty rights, as was recommended by the Royal Proclamation (discussed earlier) and recognize, as treaties once did, that Indigenous people are sovereign people with rights as a Nation, including the right to self-determination (OISE, n.d.).

It is very important to keep in mind that before the arrival of European settlers, Indigenous people had their own complex political systems and systems of governance; they were regarded by the Crown at certain points in time as independent, sovereign Nations with whom the Crown had to negotiate and enter into bilateral arrangements. Unfortunately, the *Indian Act* undermined these diverse governance systems and imposed a band council system, whereby communities had to vote on and elect a band council chief every few years—although this chief was ultimately accountable to the federal government and had limited bylaw-making power (Indigenous Corporate Training Incorporated, 2015). This is yet another example of ethnocentrism and the imposition of Western traditions onto Indigenous people—displacing and devaluing what was in existence for thousands of years before the arrival of European settlers. Thus, it is up to all people of Canada, Indigenous and non-Indigenous, to respect the governance and political structures of Indigenous people.

Perhaps one of the most significant examples of self-determination and decolonization is the Nunavut Land Claims Agreement (NLCA), which resulted in the creation of the territory of Nunavut and the establishment of a territorial government that is predominantly Inuit and heavily based on Inuit values. The NLCA also contained provisions that mandate the participation of Inuit people in major decisions related to economic development projects. Although governance challenges remain, since the establishment of Nunavut, employment (another key determinant of health) in the region has improved and Nunavut is now the only Canadian territory to have a public service that is majority Indigenous (Rice, 2016). Another great example of self-determination within the health sector, specifically, is presented in the Case Study box.

Last, it is critical to recognize that in addition to these examples of self-determination within a colonially imposed system, Indigenous people have many well-established, large, independent governance structures that have been in existence for some time and that are once again gaining recognition. For example, the Métis National Council was founded in 1983 and is made up of various provincial bodies, including Métis Nation British Columbia, Métis Nation of Alberta, Métis Nation—Saskatchewan, Manitoba Metis Federation, and Métis Nation of Ontario. Overall, the goals of the Métis National Council are to "build a common sense of Métis identity among its constituents, to pursue the Métis' inherent Indigenous rights through the court, and to establish and maintain a nation-to-nation relationship with Canada" (Canadian Geographic, n.d.). The Assembly of First Nations (composed of First Nations chief leaders and founded in 1982) is another large organization representing the interests of 634 First Nations communities across the country, with a goal of advocating for First Nations interests with a unified voice and fostering relationships between the Crown and First Nations people (Assembly of First Nations, 2019).

CASE STUDY

British Columbia's First Nations Health Authority

Before 2011, Health Canada's First Nations and Inuit Health Branch (FNIHB) (described further below and also in Chapter 16) supported health programming for Indigenous people living on reserve in British Columbia (B.C.), as they do in many other parts of Canada. However, in 2011, the B.C. Tripartite Framework Agreement on First Nation Health Governance was signed by federal and provincial health ministers and the First Nations Health Authority (FNHA). This agreement, one of the first of its kind across Canada, empowered the FNHA (led by First Nations people) to lead the design, management, delivery, and funding of health programming for 150 000 First Nations people in B.C.

The FNHA works closely with its partners, specifically the province of B.C. and Health Canada to ensure coordination and collaboration and since 2013 has fully taken over the work that the "FNIHB" once did (Government of Canada, 2017b), including the provision of primary care, mental health and addictions services, and the administration of the noninsured health benefits program (discussed later in this chapter). The main benefit of an agreement such as this is to strengthen the involvement of First Nations people in health decision making and ensure access to all for critical health services (Office of the Auditor General of Canada, 2015).

The Idle No More Movement

Idle No More is a one of the largest social movements in Canada that draws heavily on social media platforms and is aimed at educating and garnering support for civic dissent against policies that oppress Indigenous communities. Fundamental to the ethos of Idle No More is the idea of self-determination and the realization of this right under the UN declaration. The movement began in 2012 when four women in Saskatchewan began to speak out against various pieces of federal legislation that reduced funding for Indigenous communities and reduced the need to assess the environmental impacts of various industrial processes and consult with Indigenous communities. The movement was immensely

TABLE 7.1   Determinants of Health Applied to Indigenous People of Canada

Determinant of Health	Determinant As Applied To The Indigenous Population In Canada
Income	81% of Indigenous reserves across Canada have a median income below the nation's poverty line (which is just over $22 000 for a single person) (Press, 2017).
Social support network	Indigenous people in Canada have been found to have larger relative and friend networks compared with White or immigrant Canadians but also report lower levels of a sense of belonging and trust compared with these groups (Na & Hample, 2016).
	Inuit communities, specifically, report high levels of having a sense of belonging. For example, 81% of Inuit reported a strong sense of belonging to their local community (in comparison, only 65% of non-Indigenous people reported a strong sense of self belonging) (Gionet & Roshanafshar, 2015).
Employment and working conditions	The employment rate among Indigenous people in Canada is about 7% lower than non-Indigenous Canadians, even among Indigenous people with a postsecondary education. Indigenous people are underrepresented in occupations, including professional, managerial, and technical occupations, and have a higher likelihood of working in occupations related to trades, transport, and agriculture (Statistics Canada, 2017c).
Education and literacy	Around 50% of Indigenous people in Canada have a postsecondary certificate or diploma compared with 70% of non-Indigenous Canadians (Statistics Canada, 2017c). (See In the News box about Shannen's Dream for a further description of the ways in which government policy has affected the quality of education on some Indigenous reserve communities.)
Early childhood development	Indigenous children make up almost 50% of all foster children across the country. In general, Indigenous children are twice as likely to live in a lone-parent family or to live with their grandparents (Turner, 2016).
Housing	Nearly one in five Indigenous people in Canada live in a house that requires major repairs, and 18% live in overcrowded housing (Statistics Canada, 2017d).
Healthy behaviours	Indigenous people have higher rates of physical inactivity and smoking compared with non-Indigenous Canadians, particularly First Nations people living on reserve (MacDonald, Barnes, & Middleton, 2015). This is primarily because of adoption of European lifestyles, a loss of traditional foods and ways of being, and lack of access to affordable fresh foods on rural and remote reserve communities, for example.
Access to health services	Indigenous people in Canada report greater odds of having difficulty accessing immediate care for a minor health problem, as well as ongoing, routine care compared with non-Indigenous (Clarke, 2016).

successful and led to the engagement of youth and increased awareness about the impacts of government policy on Indigenous communities (Tupper, 2014).

Other Determinants of Indigenous Health

As with all individuals and communities, health is determined by a range of factors, including education, income level, housing, and behaviours. As emphasized in earlier chapters in this book, not all determinants are equal in terms of their impact. The more influential determinants of health include policies that shape socioeconomic position, which then, in turn, influence things such as employment and housing, as well as lifestyle (e.g., alcohol consumption, nutritious diet, and smoking). Table

7.1 examines determinants of Indigenous health outside of the ones discussed earlier (i.e., racism, colonialism, and self-determination). It is important to keep in mind that this table is based on averages found in the most up-to-date data sources, but in reality, there is much diversity and variation among Indigenous communities and the experience of determinants of health that is difficult to express in tabular format. Additionally, it is essential to read the statistics with a critical and curious lens and to understand them in the context of both the distal and proximal determinants of health. Oppressive colonial policies, intergenerational trauma, and the legacy of the residential school system have resulted in a profound loss of traditional values, languages, and customs and have deeply influenced the socioeconomic position of many Indigenous communities, which in turn has affected living and working conditions, resulting in significant health inequities in most areas of health status. The root cause analysis (see Fig. 7.3, earlier) is a helpful framework to use when reading such statistics to dig deeper into the causes of these issues.

Although Table 7.1 takes an inequity-based perspective, the protective determinants of health that promote resiliency, such as self-determination, community mobilization (with Idle No More being a perfect example), social support, and others must also be weighed against the statistics presented later. For example, many Inuit communities report very high levels of social support and a sense of community belonging—much higher than the rates reported by non-Indigenous people. Additionally, in many communities, mobilization and organization have strengthened the community fabric and well-being and can be seen as protective factors when it comes to population health and fostering resiliency (see Case Study box).

Protective factors such as social support, community mobilization, and others contribute to something called resiliency. **Resiliency** can be thought of as "the ability to do well despite adversity" and must be thought of in the context of culture and history (Kirmayer et al., 2011). In other words, protective factors that foster resiliency are not only the positive determinants of health that have been mentioned many times in this book (e.g., wealth, education) but also include many other elements that are key to a group's history and ideas about self and the community. For many Indigenous people, for example, identity and personhood have for generations been tied to the land, and the natural environment is a strong source of healing. Thus, revitalizing language, culture, connection to the land, and spirituality helps with a return to ways of thinking that promote healing and a sense of identity. Last, collective political activism and involvement promote resiliency (Kirmayer et al., 2011), and there are many examples of advocacy and activism among Indigenous people (e.g., Idle No More movement, Shannen Koostachin) that you will read about in this chapter.

IN THE NEWS

Shannen's Dream

In 2007, 13-year-old Shannen Koostachin began a youth-driven movement called Shannen's Dream that brought national attention to the chronic underfunding of Indigenous schools, as well as the unsafe school environments experienced by First Nations children.

Shannen was from a small reserve in Attawapiskat, Ontario, where most of her elementary schooling occurred in government-supplied portables (as the original school building had closed years ago because of environmental contamination), with rapidly deteriorating indoor conditions. Shannen and her peers wrote thousands of letters to the federal government, demanding a safer school and equal funding for Indigenous education.

Finally, in 2014, after receiving international attention, a new school was built as a result of Shannen's campaign. Shannen also brought attention to the fact that many First Nations children on reserve have to leave their communities to attend high school. Shannen herself had to relocate to another community off her reserve to receive a secondary school education (CBC News, 2017).

Shannen is a perfect example of youth-led community mobilization—a key tenet of community health practice. She garnered national and international support, brought pride and awareness about her community, and undoubtedly brought hope to many, given what she was able to accomplish at such a young age with her drive and passion.

CASE STUDY

Community Mobilization Efforts As a Protective Determinant of Health

In Cree culture (as well as in many other Indigenous cultures), collective leadership and decision making, shared responsibility, and contribution to the community are widely held values (Public Safety Canada, 2009). These values lend themselves very well to community mobilization (discussed in Chapter 3), which is predicated on working as a collective, within a community, to move forward change. Many examples of community mobilization—which can be thought of as a strength and resource for health and its determinants—exist among Indigenous communities, which undoubtedly helps in closing the health gap.

continued

CASE STUDY—cont'd

Community Mobilization Efforts As a Protective Determinant of Health

One such example is the Community Holistic Circle Healing Program in Hollow Water First Nation, Manitoba, which was established in the 1980s as a way to heal legal offenders (particularly those involved in family violence). The goals of the program, which rely on the work of local community-based service providers, include revitalizing the family unit, reconciling offenders and victims of violence in a family, and fostering healthier communities. Through counselling and group sessions, offenders and families are encouraged to build a relationship with the spirit world, to learn traditional ways of doing and healing, and ultimately, to use healing as a way of obtaining justice. Healing is seen as communal process, and everyone participates, fostering a great sense of social support and purpose—both of which are important determinants of health. The program has not only resulted in cost savings but has also improved traditional knowledge and practices in the community (Department of Justice, 2015).

CRITICAL THINKING QUESTION 7.4: What does resiliency mean to you? Using either the example of the Community Holistic Circle Healing Program (mentioned in the Case Study box) or another example of community mobilization in an Indigenous community in your jurisdiction, discuss how the elements of a community mobilization effort might contribute to resiliency.

THE HEALTH OF CANADA'S INDIGENOUS POPULATION

Keeping in mind the determinants of health already discussed, the health of Indigenous peoples in Canada is described further in this section, focusing specifically on indicators of mortality, morbidity, perceived health and well-being, and rates of health care utilization. Although this section presents the most recent statistics and represents averages, it does not fully capture all of the variation in health status that exists among the wide range of Indigenous people spread across Canada, and, as will be emphasized further, the health status data on Canadians has many gaps (see Box 7.4 for more details). Just like in the previous section, these statistics must be contextualized and read with the determinants of health (particularly the distal determinants such as racism, colonialism, and self-determination) in mind.

CRITICAL THINKING QUESTION 7.5: Although some people advocate for the inclusion of questions related to race, ancestry, and Indigenous status on data-collection forms, others say this practice perpetuates the idea of racism (the idea being that if race is a social construct, why do we validate it by asking questions on a form about it?). Debate the merits of both arguments.

BOX 7.4 Limitations in Health Data Pertaining to Indigenous People in Canada

The information we have pertaining to the health of Indigenous people is limited, at best. Chapter 2 touches on the types of data available to health sector practitioners to inform about the health status of our communities and people, including vital statistics, surveys, and health administration data. Unfortunately, many of the major national health surveys (e.g., Canadian Community Health Survey, Canadian Health Measures Survey) do not include on-reserve First Nations communities. Additionally, not all health administration data collected by provinces and territories consistently collect information on whether someone identifies as being Indigenous or not. In particular, many data initiatives leave out specific groups of Indigenous people, particularly non-registered First Nations people or Indigenous people living in urban areas (which represents a growing subset of Indigenous people) (NCCAH, 2013a). As a result, the information presented here is somewhat limited in its scope and accuracy.

Mortality

Chapter 4 discusses the average life expectancy for the Canadian population: 79 years for men and 83 years for women. Some Indigenous people have a lower life expectancy than the overall Canadian average, although on the whole, life expectancy for Indigenous people in Canada has increased by a couple of years since 2001. Inuit life expectancy is one of the lowest in Canada (64 years for men and 73 years for women). Life expectancy for Métis and First Nations people, in comparison, is approximately 73 to 74 years for men and 78 to 80 years for women (Statistics Canada, 2015).

According to Statistics Canada, First Nations people are more likely to die prematurely (i.e., before the age of 75 years) compared with non-First Nations Canadians. When examining the rates of avoidable deaths (i.e., those that could have been avoided through provision of public health or health care services, policies, or preventive efforts), First Nations men are twice as likely to die from these avoidable causes, and First Nations women are 2.5 times more likely to die from these causes. The types of ailments First Nations men are more likely to die from compared with non–First Nations men include alcohol and substance use disorders, unintentional injuries, and diabetes mellitus. When comparing First Nations women with non–First Nations women, Statistics Canada has found that First Nations women were more likely to die from the following causes: alcohol and drug use disorders, diabetes mellitus, infections, and unintentional injuries (Park, Tjepkema, Goedhuis, & Pennock, 2015). Not only is premature and avoidable death higher for Indigenous people, but a range of studies have also determined that both First Nations and Inuit people have higher infant mortality and stillbirth rates compared with the rest of the Canadian population (Gilbert, Auger, & Tjepkema, 2015). Many of these inequities can be traced back to the *Indian Act* and to deliberate colonial policies that resulted in widespread trauma and loss of culture for Indigenous people across the land.

Morbidity

Noncommunicable Diseases

Overall, Indigenous people are at a higher risk of experiencing chronic, noncommunicable diseases when compared with non-Indigenous Canadians. A 2015 Statistics Canada report found that nearly 55% of both First Nations and Métis people reported being diagnosed with one or more chronic diseases. This compares with 48% of the general Canadian population reporting the presence of any chronic condition. The proportion of Inuit people who reported being diagnosed with a chronic disease was less than the general population, at 43%, although some have hypothesized that this may be due to poorer access to physicians to obtain a diagnosis (Gionet & Roshanafshar, 2015).

Although some noncommunicable diseases are more prevalent among Indigenous people, others are not. Respiratory conditions such as asthma tend to be higher among First Nations, Inuit, and Métis people. Additionally, in general, rates of type 2 diabetes and

the resulting complications of this condition are higher among Indigenous people compared with non-Indigenous Canadians. The rates of type 2 diabetes have also been increasing among this population over time (Mansuri & Hanley, 2017).

Because many of the risk factors for diabetes and heart disease are the same, it is not surprising, then, that they tend to go hand in hand. It is generally accepted that rates of heart diseases are higher in the Indigenous population. Large-scale surveys have shown that First Nations adults between the ages of 50 and 59 years have twice the prevalence of heart disease compared with the general Canadian population (11.5% vs 5.5%) (Reading, 2015). It is important, when reading these statistics, to keep in mind the determinants of Indigenous health, such as colonialism and how government policy and historical trauma contribute to high rates of smoking and reduced access to healthy nutritious foods, for example.

> **EXERCISE 7.3:** What are some factors that may explain the higher rates of respiratory diseases (e.g., asthma) in Indigenous communities? What about type 2 diabetes? (HINT: In your answers, consider the determinants of Indigenous health [e.g., colonialism] mentioned earlier.)

Communicable Diseases

The prevalence of tuberculosis (TB) among some groups of Indigenous people is much higher than the Canadian average (as discussed in Chapter 10). Although Indigenous people make up just 4% of the Canadian population, they account for just over one in five (or 20%) of all cases of active TB reported in Canada. Rates of TB are extremely variable, however. For example, First Nations on reserve have higher rates of TB compared with those off reserve. Métis people have lower TB rates compared with other Indigenous people in Canada, and the Inuit in some places have almost 50 times the TB rate of the general Canadian population (Public Health Agency of Canada, 2016).

Indigenous people have a long and arduous history with TB, a disease introduced to Indigenous communities by European settlers in the 1700s. It is notable that before European settlement TB was not an issue among Indigenous communities. Because of high rates of malnutrition and overcrowding on reserves, TB death rates in the 1930s and 1940s were extremely high (some of the highest ever recorded in the world, in fact). TB death rates among residential school attendees were also extremely high (at an estimated rate of 8 000 deaths per 100 000 children) for similar reasons. Notably, when Indigenous people were diagnosed with TB, they were often forcibly removed from their families and not allowed to say their goodbyes or collect any belongings and were sent to sanitoria in urban centres. Some TB patients stayed for years in these sanitoria (the average length of stay was around 2.5 years), far away from friends and family, and many times, family and friends were not notified about a TB client's death (Canadian Public Health Association, n.d.) Health care providers should be mindful and aware of this history when evaluating or treating someone with possible TB, as it may have an impact on health care decisions, trust and other factors impacting care.

In terms of other communicable diseases, it is also reported that some Indigenous people, particularly First Nations and Inuit people living in northern, remote areas have higher rates of sexually transmitted infections, including gonorrhea and chlamydia. Additionally, Indigenous people in Canada make up about 8% of all HIV cases (despite being only 4% of the Canadian population), and there has been a substantial increase in the proportion of HIV cases being reported by Indigenous people—from 19% in 1998 to just over 25% in 2003 (National Collaborating Centre for Aboriginal Health [NCCAH], 2012). Reasons for this may include poorer access to health care and alcohol and substance use disorders (including injection drug use), fuelled by issues related to poor housing, lack of employment opportunities in some areas, and trauma, among other reasons ultimately driven by colonial policies and intergenerational trauma.

Mental Health and Addictions

The concept of intergenerational trauma and exposure to the residential school system is particularly important to consider when discussing the prevalence of mental health issues (including substance misuse) among Indigenous people, which is reportedly higher than in non-Indigenous communities. For example, Indigenous populations with parents or grandparents who attended residential schools report higher rates of depression and suicidal thoughts compared with those who did not. Among Indigenous youth, rates of drug use, suicidal thoughts, and suicide completion are higher compared with non-Indigenous youth (Boksa et al., 2015). Suicide among Indigenous people, in particular, has been a heavily publicized issue in recent years. Reports have pointed to the fact that First Nations have approximately twice the risk of suicide compared with the general population, but some Inuit communities have nearly 6 to 11 times the rate, though much variation exists from community to community (Crawford, 2016). Interestingly, studies aimed at explaining the immense variation in the rates of suicide in Indigenous communities in British Columbia show that the more control a particular community has over its own services (e.g., education, health, police and fire, i.e., self-determination), the lower the rates of suicide in that community (Boksa et al., 2015). Additionally, it has been shown that communities that preserve their language and culture tend to have lower rates of suicidal thoughts and attempts, pointing towards this as a protective factor as well (Crawford, 2016). See In the News box for a recent government initiative to support Indigenous languages.

IN THE NEWS

The Indigenous Languages Act

In February 2019, in follow-up to the language- and culture-based recommendations of the Truth and Reconciliation Commission, the federal government tabled *Bill C-91: An Act Respecting Indigenous Languages*. Co-developed by Indigenous partners, this bill secures funding to recognize, preserve, revitalize, and strengthen Indigenous languages and establishes an Office of the Commissioner of Indigenous Languages to support the work.

One of the main reasons behind this piece of legislation is the fact that, according to the United Nations Educational, Scientific and Cultural Organization (UNESCO), nearly 75% of Canada's approximately 90 or so Indigenous languages are considered endangered. Much of this is a direct result of the residential school system, where pupils were not allowed to speak their own languages, and of the Sixties Scoop, where many Indigenous children were forcibly removed from their homes and adopted by non-Indigenous families, separating them from their languages and culture.

There are some criticisms of the legislation and the process that was used to develop it. For example, some groups (particularly Inuit groups) thought that the process was more consultative versus true co-development (in which Indigenous groups would have had more say in the components of the legislation) and that the bill itself lacks Inuit-specific content. The context among Inuit people is different, however, because it is estimated that around 80% of Inuit people spread across 51 communities in Canada speak Inuktuk. Other critics argue that the legislation didn't go far enough to recognize Indigenous languages as part of the official languages of Canada. Inuktuk, for example, has official language status in Nunavut and the Northwest Territories (Brake, 2019).

EXERCISE 7.4: Why might the preservation of language and culture be protective when it comes to suicide risk?

Maternal and Child Health

A number of issues facing mothers and their developing children disproportionately affect Indigenous communities. A recent Statistics Canada analysis examined the rates of adverse birth outcomes and found that Indigenous infants tend to suffer more from issues such as being preterm or large for gestational age (Sheppard et al., 2017).

Additionally, disparities in dental health among Indigenous and non-Indigenous children are being recognized, with studies pointing to higher rates of poor dental health among Indigenous children. A large-scale national survey found the rates of poor dental health to be the highest among the Inuit, compared with First Nations and Métis people (NCCAH, 2012).

An issue that has received much attention is fetal alcohol spectrum disorder (FASD), which refers to a range of conditions caused by exposure to alcohol in the womb, resulting in developmental, facial, and growth problems. It is estimated that in the general Canadian population, the prevalence of FASD is less than 1%; however, in some Indigenous communities, the prevalence is estimated to be between 10% and 19% (Rai et al., 2017). High rates of FASD can also be traced back to root causes, including mental health challenges; isolation; and inequities in accessing health services, including addictions services and educational and employment opportunities as a result of colonialism, the *Indian Act*, and the residential school system in which many endured trauma.

EXERCISE 7.5: How might a history of attending a residential school contribute to the risk of fetal alcohol spectrum disorder in one's children?

Self-Perceived Health

As outlined in Chapter 4, self-perceived health is sometimes a good indicator of overall population health and often takes into account quality of life and factors related to well-being and functionality. In general, Indigenous people tend to rate their health as being poorer than the general population. More specifically, whereas 63% of the general Canadian population rated their health as very good or excellent in large national surveys, only

44% of First Nations people on reserve, 50% of First Nations off reserve, 54% of Métis, and 55% of Inuit people rated their health in the same way. When it comes to perceived mental health, similar trends prevail: whereas 75% of non-Indigenous Canadians report their health as being very good or excellent, only 65% to 67% of Indigenous people who were surveyed considered this to be true (Public Health Agency of Canada, 2018). When interpreting these statistics, it is important to keep in mind the fact that concepts of health and mental health may differ among various Indigenous communities and also between Indigenous and non-Indigenous people, as will be discussed later.

Health Care Utilization

Health care utilization (e.g., rates of hospitalization or ED visits), although being an indicator of health, may also reflect access to health services. Thus, when considering health care utilization among Indigenous people in Canada, one must consider differential access to health care (e.g., primary care, hospital care, specialist care) and openness to attending health care institutions (which were a source of distrust historically and still may be a source of anxiety and racism), as well as the prevalence of health conditions requiring such care.

For all age groups, rates of hospitalization among Indigenous people are higher than the Canadian averages (Statistics Canada, 2016). Rates of hospitalization for Indigenous youth, in particular, are also known to be higher than for non-Indigenous youth. For children aged 0 to 9 years, the rate of hospitalization is highest for on-reserve First Nations children (at 1.8 times the rate of non-Indigenous people) followed by off-reserve First Nations children, Métis children, and Inuit children (whose rates ranged between 1.3 and 1.4 times that of non-Indigenous children of the same age). Among those aged 10 to 19 years, the hospitalization rate was highest among the Inuit (3.8 times the Canadian average) followed by on-reserve First Nations youth (3.6 times the Canadian average) and then off-reserve and Métis youth (2.0–2.3 times the Canadian average) (Statistics Canada, 2017b).

CRITICAL THINKING QUESTION 7.6: Reflect on the importance of language. How does speaking the languages you do influence your thinking and day-to-day life? What are the implications of Indigenous languages being included in Canada's "official" languages, and what is your position on whether this should be the case in Canada?

HEALTH SERVICES FOR INDIGENOUS PEOPLES IN CANADA

Now that we have discussed the determinants of health and health status of Indigenous people, we will turn our attention to health services as a determinant of health. In the next section, how health care for Indigenous peoples is financed and delivered is discussed after a brief discussions on challenges faced in providing these services; Indigenous concepts of health and well-being; and finally, how the health system can be strengthened to better care for Indigenous people across the country.

Financing and Delivery of Health Care for Inuit and First Nations People

One of the treaties negotiated between the Crown and Indigenous peoples in 1876 is treaty number 6, which included a clause to provide medicine and is known as the "Medicine Chest Clause." This clause reads as follows: "[a medicine chest] shall be kept at the house of each Indian Agent for the use and benefit of the Indians" (Burnham, 2003). This specific treaty has been interpreted widely to mean that health care services for Indigenous people are, in fact, a treaty right and thus the responsibility of the federal government (Journal of Obstetrics and Gynaecology Canada [JOGC], 2013). As such, the federal government reimburses health care providers working under the health insurance systems of their own province or territory in delivering hospital and physician care to Inuit and status First Nations people. For Inuit and First Nations people who live in isolated or remote communities where access to physician or hospital services are limited, the federal government funds nursing stations, predominantly staffed by either nurses or community health workers. People who require additional or specialized care beyond what can be offered by the nursing station staff are then transported to a nearby centre with provincial hospital or physician services (which are then reimbursed by the federal government). In addition, the First Nations and Inuit Health Branch of Health Canada provides coverage for things typically not covered by provincial health insurance plans (i.e., over and above physician and hospital care) through a program known as the **Non-Insured Health Benefits (NIHB) Program**. The NIHB program provides coverage for things such as medications, dental care, vision care, short-term mental health interventions, and medical transportation. It is important to keep in mind that the NIHB program only includes status First Nations people and registered Inuit. Métis people are not included in this program and thus cannot obtain the same access to ancillary health services, which has been a point of contention between the Métis and the Government of Canada for years (JOGC, 2013).

Although the federal government provides much of the care in rural and remote areas, as more and more Indigenous people migrate to urban areas, a number of provinces have also begun providing culturally safe care to Indigenous peoples. Alberta Health Services, for example, include a comprehensive Indigenous Health Program. The program partners with Indigenous peoples, communities, and key stakeholders to provide accessible, culturally safe health services for First Nations, Métis, and Inuit people. The responsibilities include providing an effective, patient-centred approach for improving care to First Nations, Métis, and Inuit peoples and communities through specific services; working with health zones to facilitate the development and delivery of health services for First Nations, Métis, and Inuit peoples; and facilitating accessible, culturally safe, equitable health service delivery for all First Nations, Métis, and Inuit communities and peoples. The program is guided by the advice of a Wisdom Council, a group of First Nations, Métis, and Inuit living in Alberta, who first came together in September 2012. Their goal is to help ensure that all Indigenous people living in Alberta receive the best possible health care (Alberta Health Services, 2018).

Additionally, many health systems are moving towards self-determination models through which Indigenous people lead, govern, and deliver health care and public health services for Indigenous communities, taking over from institutions such as Health Canada (as is the example of the FNHA in B.C. outlined in a Case Study earlier in the chapter). Alberta Health Services is another good example of a health system that has incorporated Indigenous traditions related to healing and well-being. In some acute care facilities, an Indigenous cultural helper provides support to Indigenous clients. The helper can facilitate and organize prayers, smudging ceremonies (described later), or any other cultural practices using hospital space (Alberta Health Services, 2017).

It is clear from the description that both provinces and territories, as well as Indigenous organizations and the federal government, are responsible for the actual delivery and, in some cases, the financing of health care.

However, it is not always clear cut *who* funds and delivers which services for Indigenous people, which can result in confusion with regard to reimbursement of payment, and ultimately can result in delays in obtaining care. This confusion of roles has had an impact on the health of Indigenous people across the country. A specific example from several years ago is an Indigenous child named Jordan, who had complicated medical needs, was hospitalized in Manitoba, and was ready to be discharged from the hospital to home. Unfortunately, a disagreement between Manitoba and the federal government regarding who was responsible for covering the cost of his home care services led to Jordan remaining in hospital unnecessarily for an additional 2 years. Sadly, Jordan died at age 5 years in the hospital in 2005 and never got to receive services in the comfort of his own home. This tragic case led to the House of Commons unanimously passing a motion in 2007 in support of what is known as Jordan's Principle (Hayes, 2017). **Jordan's Principle** states that "where a government service is available to all other children, but a jurisdictional dispute regarding services to a First Nations child arises between Canada, a province, a territory, or between government departments, the government department of first contact pays for the service and can seek reimbursement from the other government or department after the child has received the service." The goal of Jordan's principle is to prevent Indigenous people from experiencing barriers to accessing care because of disputes over roles and responsibilities of health care for Indigenous people of Canada (Government of Canada, 2018). Interestingly, even after Jordan's Principle was endorsed by the House of Commons, it was inconsistently being applied until January 2016, when the Canadian Human Rights Tribunal ordered the Government of Canada to immediately take measures to implement the principle to its fullest extent (Hayes, 2017).

Indigenous Health Care Challenges

Aside from jurisdictional disputes between the federal government and provinces and territories, a number of other challenges exist with respect to health care in Indigenous communities, particularly for those that are rural and remote.

As with many rural and remote areas, consistent access to qualified health staff can be an issue. At many First Nations reserves, for example, nurses and physicians come infrequently, and there is a high turnover of professional staff, resulting in understaffing and issues

related to the follow-through of care plans. Additionally, particularly for emergency services, there are high rates of medical air travel to major urban centres. This is not only costly but also means that individuals must access complex care outside of their home communities where their social support systems lie. As mentioned earlier, often primary health care may be provided by community health workers, who are members of the community themselves. This can present challenges to confidentiality and privacy, with those seeking care often afraid to share information for fear of community repercussions and stigma. Another main issue is that because of a lack of resources and need to address urgent and emergent issues, preventive care and addressing the determinants of health through population health services can be lacking and are often underfunded and under prioritized. Finally, barriers in achieving culturally sensitive and appropriate care continue to exist. With providers coming from outside the community and government institutions often dictating the types of services provided, care may be culturally irrelevant and may not be offered in languages native to the areas served (Oosterveer & Young, 2015).

For some Indigenous people, trust in health care and government institutions is lacking. This is not entirely surprising, given the role of the government in the residential school system, the Sixties Scoop, and other systems of oppression and colonialism and, additionally, because of the well-documented racism experienced by Indigenous people in health care institutions.

All of these factors very much highlight the need for health care providers of all disciplines to be reflective. We must all consider our own biases and perceptions of Indigenous people (perpetuated by the dominant culture and narrative), reflect on how this influences the care we provide, and think critically about what concrete steps we can take as individuals to, in an ongoing way, provide better and more sensitive, competent, and safe care.

Indigenous Views of Health

Perspectives on health, well-being, healing, and medicine vary significantly across diverse Indigenous communities, which each has its own rich tradition when it comes to traditional medicines and ceremonies to improve health and well-being (JOGC, 2013). However, some key tenets and principles tend to apply across many First Nations, Inuit, and Métis people.

One is that the concept of health is holistic. A person's physical health is thought to be closely connected

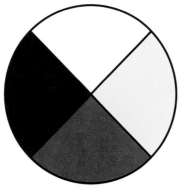

Fig. 7.4 Indigenous medicine wheel. (From Park, S., Boyle, J., Hoyeck, P., et al. [n.d.]. Indigenous health in Ontario: An introductory guide for medical students [p. 17]. Toronto: University of Toronto. Retrieved from https://medicine.utoronto.ca/sites/default/files/IndigenousHealthinOntario-compressed.pdf.)

to one's mental, emotional, and spiritual health. The **medicine wheel**, central to some Indigenous cultures but not others (depicted in Fig. 7.4) visually represents how each of these factors (white representing spiritual health, yellow representing mental [cognitive] health, blue representing emotional health, and red representing physical health) are interconnected and equally important in contributing to good health (Park et al., n.d.). In other words, all of these dimensions of a person's health must be balanced to lead a healthy life. Health is also influenced by connections to one's community and society, as well as connection to the land and broader environment (JOGC, 2013). The FNHA in B.C. has adopted a framework that visually depicts a First Nations perspective on health and wellness (FNHA, 2012) (Fig. 7.5).

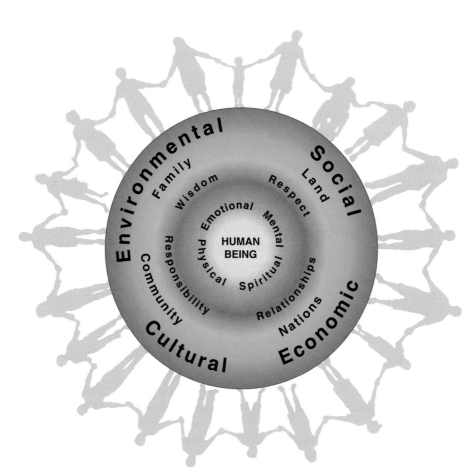

Fig. 7.5 First Nations perspective on health and wellness. (From First Nations Health Authority. [2012]. *First Nations perspective on health and wellness.* Retrieved from http://www.fnha.ca/wellness/wellness-and-the-first-nations-health-authority/first-nations-perspective-on-wellness.)

As can be seen in Fig. 7.5, the central (or first) circle represents individual human beings, emphasizing the perspective that wellness starts with an individual taking responsibility for their health and well being. The second circle shows the importance of achieving balance between mental, emotional, spiritual, and physical health. The third circle depicts key values of health, including respect, wisdom, responsibility, and relationships. The fourth circle emphasizes the importance of the people and places we come from (i.e., family, community, land, and nations). The fifth circle highlights how health is a result of broader social determinants, such as culture and the social, economic, and physical environment (FNHA, 2012).

Another broad principle that applies to Indigenous concepts of health is that decision making around health care services is often shared among family members and the broader community versus solely being a decision an individual has to make about their own care. This impacts how Indigenous people might view the sharing of information. Among the general non-Indigenous Canadian population, for example, the prevailing view is that personal health information is private and not to be shared with others (including family, friends, and community members), and decisions should be made independently without the influence of others. For many Indigenous communities, this is not how health is viewed.

The principle of mutual respect is also fundamental to Indigenous peoples and has implications on how one interacts and responds to a provider in a health care setting. Mutual respect in this regard means taking a humble, nonjudgmental, nondirective approach to health advice as a provider and respecting that a client knows themselves best and will act according to what is in their capabilities, knowledge and skill. This can be very different from European conceptualization of health care service delivery, in which often providers are seen as "knowing best" and giving direction that they expect will be followed by their clients. In the Indigenous view, providers and clients are in many ways seen as equals (JOGC, 2013).

Relating these examples back to the notions of cultural hegemony and ethnocentrism introduced earlier, providers must be careful when making assumptions regarding how clients want to receive heath information and counselling. We cannot simply approach our clients in the way we want to be approached based on our own cultural values and traditions. When in doubt, asking, learning and reflecting on encounters can support the move away from ethnocentrism and towards a more inclusive and critical view on "how things are done" in health care.

Many Indigenous people use the services of traditional healers, who provide the traditional medicines and perform healing ceremonies such as smudging ceremonies, sweat lodges, and the use of tobacco, which are discussed later. Many Indigenous health centres in Ontario provide both Western and traditional services in which physicians, nurses, dietitians, and so on work side by side with the traditional healers. Elders and learning from elder tradition, practices, and culture and improving connection to the land are also some important ways in which some Indigenous people improve and promote health—spiritually, mentally, physically, and emotionally.

> **CRITICAL THINKING QUESTION 7.7:** Reflect on an encounter with a client that did not go so well. Evaluate why it did not go well. Might this client have held other world views or values that differed from yours? How do you balance this in a clinical encounter?

Sweat Lodges

Sweat lodges are spiritual places where Indigenous people engage in ceremonies that promote the release of negative toxins and energy through exposure to heat. These ceremonies are aimed at restoring balance among physical, emotional, spiritual, and mental health. There are many different types of sweat lodge ceremonies that promote healing and well-being. Typically, participants sit in a circle inside the sweat lodge, share their personal stories, reflect, and connect with one another and nature. The *Indian Act* did not allow for the use of sweat lodges by Indigenous people until 1951. Today, they are commonly used as an important way for some to promote health and spirituality (although some Indigenous cultures, such as the Inuit and people in North-West territories, do not practice this tradition) (Gadacz, 2017). The In the News box presents an example of how one modern hospital has incorporated the use of sweat lodges into its practice.

Smudging Ceremonies

Smudging ceremonies look different across different Indigenous cultures. In general, however, smudging ceremonies are spiritual practices typically used during times of crisis or poor health for the purposes of cleansing, restoring physical health, providing clarity, and improving spiritual health. Most often during a smudging ceremony, herbs and medicines are burned, and the resulting smoke is thought to be healing for the person who is being smudged, as well as a way for prayers to be carried to the Creator. Just like with sweat lodges, many Indigenous cultural and spiritual practices, including smudging ceremonies, were outlawed until recently, and even to the present day, much controversy exists around smudging, with some private landlords and public buildings banning it. Despite this, it remains a practice that promotes health and spirituality by many, and several provinces and territories and institutions have recognized the right of Indigenous peoples to practice spiritual ceremonies and practices (Robinson, 2018). As mentioned earlier, Alberta Health Services and other acute and chronic care institutions have moved towards providing a space, and sometimes a facilitator, to support the practice of these healing ceremonies. For additional ceremonies and traditional approaches, also see Anishnawbe Health Toronto (listed in the Key Websites at the end of this chapter), which is an Aboriginal Community Health Centre.

🌐 IN THE NEWS

Use of Sweat Lodge at the Centre for Addiction and Mental Health

The Centre for Addiction and Mental Health (CAMH) is a large teaching hospital in Toronto. In 2016, as part of the hospital's journey toward offering services that are more culturally relevant for Indigenous clients, CAMH began building a sweat lodge after many of its Indigenous clientele requested such a space.

Since it opened, more than 400 people have participated in various traditional and spiritual ceremonies in the sweat lodge. In addition to opening the sweat lodge for use by Indigenous clients, CAMH has hired Indigenous social workers and an elder to assist with informing the hospital on the provision of culturally sensitive and appropriate care for those who wish this care to be incorporated into their care plans (CAMH, n.d.).

When engaging in an understanding of traditional practices, it is important to be mindful of the notion of cultural appropriation. Broadly speaking, **cultural appropriation** occurs when individuals adopt practices

related to another culture without that culture's permission and without an acknowledgement or understanding of that culture's history (Wood, 2017).

In recent years, many Indigenous practices, including smudging, have been adopted by non-Indigenous peoples. Stores are selling "smudge kits" and tools for people to use to "smudge" their homes without a deep understanding of the spiritual importance of such a ceremony (Robinson, 2018; Curtis, 2017). Thus, it is critical when learning about or engaging in traditional practices to also learn about the history and importance of the practice in various contexts and the implications of adopting or engaging in it as a settler, for example.

Tobacco

For many generations, tobacco has been used by many (but not all; the Inuit people are an exception) Indigenous peoples in ceremonies, rituals, and prayers because it is considered to be a gift from the Creator. It is often used to express gratitude to the Creator and Mother Earth, as well as to purify both the mind and body. It can be chewed, smoked, burned, or put into water during both medicinal and spiritual ceremonies (NCCAH, 2013b). Traditional tobacco products used for these purposes are separate from commercial tobacco use (e.g., smoking commercial cigarettes), introduced by the Europeans.

EXERCISE 7.6: In a health care setting, what questions might you ask every client, whether Indigenous or not, regarding their views on health and information sharing?

Improving the Health of Indigenous People: Reorienting the Health Sector

The TRC's calls to action, particularly in the area of health, represent a good starting point for making changes to close the gap between Indigenous health and the health of the general Canadian population. Healthcare CAN, an organization representing hospitals and other health care organizations across the country, recently called on the health sector to adopt "wise practices" to support the closing of this gap. Their 2018 report recommended the following three main actions.

1. Realign authorities, accountabilities, and resources back towards Indigenous communities. This represents

work towards self-determination, giving Indigenous organizations control and responsibility over resources for health.

2. Eliminate racism and increase cultural sensitivity within health care institutions.

3. Ensure equitable access to care, which entails both enhancing the quality of care and the availability of services offered to Canada's diverse Indigenous communities, both on and off reserve (Richardson & Murphy, 2018).

The report also calls on leaders of health care institutions to engage in the recommendations found in Table 7.2.

Although it is clear that the TRC calls to action in health must be realized, with the principles of community engagement embedded, action must also be taken on improving the social determinants of health for Indigenous peoples. Without also fixing issues such as housing

conditions, poverty, and inequitable access to education (as the TRC points out), the health gap cannot be sustainably reduced. Finally, at the root of these inequities lie power and decision-making authority. Indigenous peoples must be provided with more opportunities for self-determination, and the resources going towards Indigenous health and well-being must be funded at the same levels as they are for non-Indigenous programming.

CRITICAL THINKING QUESTION 7.8: Reflect on the phrase "we are all treaty people." What does it mean to you? How can you, in your own work and career trajectory, embody this principle and support the Truth and Reconciliation Commission's *Calls to Action*?

Outline two or three steps you will take in the next year to reflect on your role as a health sector participant and how you might further culturally safe care and other TRC calls to action.

TABLE 7.2 Practices for Health Leaders to Support Systems Level Change to Improve Health Care for Indigenous Peoples

Topic Area	Recommendations
Policy and systems change	Support local First Nations, Inuit, and Métis leaders in conjunction with their national counterparts at the Assembly of First Nations, Inuit Tapiriit Kanatami, and Métis National Council as they negotiate, develop, implement, and evaluate health transformation agreements and advocate for policy and systems change.
Community engagement	Identify key stakeholders for community engagement and build relationships with them. Stakeholders include representatives from local and regional First Nations, Inuit, and Métis governments and local Indigenous health service organizations, Indigenous clients, and others. When reaching out to key stakeholders, follow engagement protocols articulated by their respective organizations. Create partnership agreements that include process evaluations and accountability measures for any shared initiatives related to Indigenous health and wellness.
	Make reconciliation and Indigenous health equity part of the organization's strategic plan.
Recruitment and retention of indigenous staff and health care providers	Promote the involvement of Indigenous peoples in the organization by recruiting them for governance and leadership positions, advisory circles, community liaisons, Elders' councils, and other roles; formalize reporting and action-based accountability by the non-Indigenous leadership to prevent tokenistic or nonmeaningful engagement.
	Recruit, retain, and mentor Indigenous staff and health care providers at all levels of the organization, including procurement; create working and learning environments where they can thrive and where Indigeneity and Indigenous knowledge are valued.
Antiracism and cultural safety education	Provide antiracism and cultural safety education to all members of the organization; develop and implement safe processes for both employees and clients to debrief racist or culturally unsafe experiences in the organization; develop and implement processes to document these instances and track progress.
	Support Indigenous learners in the health professions by creating safe and respectful clinical learning environments that are free of racism and discrimination; participate in health science outreach programs for younger students.

Continued

TABLE 7.2   Practices for Health Leaders to Support Systems Level Change to Improve Health Care for Indigenous Peoples—cont'd

Topic Area	Recommendations
Indigenous client care and outcomes	Enhance the journey of Indigenous clients through the practice of trauma-informed care and programs such as Indigenous navigators, access to traditional foods and healing practices, support from Elders, and land-based healing; the specific initiatives should emerge from the recommendations made by local Indigenous communities, advisors, and clients. In jurisdictions where data related to race and ethnicity are available, track health outcomes for Indigenous versus non-Indigenous clients in the organization; appropriate Indigenous data stewardship agreements must be developed and followed. Understand and support changes to address Indigenous social determinants of health.

Source: From Richardson, L., & Murphy, T. (2018). *Bringing reconciliation to healthcare in Canada—wiser practices for healthcare leaders*. Ottawa: HealthCareCAN. Retrieved from http://www.healthcarecan.ca/2018/04/11/bringing-reconciliation-to-health-care-in-canada-wise-practices-for-healthcare-leaders/

SUMMARY

Indigenous people were the original inhabitants of North America, also known as Turtle Island. They have a long and complex history with settlers whose colonial policies had ripple effects for generations to come. In Canada, there are three main Indigenous groups—First Nations, Inuit, and Métis—with much diversity across communities in terms of traditions, language, and culture. Indigenous people make up nearly 5% of the Canadian population. As a whole, Indigenous people of Canada are younger than the general Canadian population, are increasingly living in urban environments, and are a fast-growing segment of the population. Because of social determinants of health, which include racism and colonialism, some communities face a range of health inequities compared with the general Canadian population in terms of mortality, morbidity, self perceived health, and health care utilization. Many recent developments have called to attention the legacy of colonialism and highlighted the need to respect treaty rights, enhance self-determination, and decolonize across the country in an effort to promote well being. The health sector has an important role to play in terms of offering culturally appropriate and relevant care, tackling racism in the health care sector, improving engagement with Indigenous partners, and advocating for decolonizing policies that give control of health and wellness to the Indigenous people of Canada.

KEY WEBSITES

Anishnawbe Health Toronto: http://www.aht.ca
Anishnawbe Health Toronto is a community health centre that approaches health from a traditional lens. Its goal is to: "recover, record and promote Traditional Aboriginal practices where possible and appropriate." The centre offers primary health care services, counseling, mental health and addictions, dental, chiropractic, naturopathic, and traditional counselling care.

Assembly of First Nations: http://www.afn.ca
This national organization, whose work is directed by First Nations chiefs, advocates for First Nations people across Canada and works to communicate with and build the relationship between First Nations and the Crown.

Idle No More: http://www.idlenomore.ca
Idle No More is a large-scale social movement that supports building sovereignty among Indigenous people, reframing the relationship between Indigenous people of Canada and the Canadian government, and environmental protection.

Kairos Blanket Exercise: https://www.kairosblanketexercise.org
The Kairos Blanket Exercise is a participatory and engaging history session that was developed alongside Indigenous elders for the purposes of raising awareness of Indigenous issues and fostering reconciliation efforts. This website describes the program, explains the process to book this training program, and houses some excellent resources (for both students and teachers), including reports, videos, and documentary links, to improve people's understanding of Indigenous history.

Métis National Council: http://www.metisnation.ca

Formed in 1983, the Métis National Council is made up of elected representatives and represents the voice and position of Métis Nation and Métis people across the country.

National Collaborating Centre for Aboriginal Health (NCCAH): https://www.nccah-ccnsa.ca

One of five collaborating centres, the NCCAH supports knowledge translation and exchange in order to enhance health equity and enhance inclusivity and respect of Indigenous peoples in the public health system.

National Centre for Truth and Reconciliation: https://nctr.ca/map.php

This organization now houses the materials (including statements and final report) from the Truth and Reconciliation Commission of Canada (established in 2009 by the Government of Canada), for the purposes of listening to survivors and those affected by the residential school system in Canada. The centre (housed in the University of Manitoba)'s purpose is to honour and preserve the memory of the legacy of residential schools.

National Inquiry into Missing and Murdered Indigenous Women and Girls: http://www.mmiwg-ffada.ca

This website contains the submissions and reports from the independent inquiry launched into missing and murdered Indigenous women and girls in the fall of 2016.

Native Women's Association of Canada: https://www.nwac.ca

This nonprofit organization represents an aggregate of native women's organizations across the country that works to improve the well being of Indigenous women, girls, and people who are gender diverse through the promotion of Indigenous traditions, beliefs, and languages. A sublink of this website (https://www.nwac.ca/wp-content/uploads/2018/04/The-Indian-Act-Said-WHAT-pdf-1.pdf) provides an excellent overview of the Indian Act and key historic events that have undoubtedly influenced the health and wellbeing of Indigenous people over time.

San'yas Indigenous Cultural Safety Training: http://www.sanyas.ca

This facilitated, online training program was developed by the Provincial Health Services Authority in British Columbia. It aims to increase knowledge about Indigenous health and improve the skills of people that work with Indigenous people to enhance cultural competence among service providers. Topics covered include the legacy of colonization, health inequities, history, and stereotyping, to name a few.

Secret Path: https://secretpath.ca

This website houses an album titled *The Secret Path* by Gord Downie (a Canadian music legend and late lead singer in the Canadian band the Tragically Hip). The album consists of 10 poems made into songs that were inspired by the story of Chanie Wenjack, a young boy who died in the 1960s as he was walking home from the Cecilia Jeffrey Indian Residential School, more than 400 miles away.

REFERENCES

Alberta Health Services. (2017). *How cultural ties aid healing.* Retrieved from https://www.albertahealthservices.ca/careers/Page12890.aspx.

Alberta Health Services. (2018). *Indigenous health.* Retrieved from https://www.albertahealthservices.ca/info/Page11949.aspx.

Allan, B., & Smylie, J. (2015). *First Peoples, second class treatment: The role of racism in the health and well-being of Indigenous peoples in Canada.* Toronto, ON: the Wellesley Institute.

Assembly of First Nations. (2019). *About AFN.* Retrieved from http://www.afn.ca/about-afn/.

Auger, M., Howell, T., & Gomes, T. (2016). Moving toward holistic wellness, empowerment and self-determination for Indigenous peoples in Canada: Can traditional Indigenous health care practices increase ownership over health and health care decisions? *Canadian Journal of Public Health, 107*(4-5), e393–e398.

Boksa, P., Joober, R., & Kirmayer, L. J. (2015). Mental wellness in Canada's Aboriginal communities: Striving toward reconciliation. *Journal of Psychiatry and Neuroscience, 40*(6), 363–365.

Brake, J. (2019). *Canada unveils Indigenous Languages bill to fanfare, criticism.* APTV News. Retrieved from https://aptnnews.ca/2019/02/05/canada-unveils-indigenous-languages-bill-to-fanfare-criticism/.

Burnham, P. (2003). *UN special report: Inside the medicine chest.* Indian Country Today. Retrieved from https://newsmaven.io/indiancountrytoday/archive/un-special-report-inside-the-medicine-chest-GDfORXrMREyqtH0FEFKXVg/.

Cambridge Dictionary. (2019). *Ethnocentric.* Retrieved from https://dictionary.cambridge.org/dictionary/english/ethnocentric.

Canadian Geographic. (n.d.). Indigenous governance (educational activity). Retrieved from http://www.canadiangeographic.com/educational_products/activities/ipac_gfm/IndigenousGovernance_EN.pdf.

Canadian Public Health Association. (n.d.). TB and aboriginal people. Retrieved from https://www.cpha.ca/tb-and-aboriginal-people.

Canadian Race Relations Foundation. (2019). *150 Stories: Dr. Chandrakant Shah.* Retrieved from https://www.crrf-fcrr.ca/en/programs/our-canada/150-stories/search-150-stories/item/26843-canada-129-150-dr-chandrakant-shah.

CBC News. (2017). *Shannen Koostachin, Indigenous education advocate, named one of 150 greatest Canadians*. Retrieved from https://www.cbc.ca/news/canada/sudbury/shannon-dream-legacy-150-canada-1.3981858.

Centre for Addiction and Mental Health. (n.d.). *Creating ceremony grounds at CAMH*. Retrieved from https://www.camh.ca/en/camh-news-and-stories/creating-ceremony-grounds-at-camh.

Clarke, J. (2016). *Health at a Glance: Difficulty accessing health care services in Canada*. Ottawa: Statistics Canada. Retrieved from https://www150.statcan.gc.ca/n1/pub/82-624-x/2016001/article/14683-eng.htm#fcs.

Clemens, C. (2017). Ally or accomplice? The language of activism. *Teaching Tolerance*. Retrieved from https://www.tolerance.org/magazine/ally-or-accomplice-the-language-of-activism.

Cole, N. L. (2019). *What is cultural hegemony? Thought Co.* Retrieved from https://www.thoughtco.com/cultural-hegemony-3026121.

Crawford, A. (2016). Suicide among indigenous peoples in Canada. *The Canadian encyclopedia*. Retrieved from https://www.thecanadianencyclopedia.ca/en/article/suicide-among-indigenous-peoples-in-canada.

Curtis, K. (2017). *Smudging & cultural appropriation*. Retrieved from https://kaitlincurtice.com/2017/11/04/day-4-smudging-cultural-appropriation/.

Department of Justice. (2015). *Family violence initiative*. Retrieved from https://www.justice.gc.ca/eng/rp-pr/cj-jp/fv-vf/annex-annexe/p132.html.

First Nations Health Authority. (n.d.). About us: Healthy, self-determining and vibrant BC First Nations children, families and communities. Retrieved from http://www.fnha.ca/Documents/FNHA_AboutUS.pdf.

First Nations Health Authority. (2012). *First nations perspective on health and wellness*. Retrieved from http://www.fnha.ca/wellness/wellness-and-the-first-nations-health-authority/first-nations-perspective-on-wellness.

Gadacz, R. (2017). Sweat lodge. *The Canadian Encyclopedia*. Retrieved from https://www.thecanadianencyclopedia.ca/en/article/sweat-lodge.

Gilbert, N., Auger, N., & Tjepkema, M. (2015). *Stillbirth and infant mortality in aboriginal communities in quebec*. Ottawa: Statistics Canada. Retrieved from https://www150.statcan.gc.ca/n1/pub/82-003-x/2015002/article/14139-eng.htm.

Gionet, L., & Roshanafshar, S. (2015). *Select health indicators of first nations people living off reserve, Métis and Inuit*. Ottawa: Statistics Canada. Retrieved from https://www150.statcan.gc.ca/n1/pub/82-624-x/2013001/article/11763-eng.htm.

Government of Canada. (2016). *Renewing the relationship: Key documents*. Retrieved from https://www.rcaanc-cirnac.gc.ca/eng/1307458586498/1534857991723.

Government of Canada. (2017a). *First nations in Canada*. Retrieved from https://www.rcaanc-cirnac.gc.ca/eng/1307460755710/1536862806124.

Government of Canada. (2017b). *Evaluation of Health Canada's role in supporting B.C. First nations health Authority as a governance partner*. Retrieved from https://www.canada.ca/en/public-health/corporate/transparency/corporate-management-reporting/evaluation/health-canada-role-supporting-british-columbia-first-nations-health-authority-governance-partner.html.

Government of Canada. (2018). *Definition of Jordan's principle from the Canadian human rights tribunal*. Retrieved from https://www.canada.ca/en/indigenous-services-canada/services/jordans-principle/definition-jordans-principle-canadian-human-rights-tribunal.html.

Hall, A. (2017). Treaties with indigenous peoples in Canada. *The Canadian Encyclopedia*. Retrieved from https://www.thecanadianencyclopedia.ca/en/article/aboriginal-treaties.

Hayes, A. (2017). What is Jordan's principle and why does it matter? *Indigenous perspectives society*. Retrieved from http://ipsociety.ca/2017/03/.

Indigenous Corporate Training Inc. (2015). *Indian Act and elected chief and band council system*. Retrieved from https://www.ictinc.ca/blog/indian-act-and-elected-chief-and-band-council-system.

Journal of Obstetrics and Gynaecology Canada. (2013). Clinical practice guidelines: Chapter 4: Health systems, policies, and services for first nations, Inuit, and Métis. *Journal of Obstetrics and Gynaecology Canada*, 35(6), S24–S27. Retrieved from https://www.jogc.com/article/S1701-2163(15)30704-0/pdf.

Kirmayer, L. J., Dandeneau, S., Marshall, E., et al. (2011). Rethinking resilience from Indigenous perspectives. *The Canadian Journal of Psychiatry*, 56(2), 84–91.

Loppie, S., Reading, C., & de Leeuw, S. (2014). Aboriginal experiences with racism and its impacts. *National Collaborating Centre for Aboriginal Health*. Retrieved from https://www.ccnsa-nccah.ca/docs/determinants/FS-AboriginalExperiencesRacismImpacts-Loppie-Reading-deLeeuw-EN.pdf.

MacDonald, J. P., Barnes, D., & Middleton, L. (2015). Implications of risk factors for Alzheimer's disease in Canada's Indigenous population. *Canadian Geriatrics Journal*, 18(3), 152–158.

Mansuri, S., & Hanley, A. J. (2017). Diabetes among Indigenous Canadians. In Dagogo-Jack S. (Eds.), *Diabetes mellitus in developing countries and underserved communities*. Cham: Springer.

McGhee, R. (2013). Inuvialuit. *The Canadian Encyclopedia*. Retrieved from https://www.thecanadianencyclopedia.ca/en/article/mackenzie-inuit.

Na, L., & Hample, D. (2016). Psychological pathways from social integration to health: An examination of different demographic groups in Canada. *Social Science & Medicine, 151,* 196–205.

National Collaborating Centre for Aboriginal Health. (2012). *The state of knowledge of aboriginal health: A review of aboriginal public health in Canada.* Price George, BC: Author.

National Collaborating Centre for Aboriginal Health. (2013a). *An overview of Aboriginal health in Canada.* Retrieved from https://www.ccnsa-nccah.ca/docs/context/FS-OverviewAbororiginalHealth-EN.pdf.

National Collaborating Centre for Aboriginal Health. (2013b). *Tobacco fact sheet.* Retrieved from https://www.ccnsa-nccah.ca/docs/health/FS-Tobacco-EN.pdf.

National Inquiry into Missing and Murdered Indigenous Women and Girls. (2017). *Interim report: Our women and girls are sacred.* Retrieved from http://www.mmiwg-ffada.ca/wp-content/uploads/2018/03/ni-mmiwg-interim-report.pdf.

Niigaanwewidam, J., & Dainard, S. (2017). Sixties scoop. *The Canadian Encyclopedia.* Retrieved from https://www.thecanadianencyclopedia.ca/en/article/sixties-scoop.

Office of the Auditor General of Canada. (2015). *Report 7– Establishing the first nations health authority in British Columbia.* Retrieved from http://www.oag-bvg.gc.ca/internet/English/parl_oag_201602_07_e_41064.html.

Ontario Institute for Studies in Education. (n.d.). We are all treaty people. Toronto: University of Toronto. Retrieved from https://www.oise.utoronto.ca/abed101/we-are-all-treaty-people/

Oosterveer, T. M., & Young, T. K. (2015). Primary health care accessibility challenges in remote indigenous communities in Canada's North. *International Journal of Circumpolar Health, 74*(1), 1–7.

Park, S., Boyle, J., Hoyeck, P., et al. (n.d.). Indigenous health in Ontario An introductory guide for medical students. Toronto: University of Toronto. Retrieved from https://medicine.utoronto.ca/sites/default/files/IndigenousHealthinOntario-compressed.pdf

Park, J., Tjepkema, M., Goedhuis, N., & Pennock, J. (2015). *Avoidable mortality among first nations adults in Canada: A cohort analysis.* Ottawa: Statistics Canada. Retrieved from https://www150.statcan.gc.ca/n1/pub/82-003-x/2015008/article/14216-eng.htm.

Press, J. (2017). *Census figures show depth of low incomes in Indigenous communities. CTV News (October 10).* Retrieved from https://www.ctvnews.ca/politics/census-figures-show-depth-of-low-incomes-in-indigenous-communities-1.3626488.

Public Health Agency of Canada. (2016). *Health status of canadians 2016: Report of the chief public health officer.* Retrieved from https://www.canada.ca/en/public-health/corporate/publications/chief-public-health-officer-reports-state-public-health-canada/2016-health-status-canadians.html.

Public Health Agency of Canada. (2018). *The chief public health officer's report on the state of public health in Canada 2018: Preventing problematic substance use in youth.* Retrieved from https://www.canada.ca/content/dam/phac-aspc/documents/corporate/publications/chief-public-health-officer-reports-state-public-health-canada/2018-preventing-problematic-substance-use-youth/2018-preventing-problematic-substance-use-youth.pdf.

Public Safety Canada. (2009). *Community mobilisation dialogue with Aboriginal communities.* Retrieved from https://www.publicsafety.gc.ca/cnt/rsrcs/pblctns/cmmnt-mblstn/index-en.aspx.

Rai, J., Abecassis, M., Casey, J., et al. (2017). Parent rating of executive function in fetal alcohol spectrum disorder: A review of the literature and new data on Aboriginal Canadian children. *Child Neuropsychology, 23*(6), 713–732.

Reading, J. (2015). Confronting the growing crisis of cardiovascular disease and heart health among Aboriginal peoples in Canada. *Canadian Journal of Cardiology, 31*(9), 1077–1080.

Reading, C. L., & Wien, F. (2009). *Health inequalities and social determinants of aboriginal people's health.* Prince George, BC: National Collaborating Centre for Aboriginal Health.

Rice, R. (2016). How to decolonize democracy: Indigenous governance innovation in Bolivia and Nunavut, Canada. *Bolivian Studies Journal, 22,* 220–242.

Richardson, L., & Murphy, T. (2018). *Bringing reconciliation to healthcare in Canada—wiser practices for healthcare leaders.* Ottawa: HealthCareCan. Retrieved from http://www.healthcarecan.ca/2018/04/11/bringing-reconciliation-to-healthcare-in-canada-wise-practices-for-healthcare-leaders/.

Robinson, A. (2018). Smudging. *The Canadian Encyclopedia.* Retrieved from https://www.thecanadianencyclopedia.ca/en/article/smudging.

Sheppard, A., Shapiro, G., Bushnik, T., et al. (2017). *Birth outcomes among first nations, Inuit and Métis populations.* Ottawa: Statistics Canada. Retrieved from https://www150.statcan.gc.ca/n1/pub/82-003-x/2017011/article/54886-eng.htm.

Smith, J. A., Puckett, C., & Simon, W. (2015). *Indigenous allyship: An overview.* Waterloo: Office of Aboriginal Initiatives, Wilfrid Laurier University.

Smylie, J., & Firestone, M. (2016). The health of Indigenous Peoples. In D. Raphael (Ed.), *Social determinants of health* (3rd ed.) (pp. 434–466). Toronto: Canadian Scholars' Press.

Statistics Canada. (2015). *Life expectancy*. Retrieved from https://www150.statcan.gc.ca/n1/pub/89-645-x/2010001/life-expectancy-esperance-vie-eng.htm.

Statistics Canada. (2016). *Health reports—acute care hospitalization by aboriginal identity, Canada, 2006 through 2008*. Retrieved from https://www150.statcan.gc.ca/n1/pub/82-003-x/2016008/article/14647-eng.htm.

Statistics Canada. (2017a). *Aboriginal peoples in Canada: Key results from the 2016 census*. Retrieved from https://www150.statcan.gc.ca/n1/daily-quotidien/171025/dq171025a-eng.htm.

Statistics Canada. (2017b). *Acute care hospitalization of aboriginal children and youth*. Retrieved from https://www150.statcan.gc.ca/n1/pub/82-003-x/2017007/article/14844-eng.htm.

Statistics Canada. (2017c). *Aboriginal people and the labour market*. Retrieved from https://www150.statcan.gc.ca/n1/daily-quotidien/170316/dq170316d-eng.htm.

Statistics Canada. (2017d). *The housing conditions of aboriginal people in Canada*. Retrieved from https://www12.statcan.gc.ca/census-recensement/2016/as-sa/98-200-x/2016021/98-200-x2016021-eng.cfm.

The Truth and Reconciliation Commission of Canada. (2015). *Honouring the truth, reconciling for the future: Summary of the final report of the truth and reconciliation commission of Canada*. Retrieved from http://www.trc.ca/websites/trcinstitution/File/2015/Honouring_the_Truth_Reconciling_for_the_Future_July_23_2015.pdf.

Tupper, J. (2014). Social media and the Idle No More Movement: Citizenship, activism and dissent in Canada. *Journal of Social Science Education, 13*(4), 87–94.

Turner, A. (2016). *Insights on canadian society: Living arrangements of aboriginal children aged 14 and under*. Ottawa: Statistics Canada. Retrieved from https://www150.statcan.gc.ca/n1/pub/75-006-x/2016001/article/14547-eng.htm.

United Nations. (2008). *United nations declaration on the rights of indigenous peoples*. Retrieved from https://www.un.org/esa/socdev/unpfii/documents/DRIPS_en.pdf.

UNDESA Division for Inclusive Social Development. (n.d.). United Nations declaration on the rights of indigenous peoples. Retrieved from https://www.un.org/development/desa/indigenouspeoples/declaration-on-the-rights-of-indigenous-peoples.html.

University of Calgary. (2012). *Intervention to address intergenerational trauma: Overcoming, resisting and preventing structural violence*. Retrieved from https://www.ucalgary.ca/wethurston/files/wethurston/Report_InterventionToAddressIntergenerationalTrauma.pdf.

University of Toronto Ontario Institute for Studies in Education. (n.d.). Indigenous ways of knowing. Retrieved from https://www.oise.utoronto.ca/abed101/indigenous-ways-of-knowing/.

Wood, M. (2017). Cultural appropriation and the Plains' Indian Headdress. *VCU's Journal of Undergraduate Research and Creativity*, 1–11.

8

Noncommunicable Diseases

Additional resources are available online at http://evolve.elsevier.com/Canada/Shah/publichealth/

LEARNING OBJECTIVES

- Be able to describe the burden, risk factors, and key individual and community-level prevention strategies for the four main risk factors for noncommunicable diseases (NCDs) globally and in Canada.
- List some of the determinants of key NCDs of interest in Canada, including heart disease, cancer, chronic respiratory disease, diabetes, dementia, and chronic pain.
- Describe primary, secondary, and tertiary prevention strategies related to the aforementioned conditions, including screening recommendations

- set forth by the Canadian Task Force on Preventive Health Care.
- Apply a health promotion lens to describe various strategies to address the root causes of NCDs at the community level.
- Be able to name some of the top leading causes of death and disability in Canada.
- Be familiar with the burden, risk factors, and prevention strategies associated with common unintentional and intentional injuries in Canada.
- Describe and apply the Haddon's matrix framework for injury prevention.

CHAPTER OUTLINE

KEY TERMS

chronic disease
intentional injury
noncommunicable diseases

primary prevention
secondary prevention
sedentary behaviour

tertiary prevention
unintentional injuries

INTRODUCTION

The major causes of mortality, morbidity, and the burden of illness in the Canadian population are described in Chapter 4. In high-, middle-, and increasingly now, low-income countries alike, noncommunicable diseases (NCDs) make up a large part of the burden of disease. According to the World Health Organization (WHO), in 2016, 71% of global deaths were attributable to NCDs (WHO, 2016). **Noncommunicable diseases** are disease states that cannot be transmitted or passed on between people or between people and animals. The four main NCDs, as per the WHO, are cardiovascular diseases (CVDs), cancers, diabetes, and chronic respiratory disease (WHO, 2016). Previously, the term **chronic disease** (which is usually defined as a condition lasting 3 months or longer) was used to describe such conditions. However, it is now well recognized that many communicable diseases can also be chronic in duration. HIV, for example, is no longer a disease that people die from quickly. It is a condition with which many people now live very long lives, classifying it as a chronic disease. The term NCD can also refer to injuries—either intentional or unintentional—that may or may not be chronic in nature.

There is a clear link between NCDs and disability (disability and the health of people living with disabilities are described further in Chapters 1 and 6). As introduced in Chapter 1, disability is really conceptualized based on functionality—whether people with ailments are able to participate in their communities and perform day-to-day activities. Many NCDs put people at risk for disability and may act as a precursor to a disability. For example, people living with advanced chronic lung disease may have trouble performing day-to-day activities as a result of challenges with breathing, and people with arthritis may have significant mobility issues (Hung, Ross, Boockvar, & Siu, 2012). Thus, the immense prevalence of NCDs in our society should also prompt us to think about how to design and create communities that are inclusive for people who experience activity limitations or barriers to full participation in the community.

In the Canadian context, CVD and cancer are the leading causes of NCDs. A significant proportion of NCDs are also the result of injuries, either unintentional (e.g., traffic related) or intentional (e.g., homicide). See Fig. 8.1 for a listing of the most common reasons for premature death in Canada, comparing rates in 2007 with 2017.

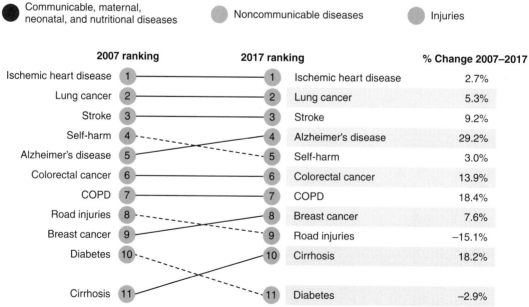

Fig. 8.1 What causes the most premature death? *COPD,* Chronic obstructive pulmonary disease. (From Healthdata.org. [2019]. Top 10 causes of years of life lost [YLLs] in 2017 and percent change, 2007-2017, all ages, number. Retrieved from http://www.healthdata.org/canada.)

From 2007 to 2017 there was no change in the top three diseases that caused premature deaths—ischemic heart disease, lung cancer, and stroke (Healthdata, 2019).

The economic and personal burden of NCDs is substantial. A number of risk factors influence the development of NCDs. Some of these are modifiable, such as those related to lifestyles, whereas others such as age, sex, or genetic makeup are not amenable to change. Substance misuse (predominantly tobacco use and excessive alcohol use), poor nutrition, and physical inactivity are the major risk factors for NCDs and play a part in several diseases; hence, they are discussed first to avoid repetition in terms of preventive strategies.

This chapter presents detailed information on the burden of illness caused by NCDs, emphasizing current approaches to prevention and control. Because many NCDs are preventable, primary and secondary prevention and, more recently, health promotion have emerged as being increasingly important. The underlying principles of disease prevention and health promotion that provide the framework are discussed in Chapter 3.

Most of the data presented here come from published studies, government sources, and nongovernmental organizations. Data, particularly percentage figures for risk factors and economic estimates of the burden of illness, quickly become out of date. Also, because of differences in methods, definitions, and time of data collection, incidence and cost figures vary slightly from report to report. The methods section of the reports cited explain how their estimates were made. The organizations cited, such as the Heart and Stroke Foundation, Canadian Cancer Society, Statistics Canada, Health Canada, and Canadian Institute for Health Information, produce annual or semiannual compilations of statistics. Updates can be found on their websites.

It is very important to keep in mind that significant inequities exist when it comes to the rates of NCDs in the population. In Canada and across the world, research has consistently shown that people with low socioeconomic status (SES) have a greater risk for developing a range of NCDs, including heart disease, diabetes, some types of cancer, and chronic obstructive lung disease, among others (Sommer et al., 2015). Research has also shown the link between SES and modifiable risk factors that contribute to NCDs (e.g., tobacco and alcohol use, physical activity, and diet). But it is very important not to stop there and simply conclude that people with lower incomes, for example, smoke more and therefore are at greater risk for NCDs. We need to dig deeper and ask: Why do people with lower incomes have higher smoking rates than people with higher incomes? Beyond modifiable lifestyle factors, at their root inequities in NCD rates are explained by differences in the social determinants of health across various groups. For example, some groups have worse living and working conditions than others because of political, economic, social, and cultural forces and this results in differing opportunities to engage in health promoting behaviours like exercising and eating healthy for example. This must be kept in mind when discussing major lifestyle issues and, more important, when developing health promotion interventions to address the high rates of NCDs we see across the globe.

Using the example of smoking, health promotion strategies (e.g., educating people about the health risks of smoking, offering smoking cessation assistance) have significantly reduced the national smoking rate. However, it is clear based on analyzing the data that people with lower levels of education and lower income haven't experienced the same decline in smoking as the general population. This is because of a phenomenon known as the inverse care law, in which people with a higher SES are able to adopt and take advantage of these interventions better and more quickly than those with a lower SES (Frohlich et al., 2010). The key lesson here is that when thinking through risk factors for NCDs, we need to be mindful of the larger forces at play (e.g., income, education, living conditions, and working conditions) and be mindful of the impact our interventions are having on equity.

Perhaps using more targeted approaches when working with low SES communities to foster agency and empowerment would be more suitable. Additionally, many are calling for all different sectors of government (e.g., transport, financing, health, social services) to work together to develop policy and regulatory interventions (e.g., advertising bans) that don't rely as much on individual action but that foster an environment that is more conducive to adopting a healthier lifestyle for all (Shilton & Robertson, 2018).

MAJOR MODIFIABLE LIFESTYLE ISSUES

As discussed, behavioural or lifestyle issues (e.g., level of physical activity or smoking status) are driven by structural determinants of health, such as the public policy environment, the physical and social environment, and socioeconomic position, for example. As such, although this chapter focuses on major modifiable lifestyle issues that influence the development of NCDs, the broader context in which these behavioural and lifestyle factors exist must also be kept in mind.

The four major underlying lifestyle or behavioural causes of many NCDs are tobacco use, excessive alcohol use, improper diet, and physical inactivity. Chronic toxic stress (discussed in the Research Perspective box) is an increasingly recognized risk factor for the development of long-term physical and mental health issues and is also linked to the four main risk factors mentioned earlier.

RESEARCH PERSPECTIVE

Chronic Toxic Stress

Activation of the body's stress response system is a normal part of day-to-day human functioning and confers survival advantages. Whenever humans are threatened in any way, the body responds with an increase in heart rate and blood pressure, release of a stress hormone called cortisol, opening of the airways, and better vision and hearing. This constellation of signs and symptoms is often called the "flight-or-fight response" which allows your body to flee or defend itself against a threat. Toxic chronic stress occurs when this stress response system is activated excessively or inappropriately over a long period and during times when there is no actual physical or immediate threat (e.g., stress that is experienced because of work or school, financial situations, or relationship difficulties).

Trauma or household dysfunction in early childhood and the absence of healthy attachments while growing up are now also recognized as important factors that can predispose people to chronic activation of the stress response system as a result of situational or life stressors (Center on the Developing Child, Harvard University, n.d.). These Adverse Childhood Experiences, further defined and described in Chapter 9, are also influential risk factors in the development of mental health and substance use problems. Whatever the cause or trigger of negative childhood events, the constant activation of the stress response system can result in changes to the brain and organ systems that lead to a range of chronic diseases, such as heart disease, diabetes, cognitive impairment, and depression.

Chronic stress also increases the risks of overeating, smoking, and alcohol consumption. According to the most recent Statistics Canada data, 22% of Canadians 12 years old and older report finding most days stressful. Females tend to experience more stress than males, and people between the ages of 35 and 54 years tend to report more stress than others (Statistics Canada, 2018).

Given the importance of early childhood experiences for predisposing or protecting people from the risk of chronic toxic stress, community and public health nurses, social workers, and others have a very critical role to play. Often these health care professionals, along with peer (nonprofessional but trained) home visitors, lead home visitation programs for high-risk families. In Manitoba, for example, the Families First program (run by community public health staff) offers intensive home visits to pregnant mothers and families with children up to kindergarten age. The goal of this program is to link higher risk families with social, health, and other community supports, promote learning of problem-solving skills, and strengthen family relationships (Government of Manitoba, n.d.), thus reducing the risk of trauma and household dysfunction.

Tobacco

Tobacco smoking is the most important preventable cause of death in Canada. The trends and prevalence rate of smoking are described further in Chapter 9. However, this chapter focuses on the effects of tobacco smoke, including the increased risk of death, health care utilization, and morbidity caused by NCDs that result from tobacco exposure.

Deaths

In Canada, nearly one in five deaths (or 45 000 deaths each year) are a result of the use of tobacco products (Dobrescu, Bhandari, Sutherland, & Dinh, 2017). According to a 2017 report published by the Conference Board of Canada, tobacco use accounted for nearly 600 000 potential years of life lost (PYLL) across the country (Dobrescu et al., 2017), mainly as a result of deaths from cancer, heart disease, and respiratory disease.

Noncommunicable Diseases Related to Smoking

Smoking is the primary cause of lung cancer and is thought to cause around 85% of all lung cancers (Lung Cancer Canada, n.d.). Lung cancer is the leading cause of cancer death in Canada and it is expected that 1 in 12 Canadians will get lung cancer over the course of their lifetime.

Smoking is thought to increase the risk of lung cancer because it causes genetic changes to lung cells as well as inhibits the process whereby the lungs get rid of toxic particles that enter them from the environment. Therefore, quitting smoking can greatly reduce the risk of lung cancer. The risk of lung cancer in those who have quit 20 or more years ago is virtually the same as those who have never smoked a day in their lives (Lung Cancer Canada, n.d.).

Aside from its association with lung cancer, smoking is also a risk factor for a number of other cancers, including cancer of the esophagus, larynx, mouth, throat, kidney, bladder, liver, pancreas, stomach, cervix, colon, and rectum (National Institute of Health [NIH], 2017). In addition to cancer, tobacco use can also increase the risk of a host of other NCDs, including the following:

- Heart disease
- Stroke
- Chronic obstructive pulmonary disease (COPD)
- Diabetes
- Osteoporosis
- Cataracts
- Rheumatoid arthritis
- Pneumonia
- Tuberculosis (TB)
- Influenza
- Erectile dysfunction
- Miscarriage (in pregnant women)
- Ectopic pregnancies (in pregnant women)
- Risk of low birth weight babies (in pregnant women)
- Sudden infant death syndrome (in newborns whose mothers smoke)

Health Care Utilization

Smoking results in an immense cost to the health care system. In 2012, smoking was estimated to directly cost the Canadian health care system $6.5 billion because of the costs associated with hospitalizations, drugs, and physician billing (Dobrescu et al., 2017). When we consider the breadth of NCDs caused by smoking, it is not surprising that this figure is as high as it is. Hospitalizations caused by smoking include people being admitted for causes or disease states directly resulting from tobacco smoking, such as cancer, heart disease, and pneumonia.

Environmental Tobacco Smoke

Smoking is a hazard not only to those who smoke but also to nonsmokers who are exposed to environmental tobacco smoke (ETS). The relationship between ETS and adverse health effects is now well accepted. ETS is a mixture of exhaled smoke (mainstream) and smoke emitted from the smouldering tobacco (side stream). It contains more than 4 000 chemicals, of which 42 are known carcinogens. Besides ETS being a known mucous membrane irritant, exposure is linked to increases in mortality from lung cancer and CVD among nonsmokers and has serious consequences for children.

For children, exposure to ETS is a risk factor for respiratory symptoms; middle ear disease; sudden infant death syndrome; and bronchitis, pneumonia, and other lower respiratory tract infections, and asthma. It is also thought to have adverse impacts on cognition and behaviour and to decrease lung function and induce and exacerbate asthma. In adults, ETS causes heart disease, lung cancer, and nasal sinus cancer and has also been linked to stroke, breast cancer, cervical cancer, and miscarriages (Johnson, 2010). ETS causes about 800 deaths from lung cancer and heart disease for nonsmoking Canadians each year (Health Canada, 2015).

Tobacco Control

A person's decision to use tobacco is the result of a complex interaction of factors that varies from one individual to another. Reducing tobacco use requires a comprehensive, multifaceted approach that targets different groups in different settings and mixes individual-level interventions with population-based interventions. Interventions also have to be culturally appropriate and relevant.

Smoking rates among Indigenous people in Canada are higher than in the general population. Much of this has its root in colonial policies and intergenerational trauma, which resulted in poorer living and working conditions for many (but not all) communities. Although Indigenous people also use tobacco ceremoniously (as discussed more in Chapter 7), commercial tobacco use remains a large issue in many Indigenous communities and thus, a multifaceted, culturally appropriate, and equity-focused approach to tobacco control is needed.

Throughout this chapter, regulatory approaches will be considered (e.g., laws that ban smoking in public). This is because they apply to the whole population (thus having a broad impact); strengthen the environment, which we know is so important in influencing health; and reduce the emphasis on working one on one with a person to alter their behaviour without changing the driving factors that put them at risk for smoking, for example. They may in many ways also be helpful in reducing the gap between the worst-off and best-off in our societies because they do not rely on having intensive individual services available but instead work to improve environments and social and economic contexts. These regulatory types of changes make it easier for communities to embrace healthier options, particularly for those who have a harder time doing so because of inequitable access to the social determinants of health. An example of this type of regulatory measure is presented next.

In February 2005, the WHO's Framework Convention on Tobacco Control (FCTC) came into effect. It was the very first treaty developed by the WHO. The FCTC came about as a result of the widespread use and harms of tobacco use across the globe and is intended to be an evidence-based framework for countries to use in trying to curb tobacco use (WHO, 2003). The FCTC requires countries to put into place strategies that both reduce the demand for tobacco among the population and reduce the supply of tobacco products. The MPOWER package is a set of six technical strategies or tobacco control measures developed by the WHO that countries can adopt to help them address the demand reduction provisions of the FCTC. MPOWER stands for:

M = Monitoring tobacco use and the existence of policies to curb it.

Conducting surveillance for countries to understand rates of tobacco use among different segments of their population is key to developing successful interventions. For example, surveillance may identify a disproportionate or high rate of tobacco use among youth, which can support evidence-based policy making for this segment of the population (Aldrich et al., 2015).

P = Protecting people from tobacco smoke

A common and effective way to protect others from tobacco smoke is to develop smoke-free policies and designate places such as outdoor public places, workplaces, and indoor commercial areas as being smoke free. These types of policies not only have the benefit of protecting others from secondhand smoke but also tend to change social norms because youth less often see people smoking as a regular and normal part of adult behaviour (Nuyts, Kuijpers, Willemsen,

& Kunst, 2018; Hawkins, Bach, & Baum, 2016).

O = Offering quit assistance to those who smoke

Smoking cessation counselling is widely recognized as an effective clinical practice. Even a brief intervention by a health care professional significantly increases the cessation rate. A smoker's likelihood of quitting increases when he or she hears the message from a number of health care providers from a variety of disciplines (Lavery, Nair, Bass, & Collins, 2016; The Role of Health Professionals in Tobacco Cessation [Joint Position Statement], 2011).

W = Warning about the dangers of tobacco

Warning about the harms of tobacco can take multiple forms. Educating the public through health messaging and social marketing can be effective. Additionally, increasingly more research is revealing how warning labels, particularly those that contain graphic images, deter tobacco use among adolescents and young adults (Roberts, Peters, Ferketich, & Klein, 2016).

E = Enforcing bans on the promotion of tobacco products

A wealth of literature has shown the link between tobacco advertising and the risk of smoking initiation among youth, in particular (Shang, Huang, Li, & Chaloupka, 2015). For decades, tobacco companies used marketing principles to sell tobacco as a desirable product (refer to Fig. 8.2 for a historical example). A recent study drawing on the Global Youth Tobacco Survey has shown that among 130 countries, those that had a ban on point-of-sale advertising to youth had significantly lower rates of youth experimenting with smoking compared with countries without such a ban (Shang et al., 2015).

R = Raising taxes on tobacco products

One of the most effective interventions to curb tobacco use is the introduction of taxes on tobacco products. The WHO cites this strategy as being the most cost effective one, particularly in low-income countries. It has been estimated that with every 10% increase in the price of cigarettes (because of increased taxes), 4% fewer people consume tobacco (Savedoff & Alwang, 2015).

In Canada, many of the MPOWER principles have been adopted at various levels of government. The federal government has committed to continuing strategies that have been successful in the past, including a pan-Canadian Quitline, requiring that pictorial health warnings must take up at least 75% of tobacco packages, banning most forms of tobacco sponsorship and promotion, and encouraging that

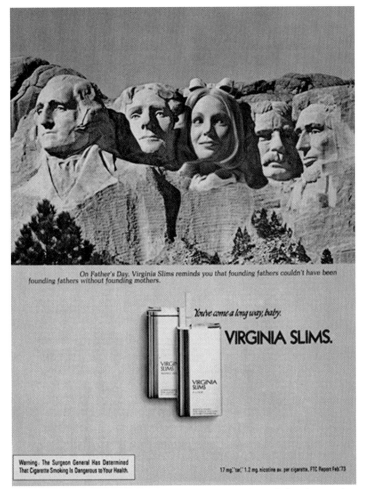

Fig. 8.2 A historic (1970s) tobacco advertisement (From Stine, J. K. [2014]. Smoke gets in your eyes: 20th century tobacco advertisements. Retrieved from http://americanhistory.si.edu/blog/2014/03/smoke-gets-in-your-eyes-20th-century-tobacco-advertisements.html.)

provinces and territories restrict where people can smoke cigarettes(Canadian Cancer Society, 2017).

Provinces and territories also have a lot of leeway when it comes to implementing tobacco policies. Ontario, for example, has the *Smoke-Free Ontario Act,* which bans smoking in all enclosed workplaces, all enclosed public spaces, and all specifically dedicated outdoor places (e.g., patios). Additionally, in retail stores, tobacco products must be stored where customers can't handle them before purchase (e.g., behind a counter), and retailers are strictly prohibited from selling tobacco to people younger than 19 years of age. Inspectors typically check whether retail stores are complying with the provisions set out in the Act, and store owners can be fined if they do not comply (Government of Ontario, 2014). Various jurisdictions, including the federal government, are also looking at regulating the availability and promotion of nicotine-containing vaping products, described in the Research Perspective box.

Although the regulatory and enforcement measures mentioned typically are led by governments at various levels, community providers have a very important role to play when it comes to fostering empowerment of people, at the community level, to not smoke. Research has shown

---

EXERCISE 8.1: Who is the target audience for the tobacco advertisement depicted in Fig. 8.2? What does the advertisement indirectly communicate to women? What are the potential harmful implications of a communication such as this?

that when it comes to prevention of tobacco use among youth, the more actively engaged youth are in these prevention initiatives, the better the result. Researchers in the United States analyzed the results of a youth-driven participatory digital media production in which a group of children in grades 4 to 8 researched the factors that lead to smoking, as well as its health effects, and scripted and produced an educational video to share with their peers. The program resulted in an increase in the intention not to smoke after people participated in the program. In addition, youth felt empowered to act as advocates in the area of tobacco control (Park et al., 2017).

As discussed earlier, when developing such programs or interventions, it is extremely important to pay attention to health inequities and whether such an intervention may lend itself to the inverse care law. For this particular example, then, one must think about whether lower SES groups may be less able to "take up" the preventive messages in the video compared with higher SES groups and what other activities the community could engage in to ensure that the gap in smoking between high and low SES groups can be closed. Perhaps engaging low-income youth, in particular, to target messaging in a way that resonates with a particular vulnerable group's unique values and priorities might be a way to address any unintended consequences (i.e., the worsening of health inequities) as a result of this initiative.

RESEARCH PERSPECTIVE

Vaping: A Harm-Reduction Tool?

Much controversy surrounds vaping or e-cigarettes—the consumption of nicotine through heating a liquid solution as opposed to smoking (i.e., combusting) tobacco. Although some people believe vaping represents a much safer alternative to cigarette smoking (because of the reduction in exposure to harmful byproducts of combustion when vaping instead of smoking), others believe that evidence for vaping as a strategy to reduce the harmful effects of tobacco smoke is lacking and that because vaping still exposes a person to nicotine, it may not be a very effective way to get people to quit smoking or smoke less.

A variety of systematic reviews have been undertaken, but many cite that the number of studies conducted to date is still small, that the studies contradict each other, and that they do not use consistent methodologies, which makes it difficult to pool them together (Pisinger & Døssing, 2014). Although some reviews point to the flaws in the evidence and conclude that e-cigarettes cannot be considered safe (Pisinger & Døssing, 2014), others conclude that e-cigarettes are more safe than conventional cigarettes and may be used successfully to help people quit smoking (Glasser et al., 2017).

This was the rationale used by Health Canada in the spring of 2018, when it introduced Bill S-5, An Act to amend the Tobacco Act and the Non-smokers' Health Act. Under this legislation, vaping products that contain nicotine (because vaping can be used in the consumption of things such as marijuana as well) can be sold by retailers according to provincial and territorial legislation, providing that retailers do not sell these products to anyone younger than 18 years. Other provisions included in the bill to protect public health (given that not much is known about the harms of vaping) include regulating how e-cigarettes are promoted to people and banning vaping in federal workplaces (Government of Canada, 2018b).

Alcohol

Alcohol is known to increase the risk of a number of diseases, both communicable and noncommunicable, including injuries. Trend and prevalence rates for drinking are discussed in Chapter 9. This section focuses on the effects of alcohol as it relates to death, health care utilization, and morbidity.

Deaths

In 2015, approximately 3076 deaths were directly attributable to alcohol use across the country, more than half of them being a result of chronic alcoholic liver disease.

It is estimated that deaths related to alcohol (for all causes such as injuries, liver disease, and suicide, for example) make up almost 4% of all avoidable deaths in Canada. Interestingly, although rates of deaths caused by alcohol have increased for both sexes since 2001, the percentage increase has been greater for women than for men (Canadian Institute for Health Information [CIHI], 2018a).

> **EXERCISE 8.2:** What are some reasons for the death rate in women caused by alcohol increasing more than for men?

Noncommunicable Diseases Related to Alcohol

Alcohol has both acute and chronic effects on health. The acute effects of heavy drinking include increases in blood pressure and an increased risk of cardiac arrhythmia. As little as one drink affects cognition, neuromotor function, and judgement and attenuates performance of skilled tasks. Acute alcohol intoxication results when a person has consumed a large amount of alcohol compared with what their body is able to metabolize. It usually presents as a constellation of signs and symptoms, including vomiting, reduced level of consciousness, and decreased breathing rate, among others (Mayo Clinic, 2018). Blood alcohol concentration (BAC) is very closely associated with risk of injury and severity of injury; risk of motor vehicle collisions increases with increasing BAC. Cross-sectional surveys show that drinking as many as five drinks per day is highly correlated with reported social problems (home life, work, legal, financial) as well. Alcohol use may also accompany suicide attempts and criminal activities. A link has also been drawn between alcohol use and engaging in risky sexual activity (e.g., unprotected sex), resulting in increased rates of sexually transmitted infections such as chlamydia and gonorrhea (Dir et al., 2018).

Excessive long-term alcohol use can also lead to chronic health problems. There is no threshold level for many health problems (i.e., risk is lowest for nondrinkers, occurs at all levels, and increases with levels of intake). Chronic alcohol-related problems include diseases of the liver (hepatitis, cirrhosis), pancreas (pancreatitis), and nervous system (neuropathy, dementia, stroke, mental health, and addiction to other substances); cancer of the colon, rectum, breast, central nervous system, larynx, pharynx, esophagus, and liver, gastritis and peptic ulcers; cardiac conditions (e.g., high blood pressure and heart disease), nutritional deficiencies (e.g., thiamine deficiency), and problems with fertility (Public Health Agency of Canada [PHAC], 2016).

Alcohol use during pregnancy can impair physical and mental development of fetuses and increase the risk of congenital defects. The most severe but uncommon example is fetal alcohol syndrome, which usually occurs in children of mothers with serious alcohol problems or who are alcohol dependent. However, measurable effects on child growth, development, and behaviour can occur with use below levels associated with dependence. (PHAC, 2016).

For many decades, it was thought that consuming small amounts of alcohol, particularly red wine, actually protected against heart disease. However, increasingly more research is now discrediting this hypothesis. In fact, more evidence is emerging about the harmful effects of even a small amount of alcohol on heart health (e.g., the risk of irregular heart rhythms), and it is now believed that previous studies showing cardioprotective effects may have been overstated (Toma, Paré, & Leong, 2017). Furthermore, these benefits (if they exist) only apply to middle-aged populations, not to children or youth (Butt et al., 2011).

Health Care Utilization as a Result of Alcohol Use

Hospitalizations because of alcohol are quite significant. In 2017, it was estimated that 217 people a day in Canada were hospitalized because of conditions directly related to alcohol consumption (CIHI, 2018b). Overall, alcohol-related harms have been estimated to cost the Canadian economy more than $3 billion in direct health care costs alone and just over $14 billion if one also accounts for all of the indirect costs (e.g., lost productivity) (CIHI, 2017).

Individual-Level Interventions

Early Detection and Brief Interventions by Health Care Professionals. Similar to interventions designed to curb tobacco use, reducing alcohol consumption in the population can take the form of individual-level interventions (which most often occur in a health care setting such as a primary care provider's office) or broader, population-level interventions (described in the next section).

Primary health care providers are well positioned to identify problem drinking and alcohol dependence quickly and offer early intervention for patients whose alcohol use is increasing their risks for medical and psychosocial consequences. Short questionnaires, such as the CAGE questionnaire (Ewing, 1984; see https://www.researchgate.net/publication/23452153_The_CAGE_Questionnaire_for_Detection_of_Alcoholism/link/5bbb5b2ca6fdcc9552d98e04/download, are often used to detect problematic alcohol intake (Davoren, Demant, Shiely, & Perry, 2016). Other, newer instruments such as the Alcohol Use Disorders Identification Test (AUDIT) are also validated and can be used. The AUDIT tool is described further in Chapter 9.

Sensitive and nonconfrontational brief intervention programs such as health care provider advice to reduce alcohol consumption for those at an early stage of problem drinking have been shown to be effective (New South Wales [NSW] Department of Health, 2008).

Other evidence-based individual level, clinical strategies to address alcohol use include the following:

- Cognitive behavioural therapy (which helps a client identify problematic thoughts regarding the use of alcohol and teaches skills related to coping with addiction, including relapse and cravings)
- Mindfulness-based stress reduction (an increasingly popular strategy that focuses on drawing one's attention to present experiences, physical, emotional, psychological, and cognitive)
- Motivational interviewing (a client-centred approach that helps people work through ambivalence regarding a specific behaviour change, e.g., reducing their alcohol consumption)
- Family therapy (to draw on available social supports and address the impact alcohol use can have on couples and families)
- Teaching emotional regulation
- Participating in group therapy such as self-help groups and others (e.g., Alcoholics Anonymous) (NSW Department of Health, 2008).

Population-Based Health Promotion Strategies

Increases in overall or per capita consumption are associated with higher rates of heavy drinking and with increased frequencies of alcohol-related problems. Therefore, an important population-based approach to preventing hazardous drinking and alcohol-related problems is to decrease overall alcohol consumption. Comprehensively, this can be done by paying attention to the 4 Es (Cook & Abreu, 1998):

- **Economic accessibility:** Just like with tobacco, pricing and taxation have a major influence on rates of consumption. Perhaps the most effective intervention for curbing alcohol use and associated harms is increasing the minimum price of alcohol (PHAC, 2016).
- **Environmental or physical availability:** Another evidence-based intervention is to reduce the number or density of alcohol outlets in a community and further to limit the number of hours or days of the week when such outlets can be open. When governments take steps to reduce the number of places where alcohol can be sold (e.g., banning the sale in grocery stores or convenience stores), usage and associated harms go down (PHAC, 2016).
- **Enforcement of laws affecting use by youth and promotion and advertising:** There is much evidence

that lowering the minimum drinking age is correlated with higher consumption of alcohol and incidence of alcohol-related problems, especially among teens. Putting into place minimum age laws has been shown to reduce underage drinking (PHAC, 2016). Laws that limit the ability of the alcohol industry to sponsor events and advertise to youth may also be effective in reducing consumption, particularly among youth. Several US studies have shown that the more youth are exposed to alcohol-related advertising, the more alcohol they consume (PHAC, 2016).

- **Education:** Public education is essential to increase awareness of the harms associated with alcohol use and equip people with the skills to implement the actions needed to reduce the risks of their alcohol use to themselves and others.

One tool that has been designed and promoted to assist with public awareness of how much alcohol might be "safe" to drink is Canada's Low-Risk Alcohol Drinking Guidelines (which are depicted in Fig. 8.3).

Education about alcohol in schools can also be very effective in delaying when people begin consuming alcohol (PHAC, 2016).

EXERCISE 8.3: What are some of the limitations of guidelines such as Canada's Low-Risk Alcohol Drinking Guidelines?

Nutrition and Physical Activity
Nutrition

Chapter 5 provides information on the nutritional and dietary status of Canadians and highlights the importance of the food environment and public policy environment for influencing the dietary status of Canadians. Diet, particularly excessive fat intake and insufficient intake of fruits and vegetables, is a major factor in the development of many chronic diseases, including the two leading killers, CVD and cancer (Valenzuela, Das, Videla, & Llorente, 2018). Cancers that are linked to consuming an unhealthy diet include esophageal, colorectal, kidney, endometrial, pancreatic, and breast cancer (Patel, Pathak, Patel, & Sutariya, 2018). Eating a diet that is high in fats, sugars, and salt also results in chronic kidney disease, stroke, oral health problems, osteoporosis, dementia, and type 2 diabetes, among other diseases (Hyseni et al., 2017; Krishnaswamy, 2016). In terms of

Canada's Low-risk Alcohol Drinking Guidelines

Drinking is a personal choice.
If you choose to drink, these guidelines can help you decide when, where, why and how.

For these guidelines, "a drink" means: ▶ ▶ ▶

Beer
341 ml (12 oz.)
5% alcohol content

Cider/ Cooler
341 ml (12 oz.)
5% alcohol content

Wine
142 ml (5 oz.)
12% alcohol content

Distilled Alcohol
(rye, gin, rum, etc.)
43 ml (1.5 oz.)
40% alcohol content

▶ YOUR LIMITS

Reduce your long-term health risks by drinking no more than:

- 10 drinks a week for women, with no more than 2 drinks a day most days
- 15 drinks a week for men, with no more than 3 drinks a day most days

Plan non-drinking days every week to avoid developing a habit.

▶ SPECIAL OCCASIONS

Reduce your risk of injury and harm by drinking no more than 3 drinks (for women) or 4 drinks (for men) on any single occasion.

Plan to drink in a safe environment. Stay within the weekly limits outlined above in **Your limits**.

▶ SAFER DRINKING TIPS

- Set limits for yourself and stick to them.
- Drink slowly. Have no more than 2 drinks in any 3 hours.
- For every drink of alcohol, have one non-alcoholic drink.
- Eat before and while you are drinking.
- Always consider your age, body weight and health problems that might suggest lower limits.
- While drinking may provide health benefits for certain groups of people, do not start to drink or increase your drinking for health benefits.

Low-risk drinking helps to promote a culture of moderation.
Low-risk drinking supports healthy lifestyles.

▶ WHEN ZERO'S THE LIMIT

- Do not drink when you are: driving a vehicle or using machinery and tools
- taking medicine or other drugs that interact with alcohol
- Doing any kind of dangerous physical activity
- living with mental or physical health problems
- living with alcohol dependence
- pregnant or planning to be pregnant
- responsible for the safety of others
- making important decisions

▶ PREGNANT? ZERO IS SAFEST

If you are pregnant or planning to become pregnant, or about to breastfeed, the safest choice is to drink no alcohol at all.

▶ DELAY YOUR DRINKING

Alcohol can harm the way the body and brain develop. Teens should speak with their parents about drinking. If they choose to drink, they should do so under parental guidance; never more than 1–2 drinks at a time, and never more than 1–2 times per week. They should plan ahead, follow local alcohol laws and consider the **Safer drinking tips** listed in this brochure.

Youth in their late teens to age 24 years should never exceed the daily and weekly limits outlined in **Your limits**.

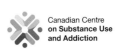

Canadian Centre on Substance Use and Addiction

Evidence. Engagement. Impact.

The Canadian Centre on Substance Use and Addiction changes lives by bringing people and knowledge together to reduce the harm of alcohol and other drugs on society. We partner with public, private and non-governmental organizations to improve the health and safety of Canadians.

CCSA wishes to thank the partners who supported development of Canada's Low-Risk Alcohol Drinking Guidelines. For a complete list of the organizations supporting the guidelines, please visit www.ccsa.ca/Eng/Priorities/Alcohol/Canada-Low-Risk-Alcohol-Drinking-Guidelines/Pages/default.aspx

Reference:
Butt, P., Beirness, D., Gliksman, L., Paradis, C. & Stockwell, T. (2011). Alcohol and health in Canada: A summary of evidence and guidelines for low-risk drinking. Ottawa, Ont.: Canadian Centre on Substance Abuse.

500–75 Albert Street, Ottawa, ON K1P 5E7
Tel: 613-235-4048 | Fax: 613-235-8101
ISBN 978-1-77178-010-0

Developed on behalf of the National Alcohol Strategy Advisory Committee

© Canadian Centre on Substance Use and Addiction 2017
Cette publication est également disponible en français.

VISIT OUR WEBSITE TO FIND OUT MORE!

www.ccsa.ca

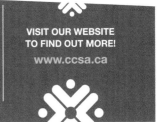

Fig. 8.3 Canada's low-risk drinking guidelines. (Butt, P., Beirness, D., Gliksman, L., Paradis, C., & Stockwell, T. (2011). Alcohol and health in Canada: A summary of evidence and guidelines for low risk drinking. Ottawa, ON: Canadian Centre on Substance Abuse.)

death data, a study has shown that between 2009 and 2010, 12% of all deaths in Canada were a result of consuming a poor diet (i.e., a diet that is high in sugar, salt, and fat) (Manuel et al., 2016). Furthermore, other studies have estimated that nearly 30 000 deaths could be prevented every year in Canada if everyone complied with dietary recommendations to eat a healthy and balanced diet (Kaczorowski et al., 2016).

More and more literature is now being published to estimate the economic burden of consuming a poor diet in Canada. A 2018 study estimated the cost of eating few protective foods and more risky foods to be equal to $13.8 billion a year, with the direct costs of health care equalling $5.1 billion (Lieffers, Ekwaru, Ohinmaa, & Veugelers, 2018). Interestingly, this is similar to the estimated economic burden of smoking and greater than the economic burden associated with being physically inactive (discussed later) (Lieffers et al., 2018).

As discussed in Chapter 5, it is important to keep in mind the larger forces behind people's eating habits. In many low-income communities, there is a lack of access to affordable, healthy foods outlets (e.g., grocery stores that sell fresh produce). Although this is true for urban communities, it is also an issue in rural Canada, where food outlets may be far away, transportation is expensive, and food itself may be much more expensive than "in the city" (Lebel et al., 2016). Fast food outlets, on the other hand, tend to be in closer proximity and provide filling foods high in sugar, fat, and salt. These foods are often more affordable and more accessible to many, further disadvantaging those who struggle to find time to cook, don't have the skills to do so, or don't have the income to access nutritious foods. These larger forces must be accounted for when reading statistics, analyzing health inequities in NCDs, and developing interventions to equitably address the high rates of NCDs we see across Canada. Interventions such as equity-oriented social and nutrition policies are required to improve the quality of Canadians' diets. This can be done through intersectoral partnerships with nonhealth actors to address the social determinants of health (e.g., improve economic security, reduce precarious employment, and ensure access to postsecondary education regardless of ability to pay), combined with equity-oriented nutrition policies (address the root causes of poor diet quality) (Olstad, Campbell, & Raine, 2019).

Physical Activity

Physical inactivity creates a significant health and economic burden in Canada. Because both poor diet and physical inactivity contribute to obesity (which is a more direct risk factor for many NCDs), many of the same diseases that are caused by poor eating habits are also caused by low levels of physical activity. Physical inactivity is linked to conditions such as heart disease, stroke, type 2 diabetes, high blood pressure, and cancers. Some health risks that are more uniquely associated with physical inactivity rather than poor diet include mental health problems such as depression and anxiety (Rebar et al., 2015), as well as injuries (particularly falls among elderly people (Bauman et al., 2016). A new category of physical inactivity is emerging in the literature: **sedentary behaviour**, defined as the time spent seated, reclined, or lying down (when one expends very little energy) during waking hours is thought to be almost as risky as tobacco smoke and is linked to the risk of death, CVD, and type 2 diabetes. More research is being called for to help better understand these links and examine the link between cancer mortality and other NCDs of interest (Patterson et al., 2018).

In terms of both direct and indirect costs to the Canadian economy, the Conference Board of Canada estimated that in 2009 physical inactivity cost around $6.8 billion (Bounajm, Dinh, & Thériault, 2014). Physical inactivity is also a large influencer of mortality. It is estimated that people who stand or walk often during the day have a 30% lower risk of death compared with those who do not (Bounajm et al., 2014).

Health Promotion Strategies for Nutrition and Physical Activity

The pillars of the Ottawa Charter for Health Promotion (i.e., develop personal skills, reorient health services, strengthen community action, create supportive environments, and build healthy public policy, as described in Chapter 3) can be applied to improving diets and physical activity and reducing the burden of illness. For example, several tools exist to provide education and information that can assist people to make healthier choices when it comes to eating nutritious foods and exercising (development of personal skills). Since 1942, the federal government (namely Health Canada) has published and periodically updated the Canada Food Guide (originally titled "Canada's Official Food Rules") to advise people on how to maintain a healthy diet. In 2019, the food guide was updated to give Canadians general advice on what foods to avoid (e.g., foods high in sugar, salt, and saturated fat) and which to consume more of (e.g., fruits, vegetables, water, plant-based foods). The 2019 food guide also gives suggestions such as taking more time to eat, cooking more often, eating with others, and being aware of the influence of food advertising. This latter point is new to the food guide repertoire and makes a conscious effort to alert people to the fact that food choices are also heavily influenced by industry marketing and promotion (Government of Canada, 2018a, 2019).

EXERCISE 8.4: Take a look at the 2019 edition of Canada's Food Guide. What are some of its limitations? What are some advantages?

CRITICAL THINKING QUESTION 8.1: Review the evidence around how the food industry influences consumer choices. Is there much evidence available to support this? Can you think of an example of an influential food marketing strategy in your community? How might you as a health care provider tackle the issue of for-profit companies trying to market unhealthy food products?

In terms of physical activity, the Canadian Society for Exercise Physiology (CSEP) has produced evidence-based physical activity targets for children, youth, adults, and older adults, as well as sedentary behaviour targets for children and youth. Table 8.1 summarizes these guidelines. Many nonprofit community-based organizations have promoted these guidelines among their communities and beneficiaries, and often it is this type of community-driven mobilization that strengthens and reinforces the described interventions.

In addition to education and raising awareness, the Ottawa Charter for Health Promotion has emphasized the value of creating environments that are conducive to eating healthy and being physically active, which may benefit vulnerable groups at higher risk of NCDs the most. When designing interventions, it is important to be mindful of the fact that being physically active is more challenging in some communities, perhaps because there is a high degree of crime and families feel less certain about letting their children

go out to play and be active, or perhaps because they live in an environment that makes it challenging to walk place to place or that has a harsh climate that does not allow for that. The following are just a few examples of interventions that municipal, provincial, and federal governments can or have implemented to advance the goal of improving the environment and making it more conducive to activity and healthier eating for all:

- Reduce the geographic density of fast food outlets
- Invest in public transportation systems
- Build bicycle lanes
- Increase the number of public parks, and accessible recreational facilities

---

EXERCISE 8.5: What other interventions can you think of that can help make a city or town more conducive to physical activity?

One program that was launched by the federal government in 2011, which specifically assists with nutrition affordability in isolated rural communities is known as the Nutrition North Program. Through this program, the government provides subsidies to the food suppliers in Northern Canada (to cover the cost of transporting food to the North). The food suppliers (i.e., grocery stores) then have to pass the subsidy on to the consumer, which means that perishable nutritious foods can be purchased for a cheaper price, making these types of foods accessible to more people (Government of Canada, 2018c). However, food in the North, particularly in rural and isolated reserve communities, can still be extremely expensive and this contributes to the health inequities we see in Indigenous communities. (This topic is analyzed further in Chapter 7.)

Reorienting health services (another pillar of the Ottawa Charter) often means investing more in preventive care and multidisciplinary approaches. When it comes to improving physical activity and healthy eating, the health care system at large can do things such as ensure that clients have access to dietitians and train and incentivize providers to spend time counselling clients on a one-to-one basis about healthy eating and active living.

Lastly, promoting policies in schools, workplaces, and the community at large that tackle physical inactivity and inadequate diets can have a large impact on reducing the incidence of chronic disease in the population, and it is important to do so in a way that promotes health

TABLE 8.1   Guidelines for Physical Activity and Sedentary Behaviour

Age Category	Recommended Physical Activity Guidance	Recommended Guidance About Sedentary Behaviour
0–4 years	Infants: Engage in physical activity several times a day Children 1–4 years of age: 180 minutes of physical activity spread throughout the day	<2 years: Screen time (e.g., TV, computer, electronic games) is not recommended 2–4 years: Screen time should be limited to <1 hour per day; less time is better Caregivers should minimize time spent being sedentary
5–11 years	60 minutes of moderate- to vigorous-intensity physical activity daily Vigorous-intensity activities at least 3 days per week Activities that strengthen muscle and bone at least 3 days per week	Limit recreational screen time to no more than 2 hours per day Limit sedentary (motorized) transport, extended sitting, and time spent indoors throughout the day
12–17 years	60 minutes of moderate- to vigorous-intensity physical activity daily. Vigorous-intensity activities at least 3 days per week Activities that strengthen muscle and bone at least 3 days per week	Limit recreational screen time to no more than 2 hours per day Limit sedentary (motorized) transport, extended sitting, and time spent indoors throughout the day
18–64 years	150 minutes of moderate to vigorous aerobic activity per week in bouts of 10 minutes or more Muscle- and bone-strengthening activities 2 days/week	N/A
65+ years	150 minutes of moderate to vigorous aerobic activity per week in bouts of 10 minutes or more Muscle- and bone-strengthening activities 2 days/week	N/A

equity rather than increasing the health gap between the best-off and worse-off in our societies. Some examples of policies that have proven effective include:

- Restricting the marketing of unhealthy foods to children (e.g., in Quebec)
- Regulating how much sugar, salt, and trans fats are added to commercial food products
- Implementing easy to read and understand nutrition labelling
- Banning vending machines containing unhealthy foods in schools and hospitals (Kaczorowski et al., 2016).

Health Canada's Healthy Eating Strategy includes some of these strategies, as well as the following additional policies:

- Introducing front-of-package (FOP) labelling: FOP labelling uses clear symbols to more quickly identify (without having to look at detailed nutritional

information on the back of a food product) whether a food is high in fat, sugar, or salt, for example.
- Banning the addition of artificially produced trans fats in foods by manufacturers: Trans fats are used to extend the shelf life of food and add extra flavour. They are mostly present in baked goods and are a strong contributor to NCDs such as heart disease (Health Canada 2018).

Examples of how two different jurisdictions have regulated the consumption of healthier options are presented in the News boxes.

It is now becoming widely accepted that the prevention and control of chronic diseases requires multilevel and comprehensive approaches (Canadian Best Practices Portal, 2016). As a result, there has been a growing movement in Canada to develop a single, coordinated strategy to address the common risk factors shared by multiple chronic diseases.

⊕ IN THE NEWS

Montreal Takes Action on Sugar-Sweetened Beverages

The consumption of sugar-sweetened beverages (SSBs)—which include drinks such as soda, fruit drinks, sports drinks, tea and coffee drinks, energy drinks, and any other beverage where sugar is added—has increased in Canada. SSBs are thought to account for nearly 8% of the daily caloric intake of Canadian adolescents. Furthermore, SSB consumption is linked to the development of obesity in children and adults (Dietitians of Canada, 2016).

In December 2017, in a landmark move, city officials in Montreal passed a motion to ban the sale of SSBs in all municipal buildings, including libraries and arenas. The same motion also calls on the federal government to introduce a tax on SSBs, a move that many public health officials have been requesting for a long time, given the benefits of taxation on curbing the intake of other harmful substances such as tobacco and alcohol (Canadian Press, 2017).

⊕ IN THE NEWS

Banning Energy Drinks in the Arctic

Energy drinks claim to boost energy, decrease fatigue, and enhance concentration. They are sold in Canada with caffeine from either pure or synthetic caffeine or herbal ingredients, such as guarana or yerba mate. Energy drinks may also be sweetened with various types of sugar, such as glucose–fructose or sucrose and amounts range between 1 g and 43 g per 237 mL/8oz serving (up to 10 teaspoons).

In 2016, the Hamlet of Aklavik in the Northwest Territories, a remote and isolated community, banned the sale of energy drinks in all municipal buildings. Instead of sugary drinks, the hamlet now stocks bottles of water at the community's recreational complex. "We feel that by providing healthy drinks, and letting our residents get more information on healthy living, we'll see positive results all around," said Fred Behrens, Aklavik's senior administrative advisor. After the ban, the hamlet challenged other communities to pass similar motions (Zelniker, 2016).

CRITICAL THINKING QUESTION 8.2: With many risk factors existing for NCDs (e.g., smoking, physical inactivity, and non-nutritious food consumption), we see a trend whereby people who have lower incomes bear a greater burden of exposure (e.g., their smoking rates are higher compared with higher income groups). Using the Social Determinants of Health framework(s) (presented in Chapter 5), discuss why this may be the case. What factors might explain why smoking is higher in low-income groups than in higher income groups?

SPECIFIC DISEASES

The top 10 leading causes of death (or mortality) in Canada in 2016 are depicted in Table 8.2. Table 8.3 shows the top 10 causes of disability (or morbidity). Note how many are caused by NCDs. In this section, we discuss a few of the more common NCDs contributing to morbidity and mortality in Canada and review major trends in their contribution to death and disability, risk factors for developing these conditions, and prevention strategies (primary, secondary, and tertiary prevention).

Heart Disease

Heart disease is a broad term that most often refers to a range of conditions that result from the buildup of plaque in the arteries of the heart, leading to reduced blood flow to this vital organ. Heart disease (also called *ischemic heart disease* or *coronary heart disease*) can result in myocardial infarction (i.e., a heart attack), angina (chest pain caused by a lack of blood flow to the heart) (PHAC, 2017a), heart failure (when the heart fails to adequately pump blood to the rest of the body), or issues with heart rhythm or heart valves.

Mortality and Morbidity

Nearly 8.5% of Canadians older than 20 years of age live with ischemic heart disease. Heart disease is the second leading cause of death in Canada and the leading cause of hospitalizations. Each year, more than 150, 000 Canadians are newly diagnosed with ischemic heart disease

TABLE 8.2   Top 10 Leading Causes of Death in Canada

Rank	Disease
1	Cancer (malignant neoplasms)
2	Heart disease (ischemic heart disease)
3	Cerebrovascular disease
4	Unintentional injuries
5	Chronic lower respiratory diseases
6	Diabetes
7	Alzheimer's disease
8	Influenza and pneumonia
9	Intentional self harm
10	Chronic liver disease

From Statistics Canada. (2018). Table 13-10-0394-01 Leading causes of death, total population, by age group. Retrieved from https://www150.statcan.gc.ca/t1/tbl1/en/tv.action?pid=1310039401

TABLE 8.3   Top 10 Leading Causes of Disability in Canada

Rank	Cause of Disability
1	Ischemic heart disease
2	Low back pain
3	Lung cancer
4	Diabetes
5	Stroke
6	Headache disorders
7	Chronic obstructive pulmonary disease (COPD)
8	Drug use disorders
9	Alzheimer's disease
10	Other musculoskeletal disorders

From Institute for Health Metrics and Evaluation. (2017). Canada. © University of Washington. Retrieved from http://www.healthdata.org/canada

(PHAC, 2017a). Heart failure has been estimated by the Heart and Stroke Foundation to cost the Canadian economy about $2.8 billion per year (Heart & Stroke Foundation, 2016). Over the past couple of decades, both the incidence of heart disease and the chance of dying because of heart disease have declined (PHAC, 2017b).

Risk Factors

The major risk factors for heart diseases can be divided into modifiable and nonmodifiable. Nonmodifiable risk factors include:

- Age: The risk of developing heart disease increases with age

- Sex: Risk of developing and dying from heart disease is greater in men compared with women, though this gap is slowly closing. Interestingly, women who have had a heart attack are 30% more likely to die than men who have had a heart attack (PHAC, 2017b).
- Family history: Having a first-degree relative with heart disease increases risk.

Modifiable factors include:
- Smoking
- Physical inactivity
- Poor diet
- Obesity
- The presence of diabetes
- High blood pressure
- High cholesterol levels
- Stress

It is estimated that 90% of adults older than 20 years of age have at least one of the aforementioned risk factors, and 40% have at least three or more risk factors (Health Canada, 2017).

A range of socially determined factors strongly influence the development of heart disease in the Canadian context. A recent publication in the *Canadian Journal of Cardiology* points to the increased risk of heart disease among vulnerable populations, which they define as those groups who are "socially or economically disadvantaged." They highlight the need to consider factors outside of the traditional ones listed above (e.g., income, racism, precarious employment status) and also think of the increased risk of heart disease in specific Canadian groups (i.e., among those who have low income and those who are nonwhite; specifically, higher rates of disease exist in Indigenous populations, as well as among South Asians) (Kandasamy & Anand, 2018).

EXERCISE 8.6: Why do you think women who have had a heart attack are more likely to die than men?

Prevention

In Chapters 1 and 3, the concept of health promotion, primary, secondary, and tertiary prevention is discussed. As a brief review, **primary prevention** refers to interventions that prevent new cases of disease from developing; **secondary prevention** refers to strategies that detect a disease in its very early stages to intervene quicker and therefore reduce the associated morbidity and mortality; and **tertiary prevention** refers to strategies that stop the advancement of an already well-established disease (University of Ottawa, 2015). Health promotion strategies (defined as the processes and actions that enable people to increase control over and improve their health through implementing healthy public policies and creating health supporting environments) are broader in nature compared to prevention strategies (because health promotion may also include primary prevention as well).

In the context of preventing heart disease, primary prevention strategies would include tackling some of the modifiable risk factors for heart disease. These might include smoking cessation for those that smoke, lowering blood pressure and cholesterol, losing weight (for people who are overweight or obese), eating a healthier diet, and exercising more. Refer to the Clinical Example box for a description of one of the landmark studies that identified key risk factors for heart disease.

 CLINICAL EXAMPLE

The Framingham Study and Risk of Heart Disease

In 1948, one of the most landmark studies in the area of heart disease began. The Framingham Heart Study followed a large cohort of people in the United States to study the effects of various factors in the development of heart disease (and is one of the reasons we are able to list the factors associated with heart disease today). Based on the results of this study, the Framingham Risk Score was developed in 1976 and is still widely used today by clinicians as a tool to estimate a client's risk of developing heart disease over the next 10 years. Using a points system, the tool helps estimate 10-year risk for developing heart disease based on the degree to which the following risk factors are present: sex, age, total cholesterol, high-density lipoprotein (a type of cholesterol), systolic blood pressure, whether or not one is treated for high blood pressure, and smoking status (Hermansson & Kahan, 2018). Using the risk score can help health care providers to identify those at high risk of heart disease and begin treating the relevant risk factors before the disease develops. It's a tool to help with primary prevention.

Secondary prevention strategies in the context of heart disease mean detecting heart disease early (because of manifestations such as angina) and aggressively controlling risk factors that prevent the development of a major event such as a heart attack. Examples of tertiary prevention are things such as surgery (coronary artery bypass grafting) or cardiac rehabilitation to reduce the risk of future heart attacks in those with established disease.

Although the medical community has gotten better at treating risk factors such as high blood pressure, high cholesterol, and diabetes, risk factors for heart disease remain rampant in the population. Health promotion interventions are what is needed to allow for communities of people to lead healthier lives, including being more physically active and eating better. Interventions such as supporting active transport, reducing the geographic density of fast food outlets, and suspending the marketing of unhealthy snacks to kids (as described earlier) can shift the distribution of risk factors and protective factors in a population.

Community-based interventions for CVD prevention have traditionally targeted educated, middle-class people who are already highly motivated to change their lives, mainly through the dissemination of messages about modifying lifestyle behaviour. However, these methods have been largely ineffective in reaching people who live in disadvantaged circumstances. Inadequate financial resources, limited education and illiteracy, unemployment or underemployment, and isolation make people less easy to reach through conventional health education methods, and their circumstances rarely provide enabling environments for behaviour change. Thus, policy level changes that enable supportive environments for all are the best way forward when it comes to closing the gap in heart disease between the advantaged and disadvantaged (see Chapter 3).

Cancer
Mortality and Morbidity
Cancer is the leading cause of death in Canada. Nearly one in two Canadians will develop cancer in their lifetime, and one in four will die from it. Excluding non-melanoma skin cancers (which are relatively common but do not cause significant morbidity or mortality), the most common cancers among Canadians are lung, breast, colorectal, and prostate cancers. In women, the most common cancer is breast cancer followed by lung

cancer and colorectal cancer. In men, the most common cancer is prostate cancer followed by lung cancer and colorectal cancer.

In general, the incidence rates of many cancers are on the decline, though the risk of developing some specific types of cancers seem to be increasing. More specifically, the incidences of melanoma, liver cancer, and thyroid cancer are increasing. In terms of cancer deaths, more than 25% are caused by lung cancer. The majority of cancer deaths occur among men and people aged 50 years or older. In general, the rates of death from cancers are declining for most cancers, with the exception of liver cancer and uterine cancer (in women) (PHAC, 2017c). An economic analysis estimated the direct cost of cancer care across Canada to be approximately $7.5 billion in 2012, a significant rise from the cost of $2.9 billion in 2005 billion (de Oliveira et al., 2018). The rise in costs mostly reflects the increasing cost of hospital-based care (vs outpatient, clinical care) and new therapies and advances that tend to be human resource intensive.

Risk Factors for Cancer

Similar to heart disease, there are some nonmodifiable factors that increase people's risk of cancer, including age. Additionally, although a few cancers may be associated with inherited genetic factors (e.g., some types of colorectal cancers and some forms of breast and ovarian cancers), behavioural and environmental factors are considered important determinants. Examples of these factors include alcohol consumption, diet, smoking, exposure to some infectious agents, and obesity (NIH, 2015).

EXERCISE 8.7: Although we often don't think of a communicable or infectious disease causing cancer, there are a few instances in which it does. Can you think of any examples in which infection with a particular pathogen (e.g., virus, bacteria, fungus) can cause cancer?

A study published by Cancer Care Ontario and Public Health Ontario emphasized the role that environmental exposures play in cancer development. According to the researchers, more than 90% of all cancers related to environmental exposures are the result of exposure to three main things: ultraviolet radiation, radon, and air pollution (more specifically, a pollutant known as $PM_{2.5}$) (Cancer Care Ontario & Ontario Agency for Health Protection and Promotion [Public Health Ontario], 2016). These are discussed in more detail in Chapter 11.

Workplace and environmental exposures to high concentrations of certain chemicals increase risks of some cancers. For example, inhalation of asbestos and chromium is associated with cancer of the lung, and benzidine and beta-naphthylamine is associated with bladder cancer. Occupational hazards are discussed further in Chapter 12.

Although the Canada-wide data shows that around 60% of people with a cancer diagnosis will live at least 5 years after the time at which they were diagnosed, mortality from cancer differs according to some important determinants of health, including Indigenous status. A landmark study published in 2016 studied more than 2 million people to compare cancer survival rates among Indigenous and non-Indigenous people in Canada. Being the first study of its kind to look at this information across Canada, the study's surprising results received significant media attention. It was found that for 14 of the 15 most common cancers, including cancer of the colon, rectum, lung, breast, oral cavity, and cervix, Indigenous people had lower survival rates compared with the general Canadian population, even when income level and geography (i.e., living in a rural, underserviced area) were accounted for (Withrow et al., 2016). The cancers with the most significant gap in survival between Indigenous people and other Canadians were prostate cancer and breast cancer. Some reasons the authors cited to explain this gap include discrimination faced by Indigenous people in the health system, leading to a delay in accessing care; Indigenous people having higher rates of other comorbid NCDs in addition to cancer (making the cancer harder to treat); and lower rates of cancer-related screening practices among Indigenous peoples and other Canadians (also partially a result of barriers accessing the health care system). It is important to keep in mind, however, that at the root of all these reasons (i.e., higher rates of comorbid NCDs, discrimination faced in the health care sector) is the colonial policies such as the *Indian Act* (described further in Chapter 7).

Prevention of Cancer

Similar to heart disease, primary prevention of many cancers includes tackling behavioural and environmental causes of cancer. For example, smoking cessation, reducing alcohol intake, practising safer sex, eating healthier, being more physically active, and protecting one's self from the sun are all primary prevention strategies.

In terms of secondary prevention, a host of accepted and evidence-based screening tools exist for various cancers. Table 8.4 lists the Canadian Task Force on Preventive Medicine's recommendations with respect to cancer screening.

Last, tertiary prevention in the context of cancer focuses on reducing some of the more major or life-threatening complications of cancer. Engaging in physiotherapy, using chemotherapy and radiation therapy techniques to shrink tumour size, and using supplementary medications to boost one's immune system after chemotherapy are all examples of tertiary prevention strategies.

> **EXERCISE 8.8:** Using the Population Health Promotion Model discussed in Chapter 3 as a guide, list some strategies that may prevent cancer while also addressing some of the structural determinants of health (e.g., income) and embodying principles of community development such as empowerment.

Chronic Respiratory Diseases

Common chronic respiratory diseases include asthma, chronic obstructive pulmonary disease (COPD), TB, emphysema, cystic fibrosis, lung cancer, and occupational lung disease. Although most chronic respiratory diseases are NCDs, a few are the result of communicable diseases (e.g., TB). This section focuses primarily on NCD related respiratory conditions. Two of the most common chronic lower respiratory diseases (meaning they affect the lower respiratory tract) are asthma and COPD.

Mortality and Morbidity Related to Lower Respiratory Disease

Lower respiratory diseases are the third leading cause of death in Canada (after cancer and heart disease), and chronic respiratory conditions (in general) are thought to be the third leading cause of hospitalizations. It is estimated that more than 3 million Canadians are living with a serious respiratory disease. Canada is seeing an increase in chronic respiratory diseases as the population ages. Between 2009 and 2011, death rates from respiratory diseases were 63.1 per 100, 000 population. COPD and asthma accounted for more than half of these deaths (Conference Board of Canada, 2015). In terms of economic burden, lung cancer, asthma, and COPD together cost the Canadian economy nearly $12 billion in 2010, $3.4 billion of which was a direct result of health care expenditures (Theriault et al., 2012).

Risk Factors for Chronic Respiratory Diseases

The two most important risk factors for chronic respiratory diseases are tobacco smoke (including exposure to ETS or secondhand smoke), as well as air

TABLE 8.4 Summary of the Canadian Task Force on Preventive Health Care's Recommendations for Cancer Screening

Cancer Type	Screening Test	Screening Eligibility	Screening Interval
Cervical	Pap test	Asymptomatic women with a cervix who are or have been sexually active and are currently between the ages of 25 and 69 years	Every 3 years
Breast	Mammogram	Asymptomatic women at average risk of breast cancer and between the ages of 50 and 74 years	Every 2–3 years
Lung	Low-dose CT scan	Asymptomatic adults not suspected to have lung cancer, between the ages of 55 and 74 years with at least a 30 pack-year smoking history who currently smoke or quit less than 15 years ago	Every year up to three consecutive times
Colorectal	FOBT or flexible sigmoidoscopy	Asymptomatic adults at average risk of colorectal cancer and between the ages of 50 and 74 years	FOBT every 2 years Flexible sigmoidoscopy every 10 years
Prostate	Prostate specific antigen	Recommended against	Recommended against

CT, Computed tomography; *FOBT*, Fecal occult blood testing.

pollution. Air pollution is described more in Chapter 11 and includes both indoor and outdoor air quality. Exposure to other environmental agents, such as asbestos, coal, and silicon, often occur in the workplace among certain occupations and are discussed more in Chapter 12.

Prevention of Respiratory Diseases

Primary prevention strategies for respiratory diseases include smoking cessation, ventilating workplaces that could expose workers to things such as asbestos, and encouraging the use of masks for workers working with chemicals or agents that cause chronic respiratory disease.

Secondary prevention strategies include screening for conditions such as lung cancer and COPD to detect them early in an attempt to improve outcomes for individual patients, and tertiary prevention strategies might include ensuring that people with established COPD are vaccinated (for influenza, for example, because they are at higher risk of contracting the flu and having significant complications as a result). Finally, better adherence to clinical management guidelines by both health care providers and patients for asthma is needed and will likely lead to reduced fatality, hospitalization, and health care utilization related to asthma.

> **EXERCISE 8.9:** Brainstorm three health promotion strategies to reduce the burden of chronic respiratory diseases.

Diabetes

Diabetes mellitus is a chronic condition that results from the body's inability to produce sufficient insulin or use it properly, leading to chronically high blood sugar levels. High blood sugar, if untreated, ends up affecting many parts of the body, including the heart, kidneys, eyes, nerves, and blood vessels. There are two types of diabetes: type 1, also known as insulin-dependent diabetes, with onset mainly in childhood or adolescence, and type 2, also known as non–insulin-dependent diabetes, which occurs primarily in the older population (typically after age 40 years). Type 2 diabetes is the most common, accounting for 90% to 95% of diagnosed cases of diabetes.

Mortality and Morbidity Resulting from Diabetes

In 2015, around 7% of the Canadian population older than 12 years of age was living with diabetes (Statistics Canada, 2017), and it is expected that by 2025, the prevalence will be closer to 12% (Diabetes Canada, n.d.). One in 10 deaths can be attributed to diabetes, and diabetes is a major risk factor for hospitalization. In fact, compared with the general Canadian population, people living with diabetes are three times more likely to be hospitalized for heart disease (Diabetes Canada, n.d.). The direct health care costs associated with diabetes totalled just over $2 billion in 2008 and are expected to rise to just over $3 billion by 2020 (Anja & Laura, 2017).

Risk Factors for Diabetes

Important risk factors for type 2 diabetes include the following:

- Age: Age of onset of diabetes typically occurs after 40.
- Genetics: There is an increased risk of diabetes in people who have a family history of diabetes
- Obesity
- Physical inactivity
- Poor diet
- Indigenous people (because of a history of colonial policies, discussed further in Chapter 7)
- Ethnicity has been accepted as an independent risk factor for type 2 diabetes. Certain ethnic groups such as Indigenous, African, Hispanic, and Asian have a higher rate of type 2 diabetes (Panagiotopoulos, Riddell, & Sellers, 2018).

Prevention of Diabetes

Prevention of type 2 diabetes takes three forms: primary, secondary, and tertiary prevention. Primary prevention of type 2 diabetes often focuses on weight loss and improving diet and physical activity.

Secondary prevention involves screening to identify diabetes in asymptomatic people. In 2012, the Canadian Task Force on Preventive Health Care did a thorough review of the evidence and recommended only screening asymptomatic individuals at high risk or very high risk of type 2 diabetes with a simple blood test. They recommended screening those at high risk every 3 to 5 years and those at very high risk every year, with the same blood test, called hemoglobin A1c (which measures average blood sugar level over the past 3 months). The idea behind screening, of course, is to detect and control diabetes early to prevent it from advancing (Canadian Task Force on Preventive Health Care, 2012).

Tertiary prevention tries to delay or prevent the complications of diabetes. Tight control of blood sugar and blood pressure levels has been shown to reduce many of the complications associated with diabetes, such as heart disease and stroke). In those with diabetes, the treatment of high blood pressure and high cholesterol also reduces risks of heart disease and stroke. For all people with diabetes, regular foot and eye examinations with early treatment can help to prevent limb amputations and progression of retinopathy of the eye.

Health promotion strategies for diabetes would include population-level interventions that facilitate healthy eating and active living in the community (e.g., creating bike lanes). Prevention of toxic stress by reducing the incidence of childhood traumatic events through parenting support programs or home visitation programs, for example, should also be considered among ways to action prevention.

Major Neurocognitive Disorder

Major neurocognitive disorder is the term used to describe what was previously known as dementia. It is an umbrella term that does not refer to a specific disease or condition but rather to a set of signs and symptoms, often including loss of memory and changes in mood, judgement, and communication, caused by a slow deterioration of cognitive functioning. Major neurocognitive disorder is caused by a number of different disease processes, the most common being Alzheimer's disease, Lewy body dementia, vascular dementia (which is caused by many of the same risk factors for stroke and heart disease), and frontotemporal dementia.

Mortality and Morbidity Resulting from Dementia

Dementia is a growing concern in Canada and currently affects around 7% of all adults older than 65 years of age. The prevalence of dementia has increased by 85% between 2002 and 2013. The incidence, however, has remained relatively stable with 76 000 new cases being diagnosed each year.

In terms of economic costs, a recent estimate by the National Population Health Study of Neurological Conditions projects that by 2031, health care costs associated with dementia will rise to $16.6 billion (CIHI, 2018c).

EXERCISE 8.10: How can one explain the fact that prevalence (or proportion of people living with dementia) is increasing while the incidence (number of new cases per year) is remaining stable?

Risk Factors for Dementia

The most important risk factor for dementia is advancing age. Women also seem to be more affected than men. Other risk factors include smoking, alcohol, high blood pressure, high cholesterol, physical inactivity, poor diet, diabetes, family history (particularly for early onset dementia), and depression (Alzheimer Society of Canada, 2018). Interestingly, some groups also suggest that low levels of education may be associated with dementia, although this relationship remains controversial. Although a number of studies have found the prevalence of dementia to be higher among those with lower education levels, other studies have contested this association. Some researchers believe that people with higher education levels may just be better at tests of cognition, but others suggest that people with higher education levels have alternative neural networks in their brain that allow them to cope with things such as brain injuries and other insults better, delaying the onset of dementia-like symptoms (Contador et al., 2017).

Prevention of Dementia

For some types of dementia, primary prevention includes smoking cessation, controlling blood pressure and cholesterol, eating healthier, and being more physically active. These measures can be supported by health promotion strategies such as ensuring road infrastructure that is conducive to walking and biking. Secondary prevention typically consists of practitioners using validated tools to screen for early cognitive decline and trying to slow down progression of the disease. Tertiary prevention includes strategies that help people living with dementia continue to function as independently as possible. Things such as exercise can help prevent falls and related complications.

Chronic Pain

Chronic pain is defined as pain that lasts several months. Similar to dementia, chronic pain is a symptom rather than a disease state and can be caused by a number of different disease entities, such as arthritis, disc herniations, and nerve damage caused by diabetes, to name a few. Taking a closer look at Table 8.2 demonstrates that chronic pain has links to many of the leading causes of morbidity. The most common types of chronic pain include chronic low back pain, migraine headaches, and arthritis (inflammation of the joints).

Fibromyalgia, a condition which causes widespread chronic pain along with fatigue, morning stiffness, and mental health issues such as depression, is being written about more and more (Andrade et al., 2017). It is a condition whose etiology is not yet well understood but remains a significant cause of disability in Canada. The case of fibromyalgia highlights how chronic pain often goes hand in hand with depression, anxiety, and substance abuse (as described more in Chapter 9).

Mortality and Morbidity Resulting from Chronic Pain

Around 9% of males and 12% of females report having chronic pain. The majority of people living with chronic pain (>60%) report that their pain limits their daily activities and functioning in almost all domains of life, including family life, social life, work life, and leisure. People with chronic pain also report greater rates of unemployment and higher rates of stress associated with work. They are also much more likely to access health care for a variety of different reasons, as well as report lower levels of life satisfaction (Statistics Canada, 2015). Recently, there has been much discussion about chronic pain leading to abuse of prescribed medicine such as oxycontin and illegal substances such as fentanyl analogues. The complexities that link chronic pain with the opioid epidemic are described in more detail in Chapter 9. Marijuana is also a substance used by many to deal with pain, including chronic pain (also discussed in Chapter 9).

Risk Factors for Chronic Pain

According to the Canadian Community Health Survey, the prevalence of chronic pain increases with age. The odds of women experiencing chronic pain are higher than men, and when comparing men and women with chronic pain, women tend to report more limitations in their activities of daily living than men. Interestingly, however, when the analysis accounted for the presence of a chronic disease, the odds of developing chronic pain were no different among men and women, suggesting that the reason women seem like they are at a greater risk for experiencing chronic pain is because they are more often diagnosed with NCDs that result in pain symptoms (Statistics Canada, 2015).

Prevention of Chronic Pain

Prevention of chronic pain depends on the specific cause of the pain, if one can be deciphered. However, addressing pain both when considering treatment strategies and prevention strategies requires one to understand how various psychosocial factors influence the extent of someone's pain. Pain is a very subjective experience, and for years, practitioners have struggled to explain why two individuals with the same disease process may have very different pain experiences. Many practitioners also fail to effectively address the needs of clients whose pain cannot be fully attributed to medically understood pathologies. Factors such as low mood, exposure to stress, adverse childhood experiences, trauma, coping techniques such as catastrophizing, and avoiding situations can influence the experience of chronic pain. In turn, chronic pain also tends to worsen mood, stress, and resiliency in the face of traumatic events—leading to a self-perpetuating cycle. Because the factors that put people at a higher risk of chronic pain are now becoming better understood, as are more effective ways to address these factors, it can be argued that working on mindfulness, cognitive behavioural therapy, and resiliency strategies, for example, may actually represent primary prevention (preventing the chronicity of pain), as well as secondary and tertiary prevention (preventing pain from interfering significantly with functioning) (Linton, Flink, & Vlaeyen, 2018). Supporting people with chronic pain to maintain activities such as employment (through various supports and accommodations) and prevent misuse and addiction to opioid painkillers can improve mood and coping, which in turn can have a positive effect on pain. In summary, although traditional prevention strategies (e.g., weight loss, exercise, healthy diets, smoking cessation) still apply to pain, chronic pain prevention and treatment require a holistic and multimodal approach.

CRITICAL THINKING QUESTION 8.3: Look up the Health Impact Pyramid. How do the five levels of the Health Impact Pyramid correspond and relate to the levels of prevention mentioned in this section (i.e., primary, secondary, and tertiary prevention)? If you were a health system planner who is worried about growing health care expenditures, which of these levels might you invest in to get the most value for your money?

INJURIES

Injuries are extremely common but can range significantly in terms of severity. For some injuries (e.g., a minor scrape), most people do not seek medical attention. For others (e.g., strains or fractures), however, people do seek attention, and some of these people will end up being permanently affected by such an injury (i.e., unable to function as they could before the injury). Finally, some types of injuries can result in significant damage, disability, and even death.

In general, injuries can be categorized as being intentional or unintentional. It is important, when conceptualizing and writing about injuries that one pays attention to terminology. Historically, **unintentional injuries** were used interchangeably with the word "accident." However, the term "accident" implies that it is a fluke chance when, in fact, many injuries Canada wide can very much be prevented.

Mortality and Morbidity Resulting from Injuries

Injuries are the leading cause of death for people between the ages of 1 and 34 years. In Canada, injuries account for around 6% of all deaths. Most deaths related to injuries are a result of suicide, transportation-related injuries (e.g., motor vehicle collisions), and falls.

In terms of morbidity, around 15% of Canadians older than 12 years of age sustain an injury that prevents them from being able to perform their day-to-day activities, and this proportion has risen over the past decade (Billette & Janz, 2015). The most common injuries among Canadians are sprains and strains, which account for just over half of all injuries, as well as fractures (broken bones), which account for nearly one in five injuries (Billette & Janz, 2015).

The economic burden of injuries is enormous. A report by Parachute Canada estimated that injuries cost the economy approximately $26 billion a year because of the number of deaths, hospitalizations, premature life lost, and resulting physical and psychosocial aftereffects of some injuries (Parachute, 2015). For a detailed example of how head injuries can result in year-long struggles with fatigue and other symptoms, see the Case Study box.

CASE STUDY

Concussions and Their Aftereffects

A concussion is a type of brain injury (for which you cannot see the impacts on radiographs or computed tomography scans) that most commonly happens because of sustaining a force to one's head. Concussions are often talked about in the context of contact sports, and in fact, almost 40% of children between the ages of 10 and 18 years who present to the emergency department (ED) because of a sports-related head injury are diagnosed with a concussion (Canadian Heritage, 2018). In Ontario, alone, it is estimated that around 80 000 people per year sustain a concussion (Stoddard, 2016). Although the symptoms of a concussion—including headaches, confusion, drowsiness, irritability, anxiety—may last for days to weeks, in some people, they can last much longer: for months or even up to a year or more. This latter situation is called postconcussion syndrome and may have devastating impacts on a person and family, including an inability to return to work or school for a long time. An Ontario-based study has estimated that around 20% of people with concussions experience postconcussion syndrome (Stoddard, 2016).

To take steps to reduce the risk of concussions, including the risk of further damage (or risk of a second injury) after a concussion, Ontario became the first province to pass a concussion law known as Rowan's Law in 2017. This law ensures that teachers and coaches are educated about recognizing and managing concussions, spells out a code of conduct for sports players to reduce the risk of concussion (e.g., strategies that encourage playing "less rough"), and enforces return to sports protocols that ensure that if a player is suspected of having a concussion, they are taken out of the game.

Risk Factors for Injuries

Age is an important risk factor for injury. People aged 12 to 19 years have the highest risk of injury, and this risk has risen over the past decade, especially among female adolescents. As mentioned earlier, injuries are the leading cause of death among children, accounting for a significant amount of PYLL. Men are more likely to sustain injuries than women. Other vulnerable populations include seniors, who are much more likely to be hospitalized and experience disability and complications after injuries (most commonly, falls), and Indigenous people, whose death rates from injuries exceed those of other Canadians.

> **EXERCISE 8.11:** What are some reasons to explain the higher mortality rate associated with injury among Indigenous people?

Prevention of Injuries

Prevention of injuries requires a multimodal approach. The Haddon matrix (Fig. 8.4), commonly used in injury prevention, is a useful framework that is similar to the epidemiological triangle discussed in Chapter 1. It conceptualizes unintentional injuries as resulting from interactions between host (person), agent or vector (e.g., a car), and environment. Within this framework, the environment consists of both the physical environment (e.g., the setting where an injury can or does take place, e.g., a roadway) as well as the socioeconomic environment (e.g., social norms and practices which can affect injury risk, such as how common alcohol consumption is). Interventions directed toward the host, agent, or environment may reduce the onset or extent of injury sustained (Runyan, 2015). Preventive injury interventions are organized in a two-dimensional matrix in which preinjury, time of impact, and postinjury preventive measures are considered in relation to the person, the agent causing the injury, or the environment.

In the preinjury phase, attention should be directed at eliminating the source of the injury, reducing exposure to it, or increasing the magnitude of resistance to it. Attention directed at the injury should reduce the magnitude and duration of exposure and decrease the host's susceptibility to injury. In the postinjury phase, the environment can be altered to reduce the source of the injury in the future and facilitate the rescue and resuscitation of victims in the short term.

Unintentional Injuries

The most common unintentional injuries causing death include transport-related injuries (which account for about 21% of injury deaths) and falls (which account for 18% of injury deaths).

Transport-Related Injuries

Although the number of traffic fatalities and serious injuries has declined over the past decade, they still represent a grave population-level health concern, particularly among young drivers, who are at the highest risk of being killed in motor vehicle collisions. When thinking of prevention strategies, one must be particularly mindful of protecting vulnerable road users (i.e., users who do not have physical protections if struck, including pedestrians and cyclists) as well as some of the emerging risk factors for harm related to transportation injuries, including:

- **Driving under the influence of drugs and alcohol:** Almost 40% of fatalities on the road involve alcohol consumption, and another one third of those who are tested in fatal collisions are found to have a drug on board. These drugs not only include illicit drugs but also prescribed drugs and over-the-counter medications that can make someone drowsy and affect their reaction time. (NOTE: Cannabis legalization has presented significant challenges with regard to the risk of injury on the road and, as such, law enforcement agencies are investing in better cannabis roadside testing and advocating for stricter laws when it comes to driving under the influence. Cannabis legalization is discussed further in Chapter 9.)
- **Distracted driving:** Distracted driving has received much attention over the past several years and is discussed in more detail in Chapter 5.
- **Driving when fatigued:** More and more attention is now being paid to the risks of driving when tired. It is estimated that nearly 20% of all fatal collisions are related to driver fatigue. Driving while fatigued is very common among the Canadian population—60% of drivers admit to driving while tired, and a shocking 15% of people admit to falling asleep while driving at least once during the past year (Transport Canada, 2011).

	Host	Agent	Environment	
			Physical	Social
Pre-event				
Event				
Post-event				

Fig. 8.4 The Haddon matrix. (Modified from Runyan, C. W. [2015]. Using the Haddon matrix: introducing the third dimension. *Injury Prevention, 21*(2), 126-130. https://doi.org/10.1136/ip.4.4.302.)

Prevention strategies must be context specific and consider the differences in traffic-related injuries in different parts of Canada. Traffic fatality rates are higher in the Yukon and Northwest Territories and lowest in Ontario (Transport Canada, 2011). Road infrastructure, access to emergency personnel, weather conditions, laws, regulations, and enforcement practices all help to account for the differences in fatalities in rural versus urban environments.

Primary prevention methods for transport-related injuries include environmental as well as individual measures. Evidence-based environmental methods include public education, improved vehicle and roadway design (e.g., separate and wide bike lanes as well as sidewalks to protect pedestrians and cyclists alike), speed controls, random breath testing for alcohol, decreasing public tolerance for drinking and driving, improved emergency response and trauma care, graduated licensing of new drivers, and other legislative and enforcement measures, such as banning use of cellular phones while driving (Ontario Injury Prevention Resource Centre, 2013). Secondary and tertiary prevention methods can include the use of seatbelts and airbags (to reduce the risk of bodily harm if a collision does occur), as well as timely access to emergency and critical medical services (if bodily harm occurs).

In December 2018, changes to the Criminal Code resulted in police officers across Canada having more authority with regard to asking drivers to provide a breath sample to detect alcohol levels in their body. Before this law came into effect, police officers needed to have grounds to be suspicious that a person was intoxicated before requesting that a breath test be provided. Now this requirement to have "reasonable suspicion" no longer exists. Although many believe this was a good move by the federal government to reduce impaired driving, others think it violates Charter rights (e.g., the right to be free from unreasonable search or seizure) and may result in a disproportionate number of people from racialized communities being stopped and asked to provide a breath sample (Swan, 2018).

EXERCISE 8.12: Apply the Haddon matrix to determine possible factors and strategies to prevent injury among bicyclists.

Falls

In 2016 and 2017, falls were the most common cause of injury in Canada. During that time period, 1800 people went to the ED, and just over 400 people were hospitalized each and every day as a result of a fall. Among seniors, falls are the leading cause of hospitalizations. Unintentional falls accounted for just over half of all injury-related ED visits in 2017. Falls that take place in a private home or dwelling are most common, and women present more often to the ED with fall injuries than men. Hip fracture is the most common type of injury resulting in hospitalization after a fall (CIHI, 2018d) and can cause significant distress for older adults, liming their mobility and predisposing them to complications such as pneumonia that increase the length of their hospital stay. Every year, it is estimated that between 20% and 30% of seniors sustain a fall (PHAC, 2014); like most injuries, falls are preventable.

Primary fall-prevention strategies targeted at seniors include:

- Equipping seniors with necessary assistive devices (e.g., cane, walker)
- Managing chronic diseases (e.g., optimizing medications to avoid side effects such as drowsiness, managing pain, controlling blood sugars)
- Educating seniors and caregivers about fall-prevention strategies
- Exercise programs to improve strength and balance
- Optimizing hearing and vision
- Taking appropriate amounts of vitamin D and calcium
- Improving the environment (ensuring adequate lighting, handrails in bathrooms)

Secondary prevention often includes screening and early treatment for osteoporosis (decreased bone density that often accompanies age and some NCDs) to prevent fall-related fractures. Last, tertiary prevention can include early mobilization after sustaining a hip fracture to prevent complications of being immobile, such as pneumonia and muscle wasting.

Intentional Injuries

Intentional injury includes suicide and self-harm (which are addressed in Chapter 9), and homicide.

Homicides

Over the past decade, the homicide rate in Canada has averaged around 1.7 per 100, 000 population. In 2016, for example, there were 611 homicide victims across the country. As a whole, however, the risk of homicide in Canada has been decreasing over the years, consistent with other countries like Australia, the United Kingdom, and the United States, though some urban centres such as Toronto have been experiencing higher levels of homicide than in the past (2018 was said to be the "deadliest year on record" for Toronto, according to news outlets) (Flanagan, 2018). Most homicide victims in Canada are young males. It seems that in recent years, gang-related homicides specifically, are on the rise. Of the 611 homicides in 2016, just over 200 of them involved firearms. Toronto, Edmonton, and Montreal had the highest proportions of firearm-related homicides among big cities in Canada. Indigenous people in Canada represented about one quarter of homicide victims, and the rate of homicide among Indigenous people is thought to be about six times higher than among non-Indigenous people in Canada (David, 2017; refer to Chapter 7 for more details on Missing and Murdered Indigenous Women and the role of intergenerational trauma and colonialism in explaining statistics such as these). The Indian Act is an important piece of legislation that set the stage for the inequities we see today regarding homicide in Indigenous versus non-Indigenous people (described further in Chapter 7).

It is well recognized that the majority of homicides are committed by someone that is known to the victim, such as a family member or intimate partner. In 2016, for example, 72 of the 611 homicides were a result of intimate partner violence.

Violence prevention is increasingly being recognized as a population health issue of importance by large credible organizations such as the Centers for Disease Control and Prevention and WHO, and community violence is discussed further in Chapter 18. Although violence can include self-harm and interpersonal violence (or harm to others) resulting in injury,

it also can refer to structural violence, which has been defined as social structures and ways of organizing societies such that some groups are inhibited from reaching their full potential—a social justice argument closely linked to the idea of health inequities described in Chapter 3. Preventing all forms of violence is a societal responsibility, with public health playing a part, particularly because of the role of both intentional and unintentional injuries in causing significant amounts of disease and death.

Interpersonal violence-prevention strategies include things such as the following:

- Gun control (which includes reducing access to firearms, ensuring owners of firearms are licensed, and ensuring background checks so those with a violent history are not permitted to own firearms)
- Limiting access to alcohol
- Accessible anger management programs
- Improved accessibility of mental health treatment
- Parenting skills
- Nurse home visitation programs
- Crisis teams
- Extended hours for after-school activities
- Promoting gender equality to reduce violence against women
- Changing social norms to reduce the acceptability of violence in our communities

> **CRITICAL THINKING QUESTION 8.4:** Consider the merits of calling violence a "public health problem." Should the health sector be a leader in the fight against gun violence, for example? Look up the concept of *health imperialism*. Keeping this notion of health imperialism in mind, what are the advantages and disadvantages of labelling an issue such as gun violence as a public health or health sector issue?

SUMMARY

This chapter surveyed the current approaches in disease prevention and health promotion in relation to major noncommunicable chronic diseases and injuries in Canada. NCDs are the cause of the major burdens of illness and death in Canada.

These illnesses are preventable, and hence there is increasing emphasis on the role of primary and secondary prevention. Many NCDs have substance abuse

(alcohol and tobacco), poor quality diet, and physical inactivity as major underlying causes.

Smoking is the number one preventable cause of death in Canada and is responsible for causing a significant proportion of heart disease, cancer, lung disease, and other diseases. There is strong evidence of an association between residential and workplace exposure to ETS, or secondhand smoke, and ill health. For children, exposure to ETS causes respiratory symptoms; middle ear disease; sudden infant death syndrome; and bronchitis, pneumonia, and other lower respiratory tract infections; it also impairs fetal growth, causing low birth weight and babies who are small for their gestational age, and it exacerbates asthma. In adults, ETS causes heart disease, lung cancer, and nasal sinus cancer and has also been linked to stroke, breast cancer, cervical cancer, and miscarriages.

There is good evidence that health care providers, can be effective in motivating people to quit smoking using brief interventions by incorporating smoking cessation messages that are repeated on multiple occasions and reinforced. Educational strategies, in conjunction with community- and media-based activities, can postpone or prevent smoking onset in adolescents. Regulation of advertising and promotion, particularly aimed at young people, is very likely to reduce both uptake and prevalence of smoking. Clean air regulations (i.e., smoking bans and restrictions) and restricting minors' access to tobacco contribute to changing social norms and may influence prevalence directly. The most effective intervention on tobacco control is raising the price.

Various diseases and injuries are associated with alcohol consumption, such as liver cirrhosis, suicide, breast cancer, upper respiratory and gastrointestinal tract cancers, and motor vehicle and other injuries. Physicians and primary health care providers are in a good position to quickly identify problem drinking and alcohol dependence using questionnaires such as CAGE. For treatment, good evidence exists for the effectiveness of brief intervention programs for those at an early stage of problem drinking. Effective health promotion programs in relation to substance abuse should be comprehensive, coordinated, and participatory. A comprehensive approach should focus on education, environmental controls, economic levers, and enforcement of legislation and regulations.

Diet, particularly excessive caloric intake and insufficient intake of fruits and vegetables, is a major factor in the development of many chronic diseases, including the two leading killers, CVD and cancer. Canada's Healthy Eating strategy aims to improve the nutrition of all Canadians using a regulatory approach (banning trans fats and introducing front of package labelling) and education-based approach (updating Canada's food guide).

Physical inactivity creates a significant population health burden in Canada. Risks of coronary artery disease, stroke, colon cancer, breast cancer, osteoporosis, and type 2 diabetes are all increased with physical inactivity. Physical activity is important in maintaining a healthy body weight and improving serum lipids and cholesterol and blood pressure. There is evidence that physical inactivity and body mass index exert independent effects on health. Canadian guidelines for physical activity have been developed across the lifespan.

The most common and burdensome NCDs in Canada include cancer, heart disease, lung disease, dementia, diabetes, and chronic pain. Risk factors for these conditions were described, as were various primary, secondary, and tertiary prevention strategies.

Injuries are the leading cause of death during the first half of the human lifespan. Injuries can be classified as unintentional or intentional and are avoidable. Some of the leading causes of injury include traffic-related injuries, falls (especially among seniors), suicide, and homicide.

Most injuries are the result of many complex factors, and therefore any effort to prevent and reduce the severity of injuries must involve multiple sectors, disciplines, jurisdictions, and approaches. Haddon's matrix is a useful framework for analyzing injuries and their prevention.

KEY WEBSITES

Cancer Care Ontario (CCO). https://www.cancercareontario.ca.
The CCO is the Ontario government's principal cancer advisor. The organization focuses on collecting and analyzing data about cancer services to share as guidelines for the health care community, as well as monitoring and measuring performance of the cancer care system. The CCO also oversees a funding and governance model in health care to ensure provider accountability and engages cancer patients and their families in the cancer care system. Follow the link to learn more about CCO and cancer care resources.

Canadian Cancer Society (CCS). http://www.cancer.ca.
As a national, community-based organization of volunteers, the CCS aims to eradicate cancer and enhance the quality of life for patients with cancer. The organization is committed to fundraising for research, educating people on risk factors for cancer, providing support services for cancer patients and their families, and advocating to governments on cancer-related issues.

Canadian Lung Association (CLA), https://www.lung.ca.

The CLA is a leading Canadian organization for promoting lung health as well as preventing and managing lung disease by funding vital research, pushing for improved treatments, smarter policies, or supporting patients in managing their health. Visit the link to learn more about the CLA's community of physicians, scientists, clinicians, educators, administrators, volunteers, and donors.

Canadian Task Force for Preventive Health Care (CTF-PHC). https://canadiantaskforce.ca.

Established by the Public Health Agency of Canada, the CTFPHC is composed of 15 primary care and prevention experts who develop clinical practice guidelines to support primary care providers in delivering preventive health care. The CTFPHC also targets community and public health professionals (public health nurses, nutritionists), physician specialists, other health care and allied health professionals, program developers, policy makers, and the Canadian public to connect them with research evidence, e-learning tools, and other resources. Follow the link to learn more about the CTFPHC and access resources on preventive health care.

Diabetes Canada. https://www.diabetes.ca.

Established by Dr. Charles Best in 1953, Diabetes Canada (formerly the Canadian Diabetes Association) was established to help Canadians combat the epidemic of diabetes. Today, Diabetes Canada provides a variety of educational resources, research evidence, community programs and support services.

Finding Balance. https://findingbalancealberta.ca.

Finding Balance is a pan Canadian fall prevention program, developed by Alberta's Injury Prevention Centre. It provides resources and information support to both seniors and health care providers in the area of falls prevention.

Heart and Stroke Foundation. http://www.heartandstroke.ca.

Did you know that since 1952, the Heart and Stroke Foundation has invested $1.52 billion dollars into research, funding more than 800 researchers? This organization has ambitious targets for fighting heart disease and stroke and focuses on new frameworks for disease prevention, transformative recovery strategies, and life-saving research. Follow the link to learn more and find out how to get involved.

Mothers Against Drunk Driving (MADD). https://madd.ca.

As a charitable, grassroot organization, MADD is dedicated to fight against impaired driving and support victims and survivors. MADD organizes a variety of aware-ness events and coordinates many victim and survivor services. Please visit the weblink to access information about impaired driving and learn about how to get involved with MADD.

Parachute Canada. http://www.parachutecanada.org.

Parachute is a national, charitable organization dedicated to preventing serious and fatal injuries by promoting research and evidence-based resources. The organization campaigns to support initiatives that help Canadians understand the effectiveness of injury prevention and adopt sound evidence-based measures. Click on the link to learn about injury-related topics and access e-learning tools as well as other knowledge translation resources.

REFERENCES

Aldrich, M. C., Hidalgo, B., Widome, R., et al. (2015). The role of epidemiology in evidence-based policy making: A case study of tobacco use in youth. *Annals of Epidemiology*, *25*(5), 360–365. https://doi.org/10.1016/j.annepidem.2014.03.005.

Alzheimer Society of Canada. (2018). *Risk factors*. Retrieved from http://alzheimer.ca/en/Home/About-dementia/Alzheimer-s-disease/Risk-factors.

Andrade, A., Steffens, R. D. A. K., Vilarino, G. T., et al. (2017). Does volume of physical exercise have an effect on depression in patients with fibromyalgia? *Journal of Affective Disorders*, *208*, 214–217. https://doi.org/10.1016/j.jad.2016.10.003.

Anja, B., & Laura, R. (2017). The cost of diabetes in Canada over 10 years: Applying attributable health care costs to a diabetes incidence prediction model. *Health Promotion and Chronic Disease Prevention in Canada: Research, Policy and Practice*, *37*(2), 49–53.

Bauman, A., Merom, D., Bull, F. C., et al. (2016). Updating the evidence for physical activity: Summative reviews of the epidemiological evidence, prevalence, and interventions to promote "active aging". *The Gerontologist*, *56*(Suppl. 2), S268–S280. https://doi.org/10.1093/geront/gnw031.

Billette, J., & Janz, T. (2015). *Injuries in Canada: Insights from the Canadian Community Health Survey*. Ottawa: Statistics Canada. Retrieved from https://www150.statcan.gc.ca/n1/pub/82-624-x/2011001/article/11506-eng.htm.

Bounajm, F., Dinh, T., & Thériault, L. (2014). *Moving ahead: The economic impact of reducing physical inactivity and sedentary behaviour*. Retrieved from http://sportmatters.ca/sites/default/files/content/moving_ahead_economic_impact_en.pdf.

Butt, P., Beirness, D., Gliksman, L., et al. (2011). *Alcohol and health in Canada: A summary of evidence and guidelines for low risk drinking*. Ottawa: Canadian Centre on Substance Abuse. Retrieved from http://www.ccdus.ca/Resource%20Library/2011-Summary-of-Evidence-and-Guidelines-for-Low-Risk%20Drinking-en.pdf.

Canadian Best Practices Portal. (2016). *Integrated approaches to chronic diseases*. Ottawa: Public Health Agency of Canada. Retrieved from http://cbpp-pcpe.phac-aspc.gc.ca/public-health-topics/integrated-approaches-to-chronic-diseases/.

Canadian Cancer Society. (2017). *Overview summary of Federal/Provincial/Territorial tobacco control legislation in Canada*. Retrieved from http://convio.cancer.ca/documents/Legislative_Overview-Tobacco_Control-F-P-T-2017-final.pdf.

Canadian Heritage. (2018). *Concussions in sport*. Ottawa: Government of Canada. Retrieved from https://www.canada.ca/en/canadian-heritage/services/concussions.html.

Canadian Institute for Health Information. (2017). *Alcohol harm in Canada: Examining hospitalizations entirely caused by alcohol and strategies to reduce alcohol harm*. Retrieved from https://www.cihi.ca/sites/default/files/document/report-alcohol-hospitalizations-en-web.pdf.

Canadian Institute for Health Information. (2018a). *Alcohol harm on the rise for Canadian women*. Retrieved from https://www.cihi.ca/en/alcohol-harm-on-the-rise-for-canadian-women.

Canadian Institute for Health Information. (2018b). *Alcohol harm on the rise for Canadian women*. Retrieved from https://www.cihi.ca/en/alcohol-harm-on-the-rise-for-canadian-women.

Canadian Institute for Health Information. (2018c). *How dementia impacts Canadians*. Retrieved from https://www.cihi.ca/en/dementia-in-canada/how-dementia-impacts-canadians.

Canadian Institute for Health Information. (2018d). *Watch your step! Falls are sending more Canadians to the hospital than ever before*. Retrieved from https://www.cihi.ca/en/watch-your-step-falls-are-sending-more-canadians-to-the-hospital-than-ever-before.

Canadian Press. (2017). *Montreal moves to ban sale of sugary drinks inside city buildings*. Retrieved from https://globalnews.ca/news/3914861/montreal-moves-to-ban-sale-of-sugary-drinks-inside-city-buildings/.

Canadian Task Force on Preventive Health Care. (2012). *Diabetes, type 2 (2012)*. Retrieved from https://canadiantaskforce.ca/guidelines/published-guidelines/type-2-diabetes/.

Cancer Care Ontario & Ontario Agency for Health Protection and Promotion (Public Health Ontario). (2016). *Environmental burden of cancer in Ontario*. Retrieved from https://www.publichealthontario.ca/en/eRepository/Environmental_Burden_of_Cancer_Technical_2016.pdf.

Center on the Developing Child, & Harvard University. (n.d.). Tackling toxic stress. Retrieved from https://developingchild.harvard.edu/science/key-concepts/toxic-stress/tackling-toxic-stress/.

Conference Board of Canada. (2015). *Mortality due to respiratory diseases*. Retrieved from https://www.conferenceboard.ca/hcp/provincial/health/resp.aspx.

Contador, I., del Ser, T., Llamas, S., et al. (2017). Impact of literacy and years of education on the diagnosis of dementia: A population-based study. *Journal of Clinical and Experimental Neuropsychology, 39*(2), 112–119. https://doi.org/10.1080/13803395.2016.1204992.

Cook, B., & Abreu, J. (1998). Alcohol-related health problems. In R. Wallace (Ed.), *Maxey-Rosenau-Last Public Health and Preventive Medicine* (14th ed.) (pp. 847–860). Stamford, CT: Appleton & Lange.

David, J. (2017). *Homicide in Canada, 2016*. Ottawa: Statistics Canada. Retrieved from https://www150.statcan.gc.ca/n1/pub/85-002-x/2017001/article/54879-eng.htm.

Davoren, M. P., Demant, J., Shiely, F., et al. (2016). Alcohol consumption among university students in Ireland and the United Kingdom from 2002 to 2014: a systematic review. *BMC Public Health, 16*(1), 173. https://doi.org/10.1186/s12889-016-2843-1.

de Oliveira, C., Weir, S., Rangrej, J., et al. (2018). The economic burden of cancer care in Canada: A population-based cost study. *CMAJ Open, 6*(1), E1–E10. https://doi.org/10.9778/cmajo.20170144.

Diabetes Canada. (n.d.). Diabetes statistics in Canada. Retrieved from https://www.diabetes.ca/how-you-can-help/advocate/why-federal-leadership-is-essential/diabetes-statistics-in-canada.

Dietitians of Canada. (2016). *Taxation and sugar-sweetened beverages: Position of dietitians of Canada*. Retrieved from https://www.dietitians.ca/Downloads/Public/DC-Position-SSBs-and-taxation.aspx.

Dir, A. L., Gilmore, A. K., Moreland, A. D., et al. (2018). What's the harm? Alcohol and marijuana use and perceived risks of unprotected sex among adolescents and young adults. *Addictive Behaviors, 76*, 281–284. https://doi.org/10.1016/j.addbeh.2017.08.035.

Dobrescu, A., Bhandari, A., Sutherland, G., et al. (2017). *The costs of tobacco use in Canada, 2012*. Retrieved from https://www.conferenceboard.ca/e-library/abstract.aspx?did=9185.

Ewing, J. A. (1984). Detecting alcoholism: The CAGE questionnaire. *Journal of American Medical Association, 252*(14), 1905–1907.

Flanagan, R. (2018). *Toronto breaks annual homicide record, on pace to exceed 100 in 2018*. CTV News. Retrieved from https://www.ctvnews.ca/canada/toronto-breaks-annual-homicide-record-on-pace-to-exceed-100-in-2018-1.4182828.

Frohlich, K. L., Poland, B., Mykhalovskiy, E., et al. (2010). Tobacco control and the inequitable socio-economic distribution of smoking: Smokers' discourses and implications for tobacco control. *Critical Public Health*, *20*(1), 35–46.

Glasser, A. M., Katz, L., Pearson, J. L., et al. (2017). Overview of electronic nicotine delivery systems: A systematic review. *American Journal of Preventive Medicine*, *52*(2), e33–e66. https://doi.org/10.1016/j.amepre.2016.10.036.

Government of Canada. (2018a). *Revision process for Canada's Food Guide*. Retrieved from https://www.canada.ca/en/health-canada/services/canada-food-guides/revision-process.html.

Government of Canada. (2018b). *Vaping products*. Retrieved from https://www.canada.ca/en/health-canada/news/2018/05/backgrounder-vaping-products.html.

Government of Canada. (2018c). *How Nutrition North Canada works*. Retrieved from https://www.nutritionnorthcanada.gc.ca/eng/1415538638170/1415538670874.

Government of Canada. (2019). *Canada's Food Guide resources*. Retrieved from https://www.canada.ca/en/health-canada/services/canada-food-guide/resources/resources-download.html.

Government of Manitoba. (n.d.). *Healthy Child Manitoba – Families First*. Retrieved from https://www.gov.mb.ca/healthychild/familiesfirst/index.html.

Government of Ontario. (2014). *Smoke-free Ontario*. Retrieved from https://www.ontario.ca/page/smoke-free-ontario.

Hawkins, S. S., Bach, N., & Baum, C. F. (2016). Impact of tobacco control policies on adolescent smoking. *Journal of Adolescent Health*, *58*(6), 679–685. https://doi.org/10.1016/j.jadohealth.2016.02.014.

Health Canada. (2015). *Dangers of second-hand smoke*. Retrieved from https://www.canada.ca/en/health-canada/services/smoking-tobacco/avoid-second-hand-smoke/second-hand-smoke/dangers-second-hand-smoke.html.

Health Canada. (2017). *Heart disease—heart health*. Retrieved from https://www.canada.ca/en/public-health/services/diseases/heart-disease-heart-health.html.

Health Canada. (2018). *Health Canada's healthy eating strategy*. Retrieved from https://www.canada.ca/en/services/health/campaigns/vision-healthy-canada/healthy-eating.html.

Healthdata.org. (2019). *Top 10 causes of years of life lost (YLLs) in 2017 and percent change, 2007-2017, all ages, number*. Retrieved from http://www.healthdata.org/canada.

Heart & Stroke Foundation. (2016). *2016 report on the health of Canadians*. Retrieved from https://www.heartandstroke.ca/-/media/pdf-files/canada/2017-heart-month/heartandstroke-reportonhealth-2016.ashx?la=en&hash=0478377DB7CF08A281E0D94B22BED6CD093C76DB.

Hermansson, J., & Kahan, T. (2018). Systematic review of validity assessments of Framingham risk score results in health economic modelling of lipid-modifying therapies in Europe. *Pharmacoeconomics*, *36*(2), 205–213. Retrieved from https://doi.org/10.1007/s40273-017-0578-1.

Hung, W. W., Ross, J. S., Boockvar, K. S., & Siu, A. L. (2012). Association of chronic diseases and impairments with disability in older adults: A decade of change? *Med Care*, *50*(6), 501–507.

Hyseni, L., Atkinson, M., Bromley, H., et al. (2017). The effects of policy actions to improve population dietary patterns and prevent diet-related non-communicable diseases: Scoping review. *European Journal of Clinical Nutrition*, *71*(6), 694.

Johnson, K. C. (2010). Environmental tobacco smoke (ETS). *Chronic Diseases in Canada*, *29*(2). Retrieved from https://www.canada.ca/en/public-health/services/reports-publications/health-promotion-chronic-disease-prevention-canada-research-policy-practice/vol-29-no-2-2009/supplement/environmental-tobacco-smoke.html.

Kaczorowski, J., Campbell, N. R. C., Duhaney, T., et al. (2016). Reducing deaths by diet: Call to action for a public policy agenda for chronic disease prevention. *Canadian Family Physician*, *62*(6), 469–470.

Kandasamy, S., & Anand, S. S. (2018). Cardiovascular disease among women from vulnerable populations: A review. *Canadian Journal of Cardiology*, *34*(4), 450–457. https://doi.org/10.1016/j.cjca.2018.01.017.

Krishnaswamy, K. (2016). Diet and nutrition in the prevention of non-communicable diseases. *Proceedings of the Indian National Science Academy*, *82*(5), 1477–1494.

Lavery, A. M., Nair, U., Bass, S. B., et al. (2016). The influence of health messaging source and frequency on maternal smoking and child exposure among low-income mothers. *Journal of Communication in Healthcare*, *9*(3), 200–209. https://doi.org/10.1080/17538068.2016.1231858.

Lebel, A., Noreau, D., Tremblay, L., et al. (2016). Identifying rural food deserts: Methodological considerations for food environment interventions. *Canadian Journal of Public Health*, *1*(107), S21–eS26.

Lieffers, J. R. L., Ekwaru, J. P., Ohinmaa, A., et al. (2018). The economic burden of not meeting food recommendations in Canada: The cost of doing nothing. *PLoS One, 13*(4), e0196333. https://doi.org/10.1371/journal.pone.0196333.

Linton, S. J., Flink, I. K., & Vlaeyen, J. W. (2018). Understanding the etiology of chronic pain from a psychological perspective. *Physical Therapy, 98*(5), 315–324. https://doi.org/10.1093/ptj/pzy027.

Lung Cancer Canada. (n.d.). Lung cancer. Retrieved from http://www.lungcancercanada.ca/Lung-Cancer.aspx.

Manuel, D. G., Perez, R., Sanmartin, C., et al. (2016). Measuring burden of unhealthy behaviours using a multivariable predictive approach: Life expectancy lost in Canada attributable to smoking, alcohol, physical inactivity, and diet. *PLoS Med, 13*(8), e1002082. https://doi.org/10.1371/journal.pmed.1002082.

Mayo Clinic. (2018). *Alcohol poisoning.* Retrieved from https://www.mayoclinic.org/diseases-conditions/alcohol-poisoning/symptoms-causes/syc-20354386.

National Institute of Health. (2015). *Risk factors for cancer.* Retrieved from https://www.cancer.gov/about-cancer/causes-prevention/risk.

National Institute of Health. (2017). *Harms of cigarette smoking and health benefits of quitting.* Retrieved from https://www.cancer.gov/about-cancer/causes-prevention/risk/tobacco/cessation-fact-sheet.

New South Wales Department of Health. (2008). *NSW Health Drug and Alcohol Psychosocial Interventions Professional Practice Guidelines.* Retrieved from https://www1.health.nsw.gov.au/pds/ActivePDSDocuments/GL2008_009.pdf.

Nuyts, P. A., Kuijpers, T. G., Willemsen, M. C., & Kunst, A. E. (2018). How can a ban on tobacco sales to minors be effective in changing smoking behaviour among youth?—A realist review. *Preventive Medicine, 115*, 61–67. https://doi.org/10.1016/j.ypmed.2018.08.013.

Olstad, D. L., Campbell, N. R., & Raine, K. D. (2019). Diet quality in Canada: Policy solutions for equity. *CMAJ, 191*(4), E100–E102.

Ontario Injury Prevention Resource Centre. (2013). *Ontario Regional Injury Data Report, Evidence-informed practice recommendations.* Retrieved from http://www.oninjuryresources.ca/downloads/publications/FINAL_ORIDR-EIPR.pdf.

Panagiotopoulos, C., Riddell, M. C., Sellers, E. A. C., & [Diabetes Canada Clinical Practice Guidelines Expert Committee] (2018). 2018 Clinical Practice Guidelines, Type 2 diabetes in children and adolescents. *Canadian Journal of Diabetes, 42*(suppl), S247–S254. https://doi.org/10.1016/j.jcjd.2017.10.037.

Park, E., Kulbok, P. A., Keim-Malpass, J., et al. (2017). Adolescent smoking prevention: Feasibility and effect of participatory video production. *Journal of Pediatric Nursing, 36*, 197–204.

Parachute. (2015). *About injuries.* Retrieved from http://www.parachutecanada.org/injury-topics.

Patel, A., Pathak, Y., Patel, J., & Sutariya, V. (2018). Role of nutritional factors in pathogenesis of cancer. *Food Quality and Safety, 2*(1), 27–36. https://doi.org/10.1093/fqsafe/fyx033.

Patterson, R., McNamara, E., Tainio, M., et al. (2018). Sedentary behaviour and risk of all-cause, cardiovascular and cancer mortality, and incident type 2 diabetes: A systematic review and dose response meta-analysis. *European Journal of Epidemiology, 33*(9), 811–829. https://doi.org/10.1007/s10654-018-0380-1.

Pisinger, C., & Døssing, M. (2014). A systematic review of health effects of electronic cigarettes. *Preventive Medicine, 69*, 248–260. https://doi.org/10.1016/j.ypmed.2014.10.009.

Public Health Agency of Canada. (2014). *Seniors' falls in Canada, second report.* Retrieved from https://www.canada.ca/en/public-health/services/health-promotion/aging-seniors/publications/publications-general-public/seniors-falls-canada-second-report.html.

Public Health Agency of Canada. (2016). *Alcohol consumption in Canada, The Chief Public Health Officer's Report on the State of Public Health in Canada 2015.* Retrieved from https://www.canada.ca/content/dam/canada/health-canada/migration/healthy-canadians/publications/department-ministere/state-public-health-alcohol-2015-etat-sante-publique-alcool/alt/state-phac-alcohol-2015-etat-aspc-alcool-eng.pdf.

Public Health Agency of Canada. (2017a). *Heart disease in Canada: Highlights from the Canadian Chronic Disease Surveillance System.* Retrieved from https://www.canada.ca/en/public-health/services/publications/diseases-conditions/heart-disease-canada-fact-sheet.html.

Public Health Agency of Canada. (2017b). *Heart disease in Canada.* Retrieved from https://www.canada.ca/en/public-health/services/publications/diseases-conditions/heart-disease-canada.html.

Public Health Agency of Canada. (2017c). *Canadian cancer statistics, overview.* Retrieved from https://www.canada.ca/en/public-health/services/chronic-diseases/cancer/canadian-cancer-statistics.html.

Rebar, A. L., Stanton, R., Geard, D., et al. (2015). A meta-meta-analysis of the effect of physical activity on depression and anxiety in non-clinical adult populations. *Health Psychology Review, 9*(3), 366–378. https://doi.org/10.1080/17437199.2015.1022901.

Roberts, M. E., Peters, E., Ferketich, A. K., et al. (2016). The age-related positivity effect and tobacco warning labels. *Tobacco Regulatory Science, 2*(2), 176–185. https://doi.org/10.18001/TRS.2.2.8.

The Role of Health Professionals in Tobacco Cessation [Joint Position Statement]. (2011). Retrieved from https://www.cma.ca/Assets/assets-library/document/en/advocacy/policy-research/CMA_Policy_Joint_Position_Statement_The_Role_of_Health_Professionals_in_Tobacco_Cessation_PD11-08-e.pdf.

Runyan, C. W. (2015). Using the Haddon matrix: Introducing the third dimension. *Injury Prevention, 21*(2), 126–130. https://doi.org/10.1136/ip.4.4.302.

Savedoff, W., & Alwang, A. (2015). *The single best health policy in the world: Tobacco taxes.* CGD Policy Paper 062 Washington DC: Center for Global Development. Retrieved from https://www.cgdev.org/sites/default/files/CGD-Policy-Paper-62-Savedoff-Alwang-Best-Health-Policy-Tobacco-Tax.pdf.

Shang, C., Huang, J., Li, Q., & Chaloupka, F. J. (2015). The association between point-of-sale advertising bans and youth experimental smoking: Findings from the Global Youth Tobacco Survey (GYTS). *AIMS Public Health, 2*(4), 832–843. https://doi.org/10.3934/publichealth.2015.4.832.

Shilton, T., & Robertson, G. (2018). Beating non-communicable diseases equitably—let's get serious. *Global Health Promotion, 25*(3), 3–5.

Sommer, I., Griebler, U., Mahlknecht, P., et al. (2015). Socio-economic inequalities in non-communicable diseases and their risk factors: An overview of systematic reviews. *BMC Public Health, 15*, 914.

Statistics Canada. (2015). *Chronic pain at ages 12 to 44: Findings.* Retrieved from https://www150.statcan.gc.ca/n1/pub/82-003-x/2010004/article/11389/findings-resultats-eng.htm.

Statistics Canada. (2017). *Health Fact Sheets, Diabetes, 2015.* Retrieved from https://www150.statcan.gc.ca/n1/pub/82-625-x/2017001/article/14763-eng.htm.

Statistics Canada. (2018). *Table 13-10-0096-04: Perceived life stress, by age group.* Retrieved from https://www150.statcan.gc.ca/t1/tbl1/en/tv.action?pid=1310009604.

Stoddard, D. W. (2016). *Post-concussion syndrome: Management for adults.* Retrieved from https://www.semisportmed.com/blog/post-concussion-syndrome--management-for-adults.

Swan, K. (2018). *"Most drivers" stopped by police will likely be tested for drunk driving: RCMP.* CBC News. Retrieved from https://www.cbc.ca/news/canada/nova-scotia/mandatory-alcohol-screening-nova-scotia-legislation-change-1.4949061.

Theriault, L., Hermus, G., Goldfarb, D., et al. (2012). *Cost risk analysis for chronic lung disease in Canada.* Retrieved from https://www.conferenceboard.ca/e-library/abstract.aspx?did=4585.

Toma, A., Paré, G., & Leong, D. P. (2017). Alcohol and cardiovascular disease: How much is too much? *Current Atherosclerosis Reports, 19*(3), 13. https://doi.org/10.1007/s11883-017-0647-0.

Transport Canada. (2011). *Road safety in Canada.* Ottawa: Author. Retrieved from http://www.tc.gc.ca/eng/motorvehiclesafety/tp-tp15145-1201.htm#s34.

University of Ottawa. (2015). *Categories of prevention.* Retrieved from http://www.medicine.uottawa.ca/sim/data/Prevention_e.htm.

Valenzuela, R., Das, U. N., Videla, L. A., et al. (2018). Nutrients and diet: A relationship between oxidative stress, aging, obesity, and related noncommunicable diseases. *Oxidative Medicine and Cellular Longevity, 2018*, 7460453. http://downloads.hindawi.com/journals/special-issues/920895.pdf.

Withrow, D. R., Pole, J. D., Nishri, E. D., et al. (2016). Cancer survival disparities between First Nation and non-aboriginal adults in Canada: Follow-up of the 1991 census mortality cohort. *Cancer Epidemiology and Prevention Biomarkers, 26*(1), 145–151. https://doi.org/10.1158/1055-9965.EPI-16-0706.

World Health Organization. (2003). *WHO framework convention on tobacco control.* Geneva: World Health Organization.

World Health Organization. (2016). *NCD mortality and morbidity.* Retrieved from http://www.who.int/gho/ncd/mortality_morbidity/en/.

Zelniker, R. (2016). *N.W.T. community moves ahead with energy drink ban.* CBC News. Retrieved from https://www.cbc.ca/news/canada/north/aklavik-energy-drink-ban-1.3772624.

Mental Health and Substance Use

LEARNING OBJECTIVES

- Define *mental health, mental illness,* and *mental health promotion* and differentiate among them.
- Describe the impact of stigma on people with mental health and substance use disorders.
- Summarize the epidemiology of common mental illnesses and substance use disorders.
- Discuss the burden of mental health (in terms of stigma, caregiver burden, and economic costs) and

substance use disorders (in terms of death, disease, social harm, and monetary costs).
- Recognize common risk factors for the development of mental illness and substance use disorders.
- Classify interventions to address mental illness and substance use disorders according to individual-level versus population-level action.

CHAPTER OUTLINE

KEY TERMS

adverse childhood experiences (ACEs)
decriminalization
Diagnostic and Statistical Manual of Mental Disorders (DSM)
harm reduction
Icelandic model

legalization
mental health
mental health promotion
mental illness
opioids
positive mental health
positive psychology

prohibition
recovery-oriented approaches
stigma
stimulant
stress
trauma- and violence-informed approaches (TVIAs)

INTRODUCTION

In Chapter 8, we explored many different aspects of noncommunicable diseases (NCDs) and NCD control. Some of the most significant NCDs that face the Canadian population today are mental health conditions such as depression, anxiety, and substance use disorders, to name a few. This chapter introduces readers to what is meant by mental health and mental health promotion, describes the risk factors and burden of various mental health conditions on the population (including substance use disorders), and discusses strategies to reduce the burden and severity of mental health challenges and promote positive mental health. Mental health and addictions services are discussed in Chapter 16.

Some Key Terminology

Mental health is as important to daily living as physical health and is a key determinant of overall health. **Mental health** is defined by the World Health Organization (WHO) as "a state of well-being in which every individual realizes his or her own potential, can cope with the normal stresses of life, can work productively and fruitfully, and is able to make a contribution to her or his community" (WHO, 2014). As you can see, mental health is a positive and holistic concept, similar to the WHO's definition of overall health. Mental health is not merely the absence of mental health ailments; it is possible for someone to have a mental health condition but still experience positive mental health (Canadian Mental Health Association [CMHA], 2018a).

Mental illness, on the other hand, refers to specific ailments that affect thinking, mood, or behaviour and are associated with significant distress and impaired functioning (Government of Canada, 2015). Examples of mental illness include schizophrenia, generalized anxiety disorder, bipolar disorder, and substance use disorder. The *Diagnostic and Statistical Manual of Mental Disorders (DSM)* is a guide that provides a classification of different mental illnesses to support health care professionals in the diagnosis of these illnesses. The DSM contains a description of various conditions, including their signs and symptoms and criteria for how to diagnose them. It is used in most countries around the world, and the most current version is the *DSM-5* (i.e., 5th edition), which was published in 2013 (American Psychiatric Association, 2018).

It is important to reflect on language surrounding discussions about mental health. A number of different terms are used in mental health. The terms *mental health client* and *mental health patient* are often used interchangeably. Generally speaking, whereas *client* often refers to individuals who are being seen in the community, *patient* indicates that the individual is being cared for in the hospital. However, the connotations around these words "patient" and "client," such as not having choices (patient) and having choices (client), can influence care. New concepts arose, such as *mental health consumer* or *mental health survivor*, from individuals who had suffered and endured inhumane treatment while hospitalized. Historically, individuals who were diagnosed with a mental illness were stripped of their rights and institutionalized, sometimes for their entire lives. The resistance to being labelled mentally ill for a lifetime gained momentum; as a result, the idea that recovery was possible took root, and recovery-oriented models of care (discussed later) grew across North America and Europe. As discussed in Chapter 6, labelling individuals as their disease also occurs frequently in mental health, such as the schizophrenic patient or client or "the schizophrenic." The *DSM-5* is a helpful tool for clinicians, and it may also provide relief to an individual when they have a diagnosis so that treatment can begin; however, a diagnosis can also have negative consequences. The person can experience a loss of identity if labelled as "schizophrenic" and can experience stigma related to their mental illness. Additionally, the terms "addiction," "abuse," and "dependence" are often used to refer to people with substance use disorders. However, these terms are often used judgementally. Health care providers and researchers now prefer to use the more comprehensive and less negative term "substance use disorder."

Avoiding such labels as "schizophrenic," "injection drug user," and "addict" and understanding that individuals are not a disease but a person with a mental illness (PMI) or person who injects drugs, is necessary to avoid stigmatization (discussed later), to support recovery-oriented models of care, and to improve the mental health system.

The Link Between Mental Health and Substance Use

This chapter speaks about various types of mental health conditions, including substance use disorders, and separates the discussion relating to substance use disorder

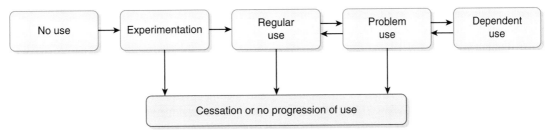

Fig. 9.1 The spectrum of substance use. (From Bonomo, Y., & Proimos, J. [2005]. Substance misuse: Alcohol, tobacco, inhalants, and other drugs. *BMJ, 330,* 777.)

where possible because it is at times a mental illness but can also be a risk factor for other mental illnesses. Although substance use disorders share many of the same characteristics and risk factors as other mental illnesses, such as depression and bipolar disorder, they are also distinct in other ways and represent an emerging issue of concern in Canada.

Although the use of substances among the Canadian population is quite common and not considered a mental illness, the *DSM-5* has "substance use disorder" in its list of mental illnesses. This category refers to a range of illnesses, based on the type of substance consumed (e.g., alcohol use disorder, opioid use disorder), all of which are categorized by similar criteria (Substance Abuse and Mental Health Services Administration [SAMSHA], 2015). Substance use disorders can range from mild to severe, but all are characterized as causing significant distress and impaired functioning. It is important to keep in mind that not everyone who uses substances has a substance use disorder. There exists a continuum of substance use (Fig. 9.1), from not using at all, to experimental use only, to occasional social use, to regular use as prescribed, to problematic use (when the substance begins to interfere with health or social and occupational responsibilities), to substance use disorders (as described earlier) (City of Toronto, n.d.).

Additionally, substance use disorder and mental illness can exist within the same person and at the same time—this is known as a *concurrent disorder.* Co-occurrence of mental illness and substance use has been associated with poor outcomes, including HIV infection, unemployment, homelessness, incarceration, and violence (Bobrowski, 2018). Historically, in Canada, there had been a separation between mental health and substance use services, which led to individuals being passed from one specialized clinician to another without information-sharing between clinicians, or service

coordination. However, during the past decade, there has been more effort across Canada to integrate the two sectors, with varying levels of collaboration.

We must be mindful of the language used to describe people experiencing substance use disorders. There has been some debate in the literature about the best term to use to describe people who experience problematic use and substance use disorders. The term "misuse" is also used; however, this term may have a negative connotation (because it is *mis*use) and does not clearly identify the fact that problematic substance use is not simply the result of individual choice but that other determinants of health also affect peoples' risk of problematic or high-risk use (Mahmoud et al., 2017). *At-risk substance use* and *substance use disorder* may be less stigmatizing terms to use; they better reflect the continuum on which use occurs, and they more clearly reflect the fact that such use is not an individual choice but rather a physiological issue influenced by many social factors (Mahmoud et al., 2017).

Mental Health Promotion

The final portion of this chapter outlines some strategies to improve mental health in the population. **Mental health promotion** is, therefore, a critical concept for readers. It refers to programs, policies, and other interventions that enable people to gain control over their lives and their mental health, in particular, and work towards the creation of an environment that supports recovery (CMHA, 2018a). Interventions can exist at the individual level in clinical or other settings, or be more population based, such as the creation of policies, and supportive physical and social environments that also address stigma.

Current Canadian Developments in Mental Health

In 2006, *Out of the Shadows at Last: Transforming Mental Health, Mental Illness, and Addiction Services in*

Canada, was produced by the Standing Senate Committee on Social Affairs, Science and Technology, and highlighted the pervasiveness of stigma in all levels of Canadian society. Subsequently, a number of reports related to mental health were published in Canada that created momentum for the creation of the Mental Health Commission of Canada (MHCC) in 2007, with support of all federal political parties. Several initiatives under the MHCC have placed mental health as an issue on the political agenda and in the public sphere. One of the first initiatives was a national research demonstration project on "housing first," a mental health and homelessness initiative, *At Home* (2008), that provided support and housing for individuals who are homeless. A second initiative of the MHCC was the 10-year anti-stigma campaign, *Opening Minds* (2009), created to bring awareness and change public attitudes towards mental illness. A key initiative was the release of Canada's first national mental health strategy, *Changing Directions, Changing Lives* (2012). However, without an implementation strategy, the national strategy lacked a clear way forward on how to take action until the release of *Advancing the Mental Health Strategy for Canada: A Framework for Action* (2017–2022), outlining specific objectives in taking action. In 2017, the federal government announced targeted funding of $5 billion over 10 years to support mental health initiatives. In 2018, new funding was also announced in the federal government's budget to support MHCC's work in studying the impact of cannabis use on the mental health of Canadians. These new federal investments in mental health will help to transform mental health in Canada and positively impact the lives of all Canadians.

> **CRITICAL THINKING QUESTION 9.1:** Look up some news stories in your province or territory that discuss the opioid crisis. How do these stories describe the issue of substance use and substance use disorders? What language is used, and how might the way the language is used impact community perceptions of people who experience substance use disorders?

EPIDEMIOLOGY AND THE BURDEN OF MENTAL ILLNESS IN CANADA

Mental illnesses are characterized by alterations in thinking, mood, or behaviour associated with significant distress and impaired functioning over an extended period. Mental illnesses may occur together; for example, an individual can have depression and anxiety disorder or addiction. A complex interplay of genetic, biological, personality, and environmental factors causes mental illnesses.

Mental illness affects people of all ages, educational and income levels, and cultures; onset of many mental illnesses occurs during adolescence and young adulthood, however, treatment often is not initiated until many years later (Malla et al., 2018; Patten, 2017). In youth, persistent negative thoughts and feelings may be related to poor mental health and well-being (Government of Canada, 2018a; Fig. 9.2). Many youth with mental health problems do not receive needed treatment from heath professionals because of barriers such as stigma, not knowing where to go, and lack of trust (British Columbia Integrated Youth Services Initiative, 2015; Butler et al., 2017).

Epidemiology of Mental Illness

The major mental illnesses in Canada are mood disorders, anxiety disorders, and schizophrenia, with suicide and suicidal behaviour being serious consequences of mental illness. The deinstitutionalization of individuals with mental illnesses who lived in hospital settings began to occur in the early 1960s and shifted their care to communities. Most bed closures in Canada occurred between 1975 (53 801 beds) and 1981 (20 301 beds)—a 62% reduction—and the average length of stay decreased from 29.5 days in 1985 to 22 days by the end of 1999, while the cost of community-based services has risen steadily (Sealy & Whitehead, 2004). The transition from hospital to community has not always been successful, particularly for some population groups, such as those diagnosed as having both mental health and developmental disabilities. Compounding this issue is the inability to meet the needs of this population in rural and remote areas.

There is now an emphasis on treating individuals with mental illness in outpatient and community clinics and the transfer of long-term care patients to residential care facilities. However, some individuals end up being admitted to the hospital several times a year. The indicator that measures what is known as the "revolving door" syndrome for many individuals with mental illness looks at how many individuals have at least three repeat hospital stays for a mental illness in a single year (Fig. 9.3). According to the Canadian Institute for Health Information (CIHI, 2016), 1 in 8 individuals with a mental illness have repeat hospital

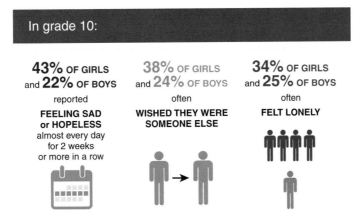

In grade 10:

43% OF GIRLS and **22%** OF BOYS reported **FEELING SAD or HOPELESS** almost every day for 2 weeks or more in a row

38% OF GIRLS and **24%** OF BOYS often **WISHED THEY WERE SOMEONE ELSE**

34% OF GIRLS and **25%** OF BOYS often **FELT LONELY**

Fig. 9.2 Mental health among youth. (From Government of Canada. [2018]. *Youth mental health infographic.* Retrieved from https://www.canada.ca/en/services/health/publications/healthy-living/youth-mental-health-infographic.html. Data are from the 2013/14 health behaviour in school-aged children. Retrieved from http://www.healthycanadians.gc.ca/publications/science-research-sciences-recherches/health-behaviour-children-canada-2015-comportements-sante-jeunes/index-eng.php. © All rights reserved. Youth Mental Health – Infographic. Public Health Agency of Canada. Adapted and reproduced with permission from the Minister of Health, 2019.)

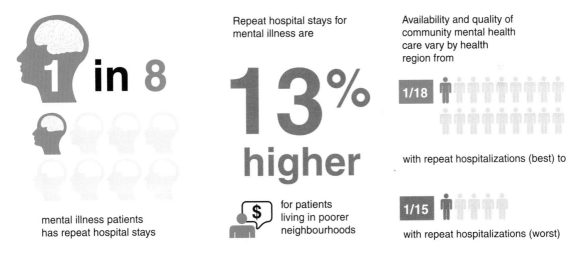

1 in 8

mental illness patients has repeat hospital stays

Repeat hospital stays for mental illness are

13% higher

for patients living in poorer neighbourhoods

Availability and quality of community mental health care vary by health region from

1/18 with repeat hospitalizations (best) to

1/15 with repeat hospitalizations (worst)

Fig. 9.3 Repeat hospital stays for mental illness. (From Canadian Institute for Health Information. [2017]. *Repeat hospital stays for mental illness.* Retrieved from https://yourhealthsystem.cihi.ca/hsp/inbrief?lang=en#!/indicators/007/repeat-hospital-stays-for-mental-illness/;mapC1;mapLevel2.)

stays, with variance from 1 in 18 to 1 in 5 individuals who have repeat hospital stays. In Quebec, individuals with a mental illness have a lower average of at least three hospital stays in a year with 10.6% of those with a mental illness having at least three hospital stays in a year. It is important to keep in mind that some hospitalizations may reflect challenges in getting appropriate care, medication, and support in the community, especially for individuals who live in poorer neighbourhoods. Readmission rates for individuals with schizophrenia and psychotic disorders are among the highest because of the chronic, highly debilitating, and refractory nature of these disorders, requiring stabilization of an individual's condition, resulting in long stays in hospital. When individuals with schizophrenia have a comorbid substance use disorder, they are 15.2% and

24.6% more likely to be readmitted within 30 days and 1 year of discharge, respectively. In the year after initial discharge, they are expected to stay in hospital 19.0% longer than individuals without comorbid substance use disorders (CIHI, 2013).

Mood and Anxiety Disorders

Mood and anxiety disorders are the most common types of mental illness in Canada, and more than 1 in 10 Canadians older than 18 years of age have reported a mood or anxiety disorder (or both) (Survey on Living with Chronic Diseases in Canada [SLCDC], 2014). Mood disorders include major depression, bipolar disorders, and dysthymia and are characterized by the lowering or elevation of a person's mood that can be classified on a continuum of being acute to chronic in nature. Anxiety disorders are, as a group, the most common mental illness and include general anxiety disorder, specific phobia, posttraumatic stress disorder (PTSD), obsessive-compulsive disorder, and panic disorder and are characterized by excessive and persistent feelings of apprehension, worry, or fear. Both types of disorders can vary from acute episodes to chronic disorders and may have a major impact on an individual's life. The onset of mood disorders usually occurs during young adulthood, although it can occur at all ages. Women are twice as likely as men to be diagnosed with depression or an anxiety disorder (O'Donnell et al., 2016). Mood and anxiety disorders often coexist with other chronic conditions; however, the bidirectional associations are poorly understood. For example, people who report having depressive or anxiety disorders are at increased risk of chronic obstructive pulmonary disease (COPD), and COPD increases the risk of depression (Atlantis, Fahey, Cochrane, & Smith, 2013). Likewise, depression and anxiety disorders have been associated with hypertension (Stein et al., 2014), causing poor physical health later in life, and conversely, living with hypertension or any other physical chronic condition may increase the risk of developing depression or anxiety disorder.

Risk Factors. The risk factors for depression are family history of mood disorder, a history of early loss (typically a parent before the age of 11 years), stress, and chronic and debilitating illness. Individuals with mood disorders are at increased risk of suicide. Anxiety risk factors are very similar and include being female, family history, genetics, chronic illnesses, stress, lower socioeconomic status, depression, and a history of self-harm (Jacobson & Newman, 2017).

Schizophrenia

Schizophrenia defines a group of disorders that is characterized by a continuum of signs and symptoms, the most prominent of which are distorted thoughts and perceptions. Schizophrenia affects approximately 7 people in 1000 over the lifetime in high income countries and 5.5 people in 1000 in low income countries (Saha et al., 2005). An individual with schizophrenia can present with various hallucinatory experiences and altered thinking, either caused by the hallucinations or the wrong interpretation of real stimuli. The group of so-called negative signs always develops in patients with schizophrenia and includes flattened affect and reduced emotions and volition or will. In many cases, the individual has difficulty thinking clearly and making decisions, managing and expressing emotions, and relating to others; therefore, a substantial part of the person is socially withdrawn. There is an increased risk of suicide in individuals who have schizophrenia. About 5% to 6% of people with schizophrenia die by suicide, about 20% make suicide attempts on more than one occasion, and many more have significant suicidal thoughts. Suicidal behaviour can be in response to hallucinations, and suicide risk remains high over the lifespan of individuals who have schizophrenia.

Risk Factors. There is a strong genetic component, with a heritability estimate around 80% (Keller, 2018). Schizophrenia has also been associated with many environmental risk factors, particularly various prenatal and perinatal stressors, infectious agents, childhood and adulthood trauma, and substance use (Matheson et al., 2011). However, many of the associations between these factors is still unknown, and the interaction effects between genetic and environmental causes can also vary from person to person. Regular cannabis use is also a risk factor for schizophrenia, particularly for those with a family history of schizophrenia (Power et al., 2014).

Suicide and Suicidal Behaviour

Unfortunately, in Canada, about 4 000 Canadians per year die by suicide—an average of 10 suicides a day (Statistics Canada, 2018; see Fig. 9.4). Suicides account for 90% of the deaths from intentional injuries in Canada. The two most important factors contributing to suicide are a recent history of mental illness and substance abuse. Whereas suicide is the voluntary and intentional act of killing oneself that results in death, referred to as completed suicide, an attempted suicide is living through the intentional act. The complexities associated

SUICIDE in Canada

CURRENT CONTEXT

An average of

10

PEOPLE
die by suicide
EACH DAY
in Canada

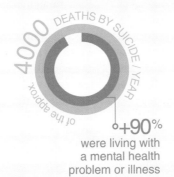

4000 DEATHS BY SUICIDE / YEAR of the approx.

+90%
were living with
a mental health
problem or illness

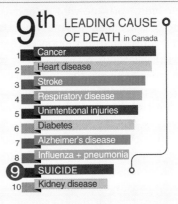

9th LEADING CAUSE
OF DEATH in Canada

1. Cancer
2. Heart disease
3. Stroke
4. Respiratory disease
5. Unintentional injuries
6. Diabetes
7. Alzheimer's disease
8. Influenza + pneumonia
9. **SUICIDE**
10. Kidney disease

ACROSS THE LIFESPAN

CHILDREN AND YOUTH
(10 to 19 years)

- Suicide 2nd leading cause of death
- Males account for 41% of suicides among 10- to 14-year-olds, increasing to 70% among 15- to 19-year-olds
- Self-harm hospitalizations: 72% females

YOUNG ADULTS
(20 to 29 years)

- Suicide 2nd leading cause of death
- Males account for 75% of suicides
- Self-harm hospitalizations: 58% females

ADULTS
(30 to 44 years)

- Suicide 3rd leading cause of death
- Males account for 75% of suicides
- Self-harm hospitalizations: 56% females

ADULTS
(45 to 64 years)

- Suicide 7th leading cause of death
- Males account for 73% of suicides
  - Highest suicide rate across lifespan observed among males 45 to 59 years
- Self-harm hospitalizations: 56% females

SENIORS
(65+ years)

- Suicide 12th leading cause of death
- Males account for 80% of suicides
  - Males aged 85+ years experience the highest rate of suicides among seniors
- Self-harm hospitalizations: 52% females

Fig. 9.4 Suicide statistics, 2016. (From Government of Canada. [2018]. *Suicide in Canada infographic*. Retrieved from https://www.canada.ca/en/public-health/services/publications/healthy-living/suicide-canada-infographic.html. © All rights reserved. Suicide in Canada. Public Health Agency of Canada. Adapted and reproduced with permission from the Minister of Health, 2019.)

with suicide are intertwined with an individual's perceptions, experiences in life, age, and gender.

Suicide is an important preventable cause of mortality and potential years of life lost (PYLLs) in Canada, especially among Canadian youth. PYLLs for suicide and self-inflicted injuries is the number of years of life "lost" when a person dies "prematurely" from suicide—before age 75 years. A person dying at age 25 years, for example, has lost 50 years of life. Suicide is the fourth cause of PYLL after cancer, circulatory diseases, and unintentional injuries (Public Health Agency of Canada [PHAC], 2014). Suicide across the lifespan (see Fig. 9.4) shows that suicide is a major concern for children as well as seniors. Men are three times more likely than women to complete suicide, but females are more likely to attempt suicide. Whereas women are more likely to attempt suicide by overdose, men are more likely to use hanging or firearms (Statistics Canada, 2017). Increases in suicide rates among Indigenous people, such as the Canadian Inuit, correlate with colonization, assimilation, forced settlement, trauma (including intergenerational trauma), and disruption of traditional social structures (King, Smith, & Gracey, 2009; see Chapter 7). Research has also shown that individuals recently discharged from psychiatric inpatient units are at extremely high risk for completed suicide (While, Bickley, Roscoe, et al., 2012).

Although not in itself a mental illness, suicidal behaviour is highly correlated with mental illness and is a risk factor for suicide. Nonfatal suicidal behaviour refers to potentially self-injurious actions in which a person intended to kill themselves and includes self-harm, suicidal ideation, suicidal threats, and risky behaviour. Suicidal behaviour is a sign of serious distress. The incidence of nonfatal suicidal behaviour is difficult to determine because many individuals do not see health professionals but are helped by family or friends or perhaps by no one at all. Individuals are sometimes hospitalized for their own protection and to address the underlying factors that precipitated the crisis. Hospitalization data provide some insight into suicide attempts, but caution is needed when interpreting these figures because they only paint part of the picture. In 2015, there were 13 438 hospitalizations associated with self-inflicted injuries in Canada—more than three times the number of suicides. Within that year, young women aged 15 to 19 years had a disproportionately high rate of hospitalizations associated with self-inflicted injuries (231.8 per 100 000; $n = 1897$), which is almost 3.5 times that of young men in the same age group. Hospitalizations of men for self-inflicted injuries are generally lower among all age groups until the 75- to 79-year-old age group, at which point the trend reverses for the subsequent age groups (PHAC, 2016).

Risk Factors. Many factors contribute directly or indirectly to suicide risk. Among them, the two most important are a recent history of mental illness and substance use disorder. People with depression are at higher risk of suicide. Alcoholism is the second most commonly reported problem, after major depression, to be associated with suicide. Certain personality disorders, such as borderline and antisocial personality disorders, increase risks of nonfatal suicidal behaviour. Childhood trauma is also a well-documented precursor of suicidal ideation and behaviour (Zatti et al., 2017).

A Public Health Approach to Suicide—Prevention and Health Promotion. Although mental health services are critical for individuals who show signs of suicidal thoughts or behaviour, community and societal strategies are also necessary to prevent someone from starting down that road. An intersectoral approach, which involves communities, government, health care, and education sectors, is required, along with building resiliency and capacity in communities and in vulnerable individuals. Strategies for suicide prevention can be categorized into five broad categories (Zalsman et al., 2016):

- Improving the identification, referral, and treatment of persons at high risk of suicide by various caretakers and "gatekeepers." Examples include training primary care physicians and health care professionals to recognize, treat, and refer patients as necessary with clinical depression and school-based screening programs to identify suicidal youth.
- Treating underlying risk factors for suicide. Examples include treating those with mental illness such as clinical depression and treating alcoholism and drug abuse through rehabilitation programs.
- Decreasing individual vulnerability to suicide through education of the general population. Examples include education to help individuals cope with problems that can lead to suicide and increasing public awareness about the resources available in the community to those who need help for specific problems. Refer to Box 9.1 for information about how the mass media reporting on suicide may influence vulnerability.
- Improving accessibility of self-referral resources for suicidal people. Examples are hotlines and walk-in crisis centres.
- Limiting access to lethal means of suicide. Examples are legislation to reduce accessibility to firearms, physical restrictions to accessing high places (e.g., buildings), and limiting amounts of potentially lethal medications dispensed to those who are depressed.

A number of protective factors have been associated with a decreased risk of suicide:
- A well-developed social support network
- Strong reasons for living

BOX 9.1 Media Reporting About Suicide

A 2018 study identified significant associations between several specific elements of media reports and suicide deaths. The findings suggest that reporting on suicide can have a meaningful impact on suicide deaths and that journalists, media outlets, and organizations should carefully consider the specific content of reports before publication.

Known as "suicide contagion," exposure to suicide within a family, within a group of friends or through media coverage may be associated with an increase in suicidal behaviours. For example, the 2017 to 2018 television series *13 Reasons Why* received controversial reviews from parents, counsellors, teachers, and youth; experts believed that the series may be romanticizing suicide and not encouraging youth to seek help from family or counsellors.

Source: From Sinyor, M., Schaffer, A., Nishikawa, Y., et al. (2018). The association between suicide deaths and putatively harmful and protective factors in media reports. *CMAJ: Canadian Medical Association Journal, 190*(30), E900–E907.

BOX 9.2 Adverse Childhood Experiences

Adverse childhood experiences include:
- Physical abuse
- Sexual abuse
- Emotional abuse
- Physical neglect
- Emotional neglect
- Intimate partner violence
- Mother treated violently
- Substance misuse within household
- Household mental illness
- Parental separation or divorce
- Incarcerated household member

- Responsibility for young children
- Religiosity (frequent attendance of religious service or personal religiosity); this may be related to religious views on suicide or to social support derived from the religious community
- Extraversion and optimism
- Effective coping and problem solving (Turecki & Brent, 2015).

Suicide Survivors. Suicide is a devastating loss that leaves behind many survivors who must cope with unique challenges, such as isolation, stigma, and the question of why the death occurred. All of these aspects can lead to negative mental health consequences for the survivors. There is evidence that survivors of suicide grieve differently than other groups. More frequent feelings of rejection, responsibility, more total grief reactions, increased levels of shame, and perceived stigmatization have been found among suicide survivors (Kõlves et al., 2019).

Risk Factors for Mental Illness

Although the mental illnesses discussed in this chapter have many unique risk factors, generally, it can be said that mental illnesses are the result of complex interactions among genetic, biological, personality, and environmental factors; however, the brain is the final common pathway for behaviour, cognition, and mood. Mental illnesses are more common in close family members of a person with mental illness, suggesting a genetic basis. For reasons that may be biological, psychosocial, or both, age and sex affect rates of mental illness. Environmental factors such as family situations, workplace pressures, and socioeconomic status can precipitate the onset or recurrence of mental illness and often determine the severity or chronicity of illness.

Stress also has a major impact on our mental health. It has been linked to increased risk for cardiovascular disease, is considered a predisposing factor for depression, and is linked to decreased work performance The level of chronic stress experienced by the Canadian population is described in Chapter 5. **Stress** can be broadly defined as the psychic or physiological disequilibrium caused by an event. Stress is a ubiquitous feature of modern life. It is part of a larger set of psychological factors that may contribute to illness. Psychological factors include internal factors, such as personality, attitudes, and reactions to events, and external factors, such as social supports and employment.

Adverse childhood experiences (ACEs) are stressful or traumatic events (Box 9.2). ACEs are strongly related to the development and prevalence of a wide range of health problems throughout a person's lifespan, including those associated with mental illness and substance misuse.

CRITICAL THINKING QUESTION 9.2: A Public Health Crisis?

The Adverse Childhood Experiences (ACEs) Study is a long-term research study following participants for the past 20 years to understand the connection between ACEs and health outcomes. The study has demonstrated an association of ACEs with health and social problems across the lifespan. As a notable landmark in epidemiological research, many scientific articles have been produced along with conference and workshop presentations that examine ACEs.

Watch the video "How Childhood Trauma Affects Health Across a Lifetime" (see https://www.youtube.com/watch?v=95ovIJ3dsNk). In the video, Dr. Robert Block states: "ACEs are the single greatest unaddressed public health threat facing our nation today." Do you agree with this statement? Explain why or why not. If you agree, what actions can be taken to address this public health issue?

BOX 9.3   Mental Illness Awareness Week

Held every year in October, the Mental Illness Awareness Week (MIAW) campaign is a national public education event coordinated by the Canadian Alliance on Mental Illness and Mental Health. It focuses on raising awareness about the reality of mental illness.

The Faces of Mental Illness campaign, in partnership with Bell Let's Talk, features personal stories from individuals who live with mental illness. These video stories are shared at events during MIAW to engage the public in conversations about mental illness.

The Burden of Mental Illness

Mental illnesses are responsible for a large and measurable burden of disease (or morbidity) in the Canadian population: 20% of Canadians will experience a mental illness during their lifetime. The burden of mental illness is more than 1.5 times that of all cancers and more than 7 times that of all infectious diseases. The burden of depression alone is more than the combined burden of lung, colorectal, breast, and prostate cancers. Stigma, caregiver burden, and the economic costs are discussed in this section.

Stigma

Stigma is a complex concept that often involves labelling, stereotyping, and displaying prejudice and discrimination against a certain group in an environment where that group has limited social, economic, or political power. Stigma is very prevalent among many groups, including Indigenous populations (see Chapter 7), individuals experiencing inequities (see Chapter 6), and individuals who experience mental health concerns. Stigma can manifest in different ways, including being fearful of or anticipating being treated unfairly, actually having this come true and being treated unfairly, feeling differently about one's self and one's condition because of internalized prejudice, and not

seeking care because of the fear of being treated differently. Studies have indeed shown that people experiencing mental health concerns may avoid seeking help because of stigma and that this is prevalent in our societies (Clement et al., 2015). Additionally, stigma can ripple out and affect all aspects of an individual's life, such as access to employment, housing, education, and relationships with friends, family, and coworkers. Media reports, television shows, and movies often depict individuals with mental illness as being dangerous or violent. These types of negative depictions are at the core of the stigma, discrimination, and social exclusion experienced by individuals who have mental health conditions (Substance Abuse and Mental Health Services Administration, 2015). Current research also shows that people with major mental illness are 2.5 times more likely to be the victims of violence than are other members of society. Interventions to promote positive mental health will only be successful if the issue of stigma against mental health conditions is also addressed.

Over the past 20 years or so, several mental health agencies have embarked on anti-stigma campaigns (see Box 9.3 for an example of an anti-stigma campaign), raising awareness, normalizing illness, and focusing on an individuals' own biases and assumptions as starting places to address stigma. In 2001, the WHO declared stigma to be the "single most important barrier to overcome in the community" (WHO, 2001). The CMHA's 2004 *Framework for Support* called on the federal government to invest in a multiyear, multilevel public campaign to reduce discrimination and stigma (see the Case Study box for an example of a public awareness campaign).

The Elephant in the Room Anti-Stigma Campaign

Mood Disorders Society of Canada created an anti-stigma campaign that involves a small blue elephant. Known as the Elephant in the Room Anti-Stigma Campaign, individuals display the elephant in their workplace, on their desk, in their classroom, or at home and use it as an artifact to signal safe spaces to talk about mental health and to start conversations about mental illness. The elephant signals a stigma-free zone.

EXERCISE 9.1 Breaking Down Stigma: Find a news article or video that reports on someone who has a mental illness. Use the STOP criteria to recognize attitudes and actions that support the stigma of mental health conditions and ask yourself:

Does what you hear do any the following?

- **S**tereotypes people with mental health conditions (i.e., assumes that they are all alike rather than individuals)
- **T**rivializes or belittles people with mental health conditions or the condition itself
- **O**ffends people with mental health conditions by insulting them
- **P**atronizes people with mental health conditions by treating them as if they were not as good as other people

If you see something in the media that does not pass the STOP criteria, speak up! Call or write to the writer or publisher of the newspaper, magazine, or book; the radio, TV, or movie producer; or the advertiser that used words that add to the misunderstanding of mental illness. Help them realize how their words affect people with mental health conditions.

Source: Exercise adapted from the Canadian Mental Health Association. (n.d.). Retrieved from https://ontario.cmha.ca/documents/stigma-and-discrimination/

Economic Costs of Mental Illness

Each year, one in five Canadians experiences some form of mental health or substance use disorder and currently this is estimated to cost the economy at least $50 billion per year (MHCC, 2010). An economic study funded by the MHCC estimated the direct costs of mental illness and substance use disorders in Canada is projected to increase to $105.6 billion in 2041. It is also predicted that by 2020, mental illness will represent the country's leading health care cost (Smetanin et al., 2011). Equally troublesome are the indirect costs to society, including the social and community costs, income support, and other services included. Half a million Canadians are unable to work each week because of disabilities caused by mental illness (Dewa, Chau, & Dermer, 2010). It is difficult to calculate absenteeism at work caused by informal caregivers' time spent caring for their family member or friend; however, it is an important indirect cost to consider. It is estimated that $5 billion Canadian every year can be attributed to providing support for those living with mental illness (MHCC, 2015).

Caregiver Burden

In the past several decades, there has been a shift of responsibility for care of individuals with a mental illness from hospitals to caregivers in the community. Caregivers can be a spouse or partner, child, parent, extended family, or friend. Approximately 8.1 million Canadians aged 15 years or older provided care to a family member with ill health (Sinha, 2013).

Many studies over the years have investigated the impact on caregivers. These include the impact on their physical and mental health and their participation in the labour force, pressures on their personal finances, and reduced time available for other activities. These adverse consequences are often referred to as caregiver burden. A study by Slaunwhite, Ronis, Sun, & Peters (2017) found that caregivers of persons with mental health or substance use problems were more likely to report that caregiving was very stressful and that they felt depressed, tired, worried or anxious, or overwhelmed; lonely or isolated; short-tempered or irritable; and resentful because of their caregiving responsibilities. Employers and governments may also be impacted, notably because of absenteeism, lost productivity, and reduced tax revenues. It is important to keep in mind that caregiving can also be rewarding and is not necessarily just a burden but also satisfying.

Mental Health Among Rural and Remote Populations

Across Canada, rural and remote communities are heterogeneous and have diverse populations. Data have shown that individual health status declines from the most urban regions to the most rural and remote ones, thus demonstrating that geography or geographic location is a determinant of health (Shah, Milosavljevic, & Bath, 2017). Individuals who live in rural and remote communities have several challenges when it comes to treating their mental illnesses and promoting their mental health. Factors that are commonly identified as interfering with the ability of rural Canadians to obtain quality mental health care include inaccessibility (e.g., too few services, not enough health care providers), costs involved in travelling for services, stigma, lack of confidentiality, and lack of anonymity or privacy. To overcome some of these barriers, multidisciplinary primary health care teams are being used in some rural and remote communities that lack psychiatric care to provide services. Collaborative care networks, intersectoral agencies such as social service agencies, law enforcement, religious groups, and education sectors are all working together as a means to build capacity and provide support for individuals with chronic mental illness who also have complex needs (DeSilva et al., 2014; Patel et al., 2013). Telepsychiatry or telemedicine initiatives are also growing across rural and remote communities to provide consultations with primary care providers as well as direct counselling and treatment for rural and remote populations.

> **CRITICAL THINKING QUESTION 9.3:** Working from a health promotion perspective, what do you think can be done to prevent suicides in rural communities?

EPIDEMIOLOGY AND THE BURDEN OF SUBSTANCE USE AND SUBSTANCE USE DISORDERS IN CANADA

Substance use is quite common around the world, and many people use a range of substances recreationally or to experiment. Some substances that people use are legal, such as alcohol or tobacco, but others are illegal, or illicit. Whether a substance is illegal or depends on government policy, and the risk of a substance cannot only be defined by whether it is legal. Essentially, just because a drug such as alcohol has legal status does not mean it is less risky from a health perspective than an illegal substance.

Epidemiology of Substance Use and Substance Disorders

According to national-level population health surveys, nearly 22% of Canadians meet the criteria for substance use disorders at some point during their lives. A greater proportion of youth meet the criteria for substance use disorders (nearly 12%) compared with people aged 45 years or older (nearly 2%) and, generally speaking, men have a higher rate of substance use disorders than women. Overall, substance use disorders related to alcohol, tobacco, and cannabis are more common than for other drugs (e.g., cocaine and opioids) (Pearson, Janz, & Ali, 2015).

Tobacco

Although legal, tobacco us is one of the most harmful substances and, as described in Chapter 8, is one of the major risk factors for other NCDs. Over the past several decades, the prevalence of smoking has been steadily decreasing. In 2015, 3.9 million or 13.0% of Canadians were smokers (10.4% women, 15.6% men), which includes 9.4% (2.8 million) daily smokers and 3.7% (1.1 million) nondaily smokers (Canadian Student Tobacco, Alcohol and Drugs Survey[CSTADS]). This represents a significant decrease from the 2001 figures of 5.4 million or 22% of Canadians. This represented the lowest overall level since regular monitoring of smoking began in 1965. British Columbia reported the lowest prevalence for current smokers 15 years of age and older at 10%; Newfoundland and Labrador, Nova Scotia, and Saskatchewan reported the highest prevalence at 18.5%, 17.8%, and 16.9%, respectively (CSTADS, 2015).

In 2015, young adults aged 20 to 24 years still had the highest smoking rate of any age group, at 18%. Over the past 10-year period, electronic cigarettes have made their mark with young Canadians. Electronic cigarettes are often flavoured and can contain nicotine. They are typically vaped, which means inhaling vapour (usually from a heated liquid), as opposed to smoked (which refers to the inhalation of smoke, a byproduct of combustion). In 2015, 13% (3.9 million) of Canadians aged 15 years and older reported having ever tried an e-cigarette, an increase from 9% (2.5 million) reported in 2013; 26% (534,000) of youth aged 15 to 19 years, and 30% (743,000) young adults aged 20 to 24 years reported having ever tried an e-cigarette. Only 11% or

2.6 million adults aged 25 years and older said they have tried an e-cigarette (CSTADS, 2015).

Smoking is closely related to unemployment, income, and education (important social determinants of health [SDHs]). Smoking rates are twice as high among those who did not complete secondary school as among those who completed university (32.7% vs 15.0%). Smoking rates increase as income decreases—42% of those in the lowest income group currently smoke, compared with 20% in the highest income group. Unemployed individuals have the highest rate of smoking (46%). Other population groups who also experience higher smoking prevalence rates are Indigenous people, whose rate is estimated to be two to five times higher than among non-Indigenous Canadians, LGBTQ+ persons (24%–45%) across different groups, and more than one third of construction workers smoked in 2015 (34%) followed by mining and oil and gas extraction workers (29%) and transportation and warehousing workers (29%) (Health Canada, 2015).

Alcohol

Alcohol use is very common in the population, as evidenced by the sale of alcohol across the country. Liquor authorities, wineries, and breweries sold 22.1 billion litres of alcoholic beverages in 2016, up 3.5% from the previous year (Statistics Canada, 2017). Beer accounted for the vast majority of sales (41.5%), and wine accounted for 31.6%, spirits 23.1%, and other alcoholic beverages 3.8%. Sales of alcoholic beverages by volume, however, should not be equated with data on consumption because consumption of alcoholic beverages also includes homemade wine and beer, wine, and beer manufactured by brew-on-premise operations and all sales to Canadian residents in duty-free shops.

In 2016, 19.0% of Canadians aged 12 years and older (~5.8 million people) reported alcohol consumption that classified them as heavy drinkers. Heavy drinking is defined as drinking five or more drinks on one occasion and drinking heavily at least 12 times in the previous 12 months (Statistics Canada, 2016). The proportion of heavy drinkers aged 12 years and older remained stable between 2015 and 2016. Overall, men were more likely (23.8%) to report heavy drinking than women (14.2%) in 2016. The highest proportion of heavy drinking for both sexes was among those aged 18 to 34 years. In this age group, 34.4% of men and 23.4% of women were heavy drinkers. Heavy

drinking follows an income gradient with the highest rates of heavy drinking observed among men in higher income groups. A similar pattern was observed in women; however, the differences were not significant (CIHI, 2016). People in the highest income group are more than twice as likely as those at the lowest level to consume alcohol; however, people at the lowest level bear a disproportionate burden of alcohol harm (Lewer et al., 2016). The potential explanation is that a people in the lower income group have a greater susceptibility to the consequences associated with alcohol use because of factors, including higher stress levels, fewer social support networks, fewer resources to cope, and other risk factors such as poorer diet and physical inactivity (Alcohol Research UK, 2015).

Cannabis

Most population health surveys assessing cannabis use were administered before 2018, when the Government of Canada introduced the *Cannabis Act* to legalize cannabis for nonmedical purposes. As such, the data are slightly limited (because people tend to underreport use of illegal substances). Nevertheless, most surveys have revealed that cannabis is the second most commonly used drug after alcohol. Nearly half of Canadians aged 15 years and older (44.5%) report having ever tried cannabis, 12.3% have used it in the past year, and 8.8% have used cannabis in the past 3 months. Recent use of cannabis is more prevalent among young people: approximately 20% of youths aged 15 to 19 years and 30% of young adults aged 20 to 24 years have used cannabis in the past year, compared with 10% of Canadians aged 25 years and older (CSTADS, 2015). Reported rates of use have also gone up over the past couple of decades. For example, in 1985, 6% of Canadians reported using cannabis at least once during the past year. In 2015, approximately 12% of Canadians reported using cannabis at least once during the past year (PHAC, 2018). In general, cannabis use tends to be greater among urban populations compared with rural and is higher for First Nations on reserve versus the general population (PHAC, 2018). Additionally, cannabis use is higher among those who smoke cigarettes (Meier & Hatsukami, 2016; Montgomery, 2015). When it comes to the prevalence of problematic use, it is estimated that nearly 3% of Canadians meet the criteria for problematic use, which includes using cannabis every day or almost every day during the previous 3 months (PHAC, 2018).

It is important to keep in mind, however, that the medical use of marijuana has been legal in Canada since 2001. Cannabis can sometimes be used to treat chronic pain, along with some other conditions. It is estimated that around 3% of Canadians report using at least some cannabis for self-defined medical reasons (which could include people who were formally prescribed cannabis by a health care provider or those who self-medicate). Around 50% of people who use cannabis for this purpose do so because of pain, and the majority of people using for self-defined medical reasons use cannabis every day or almost every day. Thus, in general, people using cannabis for medical reasons represent the minority of cannabis users and tend to use more frequently and because of pain compared with those using recreationally (Rotterman & Page, 2018).

Opioids

Opioids are substances that work on specific opioid receptors in the brain and around the body, causing euphoria, pain relief, and a number of other physiological effects. Examples of common opioids include heroin, morphine, hydromorphone, and fentanyl. Opioids can be prescribed (obtained legally) or illicit (obtained through nonregulated means). Opioids may be taken for certain medical conditions appropriately or may be used in a high-risk way (taken more often or in higher amounts than prescribed). Prescribed opioids can be diverted and bought online or off the streets by people for whom they are not prescribed, and illicit opioids (nonpharmaceutical, usually synthetic opioids, made in laboratories as opposed to by drug companies) can also be purchased in the same way. As will be discussed later in the chapter, the main issue

with nonpharmaceutical-grade opioids is that they are unregulated, with no quality checks, and they can often be mixed with very toxic and potentially lethal substances, such as fentanyl and carfentanil.

Opioids are a very commonly prescribed and used substance across Canada. In fact, after the United States, Canada is the second largest consumer of prescription opioids. In 2015, just over 20 million prescriptions were written for opioids (which equates to one prescription written for nearly every Canadian over the age of 18 years) (PHAC, 2018). Because they are highly addictive medications that relieve pain and produce a strong euphoric effect, opioids are prone to being used in a high-risk way. As described in the In the News box, in the past, pharmaceutical companies deliberately misled prescribers of opioids and heavily marketed them, contributing to the origins of the opioid crisis.

When it comes to opioid-related use disorder, the rise in the number of deaths associated with opioids (described in the next section) highlights how common it is to misuse these substances and develop opioid use disorder. Rates of opioid use disorder are likely underreported because many forms of opioids are illegal and because of stigma towards people who use or misuse substances. In 2017, a survey administered by Health Canada found that more than one third of Canadians who reported using an opioid over the past 12 months obtained it without a prescription. Additionally, a 2015 survey found that 0.3% of Canadians reported using prescription opioids in ways not intended by their prescriber—an indicator of higher risk use. High-risk use in youth is also an issue. Three percent of students in grades 7 to 12 reported using prescription opioids to get "high" over the past year (PHAC, 2018).

⊕ IN THE NEWS

The Opioid Crisis Explained

Rates of opioid prescribing (primarily to treat acute and chronic pain) are very high in both the United States and Canada. Very aggressive marketing techniques by pharmaceutical companies, high rates of chronic pain, a lack of access and funding for alternative pain treatments (like acupuncture and mindfulness, for example), and stigma towards people with mental health and addictions issues have all resulted in widespread and ongoing use of these substances (Donroe, Socias, & Marshall, 2018).

Because opioids are highly addictive, they are diverted (sold to those who do not have a prescription for them) and used by many for their euphoric effect. In an era when mental health challenges are so prevalent, alongside trauma and loneliness, it is no surprise that people turn to substances as a form of relief and self-treatment. Although some people begin using opioids to treat pain (through obtaining a prescription), others begin using them illicitly (without a prescription, or "off the streets").

The Opioid Crisis Explained

Overall, although opioid use has been on the rise since the late 1990s, the rates of opioid-related death have sky-rocketed in recent years. This is mainly because of the presence of very lethal potent opioids such as fentanyl and carfentanil in the drug supply (which make drugs easier to traffic). In British Columbia, for example, the number of illicit drug overdose deaths rose from 183 in 2008 to 1380 in 2018. In November 2018 alone, the number of illicit drug overdose deaths equalled nearly one in four people dying each day—mostly from fentanyl (B.C. Coroners Service, 2018).

Many people who take drugs such as heroin or morphine do not know that the drugs contain these toxic additive products (Donroe et al., 2018). Interestingly, as health agencies and Ministries of Health crack down on opioid overprescribing and pharmaceutical-grade opioids become more difficult to obtain, there is a growing trend towards the use of riskier forms of illicit opioids—such as heroin and fentanyl analogues made in laboratories with no quality control—which are increasingly available to users (Monico & Mitchell, 2018).

The rising death rates from opioid use have devastated many communities, causing widespread loss and grief. Front-line harm-reduction and emergency services workers also experience a considerable amount of trauma from witnessing many overdose deaths. This tragedy will likely have impacts for years to come.

Although engaging people in treatment or harm-reduction initiatives (described further in the Interventions section below) may help for a short time, the root factors that led to this crisis—high rates of opioid prescribing, high rates of childhood trauma and mental health issues, and lack of access to ancillary pain services—must also be addressed to curb the crisis.

Stimulants

Stimulant is an umbrella term that includes a range of substances that "speed" people up or increase alertness and energy by increasing the activity of one's nervous system. Stimulants can be prescribed (e.g., medications used to treat attention deficit hyperactivity disorder), over the counter or for general use (medicines used to treat cough and colds, caffeine, energy drinks), or illegal (cocaine, methamphetamines). When it comes to prescribed stimulants, just about 1% of the population is on them for medical purposes. However, they can also be used to get high or be diverted for recreational use, just like opioids. For example, just over 1% of students in grades 7 to 9 reported using prescribed stimulants to get high. Surveys of postsecondary students show that nearly 4% to 6% have used prescribed stimulants to get high (Canadian Centre on Substance Abuse [CCSA], 2016).

With respect to illicit stimulants, around 1% of the population reports using cocaine or crack (Government of Canada, 2014). Recently, more attention is being paid to methamphetamine (or "crystal meth") use. A number of recently published CBC News articles have reported a rise in its use, particularly in British Columbia and Alberta, and many experts have been saying it is a silent crisis, overshadowed by the opioid epidemic. In British Columbia's supervised consumption facility (known as Insite), for example, there has been a 600% rise in the use of crystal meth compared with 2005 rates (Merali, 2017). Furthermore, in 2017, Alberta Health Services saw a tripling in the number of people accessing services who reported using crystal meth over the past 5 years (Todd, 2017).

Other Substance Use Disorders

Other than chemical substances, addictions can also exist in the context of behaviours such as gambling, sex, Internet use, gaming, and shopping, to name a few examples. The *DSM-5*, published in 2013, included gambling disorder among a list of substance use disorders and as such highlighted its importance to the international community. At the time of developing the *DSM-5*, some experts were calling for inclusion of Internet gaming disorder because it, too, has been shown to be problematic in similar biological and cognitive ways as other addictions. The *DSM* named Internet gaming disorder as a condition requiring more study (Potenza, 2015). More recently, the problematic and compulsive use of social networking sites has drawn attention because it has been associated with poor emotional regulation and problematic alcohol use among youth (Potenza, 2015). It is estimated that about one third of the world's population uses social media sites such as Facebook, Twitter, Instagram, and others. On average, Facebook alone has just over 1 billion users every day (Hawi & Samaha, 2017). Addiction to social media is being written about more and more. Social media addiction, according to many experts, is compulsive use of social media sites that results in symptoms similar to other addictions, such as tolerance, withdrawal, conflict, and alterations in mood. Additionally, recent research has shown that compulsive use of social media tends to result in lower self-esteem among university students (Hawi & Samaha, 2017).

The Burden of Substance Use and Substance Use Disorders

In discussing the burden of substance use and substance use disorders, it is valuable to think about the various types of harms and costs that individuals and society can incur, including deaths, diseases and injuries, social costs, and economic burden. Although we have good data on things such as death and disease rates as well as hospitalizations, quantifying social and economic harm is much more difficult—mostly because people experiencing this type of harm may not have any contact with the health care or social system and because it involves types of societal harms (e.g., psychosocial trauma) that are more difficult to associate with a number value.

Deaths

Fatalities from using substances are far too common. In fact, for the first time in many decades, we may actually see a decrease in life expectancy as a result of deaths because of the opioid crisis (PHAC, 2018). In 2017, it was estimated that more than 4 000 Canadians (which equates to 11 Canadians each day) died from opioid overdoses, and in 2015, nearly 3 000 Canadians died of conditions associated with alcohol use (Government of Canada, 2018c). Sadly, deaths caused by substance use or substance use disorders affect younger people and take lives prematurely.

EXERCISE 9.2: Mohammed is a 29-year-old construction worker who lives in Halifax. He moved there after graduating from college in British Columbia and is living away from his friends and family. Two months ago, Mohammed sustained a leg injury at work and has had chronic pain ever since. He has not returned work. His health care provider recommended that he see a physiotherapist, but he could not afford to do so. A coworker of Mohammad let him try his morphine pills, and since then, Mohammed uses morphine (which he buys off the street) to help with his pain. At first, he was using two or three pills a month but now finds that he uses it almost every day, and sometimes he takes three or four pills at once because he likes how it makes him feel.

1. What are some factors that put Mohammed at risk of opioid use disorder?
2. List some reasons why loneliness may be a risk factor for high risk opioid use or opioid use disorder.
3. What could you do in practice to address some of Mohammed's risk factors for substance use disorder?

Disease and Injury

The frequent use of substances can lead to a range of physical and mental health conditions. As mentioned earlier, tobacco and alcohol are two of the four main risk factors for a number of NCDs, including heart disease and cancer. Many other substances, both legal and illegal, can also result in substance use disorders and other mental health conditions. For example, it is estimated that around 10% of adults who have ever used cannabis will go on to develop a substance use disorder of any type (PHAC, 2018). Additionally, people who start using cannabis at a young age and use frequently have been shown to have higher rates of mental health problems, including schizophrenia, mood disorders, and anxiety disorders. Alcohol is a known cause of fetal alcohol spectrum disorder, a lifelong developmental disorder affecting cognition, memory, behavior, and learning. Injuries are also a common harm resulting from substance use. In fact, almost 40% of deaths caused by motor vehicle collisions involve alcohol, and alcohol-impaired driving incidents are very common (totaling more than 65 000 events in 2017) (PHAC, 2018).

Finally, although we tend to think of substance use being most associated with NCDs, including injury, substance use disorders also have a significant impact on the rates of communicable diseases. For example, injection drug use has contributed to recent outbreaks of HIV in North American cities and a rise in the rates of infectious endocarditis (a very serious heart condition) and hepatitis C (Donroe et al., 2018).

Social Harm

From an individual-level perspective, a substance use disorder may interfere with interpersonal relationships, work or school, and a general ability to fulfill important roles (as is mentioned in the *DSM-5* criteria for substance use disorders). Often with illegal substances, involvement with an underground market or illicit substance puts people at risk of being arrested, charged, and incarcerated. The year before cannabis was legalized, nearly 48 000 cannabis-related drug offenses were reported in Canada (Government of Canada, 2018c). For those convicted, having a criminal record can then go on to affect their lives indefinitely, including challenges with finding employment, gaining access to training programs, and even restrictions on travel.

From a societal perspective, substance use and substance use disorders can, in some cases, lead to increases in crime, community violence, and even intimate partner violence. A recent report highlighted the fact that one in five violent crimes committed in Canada are attributed to alcohol (Canadian Substance Use Costs and Harms Scientific Working Group, 2018). Substance use can also result in the breakdown of families and devastation to communities that suffer trauma and constant loss because of people being affected by substance use disorders.

One challenge that should not be overlooked is the impact of the effects of substance use on those who work on the front lines: first responders, health care providers, and harm-reduction workers, for example (see Case Study box).

CASE STUDY

Impact of the Opioid Crisis on Front-Line Workers in British Columbia

In December 2017, the Central City Foundation released a report titled *On the Front Lines of the Opioid Crisis: How Community Organizations and their Staff are Coping*. The writers of the report conducted in-depth interviews with front-line workers, including shelter managers, health workers, and others, to assess the impact of the stress, loss, trauma, and grief that many of the staff of community-based organizations experience on a daily basis.

The results of the report are staggering: 71% of the organizations reported that their staff were directly affected by the opioid crisis, to the point where it was impacting their work with the clients they serve. Many were experiencing trauma and burnout, and organizations were finding that more people were going on stress leave or taking sick days.

A quote from one worker of a community-based organization is very telling and speaks to the immense stress, anxiety, and sometimes helplessness staff may feel:

This is already a sector for which burnout is rampant and high. It's already a very stressful job. The overdoses are adding a whole other element that we have never

seen before and that staff have never seen before where they are reviving women. They are administering naloxone. They are hearing about women who are being revived 10, 12, 14 times and I think we all have this feeling of who is next? What's next? (Central City Foundation, 2017)

Many front-line workers also felt helpless because they believed that the root causes of the crisis (discussed earlier in this chapter) were not being invested in adequately.

Addressing this level of trauma and grief in front-line workers is essential to prevent high rates of PTSD, and other chronic issues such as anxiety and depression. Some recommendations mentioned in the report include ensuring that counselling and mental health support services are available for all workers, allowing for adequate grieving and reflection (creating time for things such as memorial services), and exploring ways to empower affected communities to address the root causes of the crisis (Central City Foundation, 2017).

Monetary Costs

The direct and indirect costs of substance use on the Canadian economy are immense. Costs occur because of the use of health care resources (related to hospitalizations, emergency department visits, home care, visits to primary care and outpatient specialists), criminal justice resources (e.g., costs involved in policing and bringing cases to court), and indirect costs from losses in productivity (e.g., people taking time off of work). Health care costs, in particular, make up about 30% of the total costs, which is not surprising considering the increase in hospitalizations caused by opioids across the country and the fact that the rates of hospitalization for alcohol are greater than rates of hospitalizations for heart attacks (PHAC, 2018). Overall, the Canadian Centre on Substance Use and Addiction estimates that in 2014, the total costs of substance abuse in Canada was just over $38 billion. Alcohol was responsible for nearly 40% of the total costs, followed by tobacco (accounting for just over 30%), opioids (9%), and cannabis (7%). Overall, the costs associated with substance use have increased almost 5% between 2007 and 2014 (Canadian Substance Use Costs and Harms Scientific Working Group, 2018).

CRITICAL THINKING QUESTIONS 9.4: Research the state of the opioid crisis in your local area (city, town, or region). What statistics can you find related to deaths from opioids? What about harms, such as emergency department visits, 911 calls, and nonfatal overdoses? What information is missing for you to get a good sense of the "picture" of opioid harm in your community, and how might you work with partners in the community to get a better understanding of the issue to guide prevention efforts? What challenges might exist in obtaining the same information in a rural or remote community, and how might your strategies for gaining more information change if you lived in a rural or remote area in Canada?

MENTAL HEALTH PROMOTION

Although there are multiple approaches to addressing mental health, a primary focus ought to address the SDHs. It is estimated that 70% of mental health problems have their onset during childhood or adolescence (CMHA, 2014), indicating that early child and youth mental health promotion is a necessary strategy. As discussed earlier, ACEs have a major impact on our physical and mental health. Mental health promotion is the process of enhancing the capacity of individuals and communities to take control of their lives and improve their mental health. *Mental health promotion is an umbrella term that covers a variety of strategies, all aimed at having a positive effect on mental health.* Addressing the SDHs to improve the socioeconomic environment is one of these strategies.

Mental health promotion uses strategies that foster supportive environments and individual resilience while showing respect for culture, equity, social justice, interconnections, and personal dignity. The underlying principles include building on participants' and communities' competencies and strengths, demonstrating cultural humility and responsiveness, involving meaningful individual participation, addressing issues in the everyday life context of individuals, and ensuring the personal dignity of individuals (Clarke, Kuosmanen, & Barry, 2015).

Individual Interventions to Promote Mental Health

At the level of the individual, a sense of control, social support, and meaningful participation are important in helping to reduce stress, anxiety, burnout, and frustration. **Positive mental health** is distinct from mental illness. It embraces the emotional, psychological, and social components and can be viewed as the capacity to feel, think, and act in ways that enhance our ability to enjoy life and deal with the challenges we face. For example, a youth-driven web app was created by youth and for youth living in a rural community to enhance community connectedness. Use of the web app by youths was associated with higher levels of positive mental health characteristics (i.e., resilience and connectedness). Youth who helped to create the web app also reported enhanced self-concept, knowledge, and empowerment (Jenkins et al., 2018).

Social support plays an important role in the positive mental health of youth, which includes support from family, peers, schools, and communities. Thus, mental health promotion requires intersectoral action, involving a number of government sectors, such as health, employment or industry, education, environment, transport, and social and community services, as well as nongovernmental or community-based organizations, such as health support groups, places of worship, religious organizations, clubs, and other bodies. Other promising interventions include Art With Impact (see the Case Study box), Iris the Dragon (see the Case Study box), and Mental Health First Aid (see the Case Study box).

CASE STUDY

Art With Impact

Art With Impact, a nonprofit organization based in San Francisco, California, with offices in Canada, promotes mental wellness by creating spaces for young people to learn and connect through art and media. The organization's activities include assisting participants in exploring ideas related to mental health, stigma, and personal diagnosis and supporting friends and family through a 2-hour collaborative workshop that uses short films to spark dialogue that reduce stigma and encourage ear-

CASE STUDY—cont'd

Art With Impact

ly intervention for issues relating to mental health. A panel presentation provided participants an opportunity to learn about local resources available to them, specific information on what can be done to support and help loved ones, and generally improve mental health overall. The workshops are interactive, engaging experiences that encourage personal participation through the emotional connections felt through film.

See website: https://www.artwithimpact.org.

CASE STUDY

Iris the Dragon

Iris the Dragon is a registered Canadian charity that promotes positive youth development, recovery, and resilience by correcting misunderstandings and misinformation about mental illness through storytelling and using therapeutic approaches, such as solution-focused therapeutic strategies (i.e., cognitive behavioural therapy and narrative therapy). There is a series of six storybooks that deliver educational and empowering messages about mental illness, and these have been shown to change attitudes in reducing social distancing towards those with mental illness after exposure to the stories (Stuart et al., 2014).

CASE STUDY

Mental Health First Aid

Mental Health First Aid (MHFA) was initially developed in Australia but has since spread across the globe. It is a training program that teaches members of the public how to help a person who is developing a mental health problem (including a substance use problem), experiencing a worsening of an existing mental health problem, or is in a mental health crisis. Like traditional first aid, MHFA does not teach people to treat or diagnose mental health or substance use conditions. Instead, the training teaches people how to offer initial support until appropriate professional help is received or until the crisis resolves. The program has been shown to decrease stigma, increase confidence, and increase awareness among the general population who take the course (MHFA, 2019).

Trauma- and Violence-Informed Approaches

Practitioners and decision makers have recognized the impact of trauma (psychological and physical) on healthy development. In efforts to support individuals who experience trauma, the terms "trauma-informed care" or "trauma-informed approach" have gained traction among the health, social, and education fields and services across Canada. Trauma-informed care broadly refers to a set of principles that guide and direct how we view the impact of severe harm on an individual's mental, physical, and emotional health. A trauma-informed approach requires not only that practitioners understand the many impacts of trauma for the individual, family, and community but also that there is support from the organization and related services.

Trauma- and violence-informed approaches (TVIAs) have also emerged, and acknowledge the connections between violence, trauma, negative health outcomes and behaviours (see the Case Study box for an example of use of the trauma- and violence-informed approach). TVIA theory seeks to awaken in everyone the sense of having been traumatized and in which individuals are seen as an oppressed class—victims of, but potential victors over, trauma.

CASE STUDY

A Trauma- and Violence-Informed Approach: Yoga Outreach

Yoga Outreach is a nonprofit organization in British Columbia that trains volunteers to offer strength-based, trauma-sensitive yoga programs for people without resources who otherwise would be unable to participate. Its work is inspired by research conducted by the Trauma Center at the Justice Resource Institute.

In trauma-sensitive yoga, teachers adapt how they lead their classes to help participants build a sense of safety and control over their bodies. This approach is particularly important for people who have "disassociated" from their bodies after experiences of violence and trauma. There are no physical assists or touching in trauma-sensitive yoga. To minimize visual triggers, the lights are kept on, the curtains are drawn, and there are no mirrors. Teachers stay on their mats to avoid "lurking above" participants. Rather than offer direct instruction such as, "Put your hand on your hip," teachers offer an invitation to participants by saying, "If this feels good for you, I invite you to put your hand on your hip."

Although argued to increase safety, control, and resilience for people who are seeking services in relation to experiences of violence or have a history of experiencing violence (Government of Canada, 2018b), TVIA has also been criticized. Current expressions of this approach presume that trauma and violence are individual experiences rather than a collective experience. For example, many populations that disproportionately suffer from disasters such as a major flood, fire, or hurricane share a common experience that if viewed individually simply fails to capture how collective harm requires a different approach than individual harm. TVIA also provides very little insight into how we might address the root causes of trauma and violence in communities, families, and schools. If trauma is collectively experienced, this means that we must also consider the environmental context or the determinants that caused the harm in the first place. Additionally, using the concept of TVIA runs the risk of focusing on what's wrong with the individual (trauma), looking for symptoms and deficits, rather than recognizing symptoms as means of adaptation to stress. Reframing TVIA to a strengths-based approach is necessary to foster the possibility (well-being) of an individual's potential. **Positive psychology** offers insight into the limits of only "treating" symptoms and focuses on enhancing the conditions that contribute to well-being (Seligman, 2004). Without more careful consideration, trauma-informed approaches sometimes slip into rigid medical models of care that are steeped in treating the symptoms rather than strengthening the roots of well-being (Ginwright, 2018).

Population Interventions to Promote Mental Health

At a population level, strategies that create supportive environments, strengthen community action, develop personal skills, and reorient health services can help to ensure that the population has some control over the psychological and social determinants of mental health (Canadian Public Health Association & WHO, 1986). Mental Health in All Policies (MHiAP), a cross-sectoral approach, acknowledges that determinants of mental health often lie in nonhealth domains, such as social and family policies, labour policies, and education policies. MHiAP is an approach to public policies across sectors that systematically takes into account the health implications of decisions, seeks synergies, and avoids harmful health impacts in order to improve population health

and health equity. Although still a work in progress, the National Collaborating Centres are leading the way in moving this agenda forward in Canada.

Additionally, a whole-of-society approach goes beyond MHiAP to intersectoral partnerships that promote and enhance mental health. Engaging new stakeholders from across diverse sectors such as childcare, education, welfare, community, youth services, media, arts and culture, sports, urban design, local authorities, environment, and economic and social policies working together on promoting mental health supports a society to flourish. Poverty reduction is a promising intervention to promote mental health that can include a MHiAP and a whole-society approach. An example of an initiative to reduce poverty is through income security or having a sufficient income, which allows access to adequate housing, nutritious foods, safe communities, and participation in recreational, educational, and cultural opportunities, as well as other essentials for a healthy life, thus promoting mental health.

Interventions to Address Substance Use and Substance Use Disorders

Interventions to address the burden of substance use and substance use disorders are varied and can be thought about according to whether they address the issue at an individual level or a population level. Individual-level interventions typically occur on a one-to-one basis (and potentially in group settings) with the support of a community health worker or health care provider. Population-level interventions, on the other hand, work to shift norms and address environmental and policy challenges to support an overall move away from substance misuse and harm. In this section, population-level interventions are categorized according to the five Es of education, enforcement, environment, economics, and engineering.

Individual-Level interventions

A range of individual-level interventions exists for screening, diagnosing, and treating individuals with substance use disorders. Since the 1980s, screening tests (such as the AUDIT screening tool developed by the WHO and depicted in Fig. 9.5) have been validated and widely adopted to identify people who might have a substance use disorder diagnosis (Babor, Del Boca, & Bray, 2017). Often in primary care settings, screening is coupled with what is known as brief interventions. Brief

The Alcohol Use Disorders Identification Test: Interview Version

Read questions as written. Record answers carefully. Begin the AUDIT by saying "Now I am going to ask you some questions about your use of alcoholic beverages during this past year." Explain what is meant by "alcoholic beverages" by using local examples of beer, wine, vodka, etc. Code answers in terms of "standard drinks". Place the correct answer number in the box at the right.

1. How often do you have a drink containing alcohol?

   (0) Never [Skip to Qs 9–10]
   (1) Monthly or less
   (2) 2 to 4 times a month
   (3) 2 to 3 times a week
   (4) 4 or more times a week

2. How many drinks containing alcohol do you have on a typical day when you are drinking?

   (0) 1 or 2
   (1) 3 or 4
   (2) 5 or 6
   (3) 7, 8, or 9
   (4) 10 or more

3. How often do you have six or more drinks on one occasion?

   (0) Never
   (1) Less than monthly
   (2) Monthly
   (3) Weekly
   (4) Daily or almost daily

   Skip to Questions 9 and 10 if Total Score for Questions 2 and 3 = 0

4. How often during the last year have you found that you were not able to stop drinking once you had started?

   (0) Never
   (1) Less than monthly
   (2) Monthly
   (3) Weekly
   (4) Daily or almost daily

5. How often during the last year have you failed to do what was normally expected from you because of drinking?

   (0) Never
   (1) Less than monthly
   (2) Monthly
   (3) Weekly
   (4) Daily or almost daily

6. How often during the last year have you needed a first drink in the morning to get yourself going after a heavy drinking session?

   (0) Never
   (1) Less than monthly
   (2) Monthly
   (3) Weekly
   (4) Daily or almost daily

7. How often during the last year have you had a feeling of guilt or remorse after drinking?

   (0) Never
   (1) Less than monthly
   (2) Monthly
   (3) Weekly
   (4) Daily or almost daily

8. How often during the last year have you been unable to remember what happened the night before because you had been drinking?

   (0) Never
   (1) Less than monthly
   (2) Monthly
   (3) Weekly
   (4) Daily or almost daily

9. Have you or has someone else been injured as a result of your drinking?

   (0) No
   (2) Yes, but not in the last year
   (4) Yes, during the last year

10. Has a relative or friend or a doctor or another health care worker been concerned about your drinking or suggested you cut down?

    (0) No
    (2) Yes, but not in the last year
    (4) Yes, during the last year

Record total of specific items here

If total is greater than recommended cut-off, consult User's Manual.

Fig. 9.5 The AUDIT tool. (From National Institute on Drug Abuse. [2018]. *Audit* [p. 2]. Retrieved from https://www.drugabuse.gov/sites/default/files/files/AUDIT.pdf)

interventions often involve a health care provider providing the client with feedback about the risk of their behaviour, advice on how to reduce consumption, and setting goals together with the client regarding reducing consumption. Together, screening and brief interventions have shown much success when it comes to diagnosing and treating a range of substance use disorders (particularly alcohol) (Le et al., 2015).

After a diagnosis has been established, treatment may consist of medications (e.g., for opioid use disorders, substitution therapy with methadone or buprenorphine is used), counselling, group-based therapies (e.g., Alcoholics Anonymous), and detoxification (withdrawal in a supervised environment with the purpose of remaining abstinent), among others. It is important to understand and develop, along with clients, the goals of treatment. For some, the goal may include complete abstinence (not using again), but for others, it may involve a reduction in problematic or harmful use, also known as harm reduction.

Harm Reduction. **Harm reduction** is defined as an "evidence-based, client-centred approach that seeks to reduce the health and social harms associated with addiction and substance use, without necessarily requiring people who use substances from abstaining or stopping" (CMHA, 2018b). This nonjudgemental approach recognizes that complete abstinence is not possible, nor is it a desired goal, for some people. It shifts the focus towards ensuring that a person is safe when using and meets people where they are at in terms of their journey of use and recovery. When engaging people in this way, they are more likely to stay involved in treatment and often the harms associated with use (e.g., risk of overdose and acquisition of things such as hepatitis C or HIV) are reduced (CMHA, 2018b). One example of a successful, evidence-based harm-reduction intervention is the existence of supervised consumption facilities where people bring their substances to use under the supervision of trained professionals who can respond to overdoses; at the same time may receive some counselling, education, and referrals to other services and supports. Facilities such as these are opening across the country. Perhaps the best studied supervised consumption facility, Insite in Vancouver, has been open since 2003. Many studies evaluating Insite have found sites like this to be successful in terms of preventing overdose deaths, reducing health care costs, preventing bloodborne infections, and keeping people engaged in care (Young & Fairbairn,

2018). Other examples of harm-reduction interventions include needle exchange programs (to give people who inject drugs access to clean supplies to reduce bloodborne infection transmission) and using nicotine patches instead of smoking (CMHA, 2018b).

Harm reduction is recognized as a key pillar in terms of responding to the opioid crisis. In the Government of Canada's drugs and substances strategy, the four pillars for responding to the crisis are as follows:

1. Prevention (e.g., reducing opioid prescribing by providers, ensuring access to pain services)
2. Treatment (e.g., engaging people in opioid substitution therapy)
3. Harm reduction (e.g., needle exchange, supervised consumption facilities)
4. Enforcement (e.g., criminal justice interventions to curb use) (Government of Canada, 2018d).

Unfortunately, when it comes to both the opioid crisis and other drug use issues, much more attention is paid to interventions such as enforcement, harm reduction, and treatment; prevention efforts may be more limited in scope. In general, fewer one-on-one interventions exist for people at risk of substance use disorders or to address the risk factors that may lead to addictions later in life. As discussed earlier, some other interventions that could work on the individual level targeting risk factors include parenting programs and support, home visitation programs working to improve attachment and family relationships, and recovery-oriented approaches (see Case Study box). The challenge, however, is that in the face of an acute crisis such as the opioid issue, results are realized more immediately with treatment and harm-reduction actions.

CASE STUDY

A Recovery-Oriented Approach—The Role of Peer Support

Recognizing that substance use disorders are chronic ailments that require ongoing support, a recovery-oriented approach is often needed for achieving success. According to the Mental Health Commission of Canada, *recovery* refers to living a satisfying, hopeful, and contributing life; even when a person may be experiencing ongoing symptoms of a mental health problem or illness, recovery is not only possible but is also expected (MHCC, 2019). **Recovery-oriented approaches** are holistic (they address multiple needs of clients, including

CASE STUDY—cont'd

A Recovery-Oriented Approach—The Role of Peer Support

addressing the SDHs), self-directed (they allow people to take control over their healing and recovery), and person centred (they are based on the goals and values of the individual client) (Bassuk et al., 2016). These approaches espouse key values of community health, including empowerment and collaboration.

More and more, recovery-oriented approaches (in the areas of both mental health and substance use) are using peers, who are people with lived experience. Because peer workers have experiential knowledge about how substance use disorders affect one's life, they bring a unique and supportive perspective to someone who is trying to recover. These peers (who may be paid or unpaid) can work as "coaches" and operate as nonprofessional and nonclinical members of the interprofessional care team. Alcoholics Anonymous is one well-known example of this type of peer support program (Bassuk et al., 2016).

CRITICAL THINKING QUESTIONS 9.5: You are a health care provider who is working within a multidisciplinary team model in an inner-city context. Many of your patients are underhoused and have a low income. One of your clients is an older gentlemen who tells you that he suffers from alcoholism (and that it runs rampant in his family) but does not want to completely stop his use, just cut back.

Who among your multidisciplinary team members might you involve to support you in caring for this patient, and what might their roles be? How might you involve a peer worker, and what might the benefits of their involvement be?

Reflect on whether you are comfortable with this client's goals and how you might approach having a different view on what might be more effective (e.g., whether you believe abstinence programs might be more effective in reducing the harms associated with use).

Population-Based Interventions

Using the 5E approach, Table 9.1 provides some examples of evidence-based population-level interventions to minimize the burden of substance use and substance use disorders.

In general, education campaigns alone are of limited use. Although they may work to shift social norms over time, they must be coupled with other regulatory approaches that alter the environment and context of drug use.

In 2018, the entire policy context around the nonmedical (or recreational) use of cannabis shifted in Canada, and this presents a good example of how critical regulatory models are in influencing harms associated with substance use. There are three main models when it comes to the legal context of a substance: prohibition, decriminalization, and legalization.

Prohibition means that most aspects of a substance, including producing it, distributing it, and possessing it, are illegal and have associated criminal penalties (Jesseman & Payer, 2018). Many critics of prohibition as a regulatory approach point to the social harms associated with convicting people of nonviolent crimes such as simple possession. They argue that the criminal justice costs and lifelong harms that an individual with a criminal record incur do not outweigh any potential deterrence benefit from making substances illegal. Critics of prohibition also argue that substance use continues regardless of whether something is legal, and in the black market, products have no quality assurance. The recent emergence of fentanyl and carfentanil contaminated products are evidence of the potential harm associated with a completely unregulated black market.

Decriminalization, on the other hand, means that instead of issuing criminal penalties for the above activities, they are subject to warnings and fines (Jesseman & Payer, 2018). Often, decriminalization refers to applying fines and other noncriminal penalties to possession but leaving activities such as major trafficking in the criminal realm. Decriminalization addresses the issue of the social harms and criminal justice costs associated with convicting people of charges such as simple possession. However, it leaves substances in the black market, and the challenge of having an unregulated market with no quality assurance remains (Rehm, 2014). Several jurisdictions, including Portugal, have decriminalized the possession of small amounts of all drugs, including substances such as cocaine and heroin. Portugal, specifically, has invested in treatment and prevention activities at the same time and requires people who are found to be in possession of substances to appear before a panel that can refer the individual to treatment and other support services. This change in their regulatory framework has been shown to be associated with reduced social harms of substance use, reduced transmission of bloodborne infections,

TABLE 9.1	Applying the 5 Es Approach to Substance Use
Category	**Examples**
Education	• Awareness and social marketing campaigns regarding the harms of substance use
Environment	• Limiting the number and concentration of places where you can obtain substances (e.g., alcohol, tobacco) in a community
	• Locating retail outlets where you can obtain substances far away from schools, daycares, rehabilitation centres, and so on
	• Protecting the environment from secondhand smoke (limiting where people can consume various substances)
Enforcement	• Fines and criminal charges for possession, use, and trafficking of substances
	• Banning promotion of substances to those younger than a certain age
	• Minimum age of purchase of various substances (e.g., tobacco, alcohol minimum ages)
	• Prohibiting, legalizing, and decriminalizing various substances
Economics	• Raising taxes on legal products such as tobacco and alcohol to deter use
	• Imposing fines for use and consumption
Engineering	• Producing less harmful substances (e.g., vaping versus smoking)
	• Manufacturing products (e.g., opioids) that are less addictive or cannot be tampered with and misused as easily

and reduced costs to the criminal justice system. Interestingly, this model has not been shown to significantly increase drug use, as many people feared (Jesseman & Payer, 2018). Many in Canada have been calling for a similar approach to help reduce social harms and stigma associated with opioid use, but some say it doesn't go far enough to reduce harms, calling instead for legalization.

Legalization is the third regulatory option for substances. Under legalization, criminal sanctions are removed for most activities, and production and distribution can come out of the underground market and be regulated (Jesseman & Payer, 2018). This is the case for alcohol, tobacco, and now cannabis in Canada. The concern with regards to legalization is that use might increase. This issue will be studied in Canada extensively in the case of nonmedical cannabis use. Outside of Canada, Uruguay is the only other country that has, at a national level, legalized cannabis in 2017. Data from their experience are only now being analyzed and reported (Jesseman & Payer, 2018).

According to the Centre for Addiction and Mental Health (CAMH), the ideal regulatory state for cannabis is legalization, with strict regulation. Their model for cannabis, which may have applicability to other substances, is depicted in Fig. 9.6.

According to CAMH, legalization has the benefit of removing a substance from the black market and ensuring quality checks. Strict regulation can still exist to curb use. This would consist of interventions described earlier in Table 9.1, including limiting retail outlet density and putting strict controls on who can purchase a substance (e.g., minimum age), marketing to vulnerable people such as youths, limiting where a substance can be consumed (e.g., smoked), and so on (CAMH, 2014).

Through the Lens of the Social Determinants of Health. Regulatory approaches must be coupled with other mental health prevention and promotion efforts that target the root causes for why people engage in substance use and might be at risk for substance use disorders in the first place. One very interesting model for prevention of substance use at a population level is the **Icelandic model.** This community-based approach has its roots in the early 1990s and was developed by the Icelandic Centre for Social Research and Analysis (ICSRA), a not-for-profit research body. Working intersectorally, partners analyzed root causes for substance use in youth. The complex interplay of the SDHs were found to have an influence on substance use in youth, which included social support, parental support, and time spent with parents, in addition to participation in activities such as sports. As such, the goal of the model is to improve support from parents, schools, and the community at large to improve opportunities for youth in these areas and thus decrease substance use (Sigfúsdóttir et al., 2009).

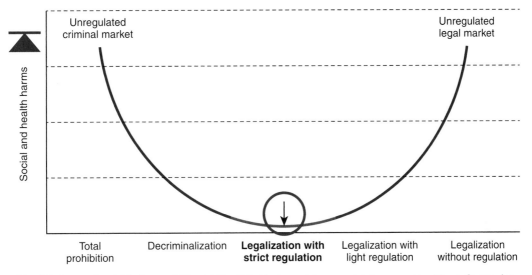

Fig. 9.6 Centre for Addiction and Mental Health's ideal regulatory model for cannabis. (From Centre for Addiction and Mental Health. [2014]. *Cannabis policy framework* [p. 11]. Retrieved from https://www.camh. ca/-/media/files/pdfs---public-policy-submissions/camhcannabispolicyframework-pdf.pdf?la=en&hash=25B17-3918327AA9FE4A11A5286B0B79495CE2797.%20P.11.)

Decreasing the barriers to accessing sports, such as giving adolescents a prepaid leisure time card so they have access to structured activities such as participation in sports teams, was one of the health promotion strategies they used in this model. Working in concert with health promotion strategies, the model also focuses on behaviour-change strategies such as media campaigns to warn about the negative effects of alcohol and tobacco use and to encourage parents to spend more time with their children (Reykjavik University, 2017). Data evaluating the initiative have shown that alcohol and tobacco use, as well as use of illicit substances, declined in youth between 1997 to 2007 (Sigfúsdóttir et al., 2009).

> **CRITICAL THINKING QUESTIONS 9.6:** Critics of community-based harm-reduction approaches often argue that harm-reduction programs (e.g., needle exchanges or supervised consumption facilities) promote substance use. Review some of the literature about this topic and develop key points that could be used to respond to this argument.
>
> Is there any validity to these claims? What does the evidence say? How might your answer differ when you specifically apply a public health, human rights, and ethical lens to this discussion?

SUMMARY

This chapter introduced readers to what is meant by mental health and mental health promotion; described the risk factors and burden of various mental health conditions on the population (including substance use disorders); and discussed strategies to reduce the burden and severity of mental health challenges, including high-risk substance use and substance use disorders, and promote positive mental health.

Mental health is as important to daily living as physical health and is a key determinant of overall health. Mental health is not merely the absence of mental health ailments, and it is possible for someone to have a mental health condition but still experience positive mental health. Mental illness, on the other hand, refers to specific ailments that affect thinking, mood, or behavior and are associated with significant distress and impaired functioning. Examples of mental illness include schizophrenia, generalized anxiety disorder, bipolar disorder, and substance use disorder. Mental illnesses are responsible for a large and measurable burden of illness in the Canadian population, more than all cancers combined.

A significant number of Canadians meet the criteria for substance use disorders at some point during their lives. Substance use disorders related to alcohol and cannabis are more common than other drugs. The frequent use of substances can lead to a range of chronic and mental health conditions. Tobacco and alcohol are two of the four main risk factors for a number of NCDs, including heart disease and cancer. Many other substances, legal and illegal, can result in substance use disorders and other mental health conditions. Substance use and substance use disorders can in some cases lead to increases in crime, community, and even intimate partner violence. Substance use can also result in the breakdown of families and devastation to communities that suffer trauma and constant loss because of people being affected by substance use disorders.

Although there are multiple approaches to addressing mental health and substance use, a primary focus is to address the SDHs. At the level of the individual, a sense of control, social support, and meaningful participation are important in helping to reduce stress, anxiety, burnout, and frustration. At a population level, strategies that create supportive environments, strengthen community action, develop personal skills, and reorient health services can help to ensure that the population has some control over the psychological and social determinants of mental health. Harm reduction is one approach that is used to reduce the health and social harms associated with addiction and substance use. Evidence-based population level interventions to minimize the burden of substance use and substance use disorders include the 5 Es approach.

KEY WEBSITES

Anxiety Canada (MindShift): https://www.anxietycanada.com/resources/mindshift-app
This application is aimed at teenagers and young adults. It provides resources and tools to support people in coping with anxiety, including helping people think differently about it, relax, and take other steps to address anxiety at its source.

Canadian Association of People Who Use Drugs (CAPUD): http://capud.ca.
CAPUD advocates for the engagement and inclusion of people who use drugs in the policy making process, with a guiding principle of: "Nothing About Us Without Us." CAPUD's website has a blog and a number of reports that describe harm reduction and inclusion.

Canadian Mental Health Association (CMHA): https://cmha.ca
The CHMA is a volunteer-based organization that provides supports and services to people with mental health challenges and their families and works to build resilience, enhance social and community integration, and support recovery for people living with mental illness.

Centre for Addiction and Mental Health (CAMH): http://www.camh.ca
CAMH is a major mental health teaching and research hospital affiliated with the University of Toronto, in addition to being a WHO collaborating centre. This organization engages in research, training, program planning, and implementation, as well as policy advocacy focused on mental health. Its website provides information on a range of mental illnesses as well as publications and reports.

REFERENCES

Alcohol Research UK. (2015). *Alcohol Research UK annual review 2015*. Retrieved from https://alcohol-change.org.uk/about-us/annual-report-and-accounts.

American Psychiatric Association. (2018). *DSM-5: Frequently asked questions*. Retrieved from https://www.psychiatry.org/psychiatrists/practice/dsm/feedback-and-questions/frequently-asked-questions.

Atlantis, E., Fahey, P., & Cochrane, B., et al. (2013). Bidirectional associations between clinically relevant depression or anxiety and COPD: A systematic review and meta-analysis. *Chest, 144*(3), 766–777.

Babor, T. F., Del Boca, F., & Bray, J. (2017). Screening, Brief Intervention and Referral to Treatment: Implications of SAMHSA's SBIRT initiative for substance abuse policy and practice. *Addiction, 112*(2), 110–117.

Bassuk, E. L., Hanson, J., Greene, R. N., et al. (2016). Peer-delivered recovery support services for addictions in the United States: A systematic review. *Journal of Substance Abuse Treatment, 63*, 1–9.

B.C. Coroners Service. (2018). *Illicit drug overdose deaths in B.C., January 1, 2008 to November 30, 2018*. Retrieved from https://www2.gov.bc.ca/assets/gov/birth-adoption-death-marriage-and-divorce/deaths/coroners-service/statistical/illicit-drug.pdf.

Bobrowski, D. (2018). Concurrent disorders: A case in point for improved interdisciplinary care between addictions and mental health systems in Canada. *University of Toronto Medical Journal, 95*(2), 54–56.

Bonomo, Y., & Proimos, J. (2005). Substance misuse: Alcohol, tobacco, inhalants, and other drugs. *BMJ, 330*, 777.

British Columbia Integrated Youth Services Initiative. (2015). *British Columbia Integrated Youth Services Initiative rationale and overview.* Retrieved from http://bciysi.ca/assets/downloads/bc-iysi-background-document.pdf.

Butler, A., Adair, C. E., Jones, W., et al. (2017). *Towards quality mental health services in Canada: A comparison of performance indicators across 5 provinces.* Vancouver: Centre for Applied Research in Mental Health & Addiction.

Canadian Centre on Substance Abuse. (2016). *Prescription stimulants.* Retrieved from http://www.ccsa.ca/Resource%20Library/CCSA-Canadian-Drug-Summary-Prescription-Stimulants-2016-en.pdf.

Canadian Institute for Health Information. (2013). *Hospital mental health services for concurrent mental illness and substance use disorders in Canada.* Retrieved from https://secure.cihi.ca/free_products/MH%20Concurrent%20Disorders%20AiB-ENweb.pdf.

Canadian Institute for Health Information. (2016). *Repeat hospital stays for mental illness.* Retrieved from https://yourhealthsystem.cihi.ca/hsp/inbrief?lang=en#!/indicators/007/repeat-hospital-stays-for-mental-illness/;mapC1;mapLevel2;/.

Canadian Mental Health Association. (2014). *Mental illness in children and youth.* Retrieved from https://cmha.bc.ca/documents/mental-illnesses-in-children-and-youth-2/.

Canadian Mental Health Association. (2018a). *Mental health promotion.* Retrieved from https://ontario.cmha.ca/documents/mental-health-promotion/.

Canadian Mental Health Association. (2018b). *Harm reduction.* Retrieved from https://ontario.cmha.ca/harm-reduction/.

Canadian Public Health Association & World Health Organization. (1986). *Ottawa Charter for Health Promotion.* Ottawa: Health and Welfare Canada.

Canadian Student Tobacco, Alcohol, and Drugs Survey. (2015). Ottawa: Health Canada. Retrieved from https://www.canada.ca/en/health-canada/services/canadian-student-tobacco-alcohol-drugs-survey.html.

Canadian Substance Use Costs and Harms Scientific Working Group. (2018). *Canadian substance use costs and harms (2007–2014).* (Prepared by the Canadian Institute for Substance Use Research and the Canadian Centre on Substance Use and Addiction.) Ottawa, ON: Canadian Centre on Substance Use and Addiction.

Central City Foundation. (2017). *On the front lines of the opioid crisis: How community organizations and their staff are coping.* Retrieved from https://www.centralcityfoundation.ca/wp-content/uploads/2017/12/CCF-Community-Report-2017_F3web.pdf.

Centre for Addiction and Mental Health. (2014). *Cannabis policy framework.* Retrieved from https://www.camh.ca/-/media/files/pdfs---public-policy-submissions/camhcannabispolicyframework-pdf.pdf?la=en&hash=25-B173918327AA9FE4A11A5286B0B79495CE2797.%20P.11.

City of Toronto. (n.d). *Continuum of use.* Retrieved from https://www.toronto.ca/community-people/health-wellness-care/health-programs-advice/overdose-prevention-and-response/get-support/continuum-of-use-2/.

Clarke, A. M., Kuosmanen, T., & Barry, M. M. (2015). A systematic review of online youth mental health promotion and prevention interventions. *Journal of Youth and Adolescence, 44*(1), 90–113.

Clement, S., Schauman, O., Graham, T., et al. (2015). What is the impact of mental health-related stigma on help-seeking? A systematic review of quantitative and qualitative studies. *Psychological Medicine, 45*(1), 11–27.

DeSilva, M., Samele, C., Saxena, S., et al. (2014). Policy actions to achieve integrated community-based mental health services. *Health Affairs, 33*(9), 1595–1602. https://doi.org/10.1377/hlthaff.2014.0365.

Dewa, C. S., Chau, N., & Dermer, S. (2010). Examining the comparative incidence and costs of physical and mental health-related disabilities in an employed population. *Journal of Occupational and Environmental Medicine, 52*(7), 758–762.

Donroe, J. H., Socias, M. E., & Marshall, B. D. L. (2018). The deepening opioid crisis in North America: Historical context and current solutions. *Curr Addict Rep*, 1–10.

Ginwright, S. (2018). *The future of healing: Shifting from trauma informed care to healing centered engagement.* Retrieved from https://medium.com/@ginwright/the-future-of-healing-shifting-from-trauma-informed-care-to-healing-centered-engagement-634f557ce69c.

Government of Canada. (2014). *Canadian alcohol and drug use monitoring survey—summary of results for 2012.* Retrieved from https://www.canada.ca/en/health-canada/services/health-concerns/drug-prevention-treatment/drug-alcohol-use-statistics/canadian-alcohol-drug-use-monitoring-survey-summary-results-2012.html.

Government of Canada. (2015). *Mental illness.* Retrieved from https://www.canada.ca/en/public-health/services/chronic-diseases/mental-illness.html.

Government of Canada. (2018a). *Youth mental health infographic.* Retrieved from https://www.canada.ca/en/services/health/publications/healthy-living/youth-mental-health-infographic.html.

Government of Canada. (2018b). *Trauma and violence informed approaches to policy and practice.* Retrieved from https://www.canada.ca/en/public-health/services/publications/health-risks-safety/trauma-violence-informed-approaches-policy-practice.html.

Government of Canada. (2018c). *Cannabis legalization and regulation*. Retrieved from http://www.justice.gc.ca/eng/cj-jp/cannabis/.

Government of Canada. (2018d). *Federal action on opioids*. Retrieved from https://www.canada.ca/en/health-canada/services/substance-use/problematic-prescription-drug-use/opioids/federal-actions.html.

Hawi, N., & Samaha, M. (2017). The relations among social media addiction, self-esteem, and life satisfaction in university students. *Social Science Computer Review, 35*(5) 676–586.

Health Canada. (2015). *Overview of Canada's Tobacco Strategy*. Retrieved from https://www.canada.ca/content/dam/hc-sc/documents/services/publications/healthy-living/canada-tobacco-strategy/overview-canada-tobacco-strategy-eng.pdf.

Jacobson, N. C., & Newman, M. G. (2017). Anxiety and depression as bidirectional risk factors for one another: A meta-analysis of longitudinal studies. *Psychological Bulletin, 143*(11), 1155.

Jenkins, E. K., Bungay, V., Patterson, A., et al. (2018). Assessing the impacts and outcomes of youth driven mental health promotion: A mixed-methods assessment of the Social Networking Action for Resilience study. *Journal of Adolescence, 67*, 1–11.

Jesseman, R., & Payer, D. (2018). *Decriminalization: Options and evidence*. Ottawa: Canadian Centre on Substance Use and Addiction. Retrieved from http://www.ccsa.ca/Resource%20Library/CCSA-Decriminalization-Controlled-Substances-Policy-Brief-2018-en.pdf

Keller, M. C. (2018). Evolutionary perspectives on genetic and environmental risk factors for psychiatric disorders. *Annual Review of Clinical Psychology, 14*, 471–493.

King, M., Smith, A., & Gracey, M. (2009). Indigenous health part 2: The underlying causes of the health gap. *Lancet, 374*(9683), 76–85.

Kõlves, K., Zhao, Q., Ross, V., et al. (2019). Suicide and other sudden death bereavement of immediate family members: An analysis of grief reactions six-months after death. *Journal of Affective Disorders, 243*, 96–102.

Le, K. B., Johnson, J. A., Seale, J. P., et al. (2015). Primary care residents lack comfort and experience with alcohol screening and brief intervention: A multi-site survey. *Journal of General Internal Medicine, 30*, 790.

Lewer, D., Meier, P., Beard, E., et al. (2016). Unravelling the alcohol harm paradox: a population-based study of social gradients across very heavy drinking thresholds. *BMC Public Health, 16*(1), 599.

Mahmoud, K. F., Finnell, D., Savage, C. L., et al. (2017). A concept analysis of substance misuse to inform contemporary terminology. *Archives of Psychiatric Nursing, 31*(6), 532–540.

Malla, A., Shah, J., Iyer, S., et al. (2018). Youth mental health should be a top priority for health care in Canada. *Canadian Journal of Psychiatry, 63*(4), 216–222.

Matheson, S. L., Shepherd, A. M., Laurens, K. R., et al. (2011). A systematic meta-review grading the evidence for non-genetic risk factors and putative antecedents of schizophrenia. *Schizophrenia Research, 133*(1–3), 133–142.

Meier, E., & Hatsukami, D. K. (2016). A review of the additive health risk of cannabis and tobacco co-use. *Drug and Alcohol Dependence, 166*, 6–12.

Mental Health Commission of Canada. (2010). *Making the case for investing in mental health in Canada*. Calgary: The Commission. Retrieved from https://www.mentalhealthcommission.ca/sites/default/files/2016-06/Investing_in_Mental_Health_FINAL_Version_ENG.pdf.

Mental Health Commission of Canada. (2015). *Caregiving*. Calgary: The Commission. Retrieved from http://www.mentalhealthcommission.ca/English/issues/caregiving.

Mental Health Commission of Canada. (2019). *What is recovery?* Calgary: The Commission. Retrieved from https://www.mentalhealthcommission.ca/English/what-we-do/recovery.

Mental Health First Aid. (2019). *Evaluated outcomes*. Retrieved from https://www.mhfa.ca/.

Merali, F. (2017). Crystal methamphetamine: The "elephant in the room" on Vancouver's downtown Eastside. *CBC News*. Retrieved from https://www.cbc.ca/news/canada/british-columbia/crystal-meth-increase-seven-fold-1.4404492

Monico, L. B., & Mitchell, S. G. (2018). Patient perspectives of transitioning from prescription opioids to heroin and the role of route of administration. *Substance Abuse Treatment, Prevention, and Policy, 13*(1), 4. https://doi.org/10.1186/s13011-017-0137-y.

Montgomery, L. (2015). Marijuana and tobacco use and co-use among African Americans: Results from the 2013, National Survey on Drug Use and Health. *Addictive Behaviors, 51*, 18–23.

O'Donnell, S., Vanderloo, S., McRae, L., et al. (2016). Comparison of the estimated prevalence of mood and/or anxiety disorders in Canada between self-report and administrative data. *Epidemiology and Psychiatric Sciences, 25*(4), 360–369.

Patel, V., Belkin, G. S., Chockalingam, A., et al. (2013). Grand challenges: Integrating mental health services into priority health care platforms. *Public Library of Science Medicine, 10*(5), e1001448. https://doi.org/10.1371/journal.pmed.1001448.

Patten, S. B. (2017). Age of onset of mental disorders. *Canadian Journal of Psychiatry/Revue Canadienne de Psychiatrie, 62*(4), 235.

Pearson, C., Janz, T., & Ali, J. (2015). *Health at a glance: Mental and substance use disorders in Canada*. Ottawa: Statistics Canada. Retrieved from https://www150.statcan.gc.ca/n1/pub/82-624-x/2013001/article/11855-eng.htm.

Potenza, M. (2015). Perspective: Behavioural addictions matter. *Nature, 522*, S62.

Power, R. A., Verweij, K. J., Zuhair, M., et al. (2014). Genetic predisposition to schizophrenia associated with increased use of cannabis. *Molecular Psychiatry, 19*(11), 1201.

Public Health Agency of Canada. (2014). *The Chief Public Health Officer's Report on the State of Public Health in Canada 2014: The health and well-being of Canadians. Appendix A*. Retrieved from https://www.canada.ca/en/public-health/corporate/publications/chief-public-health-officer-reports-state-public-health-canada/chief-public-health-officer-report-on-state-public-health-canada-2014-public-health-future/appendix-a.html.

Public Health Agency of Canada. (2016). *Suicide and self-inflicted injury hospitalizations in Canada (1979 to 2014/15): HPCDP: Volume 36-11, November 2016*. Retrieved from https://www.canada.ca/en/public-health/services/reports-publications/health-promotion-chronic-disease-prevention-canada-research-policy-practice/vol-36-no-11-2016/suicide-self-inflicted-injury-hospitalizations-canada-1979-2014-15.html

Public Health Agency of Canada. (2018). *The chief public health officer's report on the state of public health in Canada 2018: Preventing problematic substance use in youth*. Retrieved from https://www.canada.ca/content/dam/phac-aspc/documents/corporate/publications/chief-public-health-officer-reports-state-public-health-canada/2018-preventing-problematic-substance-use-youth/2018-preventing-problematic-substance-use-youth.pdf.

Rehm, J. (2014). *CAMH's cannabis policy framework: Legalization with regulation*. Toronto: Centre for Addiction and Mental Health. Retrieved from https://www.camh.ca/en/camh-news-and-stories/camhs-cannabis-policy-framework-legalization-with-regulation

Reykjavik University. (2017). *The world could learn from the "Icelandic Model."* Retrieved from https://en.ru.is/news/every-single-country-could-learn-from-the-icelandic-model.

Rotterman, M., & Page, M. (2018). *Prevalence and correlates of non-medical only compared to self-defined medical and non-medical cannabis use, Canada, 2015*. Ottawa: Statistics Canada. Retrieved from https://www150.statcan.gc.ca/n1/pub/82-003-x/2018007/article/00001-eng.htm.

Saha, S., Chant, D., Welham, J., et al. (2005). A systematic review of the prevalence of schizophrenia. *PLoS Medicine, 2*(5), e141.

Sealy, P., & Whitehead, P. C. (2004). Forty years of deinstitutionalization of psychiatric services in Canada: An empirical assessment. *Canadian Journal of Psychiatry, 49*(4), 249–257.

Seligman, M. E. (2004). *Authentic happiness: Using the new positive psychology to realize your potential for lasting fulfillment*. New York: Simon and Schuster.

Shah, T. I., Milosavljevic, S., & Bath, B. (2017). Measuring geographical accessibility to rural and remote health care services: Challenges and considerations. *Spatial and Spatio-Temporal Epidemiology, 21*, 87–96.

Sigfúsdóttir, I. D., Thorlindsson, T., Kristjánsson, A. L., et al. (2009). Substance use prevention for adolescents: The Icelandic model. *Health Promotion International, 24*(1), 16–25.

Sinha, M. (2013). *Portrait of caregivers 2012*. Statistics Canada Catalogue no. 89-652-X-No.001. Ottawa. Industry Canada. Retrieved from http://www.statcan.gc.ca/pub/89-652-x/89-652-x2013001-eng.pdf

Slaunwhite, A. K., Ronis, S. T., Sun, Y., et al. (2017). The emotional health and well-being of Canadians who care for persons with mental health or addictions problems. *Health & Social Care in the Community, 25*(3), 840–847.

Smetanin, P., Stiff, D., Briante, C., et al. (2011). *The life and economic impact of major mental illnesses in Canada: 2011 to 2041*. Toronto: RiskAnalytica, on behalf of the Mental Health Commission of Canada.

Statistics Canada. (2016). *Heavy drinking 2016*. Retrieved from https://www150.statcan.gc.ca/n1/pub/82-625-x/2017001/article/54861-eng.htm.

Statistics Canada. (2017). *Suicide rates: An overview*. Retrieved from https://www150.statcan.gc.ca/n1/pub/82-624-x/2012001/article/11696-eng.htm.

Statistics Canada. (2018). *Deaths and age-specific mortality rates, by selected grouped causes, Canada, 2016 (Table: 13-10-0392-01)*. Ottawa: Author.

Stein, D. J., Aguilar-Gaxiola, S., Alonso, J., et al. (2014). Associations between mental disorders and subsequent onset of hypertension. *General Hospital Psychiatry, 36*(2), 142–149.

Stuart, H., Chen, S.-P., Christie, R., et al. (2014). Opening minds in Canada: Background and rationale. *Canadian Journal of Psychiatry, 59*(suppl 1), 8–12. https://doi.org/10.1177/070674371405901S04.

Substance Abuse and Mental Health Services Administration. (2015). *Substance use disorders*. Retrieved from https://www.samhsa.gov/disorders/substance-use.

Survey on Living with Chronic Diseases in Canada. (2014). *Mood and anxiety disorders in Canada: Fast facts from the 2014 Survey on Living with Chronic Diseases in Canada*. Retrieved from http://www.canada.ca/en/public-health/services/publications/disease-conditions/mood-anxiety-disorders-canada.html.

Todd, Z. (2017). *Reports of crystal meth use in Alberta nearly triple in five years, AHS says*. CBC News. Retrieved from https://www.cbc.ca/news/canada/edmonton/alberta-methamphetamine-crystal-meth-drugs-rcmp-health-1.4295331.

Turecki, G., & Brent, D. A. (2015). Suicide and suicidal behaviour. *Lancet*, *387*(10024), 1227–1239.

While, D., Bickley, H., Roscoe, A., et al. (2012). Implementation of mental health service recommendations in England and Wales and suicide rates, 1997–2006: a cross-sectional and before-and-after observational study. *Lancet*, *379*(9820), 1005–1012.

World Health Organization. (2001). *The World health report: 2001: Mental health: New understanding, new hope*. Geneva: World Health Organization. Retrieved from http://www.who.int/whr/2001/chapter4/en/index2.html.

World Health Organization. (2014). *Mental health: A state of well-being*. Retrieved from http://www.who.int/features/factfiles/mental_health/en/.

Young, S., & Fairbairn, N. (2018). Expanding supervised injection facilities across Canada: Lessons from the Vancouver experience. *Canadian Journal of Public Health*, *109*(2), 227–230.

Zalsman, G., Hawton, K., Wasserman, D., et al. (2016). Suicide prevention strategies revisited: 10-year systematic review. *The Lancet Psychiatry*, *3*(7), 646–659.

Zatti, C., Rosa, V., Barros, A., et al. (2017). Childhood trauma and suicide attempt: A meta-analysis of longitudinal studies from the last decade. *Psychiatry Research*, *256*, 353–358.

Communicable Diseases

Ⓔ Additional resources are available online at http://evolve.elsevier.com/Canada/Shah/publichealth/

LEARNING OBJECTIVES

- Define key terms in the field of communicable disease control, including *attack rate, secondary attack rate, infectivity, pathogenicity, virulence, period of communicability,* and *incubation period.*
- List the main modes of transmission of microorganisms.
- Describe an approach to managing a communicable disease outbreak.
- List the benefits of vaccinations and describe the infrastructure for vaccines in Canada.
- Be familiar with some of the epidemiological trends, morbidity and mortality, and equity considerations,

as well as public health control measures for communicable diseases of concern in Canada, including sexually transmitted and bloodborne infections.
- Describe drivers of the rise in antimicrobial-resistant organisms.
- List two emerging, vector-borne diseases in Canada and be familiar with some factors leading to their spread.
- Define *bioterrorism* and list the pathogens most at risk of being used in bioterrorism events

CHAPTER OUTLINE

KEY TERMS

additional precautions
agent–host–environment
airborne transmission
antimicrobial resistance
antimicrobial stewardship
attack rate
bioterrorism
carrier
case fatality rate
cold chain
common source outbreak
communicable disease
communicable period
continuous common source
    outbreak
direct transmission

elimination
emerging infectious diseases
    (EIDs)
endemic
epidemic
epidemic curves
eradication
extinction
generation time
harm-reduction strategies
herd immunity
incubation period
indirect transmission
isolation
nosocomial infections
notifiable disease

outbreak
pandemic
pathogenicity rate
point source outbreak
propagated outbreak
quarantine
reportable disease
reservoir
routine precautions
secondary attack rate
transmission
vaccine hesitancy
vector-borne transmission
vehicle-borne transmission
vertical transmission
virulence

INTRODUCTION

Communicable disease is defined as an illness caused by a specific infectious agent or its toxic products that arises through transmission of that agent or its products from an infected person, animal, or reservoir to a susceptible host, either directly or indirectly, through an intermediate plant or animal host, vector, or the inanimate environment (Last, 2001). The beginning of the 20th century was characterized by a progressive decline in morbidity and mortality from communicable diseases in high-income countries. However, since the last two decades of the 20th century, there has been a rise in emerging and re-emerging infectious diseases; human immunodeficiency virus (HIV), Lyme disease, West Nile virus (WNV), outbreaks of viral hemorrhagic fevers (Ebola), Zika virus, hantavirus, syphilis, and tuberculosis represent examples of the new challenges to population health. Outbreaks of plague in India underscore the failure of health care systems to manage previously well-controlled diseases. Outbreaks of strains of tuberculosis that resist multiple drugs and vancomycin-resistant enterococci (VRE) have raised the spectre of bacteria not susceptible to conventional antibiotics. This prospect was inconceivable in 1967, when the US Surgeon General William H. Stewart decreed that the war against infectious agents had been won. Outbreaks of *Escherichia coli (E. coli)*, the importation of WNV,

severe acute respiratory syndrome (SARS), and anthrax (as a weapon of bioterrorism) in the United States further highlight the importance of infectious diseases.

The reasons for the persistence and emergence of new communicable diseases are as broad as the determinants of health. Behavioural factors, poverty, war, immigration, environmental degradation, health care–associated infections (i.e., diseases that result from interactions with our health care system), and increased international travel figure prominently in the causal underpinnings.

Not only do the social determinants of health (SDHs; described extensively in Chapter 5) explain the persistence and emergence of some communicable diseases, but they also underlie many of the health inequities we see in this area. For example, research from Manitoba has highlighted that the rates of infection with influenza (i.e., the "flu") are 12 times higher for Indigenous children than they are for non-Indigenous children (Clow, n.d.). When analyzing statistics such as this, we need to be mindful of why this inequity exists and, more specifically, which social determinants of health may explain such a gap. It has been theorized that poor housing conditions, greater exposure to indoor air pollution (described in Chapter 11), and a higher prevalence of chronic diseases (e.g., asthma or diabetes), which put one at risk for serious complications if one develops the flu, may help explain the higher rates of influenza among Indigenous children in Manitoba. Furthermore, inequitable access to these key SDHs (e.g., good housing, clean air) are ultimately a result of government policy that promoted colonialism and intergenerational trauma experienced by Indigenous people as a result of the residential schooling system (Clow, n.d.). Inequities such as these are highlighted throughout this chapter, and reasons for the inequities are touched upon. Readers are encouraged to apply an equity lens when reading through the statistics and to critically think about what can be done as partners and providers in our health system to remedy these inequities. For example, a clinic or hospital should be encouraged to think about how accessible their institution is for everyone, what they can do to assist certain groups that need it the most (e.g., extend open hours into the evening for those who work and cannot miss days because of financial constrictions, ensure that printed materials are available in other languages for new Canadians, ensure the space being used is accessible for people with mobility restrictions), and how they can partner with other sectors to advocate for policies that improve the SDHs across the population (e.g., provide better income support or a travel allowance for people to get to their providers to receive an influenza vaccine). These interventions become even more important as we think about the risks of new and emerging communicable diseases (e.g., Lyme disease).

Despite the fears and extensive publicity given to emerging communicable diseases, the traditional principles of communicable disease control remain effective, but they do require the application of an equity lens. In Canada, immunization programs, for example, have significantly decreased the incidence of many communicable diseases. However, discrepancies still exist in terms to who gets vaccinated. For example, a Saskatchewan-based study highlighted the fact that in low-income neighbourhoods, child immunization coverage rates were approximately half of what they were in high-income, affluent neighbourhoods (Lemstra et al., 2008). This example draws attention to some of the barriers that people living with low income experience in terms of getting to a provider to receive a vaccine (e.g., transport, parking, and taking time off of work can be significant barriers for some) and some of the ways our control measures must be adjusted to ensure accessibility for those who are most at risk.

Similarly, infection control, good hygiene, timely surveillance, and outbreak management remain essential components of the public health response to communicable diseases, and we must be mindful of equity challenges in each of these interventions as well. For example, public health agencies may recommend the closing of schools or daycares in cases when there are large-scale outbreaks in a school or childcare facility, or more commonly, they may recommend that students experiencing signs or symptoms of a communicable disease stay home. Although such measures may help to curb the outbreak or prevent spread, they may also worsen inequities because these types of closures have been shown to have a worse effect on people who are low-income earners compared with higher income earners (Clow, n.d.).

BASIC CONCEPTS AND TERMINOLOGY OF COMMUNICABLE DISEASE CONTROL

A **notifiable** or **reportable disease** is disease deemed to be of sufficient importance to public health to require that its occurrence be reported to public health officials (Last, 2001). All provinces and territories mandate reporting of certain communicable diseases. For example, like many other provinces, Nova Scotia requires by law that health care providers (including nurses, laboratory technicians, and physicians) report cases of communicable diseases, including rabies, measles, and gonorrhea, among others. Nationally there exists a list of notifiable diseases as well; however, reporting to the federal level is not mandatory (i.e., it is not required by law). As will be seen in Part III of this book, this is because health care is primarily a provincial or territorial responsibility.

Mandatory reporting is essential because it gives public health authorities the knowledge about which cases exist where and when a disease is being reported in higher amounts than normal, signalling the potential existence of an outbreak.

This type of investigation and control of communicable diseases (contagious or infectious diseases) requires some knowledge of the spectrum of infectious diseases and the relevant terminology. The spectrum of communicable disease is illustrated by Fig. 10.1.

Public health practitioners and researchers can characterize the threat of an offending organism by calculating several rates. The **attack rate** is the total number of

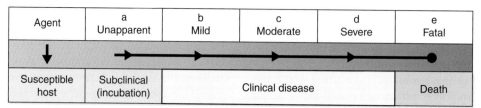

Fig. 10.1 Spectrum of infectious disease.

people who developed clinical disease divided by the population at risk (a + b + c + d + e), usually expressed as a percentage. In Fig. 10.1, therefore, the attack rate can be derived by (b + c + d + e)/(population at risk). The **secondary attack rate** is the number of contacts (e.g., household contacts or people that share a work-space) who were exposed to the primary case that developed disease within the incubation period in relation to the total exposed contacts. The denominator is thus restricted to the number of susceptible contacts that can be ascertained. This is often used to gauge contagiousness and evaluate disease control measures. The Case Study box presents a hypothetical example and a short exercise related to attack rates.

CASE STUDY

Escherichia coli at a Summer Camp

Fifty children attended a summer camp where they were served leafy greens that were contaminated with *E. coli*, a bacteria that typically causes diarrhea and stomach cramps and can lead to serious complications like kidney failure in children. Of the 40 children who ate the leafy greens, 32 got sick with fever, diarrhea, and abdominal cramping and returned home to their families.

Exercise
1. Calculate the attack rate.
2. What does this suggest?

Although the terms *infectivity, pathogenicity,* and *virulence* are often used interchangeably, they actually mean very different things. *Infectivity* refers to how easily a disease establishes infection in a person (with or without causing the person actual clinical symptoms). **Pathogenicity rate** describes the power of an organism to produce clinical disease in those who are infected (because not all who are infected will experience signs and symptoms and actually be sick); this is expressed as (b + c + d + e)/(a + b + c + d + e). **Virulence** describes

the severity of disease produced by the organism in a given host and is expressed as a ratio of the number of cases of severe and fatal infection to the total number clinically infected, or (d + e)/(b + c + d + e). The **case fatality rate** is one way to describe virulence and is the proportion of persons contracting the disease who die of it, namely e/(b + c + d + e).

A **reservoir** of infection is a person, animal, or inani-

> **EXERCISE 10.1:** Fill in the blanks below with the correct term that applies (infectivity, pathogenicity, or virulence):
> 1. Rabies has a high _____ rate because almost everyone who is infected with rabies actually dies of it.
> 2. Chlamydia has a low _____ rate because many people who harbour the infection do not have any signs or symptoms.

mate object in which infectious agents can live and multiply for extended periods of time. **Transmission** of microorganisms occurs by various means or from one host (human or animal) to another. **Direct transmission** involves the transfer of infectious agents directly from one host to another; for example, the common cold can be transmitted from person to person by one individual coughing or sneezing near others, causing droplets with the virus to land on the mucous membranes (eyes or mouth) of other susceptible hosts. **Indirect transmission** can occur through a vehicle (e.g., inanimate object), vector (e.g., organism), or the air—for example, someone with the common cold touches a doorknob and then another susceptible person touches that doorknob immediately afterwards and subsequently rubs their eyes. In **vehicle-borne transmission**, organisms are spread via inanimate materials, objects, or media (e.g., toys, clothes, milk, food). **Vector-borne transmission** may be mechanical (e.g., simple carriage of agents by animals) or biological (e.g., organisms multiplying inside insects). Malaria is an example of biological transmission of parasites from mosquito vectors to human hosts. **Airborne transmission** may occur via small droplet nuclei or dust particles suspended in the air. With airborne transmission, contacts are usually defined as anyone who has shared airspace with an infected person. The term *droplet transmission* is also used at times. Droplets are larger particles that typically fall to the ground quickly versus remaining suspended in the air. They can be projected up to a distance of 1 m through sneezing, coughing, singing, and so on. However, droplets are still thought of as being transmitted, either directly or indirectly.

A **carrier** is defined as an individual who harbours a specific infectious agent, usually without overt clinical disease. A carrier state may be of long or short duration, and it may serve as a potential source of infection because the person can pass it on to others without even realizing they themselves are sick

The **communicable period** is the time during which an infectious agent may be transferred from an infected person or vector to another host. **Generation time** is the interval between the entry of infection into the host and its maximal infectivity. **Incubation period** is the interval between infection by an agent and the appearance of the first symptom of the disease. Often generation time is equivalent to the incubation period. It is important to keep in mind that a person's communicable period may overlap with their incubation period. In this scenario, the individual has an established infection that can be passed on to others, but they themselves are not showing any clinical evidence of disease. They do not feel sick, so will continue going about their day-to-day activities, unknowingly putting others at risk. This often happens for diseases such as influenza, which can be transmitted to others in the days before a person actually becomes sick from the infection.

> Research a bit about the impact of SARS in Canada. Besides morbidity and mortality, what other societal impacts did this disease have on Canada as a whole?

Outbreaks of Infectious Diseases

An **outbreak** of disease is the occurrence of new cases clearly in excess of the baseline, or normally expected, frequency of the disease in a defined community or institutional population over a given period of time. An **epidemic** has a synonymous definition, although in common parlance, an outbreak usually means an epidemic that is localized, of acute onset, or relatively short in duration. One of the most notable examples of an outbreak that occurred in Canada was SARS in 2003, when 44

people died and about 400 people became ill. Less publicized are the outbreaks of diseases of moderate morbidity for the general population but of more severe morbidity for those already compromised in health, such as influenza among nursing home residents or viral gastroenteritis among infants and children in day care.

Two other terms are worth noting: endemic and pandemic. **Endemic** refers to the constant presence of a disease or infectious agent within a given geographic area or population subgroup. **Pandemic** refers to an epidemic occurring over a wide area, crossing international boundaries, and affecting a large number of people. For example, in 2009, the H1N1 strain of influenza was referred to as pandemic influenza because it crossed international boundaries and affected people throughout the world in large numbers, beyond what was expected.

An infectious disease outbreak investigation requires steps to establish the outbreak's existence, cause, risk factors, and modes of transmission, as well as develop, evaluate, and refine hypotheses using epidemiological methods (Centers for Disease Control and Prevention [CDC], 2016). The control of the outbreak can then be achieved by removing or neutralizing the agent, strengthening the resistance of the host, and interrupting the means of transmission in the environment. Thus, the **agent–host–environment** triad (mentioned in Chapter 1) applies. In addition, the outbreak control response must incorporate appropriate communication and sensitivity to public perceptions of risk, which may differ from expert opinions (see Chapter 3 for risk communication).

Epidemic curves, visual depictions of the number of cases of disease over time, are often used in outbreak investigations. The epidemic curve is constructed as a histogram with the number of cases plotted on the vertical axis and their dates or times of onset along the horizontal axis. The epidemic curve can visually indicate whether the outbreak has a common (or point) source or whether it is propagated. In a **common source outbreak**, individuals become ill because of exposure to a single (common) source of infection; the exposure may be of long or short duration. A **point source outbreak** is a type of common source outbreak of short exposure duration, with the number of cases rising and falling acutely because of short-term exposure to the infectious source, such as food poisoning in a group of persons eating the same contaminated item at a picnic. Hence, the epidemic curve would show a single, sharp peak (Fig. 10.2A). A **continuous common source outbreak** refers to an outbreak

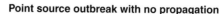

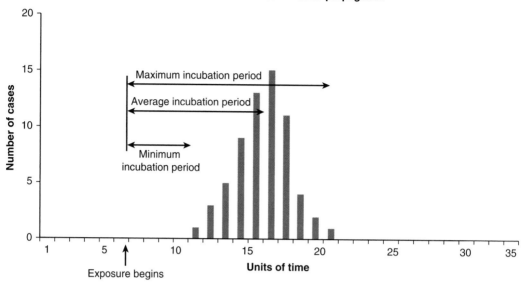

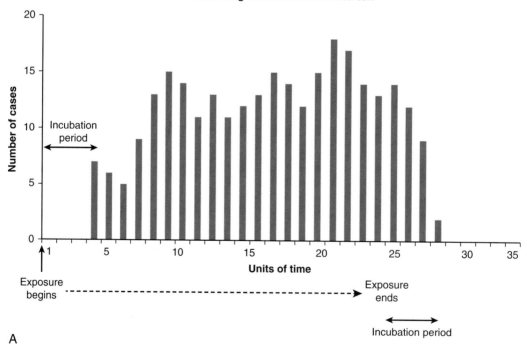

A

Fig. 10.2 A–C, Epidemiological curves. (McDowell, I. [2019]. *Epidemic curves*. Retrieved from http://www.med.uottawa.ca/sim/data/public_health_epidemic_curves_e.htm.)

Point source with index case and limited spread

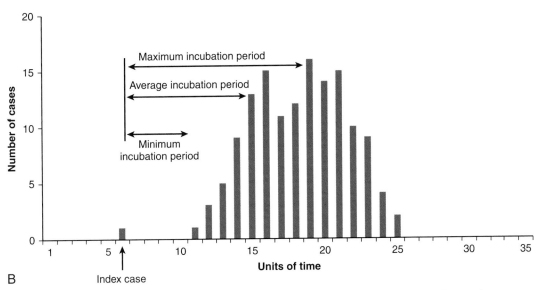

B

Disseminated outbreak originating from an index case with propagated spread

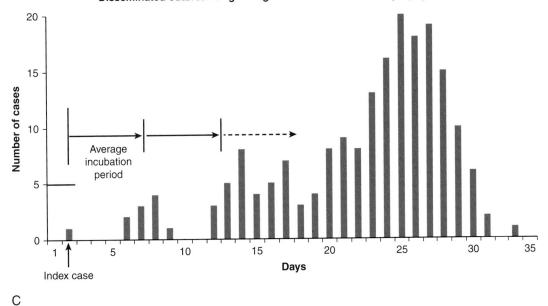

C

Fig. 10.2, cont'd

where the exposure or source of contamination is ongoing (e.g., contaminated water that people keep using over a long period of time). This type of outbreak may resemble the curve of a point source outbreak (with a rapid rise), but the peak of the curve lasts beyond one incubation period because the exposure is ever-present (Fig. 10.2B). A **propagated outbreak** may begin with only a few exposed persons but is maintained by person-to-person transmission. The epidemic curve will generally show a series of peaks (Fig. 10.2C). Norovirus infection is a good example of a gastrointestinal virus that is very easily spread from person to person, and thus in an outbreak situation, the epi curve would likely be in the shape of a propagated outbreak. When the preliminary analysis has the infectious disease risk factor(s) of interest, further investigation (e.g., case control studies) can help define the likely cause and disease transmission pattern, as described in Chapter 2.

Implementation of Initial Control Measures

Depending on the symptoms, the suspected agent, the population at risk, and the location, initial control measures will be adopted. These may include isolation of residents in a facility, augmented hand washing and cleaning, cohort nursing (using the same nursing staff in an institution for cases for the duration of the outbreak), exclusion of symptomatic staff, immunization (e.g., for influenza or measles), prophylactic medication for those exposed or at risk (e.g., antibiotics for meningococcal disease), withdrawal of contaminated food from distribution, or issuance of a boil-water advisory.

> **EXERCISE 10.2:** As mentioned in the chapter introduction, excluding children with signs and symptoms of a communicable disease from school or daycare or closing down such a facility in the event of a widespread outbreak to control the outbreak may negatively impact low-income families more than it would impact high-income families. Can you think of reasons why this might be true?

Outbreaks of **nosocomial infections** (i.e., those acquired during stay in a health care facility) require an *outbreak management team* to coordinate the efforts of many departments—such as housekeeping, maintenance, dietary, nursing, and medical staff—in implementing investigation and control measures.

Depending on the cause of the outbreak and the mode of transmission, specific control measures (e.g., immunization or specific improvements in the processes of food preparation) may be implemented.

A number of organizations have summarized the steps of an outbreak investigation and response. Most of them follow a similar set of steps, which include the following:

- Confirm the existence of an outbreak and the diagnosis.
- Assemble an outbreak team.
- Implement immediate control measures.
- Formulate a case definition as well as a line listing.

- Describe the outbreak in terms of person, place, and time (epidemiological curve).
- Conduct active surveillance to find other cases and identify those at risk.
- Generate and test hypothesis regarding the causative agent.
- Declare the outbreak over.
- Debrief the team and stakeholders, as needed (write a written report).

Although these steps are listed in sequence, in reality, many of the steps can occur at the same time, although the priority actions are always confirming the diagnosis and presence of an outbreak, implementing control measures, and creating a case definition and line list.

> **CRITICAL THINKING QUESTION 10.1:** Imagine you are a health care practitioner working at a small multi-disciplinary clinic whose clients include a high proportion of young women of reproductive age. You learn that cases of Zika virus infection are not legally mandated to be reported to public health agencies in many provinces and territories, even though many have argued for mandatory reporting of this novel virus.
>
> Refer to Canadian resources on Zika virus to better understand its epidemiology, clinical presentation (including complications), and interventions to limit its spread. Equipped with this understanding, consider some of the advantages and drawbacks of making Zika virus reportable by law. Is this something you and your team would advocate for to your provincial Ministry of Health?

IMMUNIZATION

Immunization remains the most important factor in the prevention of infectious disease. Its success in reducing morbidity and mortality from infectious diseases is unrivalled by any other medical intervention, both in terms of health benefits and cost effectiveness (Rémy, Zöllner, & Heckmann, 2015).

This effectiveness depends not only on the efficacy of individual vaccines but also on the degree of population coverage achieved. A very efficacious vaccine may exist, but if members of the public are reluctant to get it, the vaccination program will not be effective. For example, in 2006, many provinces and territories decided to publicly fund and deliver vaccination programs against human papilloma virus (HPV), a very common sexually transmitted infection (STI) that can lead to the development of various cancers. However, a recent pooled analysis showed that the uptake among the general Canadian population was only about 56% (Bird et al., 2017), meaning that the full benefit of vaccinating the public against this cancer-causing infection has still not been realized.

There are many reasons that may explain this reluctance, including the high cost of the vaccine (because many provinces and territories only publicly fund the vaccine for certain age cohorts), miseducation regarding whether the vaccine promotes promiscuity (given it is sexually transmitted), the required number of doses needed to achieve protection, and barriers to accessing health care for some groups. Vaccine uptake is very important because vaccines not only benefit the individual who receives the vaccine but can also have protective effects for the population as a whole (including those who may not have received the vaccine). This concept is known as **herd immunity** and is related to the fact that when a certain coverage is reached, a disease is much less likely to spread in a population because so many people are vaccinated against it and therefore cannot get sick and continue propagating the disease. As a result, people who may not be able to get the vaccine because of medical reasons (i.e., their immune systems are too compromised or they are pregnant) are still protected. For herd immunity to take effect, a certain percentage of the population needs to have received the vaccine. This percentage varies from disease to disease. The more communicable a disease is, the greater the number of people who need to be vaccinated for herd immunity to be realized.

Another factor that influences effectiveness is adherence with the vaccination schedule. For vaccines requiring multiple doses, compliance may be an issue because people forget to come in to finish the series. Hepatitis B and HPV-9 vaccine are examples of vaccines that require multiple doses, administered months apart.

Lastly, how easy it is for the cold chain to be maintained for a particular vaccine will also affect its effectiveness. **Cold chain** refers to all of the processes that ensure a vaccine is transported, stored, and handled optimally along the pathway from manufacturer to client (Public Health Agency of Canada [PHAC], 2015). For example, a vaccine that is to be refrigerated must always be maintained between 2° and 8°C, and many vaccines (particularly live ones, e.g., measles vaccine) should be protected from light. Detailed guidelines are available to health care providers and manufacturers alike on maintaining cold chain.

Vaccine hesitancy is a growing problem in Canada and other high-income countries and was named by the World Health Organization (WHO) as being among the top 10 threats to global health in 2019 (WHO, n.d.). **Vaccine hesitancy** is defined as a "delay in acceptance or refusal of vaccines despite availability of vaccine services" (Strategic Advisory Group of Experts [SAGE] Working Group on Vaccine Hesitancy, 2014). Although the majority of Canadian parents do vaccinate their children, a growing proportion are skeptical about safety and efficacy of vaccines and thus are choosing not to vaccinate, selectively vaccinate, or simply delay vaccination (Dubé et al., 2018). In a 2018 survey of parents, about 15% of parents did not vaccinate their children according to the recommended vaccine schedule in the province or territory where they lived (Dubé et al., 2018).

Vaccine hesitancy is a very complex phenomenon, and parents may be hesitant for a variety of reasons, including religious, cultural, or philosophical ones. The WHO has endorsed a way of conceptualizing vaccine hesitancy, known as the 3 C model (SAGE Working Group on Vaccine Hesitancy, 2014). In this model, vaccine hesitancy is described as being the result of three main factors: *confidence* (e.g., a lack of trust in the safety and efficacy of vaccines and the systems and policy makers that deliver them), *complacency* (parents believe the risk of developing a vaccine preventable disease is low and therefore that vaccinating is not necessary), and *convenience* (which speaks to the barriers parents may face in getting a vaccine administered, e.g., getting time off work, costs of travel to a clinic, affordability of the vaccine itself).

The issue of vaccine hesitancy cannot be taken lightly. Groups of people who don't believe in vaccinations (often referred to as "anti-vaxxers") have taken to social media to promote their message, share information, and encourage others to be skeptical and delay or refuse vaccination. This has had an enormous impact on population health (Jackson, Fraser, & Ash, 2014). Communities that are vaccine hesitant have seen outbreaks of preventable diseases as well as unnecessary fatalities from those diseases. This issue must be monitored and addressed by health care providers (working one on one with clients) and by public health professionals through education and awareness raising and, in some cases, enforcing legislation (see the In the News Box for an example of such legislation in the Ontario context).

The Immunization of School Pupils Act

In 1982, Ontario became the first province in Canada to enact legislation that required school-aged children to be vaccinated against specific diseases. The *Immunization of School Pupils Act (ISPA)* requires that all children (ages 4 and above) who are attending school be immunized against specific pathogens unless they have a valid medical or conscientious exemption signed off by an appropriate authority. Parents must show proof of these vaccinations to their local public health department. If a child is not up to date on the required vaccines (which include diphtheria, tetanus, polio, measles, mumps, rubella, meningococcal, pertussis, and varicella), they are at risk of being suspended from school for noncompliance and may be excluded from school during an outbreak.

Policies such as these have shown success for improving vaccine coverage in some jurisdictions, especially in the United States, although they are not without controversy (Robinson, 2018). Although some argue that such policies compromise individual freedom, others say they do not go far enough and even advocate for removing philosophical or conscientious objections and only allowing medical exemptions, in order to protect children and the public.

Many members of the public, including health care professionals, do not know how vaccine schedules are developed, how publicly funded vaccine programs are decided upon, and most important, how vaccine safety is ensured. The following section describes the key players and processes that keep our system robust.

Vaccine Safety and Recommendations in Canada

Before a manufacturer of a vaccine product can get it licensed, the vaccine must be put through a number of studies and trials. These include animal trials, followed by small human trials, and then followed by large human trials in order to demonstrate safety, quality of the product, and effectiveness in humans.

After these series of studies are complete and demonstrate positive results, the manufacturer can apply to Health Canada for licensure. Health Canada's Health Products and Food Branch (HPFB) thoroughly reviews all of these studies, and when their experts decide that the benefits of a vaccine outweigh its risks, will grant the vaccine authorization status for it to be sold in Canada. After authorization, to ensure ongoing safety and quality, the manufacturer is subject to what is known as a *lot release program*. Through this program, the manufacturer is responsible for testing each lot to be released onto the market and submitting the results of this testing to Health Canada for their review and verification. The manufacturer of a vaccine is also subject to inspections by Health Canada to ensure that it is following Good Manufacturing Practice (GMP), hygienic procedures, and safe techniques.

Lastly, postmarketing surveillance is conducted on all vaccines in Canada through the Canadian Adverse Events Following Immunization Surveillance System (CAEFISS). This surveillance system has both active and passive components (see Chapter 2 for more information about surveillance and surveillance systems). The passive component relies on health care professionals and members of the public to report any adverse events that occurred after administration of a vaccine—whether they believe the event to be related to the vaccine or not. The active component relies on members of the surveillance team going to pediatric hospitals and reviewing charts to see if any hospital admissions could have been related to vaccines. In this way, if there were any harms associated with a vaccine that were not picked up in all of the pretrial data, this postmarketing surveillance has a better chance of detecting it because millions of people will receive vaccines once they are sold on the Canadian market (MacDonald & Law, 2017).

Whereas Health Canada is the regulatory body that oversees vaccine development, an expert body called the National Advisory Committee on Immunizations (NACI) is the scientific group that reviews vaccine evidence to decide on which vaccines should be given to which groups of people, at which time intervals, to optimally protect them from disease. NACI produces statements about each type of vaccine and then informs whether a provincial or territorial government in power will decide to publicly fund or deliver that vaccine (e.g., administer hepatitis B vaccine to all grade 7 students in schools). The decisions made at the provincial and territorial level, however, factor in the science as well as the cost of vaccine, anticipated uptake, cold chain requirements, and other political priorities. Hence, each province has its own immunization schedule.

CRITICAL THINKING QUESTION 10.2: Health care providers are a reliable source of information for parents who are deciding whether and when to vaccinate their children. As a future health care provider working alongside a multidisciplinary team, what might you be able to do to address vaccine hesitancy in a skeptical parent? What about in your community at large?

SELECTED VACCINE-PREVENTABLE DISEASES

In the early part of the 20th century, vaccine-preventable diseases were a major cause of morbidity and mortality in Canada, particularly among children. Although many of these diseases are now under control in Canada, some remain major problems throughout the world and among some subgroups of the Canadian population; thus, the risk of importation and spread among Canadians still remains.

Although diseases such as tetanus and diphtheria have been almost eradicated in Canada, sporadic cases and outbreaks of certain diseases that could be prevented by vaccines are still reported. A brief overview of the recent incidence of the major vaccine-preventable diseases in Canada, as well as issues relevant to control, are discussed here. In general, most of these conditions are reportable to local public health authorities, as discussed earlier. When public health professionals receive a report of such a disease, they do the following to manage the case: (1) collect more information regarding the case history, (2) ensure that proper control strategies are in place to prevent further spread, and (3) elucidate the case's close contacts at risk of disease and implement strategies to prevent that (if they exist). If they detect that the number of cases are not only sporadic but go beyond what is expected at baseline, they will then investigate and manage the disease outbreak, as discussed earlier.

Pertussis

Pertussis (whooping cough) is an infection of the respiratory tract caused by the bacterium *Bordetella pertussis*. The incidence of pertussis has decreased by 96% since the introduction of the first vaccine for pertussis in 1943. However, vaccine coverage remains suboptimal, and it is estimated that only 77% of Canadians received the recommended doses of pertussis vaccine by age 2 years. Additionally, only 10% of the adult population has received the recommended adult booster dose. Pertussis tends to be a cyclical disease, with disease activity increasing every 2 to 5 years. Several pertussis outbreaks occurred in 2012 and again in 2015 across the country (PHAC, 2017a). Between 2011 and 2015, the average incidence of pertussis was 6.6 per 100,000 population (PHAC, 2017a).

The severity of the disease has decreased because of widespread vaccination, which affords partial protection. However, the disease has a poorer prognosis in infants younger than 1 year of age (i.e., those too young to have protection from the vaccine) (PHAC, 2018a).

When a case of pertussis is reported to Public Health, it is taken quite seriously because the attack rate among susceptible contacts (under- or nonvaccinated household contacts) is up to 90% (Heyman, 2015). Those most at risk include infants younger than 1 year of age and pregnant women in their third trimester (because exposure to pertussis can then affect the newborn baby). Public Health officials recommend giving an antibiotic to those high-risk contacts to prevent disease from developing (Heyman, 2015).

Measles

Measles is one of the most contagious vaccine-preventable diseases. It is spread person to person via airborne exposure. Complications include otitis media (ear infections), pneumonia, and diarrhea and are more frequent in young children. Encephalitis (inflammation of the brain) occurs in 1 of 1 000 cases and can result in permanent brain damage. Death is estimated to occur in 1 of every 3 000 cases in Canada. Before the vaccine, thousands of measles cases were reported every year in Canada. However, since the vaccine was introduced (and further, with the implementation of a two-dose schedule by all provinces and territories in 1996/1997), the incidence of measles declined by more than 99%. It is estimated that 89% of children in Canada have received the recommended doses of measles containing vaccine by 2 years of age. While this may seem high, it actually falls short of the national targets and the percentage required to achieve herd immunity.

Around 200 cases of measles are reported each year in Canada (PHAC, 2018a), the large majority of which stem from imported cases. In fact, since 1997, there have been no cases of measles traced back to an index case in Canada, causing Canada to achieve official elimination status in 1998. Elimination of measles means that a country has been able to interrupt transmission of measles from imported cases such that there are no secondary cases that pop up 12 months or more after a community is exposed (Sherrard, Hiebert, & Squires, 2015). The Research Perspective box presents a more detailed description of how *elimination* of a disease compares with *eradication* or *extinction* of a disease.

RESEARCH PERSPECTIVE

The Difference Between Elimination, Eradication, and Extinction of a Disease

When thinking about communicable disease control, it is important to recognize the distinction among the terms *elimination, eradication,* and *extinction*. **Elimination** often refers to stopping transmission of that disease in a specific geographic area through the use of various control measures (e.g., contact tracing, isolation). **Eradication**, on the other hand, refers to reducing worldwide incidence of a disease to zero. In such a situation, no further control measures are needed. **Extinction** is the most extreme form of this eradication—in which not only does the actual pathogen never cause disease in humans, but it also does not exist anymore in nature or in any laboratory setting.

Exercise

1. Based on your research, which pathogen has achieved eradication status, and which pathogen has almost achieved eradication status?
2. Why can smallpox not be considered extinct?

Because of the desire to maintain Canada's elimination status, cases of suspected or confirmed measles are to be reported to Public Health immediately. Public Health professionals follow up with all cases to ensure that they are isolated during their period of communicability, figure out where they have been, and find out who has shared airspace with them. At times, if a case has not been adequately isolated during the period of communicability (e.g., the person was waiting in a busy emergency department [ED] waiting room), possible contacts can number in the hundreds, and public health professionals may put out general notices to the public to inform them of their risk because often they may not be able to make individual contact with every person who was in that waiting room (especially if they cannot obtain a list of their names). Unimmunized contacts are the most at risk and should be offered either vaccine or immunoglobulin (preformed antibodies to measles) to prevent the development of measles (Heymann, 2015).

Influenza

Influenza viruses are a major cause of morbidity, mortality, and lost productivity because of work and school absences in the Canadian population. Influenza A and B circulate around the globe annually, usually during the winter months. The overall estimated mortality rate from influenza and pneumonia (a complication of influenza) exceeds that of all vaccine-preventable childhood diseases. It is estimated that every year there are around 12 000 hospitalizations and 3 500 deaths caused by influenza across the country (PHAC, 2018b). The heaviest toll occurs among those older than 65 years of age, although substantial morbidity can occur in younger patients who are immunocompromised or have chronic diseases such as asthma, chronic obstructive pulmonary disease, ischemic heart disease, or diabetes.

Periodic pandemics of influenza have occurred in the past 100 years. Landmark influenza pandemics occurred in 1918 ("Spanish flu," H1N1), 1957 ("Asian flu," H2N2), 1968 ("Hong Kong flu," H3N2), 1977 ("Russian flu," H1N1), and 2009 (H1N1). Because the influenza virus undergoes genetic changes, further pandemics are possible. Antigenic shift is a major genetic change that occurs at varying intervals. Antigenic drift is a minor change that occurs between major shifts.

An issue of global concern is that of avian influenza, or bird flu. Bird flu is a type of influenza virus that affects birds, including domestic poultry. There have been some human cases of avian influenza in humans who have close contact with birds, but luckily, this form of human bird flu is not easily passed on to others. The main concern with avian influenza is that if a person contracts both regular human influenza and avian influenza, the two strains could merge genetically, resulting in a new virus that can spread very easily from person to person. This would have global consequences because nobody would have immunity (given it is a new form of the virus), and vaccines can take several months to make (Government of Canada, 2008).

Because immunization of the entire population is the best means of controlling the impact of a pandemic, it is important to promote a high level of influenza immunization between pandemics. Ontario became the first jurisdiction in the world to introduce a universal influenza immunization program in 2000, offering the influenza vaccine free of charge to anyone aged 6 months of age and older. Such a program contributes greatly to the ability to react in the event of a pandemic because it helps to raise public awareness of the seriousness of influenza and helps to build a community-based infrastructure for vaccination delivery. However, this program was not without its criticisms. Some have argued for a more targeted program and highlighted the fact that although a vaccine for influenza is developed each year, because the virus is so apt to change, in some years, the vaccine is not very protective or efficacious. Thus, having a universal program such as Ontario's may not be the best place to invest limited resources (Scheifele et al., 2014; Advisory Committee for Ontario's Immunization System Review, 2014).

Health care workers are often a target for influenza immunization because not only are they at high risk of exposure because of their occupation, but they may also be responsible for passing on influenza to their vulnerable patients (because with influenza, you can be communicable before you actually develop signs and symptoms of infection and know you are sick). Influenza vaccine uptake among health care professionals is about 50% and, many argue, is therefore suboptimal. As a result, some Canadian jurisdictions put into place "vaccinate-or-mask policies," including British Columbia in 2012 to 2013, which required health care professionals that chose not to vaccinate themselves against influenza to wear masks during flu season. A recent analysis found that such policies did increase immunization rates by just over 10% among health care workers (Buchan & Kwong, 2016). However, these types of policies remain quite controversial for ethical reasons.

EXERCISE 10.3: What are two ethical arguments in favour of "mask-or-vaccinate policies" and two arguments against such policies?

Pneumococcal Disease

Pneumococcal infection, caused by the bacterium *Streptococcus pneumoniae* (pneumococcus), is a leading cause of death and a major cause of bacterial pneumonia and meningitis among children and older adults. Invasive pneumococcal disease (IPD)—pneumococcal disease that causes pneumonia, meningitis, and infection of the bloodstream—became nationally notifiable in 2000. The incidence rate of IPD declined from 60 cases per 100 000 population (before vaccine was widely available) to just less than 20 cases per 100 000 in children

younger than 2 years of age. However, IPD is still considered to be a vaccine-preventable disease with a "moderate incidence rate" in Canada. NACI recommends routine immunization for those younger than age 2 years and for those older than age 65 years, and childhood vaccination programs were offered in most provinces and territories by 2006. Vaccine coverage is moderate and is better for children than for older adults. In 2015, it was estimated that 80% of children had received the recommended number of doses by age 2 years, but only 37% of adults aged 65 years or older had received the recommended dose (PHAC, 2017a).

Unlike measles and pertussis, when a case of pneumococcal disease is reported to Public Health authorities, there is no vaccine or antibiotic that can be offered to close contacts to prevent those who were exposed from becoming ill (Heymann, 2015). IPD is mostly notifiable for the purposes of monitoring its incidence over time (PHAC, 2017a).

EXERCISE 10.4: If you were the federal government minister in charge of deciding which communicable diseases are nationally notifiable (i.e., reportable to public health authorities) and which ones are not, what criteria might you use to help you decide?

Varicella

Varicella disease (chickenpox) is a highly contagious viral disease that affects 95% of Canadians, generally before the age of 15 years. In healthy children, the disease is relatively benign; however, in some children, chickenpox can cause more serious complications. The occurrence of invasive group A streptococcal disease (necrotizing fasciitis or "flesh-eating disease") is increased after varicella infection and can lead to a high number of hospitalizations and deaths among children. In adolescents and adults, complications associated with varicella infection are more frequent and include higher rates of pneumonia, encephalitis, and death. Case fatality rates are 10 to 30 times higher in adults than in children. A vaccine against chickenpox was approved for use in Canada in 1998, and by 2007, most provinces and territories had implemented routine varicella immunization programs (PHAC, 2017a).

The incidence of varicella has declined by 99% since the introduction of the vaccine in Canada, and today the incidence rate of varicella is around 3 cases per 100 000 population. However, despite this, vaccine coverage remains suboptimal, with only 65% of children having received the recommended doses of varicella vaccine by age 2 years (PHAC, 2017a). Like measles, chickenpox is also spread via the airborne route, although it is not as communicable as measles. Confirmed cases do not usually have to be isolated because the disease is most communicable before the onset of symptoms, so by the time a person presents to health care with chickenpox, they are usually no longer a risk to others. (For a more thorough discussion on the merits of isolation and quarantine, and the difference between the two, refer to the Research Perspective box.) Close high-risk contacts who are not immune to chickenpox can be given vaccine and immunoglobulin (depending on their age and other risk factors) to be protected from developing chickenpox if they are exposed (Heymann, 2015).

RESEARCH PERSPECTIVE

Isolation versus Quarantine

People often use the terms *isolation* and *quarantine* interchangeably; however, they are different and require due consideration if they are to be implemented, given the restrictions that each places on individual freedoms and rights.

Isolation refers to separating a person from the general public when they develop signs and symptoms of an infection, for the purpose of reducing transmission to others. Most jurisdictions allow public health officials to order someone to be isolated to protect the public. **Quarantine**, on the other hand, refers to separating a person from the public after they have been exposed to an index case. In this situation, a person is being separated from the public when they may not even have contracted the disease—they have only been exposed to the disease. The person, therefore, is not ill with any signs or symptoms and is being separated on the premise that if they are exposed and contract the disease, they are still at risk of passing it along to others before they actually experience any signs or symptoms. Quarantine, therefore, should ideally only be used in situations when a person is communicable, before they develop any signs or symptoms, and in cases when a disease is highly infectious and so exposed contacts are likely to become infected.

Much controversy occurred when people were being quarantined during the Ebola virus outbreak in West Africa. Ebola is most communicable after the onset of signs and symptoms, and people are not communicable during their incubation period. The issue with this highly fatal disease was that relying on people to self-isolate as soon as symptoms struck was too much of a challenge, and hence some jurisdictions opted to quarantine instead.

Similarly, quarantine was used during the SARS outbreak in 2003. Follow-up studies, however, revealed some significant negative effects of quarantine on nursing staff. More specifically, nurses who were quarantined reported higher levels of frustration, anger, anxiety, social isolation, and stigmatization compared with nurses who were not quarantined (Antoniou & Cooper, 2016). Thus, it is very important to keep in mind the stigmatizing nature of quarantine and its negative effects on individuals and to use this tool cautiously and only when threats outweigh its harms.

CRITICAL THINKING QUESTIONS 10.3: The Global Polio Eradication Initiative, coordinated by the WHO, is focusing its efforts on countries where polio still poses challenges—namely, Afghanistan, Pakistan, and Nigeria. In many of the countries where polio remains an issue, cultural and religious leaders have not been supportive of vaccination efforts because of issues such as widespread misconception that the vaccine causes infertility, deploying all male immunizers to more culturally conservative groups, and a belief that the vaccine contains pig products (which are not allowed to be consumed in some religious groups) (Hussain et al., 2016).

How might you apply the principles of community health and health promotion to address some of these types cultural barriers and misconceptions? Who would you involve to help address the issue and what values and principles would guide your work?

TRENDS IN OTHER SIGNIFICANT INFECTIOUS DISEASES

Tuberculosis

Tuberculosis (TB) is an important bacterial infection, especially in at-risk populations such as those who have HIV infection, homeless persons, Indigenous people, and foreign-born individuals from areas where TB is endemic. It is important to keep in mind that about 90% of people infected with TB do not actually develop active disease (which often results in symptoms such as fever, cough, fatigue, and many others) (Government of Canada, 2016). TB infection without active disease is called *latent TB*. Latent TB is not transmitted person to person the way active TB is. In most jurisdictions in Canada, TB is reportable to public health agencies because it poses a risk to the public.

Since 1987, the previously declining TB rates in Canada have levelled off, with approximately 1 600 new active TB cases a year (PHAC, 2018c). This is because of increased immigration from countries with high TB rates, HIV, and the emergence of drug-resistant TB. Coinfection (concurrent) with HIV and TB has also been a major factor in the resurgence of TB worldwide. Although the rate of TB in Canada is one of the lowest in the world (second lowest among G7 countries) at 4.8 per 100 000 population in 2016, the rates in subpopulations still vary (Vachon, Gallant, & Siu, 2018). The incidence of TB among Canadian-born non-Indigenous people is 0.6 per 100,000 compared with 170 per 100 000 among Inuit people and 34.1 per 100 000 among Indigenous people living on reserve (Vachon et al., 2018).

Apart from the difficulties of control in traditional risk groups and HIV-infected people, many immigrants, refugees, and visitors arrive in Canada each year from countries that have high rates of TB. The risk of reactivation of disease in those who have previously had it is increased in foreign-born people. It is clear then that the two largest subgroups of interest when it comes to active TB are:

1. Foreign-born people, who account for nearly 70% of active TB cases in Canada while representing less than 20% of total population
2. Indigenous people, who account for 20% of active TB cases in Canada while representing approximately 5% of total population (Vachon et al., 2018)

See Box 10.1 for a more detailed discussion of TB rates among Canada's Indigenous people.

BOX 10.1 Tuberculosis Among Indigenous People in Canada: A Deeper Dive

In previous chapters, we have explored the social determinants of health, including those specific to Indigenous people (e.g., colonialism and historical trauma). The higher rates of tuberculosis (TB) among Indigenous people compared with non-Indigenous people that we see today exemplifies how these determinants of health continue to exert their influence. As a result of oppressive colonial policies, some Indigenous groups continue to experience challenges that include poverty, overcrowding, and poor access to health care, all of which make them more vulnerable to TB and its complications. For example, overcrowding allows for the easier spread of TB to others in the household. Moreover, the *Indian Act* (discussed in Chapter 7) allowed for the creation of the residential school system, which also influenced TB rates to a substantial degree. Children in residential schools were often exposed to harsh conditions, including poor infrastructure, overcrowding, and poor ventilation. Malnutrition was rampant among those attending residential school, which had a large impact on mortality caused by TB infection (Komarnisky et al., 2016).

The *Indian Act* also allowed for the apprehension of Indigenous people who did not seek medical treatment. In the 1940s and 1950s, for example, many Indigenous people were forcibly sent to TB sanitoria, often without adequate consent and far away from their social supports. Thus, historically, Indigenous people have had negative and traumatic experiences associated with TB treatment and care (Komarnisky et al., 2016). All of these reasons must be kept in mind when reading and reviewing statistics related to the higher rates of TB in Indigenous people in Canada.

Health care practitioners need to be sensitized to the diagnosis and management of TB, particularly as it relates to health hazards and the emergence of multiple drug-resistant strains in those noncompliant with chemotherapy. Drug resistance rates have likely increased because of the high number of people arriving in Canada from countries with a high prevalence of drug resistance but also because of inappropriate or interrupted treatment here in Canada. Drug-resistant TB is associated with high mortality rates as well as high costs because of prolonged hospitalization and the cost of second-line drugs.

A major obstacle to tuberculosis control is adherence to medication regimes. A course of therapy requires at least three medications for 6 to 9 months. Because the acute symptoms rapidly disappear after 4 to 6 weeks, it is often difficult to persuade people to remain adherent. Strategies such as directly observed therapy (DOT) are effective measures to improve adherence with TB drug therapy, particularly rates of drug resistant TB DOT involves a health care worker giving medications to a patient and making sure the patient takes the medication.

When public health officials are notified of a client with active TB, they take steps to ensure that the client is isolated until he or she is no longer communicable, the client takes their medications daily, and contacts are followed up and tested for TB after exposure to the client. Given that TB is airborne (just like measles and varicella), public health officials often have to follow up with contacts who shared air space (e.g., in an airplane) with a client who is communicable for a prolonged period of time.

However, TB is much less communicable than varicella or measles, so public health officials usually start by assessing very close contacts (those with whom the client spends a lot of time), and only if there is evidence of transmission do they begin to assess other contacts (e.g., contacts at work or school, or casual contacts who may have been on the same bus or in the same room as the client) (Heymann, 2015). The Case Study box describes an innovative approach to contact management in diseases such as TB.

While a vaccine (called bacillus Calmette–Guérin) does exist for TB, it is not routinely used in the Canadian context and is not used to help prevent TB in exposed cases.

Invasive Group A Streptococcus

Invasive group A streptococcus became a nationally notifiable disease in 2000. It is caused by the group A streptococcus bacteria and is responsible for a wide range of diseases, including strep throat, cellulitis (infection of the skin), and a range of invasive conditions (known as invasive group A streptococcus [iGAS]) such as blood infections, toxic shock syndrome, and necrotizing fasciitis (National Collaborating Centre for Infectious Diseases, 2018). iGAS is responsible for quite a bit of morbidity and mortality, given the seriousness of the conditions it causes. The

Canada-wide incidence of iGAS is 2.7 cases per 100 000 population, with higher rates reported among children, older adults, and Indigenous people (PHAC, 2006). Typically, iGAS outbreaks have been commonly reported in institutional settings such as long-term care homes or daycares; however, a number of more recent outbreaks have been documented in community settings among very vulnerable groups across North America, such as homeless individuals and people who use drugs (Dickson et al., 2018). Reasons for this are not entirely clear but may be related to drug use practices (sharing equipment) and suboptimal hygiene and overcrowding, which could result in more sustained droplet or contact transmission. Rates of community-based iGAS infection also appear to be on the rise for reasons that are unclear (Dickson et al., 2018). Although no vaccine exists, close contacts who have been significantly exposed can take an antibiotic to prevent infection (Heymann, 2015); however, this practice is more difficult to implement among vulnerable populations that are transiently housed and among people who use drugs.

ANTIMICROBIAL RESISTANCE

Antimicrobial resistance (AMR) occurs when a pathogen (a bacteria or virus, for example) no longer responds as intended to a drug that was developed to slow or kill it, such as an antibiotic or antiviral medication (Health Canada, 2017a). Thus, such pathogens become very difficult to treat. The emergence of antimicrobial resistance in the past 2 decades has become a major health care issue both in the community and hospital settings in Canada. The late 1980s and 1990s witnessed the development of antibiotic resistance of several common bacteria, including penicillin-resistant *Streptococcus pneumoniae* (PRSP), methicillin-resistant *Staphylococcus aureus* (MRSA), vancomycin-resistant enterococci (VRE), and the extended-spectrum beta lactamase-producing bacteria (ESBL) (e.g., *Klebsiella pneumoniae, Klebsiella oxytoca,* and *Escherichia coli*). Although there has been some improvement in decreasing some levels of antibiotic resistance, the prevalence of other resistant bacteria has risen dramatically. For example, the rates of drug-resistant gonorrhea (traditionally an easy-to-treat organism) have risen over the years (PHAC, 2017b).

Social Network Analysis

Social network analysis (SNA) is increasingly gaining traction in the investigation of outbreaks of public health significance, including TB, HIV, and syphilis. In SNA, a visualization of social networks is produced to better understand people's social ties and who they are most exposed to, day to day. This has most often been applied to certain vulnerable and transient populations, such as homeless or underhoused individuals (Kawatsu et al., 2015). SNA allows public health nurses (who are most often involved in outbreak investigation) to determine whether there are certain central people in a social network that link others together or that many people are most exposed to. Targeting those people for public health intervention can have a large effect on many others versus targeting an individual at the periphery of a social network. This is especially important among complex social networks, where there may not be traditional household contacts, or where the disease is one that requires understanding of more intimate relationships (e.g., in the case of syphilis or gonorrhea). The following diagram is a pictorial depiction of SNA.

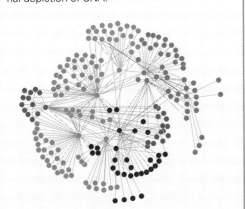

The nodes (or circles) represent individual people, and the lines between them represent the ties between the people.

The determinants of antimicrobial resistance are complex. The overprescription and inappropriate prescription of antibiotics to patients is one important factor. Over time, the rate of prescription of antimicrobials in community settings and hospitals has remained stable, which indicates that more can be done to ensure that clinicians appropriately prescribe antibiotics. One of the most common inappropriate practices among primary care providers, for example, is to prescribe antibiotics to people who present with a nonbacterial acute respiratory tract infection (i.e., the common cold). A 2017 study that was partially funded by the Ministry of Health and Long-Term Care in Ontario investigated nearly 180 000 older adults with an acute upper respiratory tract infection (of nonbacterial origin) and found that 46% of them had been prescribed an antibiotic by their primary care physicians (Silverman et al., 2017). Provider education and development of clinical guidelines and risk scores (to stratify patients that might be at higher risk of a bacterial infection) can improve **antimicrobial stewardship**—the appropriate use of antimicrobial agents.

Patient-level factors are also important in the development of AMR. For example, patients who are prescribed a several-day course of antibiotics but do not complete the full course may also foster resistance. This happens because by not taking the full dose of antibiotics prescribed, they give the organism they are infected with the opportunity to develop resistance to the drug they are taking. Because they are not finishing the course of antibiotics, this organism may thus survive and reproduce.

The use of antimicrobials in livestock is also a growing area of concern and controversy. Recent estimates suggest that nearly 80% of the world's antibiotics are used in animals in the agriculture sector (WHO, 2017). It is increasingly being recognized that using antimicrobials in excess or inappropriately for animals can also lead to the development of resistant organisms and that this resistance can then be transferred to humans through direct contact or through environmental exposure (e.g., contact with water or food contaminated with antimicrobial-resistant organisms) (PHAC, 2017b). In 2016, nearly 1.0 million kg of antibiotics used in humans were distributed with the intention to also be used in animals (e.g., livestock and pets) (PHAC, 2017b). This growing concern has led a number of countries and regions to ban the use of antibiotics in healthy animals for the sole purpose of promoting growth and preventing disease (a practice that is quite different from using the antibiotics to treat animals that are actually sick). In 2006, for example, the European Union banned this practice, and the WHO called upon all countries to do the same in 2017 (Thomson Reuters,

2017). In 2014, Health Canada announced that it was restricting the use of antibiotics for the sole purpose of promoting growth in healthy animals. Since then, the government has been looking at other strategies, such as ensuring that antibiotics that are important for human care be used in animals only if a veterinarian has prescribed them (Health Canada, 2017b).

The consequences of antibiotic resistance are sobering: persons with antibiotic-resistant infections have higher morbidity and mortality rates and have longer and more expensive hospitalizations. Antibiotic development is expensive and requires considerable time for appropriate testing. Currently, there are only a few promising new antibiotic medications on the development horizon. The control of antibiotic resistance requires some of the strategies discussed earlier, as well as enhanced epidemiological and laboratory surveillance, rational prescription practices by physicians, increased adherence by individuals requiring therapy, and adherence to infection control practices in hospitals, nursing homes, and childcare facilities.

INFECTION PREVENTION AND CONTROL

Key to most antimicrobial stewardship programs are adequate infection prevention and control (IPAC) practices. IPAC practices aim to reduce the spread of infections in all settings, including health care settings, such as long-term care homes, hospitals, and clinics, and thus can reduce how often antimicrobial-resistant organisms are passed from the environment to a susceptible host or from one person to another (Manning et al., 2018). IPAC practices can be thought of as putting into place controls at various levels, including provider controls (e.g., ensuring that providers wash their hands regularly and wear personal protective equipment), administrative controls (e.g., ensuring that staff are immunized against common communicable diseases, ensuring proper protocols for recognizing people with communicable diseases and isolating them appropriately in a health care setting, auditing practices for compliance), and environmental controls (e.g., cleaning regularly, reprocessing equipment intended to be used on multiple clients).

Infection prevention and control practices can also be categorized into *routine precautions* and *additional precautions*. **Routine precautions** are processes and procedures that should be used when interacting with all clients (regardless of their risk level) to prevent the spread of infectious agents. They are based on the notion that all clients could potentially be infectious. Examples of practices that are considered routine include hand hygiene, regular cleaning of environment, and making sure that every person who enters an institution (e.g., an ED) is screened for signs and symptoms of a communicable disease and is then treated appropriately (e.g., given a mask or sent to a separate waiting area to wait) (Public Health Ontario [PHO], 2015). **Additional precautions** or practices are interventions used to prevent the spread of specific infections when their presence is suspected or confirmed in a patient. These are also referred to as *transmission-based precautions* because they are based on knowing how a specific pathogen is spread (i.e., if it is spread via direct contact, airborne route, by droplet, or a mix of these). For example, if a health care provider suspects the presence of active TB, which we know is an airborne pathogen, any providers or visitors interacting with a case of active TB would wear a specific type of protective mask, and the client would be placed in a negative-pressure room if hospitalized (PHO, 2015). A commitment to IPAC practices is very important for keeping patients safe as they interact with the health care system, as well as for reducing the spread of dangerous organisms such as antimicrobial-resistant pathogens.

CRITICAL THINKING QUESTIONS 10.4: Imagine you are a health care provider in a busy hospital ED who has been tasked with leading the IPAC program in your department. Who might you involve in a hospital IPAC steering committee, and what are some of the ways you might assess how well your ED is doing with regard to IPAC practices? If, for example, it is found that hand hygiene compliance is low among all members of the team, what interventions might you suggest to improve it? What are some ways you might approach this specific issue (lack of hand hygiene) with a diverse group of health professionals, each with their own priorities and perhaps competing goals? (For example, although the IPAC team may have a primary goal of reducing health care–associated infections, individual practitioners may feel pressured for time and may therefore prioritize efficiency of time versus lengthy handwashing.) In other words, how can you approach these differences in a way that fosters collaboration?

VECTOR-BORNE DISEASES AND RABIES

Vectors such as mosquitoes and ticks are responsible for a small but important proportion of communicable diseases. Vector-borne illnesses such as malaria, Dengue fever, and yellow fever are major global causes of morbidity and mortality. In Canada, two important vector-borne diseases—Lyme disease and West Nile disease—are considered to be **emerging infectious diseases (EIDs)** of importance. EIDs have been defined by the WHO as representing those conditions that either newly appear in a population or that are not necessarily new but are rapidly increasing in terms of the incidence of where they are present geographically (Ogden, AbdelMalik, & Pulliam, 2017). EIDs are thought to occur because of changes in a pathogen's geographic range (e.g., dispersion of a pathogen through other vectors, travel, or trade, or change in an environment—e.g., because of climate change—that make it newly suited for a specific type of pathogen). *Adaptive emergence*, or the ability of a microorganism to genetically change in a way that makes it better suited to new environments, is another reason for emergence of new diseases (Ogden et al., 2017).

Lyme disease can affect almost every organ system and is caused by a bacteria called *Borrelia burgdorferi*. It can be transmitted to humans through the bite of an infected black-legged tick. It represents an EID of importance because in 2004, there were only about 40 reported cases across the country, and this number increased to 917 reported cases in 2015 (Aenishaenslin et al., 2017). Areas where Lyme disease is considered endemic have expanded significantly in Canada. In the 1990s, there was only one region in Ontario (Long Point) that was known to have a black-legged tick population. Today, however, black-legged ticks are prevalent in many parts of Eastern and Central Canada as well (Ripoche et al., 2018).

Climate change has been implicated in the emergence of Lyme disease in other areas across Canada. Black-legged ticks tend to latch on to deer and white-footed mice and can be carried long distances by migratory birds as well. These species may be responsible for spreading ticks across great distances, and it is thought that because of warmer weather in typically cold climates, the ticks aren't dying off as readily (Levy, 2017) and are able to establish themselves in more Northern areas where they couldn't survive before (Cheng et al., 2017).

Strategies for controlling Lyme disease in Canada include educating the public about preventive measures (e.g., using DEET insect repellent, wearing long sleeves, and doing tick checks after hikes), detecting and treating Lyme disease early (before it can spread in the body, causing more widespread disease), and ensuring ongoing surveillance of both humans and black-legged ticks.

West Nile virus, historically found in Africa, Asia, Europe, and the Middle East, was identified for the first time in the United States in 1999 and is now the leading cause of mosquito-borne diseases in Canada (Giordano, Kaur, & Hunter, 2017). Carried and spread by mosquitoes, it can cause fatal inflammation of the spinal cord and brain (encephalitis) in certain birds, horses, and humans. The first human case of WNV in Canada was reported in 2002, and since then, there have been approximately 5 000 confirmed cases (Giordano et al., 2017). Whereas cases of WNV were initially limited to Ontario and Quebec, they have now spread westwards.

West Nile virus season is typically between April and October, and the number of cases each year varies greatly based on factors such as temperature, humidity, and rainfall. Given its link to these factors, climate change has also been theorized as being responsible for some of the changing incidence and spread of WNV in Canada. Controlling WNV in Canada involves ensuring that people protect themselves from mosquitos (e.g., by wearing long sleeves and using insect repellant), surveillance of humans and animals, and larviciding and adulticiding mosquito populations.

Rabies is a universally fatal viral illness that is spread to humans via the saliva of an infected animal (usually as a result of an animal bite). Because of a combination of an effective vaccine available for postexposure prophylaxis, and excellent control of rabies in domesticated animals, human rabies cases have been a rare event over the past 2 decades. Since 1924, 25 people have died of rabies in Canada. Rabies is extremely rare in domesticated cats and dogs, and more common in Canada among raccoons, skunks, bats, and Arctic foxes (PHAC, 2018d). A range of government departments have an influence on the decline of rabies in Canada. They ensure that animals are vaccinated, can put into place trap-vaccinate-and-release programs (to vaccinate wild animals), and follow up with humans who have been bitten by high-risk animals to offer them a vaccine after exposure to prevent disease.

FOOD-BORNE AND WATER-BORNE ILLNESS

Food and water remain important and often unrecognized sources of communicable disease (see Chapter 11). In 2000, an outbreak of gastroenteritis in Walkerton, Ontario, marked the first documented outbreak of *E. coli* 0157:H7 infection associated with a treated municipal water supply in Canada. More than 2 000 cases were associated with this outbreak (Caplan, 2010). Water-borne outbreaks of *Cryptosporidium* infection affected more than 7 000 in North Battleford, Saskatchewan, in 2001 and 10 Indigenous communities between 2013 and 2014 (CTVNews, 2016). These outbreaks underscore the necessity for vigilance to ensure that municipal water supplies are maintained at the highest level of quality. Public health officials are often involved in outbreak responses such as these, in particular, with identifying the source, testing water supplies, and in some cases, ordering protective measures (e.g., issuing boil-water advisories when water is considered unsafe to drink) to ensure the prevention of such outbreaks.

Food-borne illness is a common cause of morbidity in the population. It is estimated that every year there are about 4 million episodes of foodborne illness in the country, more than 11 000 hospitalizations, and more than 200 deaths (Bélanger, et al., 2015). Common organisms associated with food-borne gastroenteritis are *E. coli, Salmonella* spp., *Staphylococcus aureus,* and *Bacillus cereus.* Reports of food-borne illness to public health authorities are underestimated. This is because the vast majority of food-borne illness does not come to medical attention, or no stool cultures are taken.

With the increased global nature of the food industry, serious illness and multiprovincial outbreaks have been associated with contaminated food. In 2018, the PHAC and the Canadian Food Inspection Agency investigated a Canada-wide outbreak of *Salmonella* in which upwards of 80 people in 10 Canadian provinces and territories were affected. One of the identified sources of illness linked to these cases included frozen raw breaded chicken products, which resulted in a food recall (PHAC, 2018e). Interestingly, these products have been implicated in several other Canadian *Salmonella* outbreaks over the years as well (Hobbs et al., 2017). Because these products typically look cooked (because they are breaded and browned),

this likely results in some people not realizing that the products still need to be handled and thoroughly cooked like any other raw meat product. An example of a tool used in foodborne illness outbreak investigations is discussed in the Evidence-Informed Practice box.

EVIDENCE-INFORMED PRACTICE

Canada's Foodbook Report

Investigating food-borne illness, especially across many jurisdictions and involving a number of infected people that are spread out, often requires a baseline understanding of what Canadians eat day to day. Implicating a particular food as the source of an outbreak involves comparing foods eaten by people who have become sick to the foods eaten by the Canadian population in general. To obtain food exposure data, the Canadian government conducted the Foodbook Study, which surveyed just more than 500 000 people, to develop a database that describes the types of foods Canadians consumed over a 7-day period in 2014 and 2015.

SEXUALLY TRANSMITTED AND BLOODBORNE INFECTIONS

Incidence

In general, socioeconomic conditions and changes in lifestyle in North America are likely to have contributed to the observed increase in STIs and bloodborne infections (BBIs) in Canada. The 1960s brought new affluence and with it more leisure time, social mobility, and changes in sexual behaviour. These changing social norms and the emergence of viral sexually transmitted infections—such as genital herpes infection in 1980s, human immunodeficiency syndrome/acquired immunodeficiency syndrome (HIV/AIDS) in the 1990s, and HPV as a cause of cervical cancer—resulted in sexually transmitted and blood borne infections being a significant cause of morbidity and mortality in adults.

Chlamydia trachomatis

Chlamydia trachomatis, a bacterial infection, is the most commonly reported STI in Canada. The number of chlamydia cases has increased steadily since the 1990s, and in 2015, upwards of 100 000 cases were reported just for that year (Choudhri et al., 2018a).

Chlamydia can result in signs and symptoms such as genital discharge but may also be asymptomatic. The fact that it can remain asymptomatic contributes to its spread because people are not prompted to seek care or use protective measures during intercourse. If not treated, chlamydia can result in significant long-term morbidity, such as arthritis, infertility, and pelvic inflammatory disease (Choudhri et al., 2018a). The rise in the number of reported cases is partly related to an increase in screening for infection, awareness of the disease, and better diagnostic techniques, resulting in increased reporting. Chlamydia infection became nationally notifiable only in 1991. Rates of infection are highest in adults aged 15 to 24 years, and risk factors other than age include sexual contact with an infected person; two or more sexual partners in the past year; a previous history of an STI; and being a member of a vulnerable socioeconomic group, such as an injected drug user, someone who is incarcerated, or someone who is involved in the sex trade (PHAC, 2010).

Gonorrhea and Syphilis

The incidence of gonorrhea (a bacterial STI caused by *Neisseria gonorrhoeae*) and syphilis has increased over the past few years. Gonorrhea is the second most commonly reported STI in the country, with nearly 20 000 cases being reported in 2015 (Choudhri et al., 2018b). Men tend to have higher rates of gonorrhea than women, and although the highest rates are among people aged 15 to 29 years, rates are increasing among people older than 60 years of age as well. In women, gonorrhea is often asymptomatic (and thus can go undetected) and, like chlamydia, untreated gonorrhea can result in chronic pelvic pain and pelvic inflammatory disease (Choudhri et al., 2018b).

After chlamydia and gonorrhea, syphilis is the third most commonly reported STI in Canada. It is caused by infection with the bacteria *Treponema pallidum*. From 2010 to 2015, rates of syphilis have risen by a shocking 85%. The highest risk of syphilis is among men aged 20 to 39. One of the most prominent risk factors for syphilis is men who have sex with men (MSM). Several outbreaks of syphilis have occurred among MSM populations who have HIV and among Indigenous people in Canada. Syphilis can be a very serious disease, and if it is not treated, it can affect organ systems, including the heart, brain, joints, and skin (Choudhri et al., 2018c).

Congenital syphilis can occur in infants of infected mothers and can be quite serious, leading to complications early in life, such as cerebral palsy, death, and hearing loss, among others. In 2015, there were six reported cases of congenital syphilis, an illness that is easily prevented by treating a mother with antibiotics (Choudhri et al., 2018c).

Both syphilis and gonorrhea are known to increase the transmission of HIV. Because early treatment and detection can have a major impact on the transmission of HIV, it is increasingly important to control the incidence and spread of bacterial STIs.

Human Papillomavirus

Although not notifiable, HPV is one of the most common STIs in Canada and worldwide. It is estimated that up to 75% of people will have HPV at some point in their lives (PHAC, 2017c), although many will clear the virus spontaneously. Unlike chlamydia and gonorrhea, HPV is a viral infection (not bacterial), and its presence isn't routinely tested for. Instead, clinicians know it is there by checking for some of its complications, which include genital warts and changes to cells in one's cervix (which, if left untreated, can cause cervical cancer) via the administration of a Papanicolaou (Pap) test. HPV is one of the few communicable diseases known to cause various cancers, including head and neck cancers, as well as anogenital cancers (e.g., cancer of the cervix, penis, anus, vulva, and vagina).

Human papillomavirus is also one of the few STIs for which a safe and effective vaccine exists to control it. NACI recommends vaccination for both men and women (PHAC, 2017c). Risk factors for HPV include multiple sexual partners, early onset of sexual activity, and smoking, among others. Condom use is somewhat effective in reducing transmission, but because HPV is spread via direct contact, condoms are not 100% preventive. Prevention includes vaccination in addition to condom use, as well as screening for cervical cancer through Pap smears.

Human Immunodeficiency Virus and Acquired Immunodeficiency Syndrome

AIDS is caused by HIV, which is transmitted by several routes: by sexual contact with an infected partner, via infected blood and blood products, from an infected mother to her unborn child perinatally, and via contaminated needles and syringes shared among people who inject drugs (PWIDs), for example.

HIV/AIDS was first identified in Canada in 1979 and became a reportable disease in Canada in 1985. Since it became reportable, just over 80 000 cases of HIV have been reported in Canada. HIV incidence steadily decreased from the 1980s to 2000 and then seemed to plateau until about 2008, when it began to decline again. In recent years, the number of new HIV cases per year has remained relatively constant at just over 2000 cases (Bourgeois et al., 2017).

For some groups, however, rates of HIV are actually on the rise, including youth and Indigenous people. Much attention has been paid recently to the rise in HIV rates among Indigenous populations across the country (Bourgeois et al., 2017). Saskatchewan, for example, has received much media attention regarding the high rates of HIV in its rural Indigenous communities—rates that are comparable to those of many low-income countries (Bellegarde, 2016). Limited access to services; high rates of intravenous drug use; and high prevalence of mental health issues, including intergenerational trauma, contribute to high rates of HIV infection among Indigenous people.

In terms of risk factors for HIV acquisition, the highest incidence of HIV infections occurs among people aged 30 to 39 years. The MSM population represents the largest proportion of HIV cases in Canada (44%), followed by sexual exposures among heterosexual groups, including those who were born in an HIV-endemic country (32%) followed by PWIDs (who account for about 15% of HIV cases in Canada) (Bourgeois et al., 2017). Men make up the large majority of HIV infections, and although historically, older men and younger women would be most at risk, the age difference among men and women acquiring HIV is beginning to close as the rates of HIV increase in people older than 50 years of age.

HIV is no longer considered an acute or life-threatening illness. In fact, with adequate treatment, people with HIV are living much longer than ever before. However, long-term complications of living with HIV are starting to be realized, including effects on the heart, kidneys, liver, nerves, and bone density (National AIDS Manual, 2017). As well, mood and mental health can be impacted (e.g., the rate of depression among people living with HIV is higher than it is for the general population) (Nanni et al., 2015).

Shifting the paradigm to think of HIV more as a chronic disease versus an acute one presents challenges when it comes to reducing the risk to others. It is no longer the case that all people with HIV should be considered infectious and, in fact, doing so contributes to stigma among those who live with HIV. The advent of new treatments has meant that the risk of passing on HIV to a sexual contact is much lower when an individual:

- Is engaged in treatment and is regularly taking antiretrovirals
- Has a suppressed viral load (meaning that high levels of the virus are not detected in that person's blood) for 6 months or more
- Has no other STIs (such as gonorrhea, chlamydia, syphilis, or herpes)
- Is undergoing regular monitoring of HIV infection.

Thus, engaging people (including those who may be living with HIV without even knowing it) in treatment is a key public health goal in reducing transmission to others. In fact, The Joint United Nations Programme on HIV/AIDS (UNAIDS) has articulated the "90-90-90 target," which aims for 90% of people living with HIV to know their status, 90% of people diagnosed with HIV to be on appropriate treatment, and 90% of people on treatment achieving viral suppression, by the year 2020 (UNAIDS, 2017).

Finally, in addition to advocating for people to be tested and treated, as well as following up with people who are potentially exposed, public health professionals are now encouraging the practice of something known as "treatment as prevention" (Amos, 2015). Treatment as prevention is the practice of people who are at high risk of HIV (but who do not yet have it) taking antiretrovirals to prevent HIV acquisition. This practice is now well supported in the literature and remains a standard of care in Canada, although the uptake of this practice has not been high across all risk groups—in large part because of issues of access to this intervention (Paperny, 2015; Knight et al., 2016).

Hepatitis B

Hepatitis B virus causes both acute and chronic liver disease in those who are infected. Most people who are infected later in life develop acute liver disease, which resolves over time and is cleared naturally by the body's immune system. However, a proportion of adults and the majority of children who acquire hepatitis B early in life end up with chronic liver infection that can then progress to cirrhosis and cancer.

The incidence of hepatitis B has declined since the mid 1990s, and in 2015, the incidence was 13.2 per 100 000 people (Canadian AIDS Treatment Information Exchange [CATIE], 2015). The major risk factors in Canada are sexual transmission and intravenous drug use. **Vertical transmission** (from mother to newborn) and medical and dental occupational transmission (patient to practitioner and vice versa) account for a small proportion of cases, reinforcing the importance of following proper IPAC practices.

Hepatitis B is the only STI for which an effective and safe vaccine is available, making vaccination a cornerstone of prevention against hepatitis B virus. Because of the high infectiousness of this virus, the expert consensus in Canada supports universal vaccination against hepatitis B. Immunization in childhood or early adolescence provides maximum protection against sexual transmission of hepatitis B. As of 1998, all provinces have universal preadolescent hepatitis B vaccination programs (Health Canada, 2017c).

Hepatitis C

Like hepatitis B virus, hepatitis C virus also affects the liver. However, unlike hepatitis B, most people who acquire hepatitis C are unable to clear the virus on their own, and 90% end up developing chronic infection, including complications such as cirrhosis (scarring of the liver) and cancer. The most recent Canadian estimates show that just over 400 000 Canadians have a history of hepatitis C infection, and the incidence rate is approximately 30 cases per 100 000 population (PHAC, 2018f). Like HIV, a number of people are unaware of their infection because a person can have hepatitis C for a long time without experiencing any signs or symptoms. In Canada, it is believed that 44% of people living with hepatitis C are unaware of their status (PHAC, 2018f).

Hepatitis C is transmitted through blood or body fluids that are contaminated with the virus. The major mode of transmission of hepatitis C is currently the sharing of drug injection equipment. Other risk factors associated with transmission include tattooing, body piercing, and needle-stick injuries if the items used in such activities are contaminated with infected blood or body fluids. There is a low but measurable rate of vertical and sexual transmission.

Currently, no vaccine exists. Prevention efforts are focused on needle- and syringe -exchange programs and opioid substitution therapy, supervised injection facilities, intervention for high-risk behaviours, risk-based screening, and testing (Høj et al., 2018; Ha & Timmerman, 2018). In recent years, newer, safer, and more affordable drugs for the treatment of hepatitis C have been made accessible to the Canadian population. As such, engaging people in treatment is another effective strategy to reduce community transmission.

Sexually Transmitted Infection and Bloodborne Infection Prevention

Public health authorities participate in primary, secondary, and tertiary prevention efforts when it comes to STIs and BBIs. Primary prevention efforts include things such as public education about the importance of things such as condom use, not sharing drug-use equipment, and taking precautions when at work (e.g., using proper procedures for handling needles). Secondary prevention includes screening some groups, encouraging regular testing, and following up with contacts of infected cases in an attempt to identify and treat those who have an STI or BBI and may not know it, early enough to prevent complications (for contacts, this may also be considered primary prevention). Lastly, tertiary prevention aims to ensure that those who have an STI are adequately treated to prevent complications such as pelvic inflammatory disease and infertility.

Specialized, sex-positive, and nonjudgemental sexual health clinics exist across the country, providing primary, secondary, and tertiary prevention. One such example is Options for Sexual Health in British Columbia, which operates clinics that offer screening and treatment for ST/BBIs and reproductive health counselling and education across the province. Their staff consists of a diverse range of health care providers, including sexual health educators who take an inclusive and rights-based approach to their work (Options for Sexual Health, 2016).

Public health officials are also involved in primary prevention of STIs and BBIs and are typically responsible for contact tracing or partner notification (i.e., ensuring that all contacts, including the sexual partners of a case, are identified, informed of their exposure, tested, and treated if appropriate). In some jurisdictions, public health law mandates that cases disclose who their partners are to ensure proper follow up. For less serious

STIs such as chlamydia, for example, public health officials may rely on the case to inform contacts themselves (partner-informed notification) and may even allow the index case to give medication to treat an STI in their partners without requiring that the partners see a medical practitioner (this is referred to as patient-delivered partner therapy). These measures are intended to reduce barriers for contacts to obtaining necessary treatment and to reduce the stigma associated with having an STI.

Because of some of the stigma associated with STIs and BBIs and the resulting legal implications in some jurisdictions, members of the public don't always feel comfortable about being tested. In addition, some do not want to know if they have a condition such as HIV, given the impact it may have on their own lives and interactions with future or current partners. Anonymous testing (most often for conditions such as HIV) is also available by some public health authorities. The idea is that even if the person's name is not attached to the testing result (and so contact tracing cannot be done consistently), the knowledge that they have an HIV infection may prompt someone to seek treatment or be careful regarding practices that might transmit the virus on to others.

Health Promotion in Sexual Health

The concept of healthy sexuality is one mode of primary prevention. Healthy sexuality is comfort with one's own sexuality, body characteristics, and self-efficacy in making decisions related to sexuality, such as contraception, pregnancy, and prevention of STIs. Developing positive sexual health involves a multifaceted approach of health education, self-esteem, and decision-making skills for behavioural change, as well as communication of specific knowledge, such as methods of birth control (oral contraception and barrier methods) and STI prevention (safer sex techniques).

Education and communication in this area must be innovative and sustain the interest of youth. Although young people appear to have adequate knowledge about STIs, they are unlikely to interpret risks personally and will take the view or optimism bias that "it cannot happen to me" (Ferguson, Topolski, & Miller, 2006; Muchiri, Odimegwu, & De Wet, 2017; Farahani et al., 2018). Public health units have developed a variety of resources on safer sex in an attempt to reach youth. Efforts to provide better communication about sexual health and services with high-risk groups have been developed and in some cases

have been integrated into school curriculums (see the In the News box for an example of the controversy surrounding Ontario's sexual education curriculum). These include more accessible clinics in schools and shopping malls, sexual and reproductive health education, counselling, and contraceptive provision (Salam et al., 2016); reaching homeless youth in the community through outreach workers; and community development.

🌐 IN THE NEWS

Ontario's Sexual Education Curriculum

In 2015, the Government in Ontario updated the 1998 sexual education curriculum to make it more relevant to contemporary teens. The 2015 curriculum included topics such as online safety, gender fluidity and identity, sexual consent, and differences in sexual orientations (including same-sex relationships), among others. The updated curriculum was praised by many public health organizations as being progressive, promoting positive sexual health, and reducing stigma for priority populations such as transgender individuals. However, the new curriculum also brought with it much controversy because many religious, conservative, and some parent groups opposed it.

In 2018, after a new provincial government was elected, the revised curriculum was cancelled, and schools were instructed to revert back to the 1998 curriculum until a new one could be developed. This prompted much backlash in the public health community and among some educator groups and required some public health units to influence public education and awareness in other ways.

Harm-reduction strategies (defined and explained in Chapter 9) are another method of primary prevention for infections such as HIV, hepatitis B, and hepatitis C. Examples of this type of strategy include the implementation of needle-exchange programs (in which clean equipment can be accessed by persons who inject drugs) and safe consumption sites (where people can bring their substances to use under the supervision of trained staff who can provide education on safer injection and inhalation practices).

Gender as an Important Determinant of Sexual Health

When looking at statistics related to STIs, it is evident that gender plays a very important role and should be considered a key determinant of sexual health. Gender, therefore, needs to be explicitly considered when developing health promotion interventions related to the area of STI prevention. (Refer to Critical Thinking Question to explore how toxic masculinity may impact STI rates and how health promotion efforts may account for this in men.)

A particularly salient example of how gender influences sexual health is among people living with HIV. As mentioned earlier, whereas women made up only 12% of people living with HIV in 1999, in 2015, they made up approximately 25% (Kaida et al., 2015). It is imperative, then, that community health practitioners ensure that risk and prevention messaging is pertinent to women as well as men when it comes to public health messaging. Often, prevention messaging involves disclosing one's HIV status to your partner and using a condom during intercourse. Given the societal power imbalances that still exist between men and women today, some women in heteronormative relationships may be less able to negotiate for condom use or disclose safely to their partners for many reasons, including fear of violence, stigma, and discrimination (Kaida et al., 2015). Thus, messaging needs to account for this, and health promotion efforts in the area of sexual health must also address societal factors, behaviours, and policies that perpetuate societal power imbalances between men and women (e.g., advocating for equal pay rules in your institution, ensuring adequate female representation in leadership positions, and advocating for policies such as affordable child care so that more women can be equal partners in the workforce if they have children).

CRITICAL THINKING QUESTION 10.5: Research the notion of toxic masculinity and be familiar with what it entails. Consider how toxic masculinity influences sexual health at the level of the individual and at the broader community or societal level. What strategies might exist to address toxic masculinity across the life course?

EMERGENCY PREPAREDNESS AND BIOTERRORISM

Bioterrorism can be described as the use of a microorganism with the deliberate intent of causing infection to achieve certain goals. With the increased availability of biological agents and the technical capacity to produce them, bioterrorism may become the weapon of choice in the future (CDC, 2017). However, the concept of biological warfare is not new, and preparations for a possible bioterrorist attack had been undertaken even before the 2001 attacks.

The US CDC has categorized pathogens according to their risk of posing a threat to national security. Category A agents, for example, are those that are easily transmitted between people and cause significant morbidity and mortality; they include pathogens such as anthrax and botulism. Category B agents are second priority and are somewhat less likely than category A agents to result in significant morbidity and mortality or to spread easily between people. Lastly, Category C agents are pathogens that have the possibility (if altered) for high morbidity and mortality and because of their wide availability and potential to disseminate could be engineered to become bioterrorism agents.

Although the probability that bioterrorism attacks will occur in Canada is low, if there is an attack, the consequences could be severe. As such, national organizations such as the PHAC, Health Canada, and the Canadian Food Inspection Agency undertake a number of emergency preparedness activities such as:
- Developing emergency response plans
- Developing lab protocols for testing bioterrorism agents at the National Microbiology Lab
- Maintaining a skilled deployable team to respond to emergencies
- Conducting surveillance activities to detect any signs of bioterrorism activities
- Stockpiling key supplies such as antibiotics (PHAC, 2012)

▮ S U M M A R Y

Despite the widespread availability of most vaccines, outbreaks of communicable diseases such as measles and meningitis continue to occur in Canada and are associated with significant mortality and morbidity.

Although vaccine-preventable diseases have declined, sporadic cases and outbreaks of a number of infectious diseases are being reported. These include pertussis, measles, influenza pneumococcal disease, varicella, and tuberculosis.

Vector-borne diseases, although rare in Canada, are important causes of morbidity and mortality worldwide, and two important vector-borne diseases (Lyme disease and WNV) are examples of EIDs of public health significance. Food-borne disease and water-borne diseases also contribute to the burden of morbidity from communicable disease in Canada. The effectiveness of vaccination in protecting individuals depends both on the efficacy, or performance of the vaccine under ideal conditions and on the degree of coverage achieved. Canada has a very robust infrastructure for ensuring the safety of vaccines and many players are involved in product safety, quality, and efficacy.

Genital chlamydia and gonorrhea are the most common causes of notifiable STIs in Canada. Risk factors for common STIs and BBIs include young age, new or multiple sexual partners, being incarcerated, being involved in sex work, and being Indigenous.

AIDS is caused by HIV and is transmitted through a range of routes, examples of which include: sexual contact with an infected partner, via infected blood and blood products, from an infected mother to her unborn child, and through the use of blood contaminated needles for injection drug use. Primary prevention strategies to control the sexual transmission of the virus include promoting behavioural change to limit the number of sexual partners and the use of condoms for safer sex, harm-reduction strategies such as needle-exchange programs, and now the use of antiretrovirals.

Bioterrorism is the use of a microorganism with the deliberate intent of causing infection to achieve certain goals. With increased availability of biological agents and the technical information required to produce them, bioterrorism may become the weapon of choice in the future.

KEY WEBSITES

Canadian AIDS Treatment Information Exchange (CATIE): https://www.catie.ca
CATIE bridges research and practice for HIV and hepatitis C by connecting with health care and community-based service providers with up-to-date and unbiased information. Follow the link to access bulletins, interactive online learning and webinars, fact sheets and guides, case studies, evidence reviews, and more.

Canadian Immunization Guide (CIG): https://www.canada.ca/en/public-health/services/canadian-immunization-guide.html
The CIG is a comprehensive resource with 54 chapters organized into five parts: key immunization information, vaccine safety, vaccine of specific populations, active vaccines, and passive immunization. This was developed for health care professionals, vaccine program decision makers, and other Canadian stakeholders based on recommendations and expertise of the National Advisory Committee on Immunization and the Committee to Advise on Tropical Medicine and Travel.

Infection Prevention and Control (IPAC) Canada: https://ipac-canada.org
IPAC Canada is a national, multidisciplinary association and a leader for promoting best practices in infection prevention and control. It aims to prevent infections and improve patient care in the health care setting by coordinating effective communication, supporting and standardizing infection control practices, promoting research in infection control, facilitating infection control education for practitioners, and more.

National Advisory Committee on Immunization (NACI): https://www.canada.ca/en/public-health/services/immunization/national-advisory-committee-on-immunization-naci.html
As a national advisory committee, the NACI reports to the Assistant Deputy Minister of Infectious Disease Prevention and Control and works with the Centre for Immunization and Respiratory Infectious Diseases of the Public Health Agency of Canada. The committee, including experts in pediatrics, infectious diseases, immunology, medical microbiology, internal medicine, and public health, works to provide timely advice and recommendations for the use of vaccines.

Options for Sexual Health (OPT): https://www.optionsforsexualhealth.org
OPT is a nonprofit sexual health organization providing inclusive and accessible clinic services and community education to British Columbia residents. OPT also offers a toll-free, confidential phone line where people can access health educators to answer questions related to sexual health, including contraception, as well as referrals to services.

The Joint United Nations Programme on HIV/AIDS (UNAIDS): http://www.unaids.org/en
UNAIDS promotes and supports delivery of HIV services by providing strategic direction, advocacy, coordination, and technical support to leadership from governments, the private sector, and communities. As part of responding to the global Sustainable Development Goals, UNAIDS aims to end AIDS as a public health threat by 2030.

REFERENCES

Advisory Committee for Ontario's Immunization System Review. (2014). *Ontario's publicly funded immunization system: building on today's strengths, innovating for the future.* Retrieved from http://www.health.gov.on.ca/en/common/ministry/publications/reports/immunization/docs/immun_sys_review_march2014_en.pdf.

Aenishaenslin, C., Bouchard, C., Koffi, J. K., et al. (2017). Exposure and preventive behaviours toward ticks and Lyme disease in Canada: Results from a first national survey. *Ticks and Tick-Borne Diseases, 8*(1), 112–118. https://doi.org/10.1016/j.ttbdis.2016.10.006.

Amos, H. (2015). What is HIV treatment as prevention? *UBC News.* Retrieved from https://news.ubc.ca/2015/07/20/what-is-hiv-treatment-as-prevention/.

Antoniou, A., & Cooper, C. (2016). *New Directions in Organizational Psychology and Behavioral Medicine.* New York, NY: Routledge.

Bélanger, P., Tanguay, F., Hamel, M., et al. (2015). Foodborne illness: An overview of foodborne outbreaks in Canada reported through outbreak summaries: 2008–2014. *Canada Communicable Disease Report, 41*(11), 254. Retrieved from https://www.canada.ca/en/public-health/services/reports-publications/canada-communicable-disease-report-ccdr/monthly-issue/2015-41/ccdr-volume-41-11-november-5-2015-foodborne-illness/ccdr-volume-41-11-november-5-2015-foodborne-illness.html.

Bellegarde, B. (2016). *Saskatchewan's high First Nations HIV numbers in the global spotlight.* The Canadian Press. Retrieved from https://globalnews.ca/news/2826436/saskatchewans-high-first-nations-hiv-numbers-in-the-global-spotlight/.

Bird, Y., Obidiya, O., Mahmood, R., et al. (2017). Human papillomavirus vaccination uptake in Canada: A systematic review and meta-analysis. *International Journal of Preventive Medicine, 8*, 71. https://doi.org/10.4103/ijpvm.IJPVM_49_17.

Bourgeois, A. C., Edmunds, M., Awan, A., et al. (2017). HIV in Canada—surveillance report, 2016. *Canada Communicable Disease Report, 43*(12), 248–256.

Buchan, S. A., & Kwong, J. C. (2016). Influenza immunization among Canadian health care personnel: A cross-sectional study. *CMAJ Open, 4*(3), E479. https://doi.org/10.9778/cmajo.20160018.

Canadian AIDS Treatment Information Exchange. (2015). *HIV in Canada: A primer for service providers.* Retrieved from https://www.catie.ca/en/hiv-canada/3/3-3.

Caplan, D. (2010). A decade after Walkerton: What still needs to be done? *The Toronto Star*, May 19. Retrieved from https://www.thestar.com/opinion/editorialopinion/2010/05/19/a_decade_after_walkerton_what_still_needs_to_be_done.html

Centers for Disease Control and Prevention. (2016). *Lesson 6: Investigating an outbreak.* Retrieved from https://www.cdc.gov/ophss/csels/dsepd/ss1978/lesson6/section2.html.

Centers for Disease Control and Prevention. (2017). *Bioterrorism.* Retrieved from https://www.cdc.gov/healthcommunication/toolstemplates/entertainmented/tips/Bioterrorism.html.

Cheng, A., Chen, D., Woodstock, K., et al. (2017). Analyzing the potential risk of climate change on Lyme disease in Eastern Ontario, Canada using time series remotely sensed temperature data and tick population modelling. *Remote Sensing, 9*(6), 609. https://doi.org/10.3390/rs9060609.

Choudhri, Y., Miller, J., Sandhu, J., et al. (2018a). Sexually transmitted infections: Chlamydia in Canada, 2010–2015. *Canada Communicable Disease Report, 44*(2), 49. Retrieved from https://www.canada.ca/en/public-health/services/reports-publications/canada-communicable-disease-report-ccdr/monthly-issue/2018-44/issue-2-february-1-2018/article-3-chlamydia-2010-2015.html.

Choudhri, Y., Miller, J., Sandhu, J., et al. (2018b). Sexually transmitted infections: Gonorrhea in Canada, 2010–2015. *Canada Communicable Disease Report, 44*(2), 37. Retrieved from https://www.canada.ca/en/public-health/services/reports-publications/canada-communicable-disease-report-ccdr/monthly-issue/2018-44/issue-2-february-1-2018/article-1-gonorrhea-2010-2015.html.

Choudhri, Y., Miller, J., Sandhu, J., et al. (2018c). Sexually transmitted infections: Infectious and congenital syphilis in Canada, 2010–2015. *Canada Communicable Disease Report, 44*(2), 43. Retrieved from https://www.canada.ca/en/public-health/services/reports-publications/canada-communicable-disease-report-ccdr/monthly-issue/2018-44/issue-2-february-1-2018/article-2-syphilis-2010-2015.html.

Clow, B. (n.d.). *Backgrounder: The relationship between burden of disease and health equity. Making evidence matter.* Retrieved from https://evidencenetwork.ca/backgrounder-the-relationship-between-burden-of-disease-and-health-equity/.

CTVNews. (2016). *Stomach parasite emerges in indigenous communities in Far North.* Retrieved from https://www.ctvnews.ca/health/stomach-parasite-emerges-in-indigenous-communities-in-far-north-1.2878669.

Dickson, C., Pham, M. T., Nguyen, V., et al. (2018). Community outbreak of invasive group A streptococcus infection in Ontario, Canada. Can we eliminate hepatitis C? *Canada Communicable Disease Report, 44*(7/8), 182. Retrieved from https://www.canada.ca/content/dam/phac-aspc/documents/services/reports-publications/canada-communicable-disease-report-ccdr/monthly-issue/2018-44/issue-7-8-july-5-2018/ccdrv44i0708-eng.pdf#page=36

Dubé, E., Gagnon, D., Ouakki, M., et al. (2018). Measuring vaccine acceptance among Canadian parents: A survey of the Canadian Immunization Research Network. *Vaccine*, 36(4), 545–552. https://doi.org/10.1016/j.vaccine.2017.12.005.

Farahani, F. K., Akhondi, M. M., Shirzad, M., et al. (2018). HIV/STI risk-taking sexual behaviours and risk perception among male university students in Tehran: Implications for HIV prevention among youth. *Journal of Biosocial Science*, 50(1), 86–101.

Ferguson, H., Topolski, R., & Miller, M. (2006). Sexually transmitted infections: Perceived knowledge versus actual knowledge. *Journal of the Georgia Public Health Association* 1,1–10.

Giordano, B. V., Kaur, S., & Hunter, F. F. (2017). West Nile virus in Ontario, Canada: A twelve-year analysis of human case prevalence, mosquito surveillance, and climate data. *PloS One*, 12(8), e0183568. https://doi.org/10.1371/journal.pone.0183568.

Government of Canada. (2008). *Avian influenza (bird flu)*. Retrieved from https://www.canada.ca/en/health-canada/services/healthy-living/your-health/diseases/avian-influenza-bird-flu.html.

Government of Canada. (2016). *Symptoms of tuberculosis (TB)*. Retrieved from https://www.canada.ca/en/public-health/services/diseases/tuberculosis-tb/symptoms-tuberculosis-tb.html.

Ha, S., & Timmerman, K. (2018). Awareness and knowledge of hepatitis C among health care providers and the public: A scoping. Can we eliminate hepatitis C? *Canada Communicable Disease Report*, 44(7/8), 157. Retrieved from https://www.canada.ca/en/public-health/services/reports-publications/canada-communicable-disease-report-ccdr/monthly-issue/2018-44/issue-7-8-july-5-2018/article-2-awareness-hep-c-among-health-care-providers.html

Health Canada. (2017a). *About antibiotic resistance*. Retrieved from https://www.canada.ca/en/public-health/services/antibiotic-antimicrobial-resistance/about-antibiotic-resistance.html.

Health Canada. (2017b). *Antimicrobial resistance and animals—Actions*. Retrieved from https://www.canada.ca/en/public-health/services/antibiotic-antimicrobial-resistance/animals/actions.html.

Health Canada. (2017c). *Hepatitis B vaccine*. Retrieved from https://www.canada.ca/en/public-health/services/publications/healthy-living/canadian-immunization-guide-part-4-active-vaccines/page-7-hepatitis-b-vaccine.html.

Heymann, D. (Ed.). (2015). *Control of Communicable Diseases Manual* (20th Ed.) Washington, DC: American Public Health Association.

Hobbs, J. L., Warshawsky, B., Maki, A., et al. (2017). Nuggets of wisdom: Salmonella enteritidis outbreaks and the case for new rules on uncooked frozen processed chicken.

Journal of Food Protection, 80(4), 703–709. https://doi.org/10.4315/0362-028X.JFP-16-431.

Høj, S. B., Minoyan, N., Artenie, A. A., et al. (2018). The role of prevention strategies in achieving HCV elimination in Canada: What are the remaining challenges? *Canadian Liver Journal*, 1(2), 4–13. https://doi.org/10.3138/canlivj.1.2.003.

Hussain, S. F., Boyle, P., Patel, P., et al. (2016). Eradicating polio in Pakistan: An analysis of the challenges and solutions to this security and health issue. *Globalization and Health*, 12, 63.

Jackson, J., Fraser, R., & Ash, P. (2014). Social media and nurses: Insights for promoting health for individual and professional Use. *Online Journal of Issues in Nursing*, 19(3).

The Joint United Nations Programme on HIV/AIDS. (2017). *90–90–90: An ambitious treatment target to help end the AIDS epidemic*. Retrieved from http://www.unaids.org/en/resources/documents/2017/90-90-90.

Kaida, A., Carter, A., De Pokomandy, A., et al. (2015). Sexual inactivity and sexual satisfaction among women living with HIV in Canada in the context of growing social, legal and public health surveillance. *Sexual and Reproductive Health and Human Rights of Women Living with HIV*, 18, 6S5.

Kawatsu, L., Izumi, K., Uchimura, K., et al. (2015). Can social network analysis assist in the prioritisation of contacts in a tuberculosis contact investigation? *International Journal of Tuberculosis and Lung Disease*, 19(11), 1293–1299. https://doi.org/10.5588/ijtld.15.0378.

Knight, R., Small, W., Thomson, K., et al. (2016). Implementation challenges and opportunities for HIV Treatment as Prevention (TasP) among young men in Vancouver, Canada: A qualitative study. *BMC Public Health*, 16(1), 262. https://doi.org/10.1186/s12889-016-2943-y.

Komarnisky, S., Hackett, P., Abonyi, S., et al. (2016). "Years ago": Reconciliation and First Nations narratives of tuberculosis in the Canadian Prairie Provinces. *Critical Public Health*, 26(4), 381–393.

Last, J. (2001). *A Dictionary of epidemiology* (4th ed.). Toronto: Oxford University Press.

Lemstra, M., Neudorf, V., Opondo, J., et al. (2008). Disparity in childhood immunizations. *Paediatrics & Child Health*, 12, 847–852.

Levy, S. (2017). Northern trek: the spread of ixodes scapularis into Canada. *Environmental Health Perspectives*, 125(7), 074002. https://doi.org/10.1289/EHP2095.

MacDonald, N. E., & Law, B. J. (2017). Canada's eight-component vaccine safety system: a primer for health care workers. *Paediatrics & Child Health*, 22(4), e13–e16. Retrieved from https://www.cps.ca/en/documents/position/vaccine-safety-system.

Manning, M. L., Septimus, E. J., Ashley, E. S. D., et al. (2018). Antimicrobial stewardship and infection prevention—leveraging the synergy: A position paper update. *Infection Control & Hospital Epidemiology*, 39(4), 467–472. https://doi.org/10.1016/j.ajic.2018.01.001.

Muchiri, E., Odimegwu, C., & De Wet, N. (2017). HIV risk perception and consistency in condom use among adolescents and young adults in urban Cape Town, South Africa: A cumulative risk analysis. *Southern African Journal of Infectious Diseases*, 32(3), 105–110.

Nanni, M. G., Caruso, R., Mitchell, A. J., et al. (2015). Depression in HIV infected patients: A review. *Current Psychiatry Reports*, 17(1), 530. https://doi.org/10.1007/s11920-014-0530-4.

National AIDS Manual. (2017). Retrieved from http://www.aidsmap.com/Longer-term-side-effects/page/1283841/

National Collaborating Centre for Infectious Diseases. (2018). *Disease debrief: Group A streptococcus*. Retrieved from https://nccid.ca/debrief/group-a-streptococcus/.

Ogden, N. H., AbdelMalik, P., & Pulliam, J. R. C. (2017). Emerging infections: Emerging infectious diseases: Prediction and detection. *Canada Communicable Disease Report*, 43(10), 206. Retrieved from https://www.canada.ca/en/public-health/services/reports-publications/canada-communicable-disease-report-ccdr/monthly-issue/2017-43/ccdr-volume-43-10-october-5-2017/commentary-emerging-infectious-diseases-prediction-detection.html.

Options for Sexual Health. (2016). *About us*. Retrieved from https://www.optionsforsexualhealth.org/about-opt.

Paperny, A.M. (2015). Made-in-Canada HIV/AIDS treatment embraced by everyone but Canada. *Global News*. Retrieved from https://globalnews.ca/news/2250681/made-in-canada-hivaids-treatment-embraced-by-every-one-but-canada/

Public Health Agency of Canada. (2006). *ARCHIVE—4.0 Epidemiology of Invasive GAS Disease in Canada*. Retrieved from https://www.canada.ca/en/public-health/services/reports-publications/canada-communicable-disease-report-ccdr/monthly-issue/2006-32/canada-communicable-disease-report/4-0-epidemiology-invasive-gas-disease-canada.html.

Public Health Agency of Canada. (2010). *Section 5-2: Canadian Guidelines on Sexually Transmitted Infections—Management and treatment of specific infections: Chlamydial infections*. Retrieved from https://www.canada.ca/en/public-health/services/infectious-diseases/sexual-health-sexually-transmitted-infections/canadian-guidelines/sexually-transmitted-infections/canadian-guidelines-sexually-transmitted-infections-30.html.

Public Health Agency of Canada. (2012). *Bioterrorism and emergency preparedness*. Retrieved from https://www.canada.ca/en/public-health/services/emergency-preparedness-response/bioterrorism-emergency-preparedness.html.

Public Health Agency of Canada. (2015). *National vaccine storage and handling guidelines for immunization providers 2015*. Retrieved from https://www.canada.ca/en/public-health/services/publications/healthy-living/national-vaccine-storage-handling-guidelines-immunization-providers-2015.html.

Public Health Agency of Canada. (2017a). *Vaccine preventable disease: Surveillance report to December 31, 2015*. Retrieved from https://www.canada.ca/en/public-health/services/publications/healthy-living/vaccine-preventable-disease-surveillance-report-december-31-2015.html.

Public Health Agency of Canada. (2017b). *Canadian Antimicrobial Resistance Surveillance System 2017 Report*. Retrieved from https://www.canada.ca/en/public-health/services/publications/drugs-health-products/canadian-antimicrobial-resistance-surveillance-system-2017-report-executive-summary.html.

Public Health Agency of Canada. (2017c). *Human papillomavirus (HPV)*. Retrieved from https://www.canada.ca/en/public-health/services/diseases/human-papillomavirus-hpv.html.

Public Health Agency of Canada. (2018a). *Pertussis vaccine*. Retrieved from the https://www.canada.ca/en/public-health/services/publications/healthy-living/canadian-immunization-guide-part-4-active-vaccines/page-15-pertussis-vaccine.html.

Public Health Agency of Canada. (2018b). *For health professionals: Flu (influenza)*. Retrieved from https://www.canada.ca/en/public-health/services/diseases/flu-influenza/health-professionals-flu-influenza.html.

Public Health Agency of Canada. (2018c). *Surveillance of tuberculosis (TB)*. Retrieved from https://www.canada.ca/en/public-health/services/diseases/tuberculosis-tb/surveillance-tuberculosis-tb.html.

Public Health Agency of Canada. (2018d). *Surveillance of rabies*. Retrieved from https://www.canada.ca/en/public-health/services/diseases/rabies/surveillance.html.

Public Health Agency of Canada. (2018e). *Public Health Notice—outbreak of Salmonella infections linked to poultry, including frozen raw breaded chicken products*. Retrieved from https://www.canada.ca/en/public-health/services/public-health-notices/2018/public-health-notice-outbreak-salmonella-infections-linked-poultry-frozen-raw-breaded-chicken-products.html.

Public Health Agency of Canada. (2018f). *Surveillance of hepatitis C*. Retrieved from https://www.canada.ca/en/public-health/services/diseases/hepatitis-c/surveillance-hepatitis-c.html.

Public Health Ontario. (2015). *Infection prevention and control for clinical office practice*. Retrieved from https://www.publichealthontario.ca/en/eRepository/IPAC_Clinical_Office_Practice_2013.pdf.

Rémy, V., Zöllner, Y., & Heckmann, U. (2015). Vaccination: The cornerstone of an efficient healthcare system. *Journal of Market Access & Health Policy*, 3. https://doi.org/10.3402/jmahp.v3.27041.

Ripoche, M., Lindsay, L. R., Ludwig, A., et al. (2018). Multiscale clustering of Lyme disease risk at the expanding leading edge of the range of Ixodes scapularis in Canada. *International Journal of Environmental Research and Public Health*, 15(4), 603. https://doi.org/10.3390/ijerph15040603.

Robinson, J. L. (2018). Potential strategies to improve childhood immunization rates in Canada. *Paediatrics & Child Health*, 23(5), 353–356. https://doi.org/10.1093/pch/pxy052.

Salam, R. A., Faqqah, A., Sajjad, N., et al. (2016). Improving adolescent sexual and reproductive health: A systematic review of potential interventions. *Journal of Adolescent Health*, 59(4), S11–S28.

Scheifele, D. W., Ward, B. J., Halperin, S. A., et al. (2014). Approved but non-funded vaccines: Accessing individual protection. *Vaccine*, 32(7), 766–770. https://doi.org/10.1016/j.vaccine.2013.12.027.

Sherrard, L., Hiebert, J., & Squires, S. (2015). Measles surveillance in Canada: Trends for 2014. *Canada Communicable Disease Report*, 41(7), 157–168.

Silverman, M., Povitz, M., Sontrop, J. M., et al. (2017). Antibiotic prescribing for nonbacterial acute upper respiratory infections in elderly persons. *Annals of Internal Medicine*, 166(11), 765–774. https://doi.org/10.7326/M16-1131.

Strategic Advisory Group of Experts Working Group on Vaccine Hesitancy. (2014). *Report of the SAGE Working Group on vaccine hesitancy*. Retrieved from http://www.who.int/immunization/sage/meetings/2014/october/1_Report_WORKING_GROUP_vaccine_hesitancy_final.pdf.

Thomson Reuters. (2017). *Stop using antibiotics in healthy farm animals, WHO warns*. Retrieved from https://www.cbc.ca/news/health/who-no-more-antibiotics-healthy-farm-animals-1.4391940.

Vachon, J., Gallant, V., & Siu, W. (2018). *Tuberculosis in Canada, 2016*. Ottawa: Public Health Agency of Canada. Retrieved from https://www.canada.ca/en/public-health/services/reports-publications/canada-communicable-disease-report-ccdr/monthly-issue/2018-44/issue-3-4-march-1-2018/article-1-tuberculosis-2016.html

World Health Organization. (2017). *Stop using antibiotics in healthy animals to prevent the spread of antibiotic resistance*. Retrieved from http://www.who.int/news-room/detail/07-11-2017-stop-using-antibiotics-in-healthy-animals-to-prevent-the-spread-of-antibiotic-resistance.

World Health Organization. (n.d.). *Ten threats to global health in 2019*. Retrieved from https://www.who.int/emergencies/ten-threats-to-global-health-in-2019.

Environmental Health

LEARNING OBJECTIVES

- Define *environmental health* and *environmental justice*.
- Define *toxicology* and list the four steps of risk assessment.
- Describe the health effects, common exposure routes, and control strategies for common health hazards, including electromagnetic radiation (ionizing and nonionizing), light, noise, and indoor and outdoor air pollution.
- Define *climate change* and list its impacts on human health.
- Explain the link between safe drinking and recreational water on human health and list strategies to ensure safe water.
- Describe the health effects, common exposure routes, and control strategies for common types of chemicals, including pesticides, heavy metals, persistent organic pollutants, and endocrine disrupters.
- Define *sustainable development* and understand its importance for the global agenda.

CHAPTER OUTLINE

KEY TERMS

biomagnification
blue-green algae
building-related illness
built environment
carcinogens
climate change

criteria air pollutants
electromagnetic radiation (EMR)
endocrine-disrupting chemicals (EDCs)
environmental health
environmental justice

global warming
maximum acceptable concentrations (MACs)
persistent organic pollutants (POPs)
precautionary principle

AN INTRODUCTION TO ENVIRONMENTAL HEALTH

In recent years, there has been increasing recognition of the interdependence of human health and the health of the global ecosystem, with its many life forms, even though this view has been a longstanding one in many Indigenous communities across the world. As mentioned in Chapters 1 and 5, the environment is very influential in shaping the health of our communities. Thus, our physical (natural and built) environment requires special attention because it shapes the conditions in which people live, work, grow, and play.

Historically, the field of environmental health has dealt with food and water safety and with the inspection and investigation of environmental hazards that may arise from inadequate sanitation. In most of Canada, provision of sanitation, potable water supply, and food free from gross contamination have been largely achieved despite tragedies such as the one that occurred in 2000 in Walkerton, Ontario (Walkerton Inquiry, 2002), where poor management of the municipal water supply and a lack of provincial safeguards resulted in several unfortunate deaths and many illnesses. However, inequities in food and water safety continue to exist, a prominent example being the number of Indigenous communities that currently have "boil water," "do not consume," and "do not use" water advisories. In fact, many Indigenous communities across Canada have had long-term advisories in place for more than a decade (Fig. 11.1). Additionally, there is growing concern over the status of the environment and the consequences of environmental pollution, particularly of chemical and biological contamination. This concern is not only limited to the effects on human health but also to the viability of ecosystems in general and of many species in particular.

Public attention has been captured by recent reports detailing the effects of acid rain on forest and aquatic ecosystems, climatic changes resulting from the greenhouse effect, the depletion of the ozone layer, and the effects of marine pollution on aquatic life. Public interest has also been heightened as a result of numerous reports linking environmental exposure to adverse human health outcomes. Environmental factors may contribute to the development of reproductive disorders, including infertility, breast cancer, and poor sperm quality or function. The negative reproductive impact of environmental factors on humans has led to increased research of the role of chemical contamination on human reproductive capacity (Sifakis et al., 2017).

The World Health Organization (WHO) and other key groups describe the field of **environmental health** as a branch of public health that addresses all "physical, chemical, and biological factors external to a person, and all the related factors impacting behaviours." It involves assessing and controlling environmental factors that may affect health. According to the WHO, the field of environmental health focuses on disease prevention and the creation of health-supporting environments. This definition of environmental health excludes behaviours related to genetic predisposition, as well as the sociocultural environment, but does include the **built environment**, or human-made physical structures where people work, live, learn, and play (including roads, buildings, parks, and other infrastructure) (Centers for Disease Control and Prevention, 2011; US National Library of Medicine & National Institutes of Health, n.d.).

Because the impact of the environment on human populations is widespread, a variety of disciplines and practitioners contribute to the field of environmental health, including clinical medicine and nursing. Whereas other disciplines assess the impact of environmental agents or hazards on the individual patient, the focus of study in environmental health is the impact of these agents on the health of the population.

In the late 1980s, the terms *environmental justice* and *environmental racism* were introduced based on the increasing recognition that vulnerable groups (often the poor and racialized) are disproportionately affected by environmental toxins because of government policy and, in some cases, government inaction. One of the more recent publicized examples of this was the

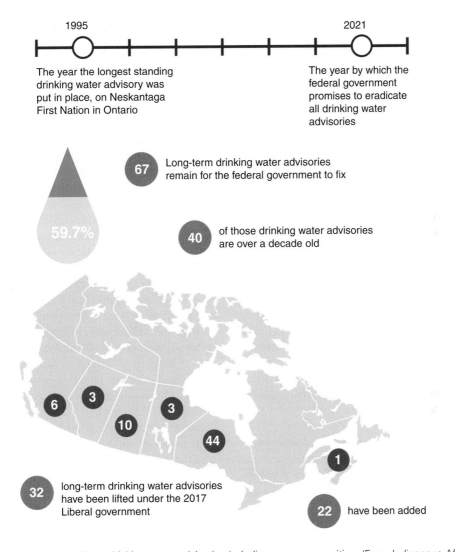

1995
The year the longest standing drinking water advisory was put in place, on Neskantaga First Nation in Ontario

2021
The year by which the federal government promises to eradicate all drinking water advisories

67 Long-term drinking water advisories remain for the federal government to fix

40 of those drinking water advisories are over a decade old

59.7%

6

3

10

3

44

1

32 long-term drinking water advisories have been lifted under the 2017 Liberal government

22 have been added

Fig. 11.1 By the numbers: drinking water advisories in Indigenous communities. (From Indigenous Affairs Canada and Health Canada. Original graphic by Nick Kirmse/CTVNews.ca (Dec 21, 2017). Retrieved from https://www.ctvnews.ca/politics/can-pm-trudeau-keep-drinkable-water-promise-to-first-nations-1.3736954.)

crisis in Grassy Narrows First Nations, where a chemical company discharged mercury waste into a river system heavily used by the Indigenous people in that area during the 1960s and 1970s. The communities in this part of Ontario are still dealing with the immense health impacts of mercury contamination, which many argue might not have occurred or been as long-lasting if the affected communities were more affluent or white. (This catastrophe is described further in the Case Study box later in the chapter.)

The environmental justice movement has grown in recent years, with many groups speaking up about the inequities that exist in terms of environmental exposures, both on a global and local level. The US Environmental Protection Agency's (EPA's) most current definition of **environmental justice** is the "fair treatment and meaningful involvement of all people with respect to development, implementation, and enforcement of environmental laws, regulations, and policies," in which *fair treatment* refers to the "reduction in inequitable consequences resulting from industrial, municipal, and commercial operations or from the execution of federal, state, and local laws; regulations; and policies" (US EPA, 2018a). Thinking about a social determinants of health approach, then, it is clear that environmental exposures can also affect health as well as its distribution.

The environment as it affects health can be divided into working and nonworking categories. The workplace environment is often associated with high-level exposure of a population predominantly of adult age and in good health. In contrast, nonworkplace environmental exposures are generally low level and may be chronic. The population at risk consists of persons at the extremes of age, developing fetuses, and ill or immunocompromised individuals. Thus, although many of the pathogenic agents are similar, there is an arbitrary distinction between working and nonworking environmental health. The specific concerns relating to the working environment (occupational health) are addressed in Chapter 12. Despite the uncertainty associated with many environmental health problems, health care providers are considered to be the most credible sources of information regarding the health effects of environmental exposures. Consequently, it is important for every health care provider to be familiar with the concepts used and the issues involved in environmental health.

This chapter explores the concepts of risk assessment (using toxicological data with exposure estimates) and risk management. Several topical issues are explored, including physical agents, climate change, air and water quality, and chemical toxicity. An approach to creating a healthy environment, which focuses on healthy public policy and managing environmental accidents, concludes the chapter.

METHODS AND TOOLS

The study of environmental health issues relies heavily on the discipline of toxicology. **Toxicology**, the science of poisons (toxins), attempts to identify adverse effects of substances on health and to predict harmful dosages. One of the fundamental tenets of toxicology is that any substance can be a poison if given in a large enough dose. By contrast, there are some substances that don't have a threshold or safe level. Most **carcinogens** (or cancer-causing agents), for example, do not have a threshold below which they no longer cause

cancer. Epidemiology, as previously defined in Chapter 2, is the study of the distribution and determinants of health and disease in human population. In the realm of environmental health, epidemiologists rely heavily on observational studies to tease out the health effects of various environmental exposures or toxic agents.

It is important to distinguish between toxins and toxicants, although these terms are often used interchangeably. Whereas the term **toxin** refers to harmful substances made by living things—cells or microorganisms (e.g., the botulism toxin made by the bacteria *Clostridium botulinum*), the term **toxicant** refers to human-made products (e.g., pesticides). This chapter mostly deals with toxicants (Chapter 10 deals with communicable diseases). Toxins are particularly important when it comes to food safety—one focus area of environmental health as it relates to public health practice.

There are a variety of problems in the measurement of specific toxic agents. Levels of some toxic agents are often difficult to determine, both in the human body and in the ambient (surrounding) environment. As technology progresses, the detection of minute quantities of chemicals is enhanced, but the interpretation of their significance to human health may remain difficult. Just because a specific toxic agent is present in the human body does not mean that it is contributing to any changes in structure or functioning. Toxicologists often don't have a good idea of what damage a specific toxic agent may cause at low levels because most toxicology data are obtained from high-dose animal experimentation. When a level is measurable, often it does not reflect the concentration in the target organ of interest; rather, it represents a crude attempt to assess dose by measuring tissue fluid levels (usually blood). For example, although clinicians can test for the presence of lead in a person's blood, this level doesn't reflect how much lead is actually affecting end organs or tissues; it is just a rough estimate of how much lead a person's cells are exposed to. The study of some adverse health outcomes, particularly mutagenic and carcinogenic (i.e., cancer-causing) effects, is complicated by the long latency period after exposure. It can take up to 20 years or more for an exposure to cause cancer. During this latency period, it is hard to pinpoint a particular exposure as being related because the exposure may have ended by then or may have been very episodic. Additionally, adverse outcomes may manifest only in a small fraction of the exposed population. Thus, rare outcomes and long latency

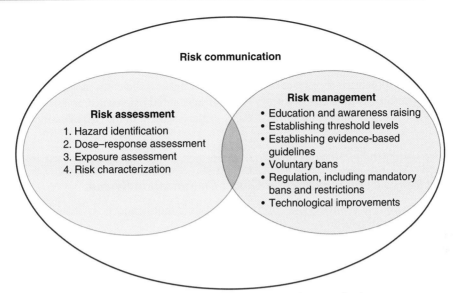

Fig. 11.2 Risk assessment, management, and communication.

periods after certain environmental exposures are challenges to epidemiological analysis (Munnangi & Boktor, 2017). Furthermore, the confounding effects of multiple exposures often mask the effects of a specific agent. The relationship between agents grows even more complex when accounting for synergistic or antagonistic relationships of multiple chemicals (Braun et al., 2016; Canadian Centre for Occupational Health and Safety, 2018). For example, although both radon exposure and tobacco smoke exposure are known causes of lung cancer, when both are present, the risk of lung cancer is increased exponentially—and beyond what would be expected if both exerted their effects independently. The study of environmental health is also complicated by the fact that many adverse outcomes are common in the population, nonspecific (i.e., that could be caused by many different pathologies), and subjective. The upper respiratory and conjunctival symptoms of the sick building syndrome, for example, are difficult to quantify objectively.

Establishing Toxicity

Every day, each of us is exposed to a variety of environmental risks. The leading authorities responsible for identifying and assessing the risks to human health posed by the environment include Health Canada, Environment Canada, the Canadian Food Inspection Agency, provincial and territorial ministries of health and environment, local and regional public health units,

the agricultural sector, and various professional groups. These bodies evaluate the political, economic, societal, and technological implications of the risk and identify the options for managing risks according to the best available evidence. They then develop the policies, regulations, and other measures for protection of the public.

Risk assessment is the first approach to assessing health risks posed by contaminants. There are four major steps in the risk assessment of any environmental contaminant: hazard identification, dose–response assessment, exposure assessment and monitoring, and risk characterization (refer to Fig. 11.2 for a visual concept of how these steps and processes fit together with risk management and risk communication as well).

Hazard Identification

Hazard identification refers to elucidating the adverse health effects linked to a particular environmental agent of concern. In identifying hazards, it is important to specify the organ system affected and the severity of potential harm. Information related to what adverse health effects a toxic agent can produce is obtained from laboratory, genetic, animal, and human epidemiological studies. The US EPA's IRIS database (Integrated Risk Information System), and the Centers for Disease Control and Prevention's (CDC's) Agency for Toxic Substances and Disease Registry are excellent information resources that contain information about human health effects that may result from exposure to various substances found in the environment. The International Agency of Cancer Research (IARC) fact sheets are also a good resource when it comes to information about the cancer-causing potential of various agents (see the Research Perspective box for an overview of the IARC classification system). It is important to keep in mind that just because a specific environmental agent is known to be causally related to a particular health effect, this does not mean that the agent poses a risk to human health. It could be that humans are not exposed to the agent sufficiently enough for there to be any type of substantial risk. Hence, assessing exposure is another critical element in the risk assessment process.

RESEARCH PERSPECTIVE

The International Agency for Research on Cancer Classification System

The IARC thoroughly reviews the scientific literature in order to classify specific agents according to their cancer-causing potential. Agents are classified as follows:

- **Group 1 agents:** These are known carcinogens based on a range of scientific studies. Examples of group 1 agents include asbestos, benzene, arsenic, outdoor air pollution, and tobacco smoke.
- **Group 2A agents:** These are agents that are "probable" carcinogens based on strong but nonconclusive evidence for their effects on humans. Examples include acrylamide and red meat.
- **Group 2B agents:** These are "possible" carcinogens, meaning there is some evidence that they may cause cancer in humans, but the evidence is far from conclusive. Notable examples include some forms of mercury and lead.
- **Group 3 agents:** Agents in this category are considered "unclassifiable" because there is a lack of evidence for their cancer-causing potential, one way or another. Examples include caffeine and ampicillin.
- **Group 4 agents:** Any agent in group 4 represents one for which there is strong evidence that it is "probably not carcinogenic" to humans. Only one substance—caprolactam (which is used to make synthetic fibres)—falls into this category.

Dose–Response Assessment

Another key step in the risk assessment process is determining how the dose of a specific health hazard corresponds to a specific health outcome. For some health hazards, there is no "safe level," but for others, there might be a safe level. Often animal studies are conducted to better define the relationship between dose and effect and to figure out what doses the population must be exposed to for harm to occur. This dose (usually calculated as a result of animal experimentation) is then compared with estimates of the dose a population is exposed to in real life (exposure assessment) to determine if there is a risk to a specific population or community.

Exposure Assessment and Monitoring

Exposure can be defined as any contact between a substance and an individual. The goal of exposure assessment is to better determine what proportion and who in the population might be exposed to an agent that is known to cause disease. An exposure pathway has five components:
- The source of contamination
- The environmental media
- The point of exposure

- The receptor populations
- The route of exposure

With this general framework in mind, it is possible to develop a model of the variety of possible exposures and their potential impact on humans. The principal environmental media for the exposure to contaminants are water, food, soil, and air. The major routes of exposure for humans are inhalation, ingestion, and dermal contact (Fig. 11.3).

Scientists and government regulatory bodies, with the help of toxicologists, often look to animal models to define exposure levels (i.e., concentration inhaled or ingested over a lifetime) at which harm can occur. Regulatory bodies then periodically monitor environmental media (e.g., air and water) to make sure that they do not contain high levels of toxicants and that humans aren't being exposed in a way that exceeds the "safe threshold." For example, Health Canada publishes *Guidelines for Canadian Drinking Water Quality*. These are designed to ensure that drinking water is free from pathogenic organisms, harmful chemicals, and radioactive matter, and that it is palatable. **Maximum acceptable concentrations (MACs)** for a wide range of chemicals, aesthetic objectives, and microbiological characteristics for water have

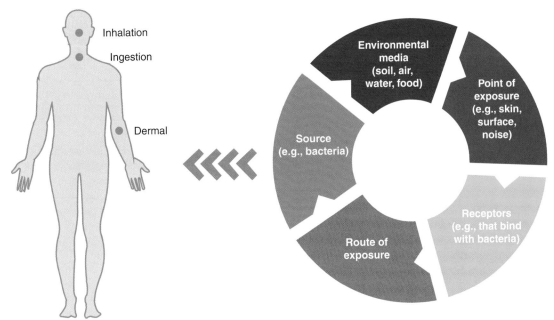

Fig. 11.3 The exposure pathway and major routes of environmental exposures.

been defined (Health Canada, 2017a). See Table 11.1 for a more detailed description of the MACs for common drinking water contaminants and their implications.

It is important to keep in mind that for some toxicants, there is no threshold or safe level, in which case toxicologists usually define a "safe" exposure level, which results in an increased risk that is very low (i.e., less than one in a million) and therefore acceptable to the population.

Risk Characterization

This step represents a summary of the hazard identification, dose–response assessment, and exposure assessment. In risk characterization, it is important to consider the following:

- The potential toxicity of the substance and the likely effects on human health
- The actual or estimated exposure and the dose–response relationship
- The measure of uncertainty inherent in this calculation

The risk characterization can be quantitative (specifying the "extra" risk of adverse health effects in an exposed population) or more qualitative (describing risk as high, medium, or low, for example). Either way, it

represents a summary statement that includes how certain the conclusion is and what major assumptions were made in the process of coming up with the conclusion (US EPA, 2017).

Whereas environmental health risk assessment is often done at a population level using these four steps, in clinical practice, health care professionals have an important role to play when assessing risks at an individual level. A thorough environmental health history is an important part of a clinical encounter that often includes the following types of inquiries:

- Location and age of the house where the client lives
- Source of drinking water
- Diet
- Drugs (prescribed, over the counter, illicit)
- Physical locations where clients spend most of their time (e.g., daycare, school, workplace)
- Type of work clients do (past and present)
- Hobbies that clients engage in (e.g., gardening, ceramics, woodworking)

Risk Management

Risk management is the series of steps that follows risk assessment and is integral to creating healthy public policy (see section titled Water Quality later in chapter)

TABLE 11.1   Common Drinking Water Contaminants and Mean Acceptable Concentrations (MACs)

Category of Contaminant	Specific Indicator	Target Level (MAC)	Implication
Microbiological	*Escherichia coli* level (measured per 100 mL)	0 per 100 mL	Any detectable levels of *E. coli* indicate fecal contamination of the water supply, prompting immediate action from public health agencies (investigation to confirm results and instituting boil water advisories).
Microbiological	Total coliforms (measured per 100 mL)	0 per 100 mL	Detectable results indicate changes in water quality and potentially integrity of the water treatment process or distribution system. Positive results need to be investigated further.
Microbiological	Turbidity (measured in units called NTU)	Various targets, depending on water system	A high level of turbidity signifies the presence of organic and inorganic particles that can interfere with the disinfection process. Typically, filtering water helps reduce turbidity level.
Chemical	Arsenic level	0.010 mg/L or as low as reasonably achievable	Long-term exposure to arsenic in the drinking water can cause cancer over many years. High arsenic levels in the water may prompt an investigation to identify the source (e.g., industrial waste vs naturally occurring from the Earth's crust) and a change in source water.
Radiological	Iodine-131	6 Bq/L	Long-term exposure can cause a range of cancers. Exposure in drinking water is usually caused by sewage effluent, and high levels would likely prompt an investigation into the cause and potential change in source water.

NTU, Nephelometric turbidity unit.

focused on reducing the impacts of environmental exposures on a population level. It involves decision making and implementation of options for management of the identified risk. For example, in the consideration of food contaminants, when there is a toxicant identified that exceeds what regulatory bodies deem to be "safe", certain risk management options may be considered. The options might include:

- Establishing guidelines or promulgating specific regulations controlling the toxic substance or substances
- Restricting the sale or distribution of food produced in an area that may have been identified as the source of the contamination
- Recommending changes in dietary habits.

Risk Communication

The communication of risk in relation to environmental hazards and to health hazards in general depends on an important concept: the perception of risk by the lay public often differs from that of scientific experts. Experts tend to express risk in terms of the actual numbers affected and numerical probabilities. The lay public tends to perceive risk according to the degree of unfamiliarity of the threat and whether there is a threat of a catastrophe involving serious adverse events (particularly death) for many people at one time. As a result, risk communication is an art and an important skill for public health professionals to develop. Key principles related to risk communication are discussed in Chapter 3.

> **CRITICAL THINKING QUESTION 11.1:** As discussed earlier, taking a thorough environmental health history is important for assessing environmental risk on an individual level. However, many health care practitioners experience barriers to doing so (e.g., time restrictions, knowledge barriers, general reluctance to delve into details of a person's occupational life). Reflect on your own practice setting. What strategies in your practice setting might you implement to encourage more thorough and regular environmental health histories or assessments?

ENVIRONMENTAL HEALTH ISSUES

In the following section, some environmental agents that have been associated with ill health are described. The sources of the agents, routes of human exposure, adverse effects, and approaches to control are included here.

Electromagnetic Radiation

Electromagnetic radiation (EMR) refers to energy emitted by things around us. Examples of EMR include ultraviolet (UV) light, x rays, and microwaves. The electromagnetic spectrum (depicted in Fig. 11.4) represents the range of EMR. There are two main types of radiation: ionizing and nonionizing.

Ionizing Radiation

Ionizing radiation is high-energy radiation (with high frequency and short wavelengths). Radiation of this nature is so high in energy that it can actually remove electrons from an atom, resulting in the atom becoming charged (i.e., ionized). It is more dangerous to human health than nonionizing radiation because of its ability to disrupt human cells. Ionizing radiation includes UV rays from the sun, as well as x rays and gamma rays. Ionizing radiation can also be in the form of particles (not represented on the electromagnetic spectrum), such as alpha particles and beta particles.

Of most concern in a health care setting is the risk of exposure to ionizing radiation as a result of medical imaging, for example, from x-rays and computed tomography (CT) scans. Members of the health care team who work in medical imaging departments must adhere to strict procedures regarding the wearing of protective equipment, for example, to protect themselves from the health effects of ionizing radiation (e.g., cancer). From a client perspective, it is notable that the dose of radiation one is exposed to after getting a chest x-ray is about 0.1 mSv (the unit of measurement that reflects the effect of radiation on human tissue). A CT scan of the chest, on the other hand, can expose a person to about 7 mSv of radiation (about 70 times that of an x-ray). It is important when counselling clients about the risk to put that risk in perspective and weigh it against the benefit and context of the procedure. For example, although receiving multiple CT scans can increase your cancer risk, it does so often by a very small amount (e.g., by 3% to 12% above a low baseline risk). Clients who are younger or who are receiving more frequent ionizing radiation from imaging are at greater risk (Harvard Health Publishing, 2018).

One of the most important types of ionizing radiation, important to human health, is UV radiation from the sun, which can cause skin cancer, eye damage, and skin changes such as aging and wrinkling. Interestingly, it can also be used as a therapeutic agent to treat various

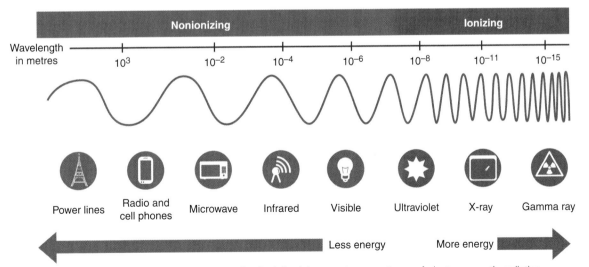

Fig. 11.4 The electromagnetic spectrum. On the left of the spectrum are types of electromagnetic radiation (EMR) that are considered high in energy (corresponding to high frequency and shorter wavelengths). On the right of the spectrum are low-energy forms of EMR (which tend to be low in frequency and long in wavelength).

chronic skin conditions such as psoriasis and is used for aesthetic purposes (e.g., tanning salons).There are two main types of UV rays that are important to human heath: UVA rays and UVB rays. It was initially thought that only UVB rays caused cancer, and UVA rays were primarily responsible for premature skin aging, but it is now well understood that both UVA and UVB rays are implicated in certain forms of skin cancer (Craig, Earnshaw, & Virós, 2018; Moan et al., 2015; Emanuele, Spencer, & Braun, 2014). UV rays also cause cataracts, eye melanoma, and skin burns. Measures to protect the population from the sun include public messaging about the importance of using sunscreen, wearing sunglasses, and reducing skin exposure to the sun (e.g., wearing light, loose-fitting long sleeves and pants, and staying in the shade during the peak daytime hours). UV indices are also used to warn the public of the strength of the sun's UV rays day to day, and recent moves to restrict the use of tanning salons of people younger than 18 years of age also help protect youth from the harmful effects of UV rays.

Humans are constantly exposed to small amounts of ionizing radiation that are emitted from the natural environment all around us. This is known as natural, background radiation. Radon is one example of this and actually represents most of the exposure we have to natural radiation.

Radon is the second leading cause of lung cancer after tobacco smoke (and the leading cause in nonsmokers). It is thought to account for 16% of lung cancer deaths and is greatly underestimated as a cause of lung cancer (Statistics Canada, 2016). Radon is a naturally occurring radioactive gas that forms as a decay product of uranium 238, a trace element found in all soil. As part of the radioactive decay process, radon produces alpha particles that, when inhaled, deposit in the lung, causing damage that can lead to lung cancer. Because of its accumulation indoors, radon is more of a concern as a form of indoor air pollution, although it is present in the ambient environment as well. Radon gas passes from porous soil into buildings through cracks in basement floors and walls. Given that most of an individual's time is spent indoors, there is a potential health risk from natural sources of radon. Health Canada has recommended that action be taken if radon concentration in the home exceeds 200 Bq/m³ (Cancer Care Ontario, 2017). When the level of radon is in doubt, houses must be individually tested for radon levels; extrapolation

from neighbouring homes is not adequate, but regional variation provides some clues.

According to recent estimates, around 25.2% of Canadian homes are exposed to equal to or greater than the WHO recommended level of 100 Bq/m³ of radon and 8.2% are exposed to equal to or greater than the Health Canada recommended level of 200 Bq/m³ (Cancer Care Ontario, 2017). Very few Canadians are aware of the risk of radon or test for radon in their private homes or in settings where they spend a lot of time. Because of the time children spend in school and the vulnerability of young children to radon exposure, some Canadian provinces and territories require schools to be tested for radon. For example, in Saskatchewan, New Brunswick, Nova Scotia, Prince Edward Island, and Yukon, all public schools are tested for radon. Prince Edward Island and Yukon actually make the test results available to the public to increase awareness and transparency (Carex Canada, 2017).

Interventions that can reduce radon levels in the home and other buildings such as schools include adequate ventilation, sealing cracks and holes in a building's foundation, and sub-slab depressurization, which actively draws radon from the soil to the outside environment, by passing the building (Health Canada, 2014).

Nonionizing Radiation

Nonionizing radiation includes types of energy that cannot actually break chemical bonds, leading to ionization. Examples include electric and magnetic fields, radio waves, and microwaves, among others (WHO, n.d.a.).

Radiofrequency Electromagnetic Radiation. Radiofrequency electromagnetic radiation (RF-EMR) is one type of nonionizing radiation that has been the source of much debate. This type of radiation has both electric and magnetic components, and common artificial sources of it include microwave ovens, mobile phones, Wi-Fi, and satellite communications.

Considerable research has been carried out on the health effects of exposure to RF-EMR. This type of radiation, although nonionizing, has the potential to cause tissue damage through heating (versus breaking chemical bonds in atoms). Generally speaking, the low levels that people are exposed to in their day-to-day lives are not thought to cause tissue damage. Certain occupational groups, however, such as those who work in telecommunications, may be in a different risk category. As well, distance from the source is a large factor in terms of predicting health effects. Very close proximity is usually needed for a significant exposure to occur (Australian Radiation Protection and Nuclear Safety Agency, n.d.). In 2011, the IARC classified radiofrequency exposures as a category 2B agent, meaning it is "possibly" carcinogenic to humans (evidence is far from conclusive based on observational studies) (Momoli et al., 2017).

With the increasing use of mobile phone technology, concerns over the health effects of RF-EMR have been raised in recent years. It was estimated that by the end of 2015, there were nearly 7 billion mobile phone subscribers around the world (Sagar et al., 2018), and the trends in Canada are no different; in fact, the number of mobile phone subscribers increased from around 6 000 in 1985 to just over 29 million in 2015 (Momoli et al., 2017). A few landmark international studies have been carried out, including the Interphone study, which specifically looked at the association between cell phone use and brain tumours. This study found that there was a small increased risk of specific types of brain tumours (e.g., gliomas) among the highest users of cell phones but not in the general population (Carlberg & Hardell, 2017). Other subsequent reviews have called into question those results, saying that the link was unlikely to be causal (Momoli et al., 2017). Either way, there are challenges with controlling for bias in these studies, so results remain largely inconclusive, but the possibility that some tumours are associated with very heavy cell phone use remains a possibility. As such, regulatory bodies such as Health Canada have set out "safe limits" for users to respect. For example, in 2015, Health Canada conducted an updated review of the scientific literature to set out exposure limits, below which exposures are not anticipated to cause any adverse health effects on the population (Health Canada, 2015). A more recent systematic review carried out in Europe found that day-to-day exposure to RF-EMR falls significantly below regulatory levels set out by government authorities and thus is unlikely to result in significant human health effects (Sagar et al., 2018).

Light Pollution

Light pollution is often defined as "excessive and inappropriate" artificial light and tends to be more of a problem in urban environments than rural environments (International Dark-Sky Association, n.d.). A 2016 World Atlas of artificial night sky brightness determined that about 80% of North Americans are unable to see the Milky Way at night, and around 99% of North American and European people experience night light pollution. In Canada, it is estimated that fewer than 1% of the population experiences a night sky that is actually dark (i.e., free of other artificial light sources) (Falchi et al., 2016). Exposure to light pollution has all sorts of effects on humans and on the ecosystem at large, including disrupting the reproductive activity of nocturnal animals, affecting the migration of birds, and interfering with sleep in humans (International Dark-Sky Association, 2018). More and more groups, such as the International Dark Sky Association and neighbourhood community groups, are taking action. For example, in the United States, the Kanab City Council in Utah passed an outdoor lighting ordinance to help the community maintain a dark sky while still keeping residents safe (e.g., during travel). Included in that ordinance are measures such as shielding bright lights and aiming lights downwards (International Dark-Sky Association, 2018).

> **EXERCISE 11.1:** In addition to the negative effects already mentioned, can you think of other, negative effects of excessive, artificial light? HINT: Think of the effects to humans and the ecosystem at large.

Noise Pollution

Noise can be thought of as unwanted sound, and chronic exposure to environmental noise has been linked with a variety of health effects, including hearing loss, sleep disturbance, annoyance, and heart disease (secondary to a lack of sleep and stress) (Hammer, Swinburn, & Neitzel, 2014). In 2009, the WHO Europe published night noise guidelines in an attempt to assist governments in regulating nighttime noise. The guidelines recommend that exposure to environmental noise at night should not exceed 40 dB (the equivalent of a quiet residential street) to safeguard against sleep disturbance and the resultant health effects. Exposure to levels over 55 dB (the equivalent of a busy street at night) can have adverse health effects, in particular heart disease (WHO, 2009).

Exposure to environmental noise (at all times of day) usually occurs in urban centres and as a result of traffic. This is becoming a growing problem as the world moves towards urbanization and as cities become more crowded. In addition to traffic, environmental noise may also be caused by aircrafts, construction equipment, and even other people. Health Canada commissioned a nationwide telephone survey to assess the level of annoyance experienced by Canadians from noise. Of those surveyed, 8% reported being highly annoyed by noise, particularly road traffic noise and noise from either people or animals outside (Government of Canada, 2006). In 2014, a study was conducted to assess exposure to traffic noise, specifically, in the City of Toronto. The researchers found that around 80% of the sites they sampled exceeded recommended sound level guidance set out by provincial authorities. Traffic noise exposure is quite widespread, particularly in urban centres (Zuo et al., 2014).

> **EXERCISE 11.2:** What types of environmental noise might one experience in a more rural and remote setting?

> **EXERCISE 11.32:** Brainstorm three interventions that may help to curb exposure to environmental noise.

Climate Change, Greenhouse Gases, and Global Warming

Climate change generally refers to changes that occur to global temperature and other aspects of climate (including precipitation and wind patterns) over a long period of time (e.g., usually decades or more). **Global warming** is the most-discussed type of climate change and generally refers to the gradual warming of the Earth's surface over many years. According to the WHO, the Earth has warmed by about 0.85°C over the past 130 years (WHO, 2018), and the human health effects of climate change are increasingly being described.

The United Nation's Intergovernmental Panel on Climate Change (IPCC) was established in 1998 to review the scientific literature on climate change and its impacts, including human health impacts. In its third assessment report, published in 2001, the IPCC described comprehensively for the first time ever how climate change can impact human health directly (e.g., through extreme weather events such as heat waves or floods) and indirectly (e.g., through altering water, food, air, and the survival and spread of vector-borne diseases as described in Chapter 10). In this landmark report, the IPCC said that heat mortality would rise and cold mortality would

decline in some places, there would be more infectious disease epidemics after floods and storms (e.g., malaria), and population displacement because of storms and rising sea levels will also impact health (WHO, 2001). (See the Case Study box for a description of recent heat waves around the world.)

CASE STUDY
Unprecedented Heat Waves

In North America and across Europe, heat waves have been among the deadliest forms of extreme weather events, especially in recent decades. For example, in 2003 a heat wave in Europe claimed the lives of an estimated 70 000 people, and in 2010, a similar type of event in Russia killed nearly 20 000 people. Heat waves in North America are increasing in frequency, duration, and intensity and will pose a challenge for the future.

Urban populations tend to be at a greater risk of death from extreme heat events because of something called the Urban Heat Island effect. This phenomenon occurs when temperatures in cities exceed that of rural surroundings because of changes in cooling land cover (e.g., vegetation that also provides shade), resurfacing with parking lots and concrete (that tend to absorb and trap heat), and the release of heat from things such as cars and air conditioners (Habeeb, Vargo, & Stone, 2015). Local governments are beginning to make efforts to protect against heat exposure in urban centres, respond to heat events by opening cooling centres, and implement warning systems for the public when heat events occur.

Inequities related to climate change are also receiving increased international attention. Climate change disproportionately affects already vulnerable groups such as children, older adults, people with underlying medical conditions, low-income and homeless individuals, and people living in low-income countries with poor infrastructure.

When it comes to addressing climate change, its main drivers must be understood. Energy from the sun drives the earth's weather and climate and heats the earth's surface; in turn, the earth radiates energy back into space. Atmospheric greenhouse gases (water vapour, carbon dioxide, and other gases) trap some of the outgoing energy, retaining heat like the glass panels of a greenhouse. Without this natural "greenhouse effect," temperatures would be much lower than they are now, and life as known today would not be possible. Instead, because of greenhouse gases, the earth's average temperature is a more hospitable 15°C. However, problems may arise when the atmospheric concentration of greenhouse gases increases.

Some greenhouse gases occur naturally in the atmosphere, but others result from human activities. Naturally occurring greenhouse gases include water vapour, carbon dioxide, methane, nitrous oxide, and ozone. Certain human activities, however, add to the levels of most of these naturally occurring gases: (1) carbon dioxide is released to the atmosphere when solid waste, fossil fuels (oil, natural gas, and coal), and wood and wood products are burned; (2) methane is emitted during the production and transport of coal, natural gas, and oil; from the decomposition of organic wastes in municipal solid waste landfills; and from the raising of livestock; and (3) nitrous oxide is emitted during agricultural and industrial activities, as well as during combustion of solid waste and fossil fuels. Very powerful greenhouse gases that are not naturally occurring include hydrofluorocarbons (HFCs), perfluorocarbons (PFCs), and sulphur hexafluoride (SF_6), which are generated in a variety of industrial processes. Carbon dioxide emissions from the combustion of fossil fuels are one of the major concerns causing global warming through the greenhouse effect. Since the beginning of the industrial revolution, atmospheric concentrations of carbon dioxide, methane, and nitrous oxides have risen substantially. Scientists generally believe that the combustion of fossil fuels and other human activities are the primary reason for the increased concentration of carbon dioxide.

Strategies to address climate change typically can be thought of as falling into one of two categories: (1) *mitigation*, which tries to slow the process of global warming (usually by reducing green house gases), and (2) *adaptation*, which involves finding ways to protect people and infrastructure and make them less vulnerable to the impacts of climate change.

EXERCISE 11.4: Brainstorm three examples of mitigation strategies and three examples of adaptation strategies to address climate change.

Shifting to cleaner sources of energy, for example, is one major way that climate change can be slowed. Renewable energy is energy produced from renewable natural sources, meaning the energy is replaced at a rate that is greater than at which its being consumed (Natural Resources Canada, 2017). Examples of renewable energy include solar power, wind power, and hydroelectricity. Nearly one fifth of Canada's energy supply consists of renewable energy sources (Natural Resources Canada, 2017). Hydroelectricity is the major form of renewable energy in Canada, with upwards of 500 hydroelectric stations existing across the country (Natural Resources Canada, 2017).

Hydraulic fracturing (also known as "fracking") has gained international attention over the years and has spurred much controversy in Canada. Fracking produces natural gas by injecting (at high pressures) a mixture of water and chemicals into deep rock formations (shale rocks) to release natural gas stored in these rocks (Olive, 2016). In the Canadian context, British Columbia, Alberta, and Saskatchewan have participated in fracking, whereas other provinces, including Nova Scotia, New Brunswick, Newfoundland, and Quebec, have banned the practice. Advocates of fracking claim that it results in fewer carbon emissions and is therefore a better alternative than fossil fuels such as coal and crude oil. They also state that fracking increases Canada's access to energy, decreasing reliance on other countries, as well as creating jobs. Those who oppose hydraulic fracturing claim that fracking can affect water stores (because much water is used in the process), water quality (because of the chemicals used in the mixture), and air quality (as a result of the transport and use of heavy equipment at sites); may result in exposure to noise; and may have occupational health hazards for workers involved in the process.

Much attention has been paid to the ways in which the health sector can slow down climate change. In 2009, for example, the Canadian Nurses Association and the Canadian Medical Association developed a *Joint Position Statement on Environmentally Responsible Activity in the Health Care Sector* (Canadian Nurses Association & Canadian Medical Association, 2009). In the position statement, the groups highlighted the role of the health sector in contributing to climate change (because the health sector is a large user of resources and energy) and developed a vision for a greener health care sector. The groups called on health care professionals, including nurses and doctors, to support reusing and recycling in health care facilities, turn down air conditioning to conserve energy, reduce waste associated with health care supplies, educate the public, model good practices, and advocate for climate change interventions.

Air Pollution

Air pollution exists when certain substances are present in the atmosphere in sufficient concentrations to cause adverse affects. Common air pollutants include sulphur oxides, nitrous oxides, carbon monoxide, ozone, ammonia, **volatile organic compounds (VOCs)**, and particulate matter (International Institute for Sustainable Development [IISD], 2017). Primary air pollutants include sulphur oxides, nitrous oxides, and carbon monoxide because they are released in the form in which they remain. Secondary air pollutants, however, include ozone, which is formed through chemical reactions with pollutants after release.

Particulate matter is unique because it is both a primary and a secondary air pollutant. It represents a mixture of solid and liquid particle compounds (e.g., aerosols, smoke, fumes, dust, pollen) suspended in the air and is often classified based on size, with PM2.5 representing PM that is less than 2.5 microns in diameter and PM 10 representing particles that range between 2.5 and 10 microns.

Air pollution occurs because of both natural phenomena, such as volcanoes, emissions from plant matter, and forest fires, and from human-made or human activity. For example, in 2016, a devastating wildfire occurred in Fort McMurray that took nearly 15 months to extinguish and resulted in the destruction of 2 400 buildings and the displacement of almost 80 000 residents. Smoke from the wildfire was shown to contribute significantly to poor air quality and high levels of air pollution in the city of Fort McMurray as well as nearby communities (Landis et al., 2018).

Generally, in Canada, air pollution results primarily from the combustion of fossil fuels, particularly by cars and some industrial processes (Environment and Climate Change Canada, 2017).

Traffic-related air pollution is a type of air pollution that results from motor vehicles and makes up a significant proportion of air pollution in urban centres. Vehicles most commonly release pollutants that include carbon monoxide, nitrogen oxides, carbon dioxide, VOCs, and particulate matter (Kim, 2015).

Since the 1990s, most common air pollutants have been decreasing, with the exception of PM2.5 (a type of particulate matter), as well as ground-level ozone (IISD).

For example, from the 1970s to 2015, the levels of nitrogen dioxide decreased by nearly 75% and the levels of carbon monoxide by 90%, despite Canadians' increasing use of energy and motor fuel consumption (McKitrick & Aliakbari, 2017). Urban areas such as city centres are more affected by air pollution, and groups that are most vulnerable to its health effects (described later) include children, older adults, those who have underlying health conditions (particularly heart and lung disease), and people who spend lots of time outdoors.

Air pollution is very closely linked to a range of human health effects. Most importantly, poor outdoor air quality is linked to both acute and chronic health issues. Acute health effects of poor air quality include shortness of breath and exacerbations of lung diseases such as asthma and chronic obstructive lung disease and allergies (Environment and Climate Change Canada, 2017). Chronic health effects of air pollution most commonly include heart disease and lung disease.

Worldwide, air pollution represents a significant risk factor for premature mortality. PM2.5 is often thought of as the most harmful of the criteria air pollutants in Canada. Because of its small size, it has the ability to be deposited deep into the lungs, causing inflammation and damage (IISD, 2017). It has been estimated that, in terms of premature death, if no action is taken to reduce levels of ozone and PM2.5 in the near future, by the middle of the century, one person will die prematurely every 5 seconds as a result of air pollution (IISD, 2017). In Canada in 2015, nearly 8 000 deaths were attributable to PM2.5 and ground-level ozone, and air pollution in that year cost the Canadian economy upwards of $36 billion (IISD, 2017).

In addition to human health effects, air pollution also affects the environment. Common environmental impacts of air pollution include smog, acid rain, and ozone depletion.

Smog

The word "smog" was coined a number of decades ago, derived from the combination of the words "smoke" and "fog," to describe the brownish yellow haze that sometimes hangs over urban areas. It is primarily a combination of ground level ozone and particulate matter. Smog may also contain acidic air pollutants, nitrogen oxides, sulphur oxides, and carbon monoxide. It usually occurs in urban areas, but suburbs and rural communities are also affected. Ground-level ozone tends to form under conditions of bright sunlight, high temperature, and a stationary air mass when VOCs and oxides of nitrogen combine. Therefore, the afternoons and early evenings of hot summer days are peak smog periods; by late in the day, the sun's rays have "baked" the exhaust from motor vehicles and industries into smog. Inhalable particulate matter concentrations depend less on temperature and can occur throughout the day, as well as result in winter smog episodes, when ozone levels are much lower. Smog can irritate the eyes, throat, and nose, may worsen respiratory conditions, and cause symptoms such as shortness of breath.

Acid Rain

Acid rain occurs when pollutants such as sulphur and nitrogen oxides react with water and oxygen to make acids before falling to the ground. Acid rain then lands and disrupts fish and other types of wildlife, buildings (eroding critical infrastructure), lakes, forests, and soil (Government of Canada, 2018).

Ozone Depletion

Air pollution also affects the thickness of the ozone layer, which protects us from the sun's harmful UV rays. Common air pollutants—as well as the release of substances causing chlorine and bromine and chlorofluorocarbons (CFCs), a substance found mainly in spray aerosols—deplete the ozone, making us much more vulnerable to UV rays (described earlier).

Strategies for Dealing with Outdoor Air Pollution

A number of strategies have been developed to minimize air pollution. The Air Quality Health Index (AQHI) is a tool developed to help the public understand variations in air quality and how that can impact health in the short term, as well as what actions people can take to protect their health at times when air quality is poor. It provides actionable advice for both the general population and those who are most vulnerable. The index itself is based on exposure to three main pollutants—nitrogen dioxide, particulate matter, and ground-level ozone—and provides a number from 1 to 10 that corresponds with the risk that the air poses at any given time. For example, an AQHI reading between 1 and 3 indicates low risk, 4 and 6 indicates moderate risk, 7 and 10 indicates high risk, and anything over 10 indicates a very high risk to human health. In addition to quantifying risk, the AQHI provides health messaging for various groups (refer to Table 11.2 for more detail).

Because the AQHI is based on research looking at the short-term health effects of air pollution in major urban environments in Canada, its generalizability to more rural environments as well as to long-term health effects is limited.

TABLE 11.2 Air Quality Health Index (AQHI) and Associated Health Messaging

Health Risk	AQHI Score	HEALTH MESSAGES	
		At-Risk Population[a]	General Population
Low	1–3	Enjoy your usual outdoor activities.	Ideal air quality for outdoor activities.
Moderate	4–6	Consider reducing or rescheduling strenuous activities outdoors if you are experiencing symptoms.	No need to modify your usual outdoor activities unless you experience symptoms such as coughing and throat irritation.
High	7–10	Reduce or reschedule strenuous activities outdoors. Children and the elderly should also take it easy.	Consider reducing or rescheduling strenuous activities outdoors if you experience symptoms such as coughing and throat irritation.
Very high	>10	Avoid strenuous activities outdoors. Children and the elderly should also avoid outdoor physical exertion.	Reduce or reschedule strenuous activities outdoors, especially if you experience symptoms such as coughing and throat irritation.

[a]People with heart or breathing problems are at greater risk. Follow your doctor's usual advice about exercising and managing your condition.
From Government of Canada. (2015). *Understanding air quality health index messages*. Ottawa: Minister of the Environment. Retrieved from http://www.canada.ca/en/environment-climate-change/services/air-quality-health-index/understanding-message.html. © Her Majesty the Queen in Right of Canada, as represented by the Minister of the Environment Canada, 2019.

In addition, the establishment of emission standards for all sources has contributed to control of air pollution, including those for cars (for which catalytic converters and other technologies have been introduced), and many industrial sources, including ferrous foundries, asphalt-paving producers, power plants, and smelters.

A number of pollution abatement technologies have been developed to address specific pollutants, and progress has been made on some emissions. Strengthening public transport systems and designing the built environment in a way that encourages active transport is another way to curb air pollution, particularly traffic-related air pollution.

With regard to acid rain, much progress has been made over the past 2 to 3 decades—so much so that it is a well-cited environmental success story in Canada. Into the early 1990s, grave concerns were raised by environmental groups about the impact of the coal industry and its contribution to producing acid rain. Many organizations and advocates drew attention to the deleterious effects of acid rain on the Great Lakes and forests in Canada. To address this complex issue, both the United States and Canada came together in the early 1990s to introduce regulatory changes to reduce air pollution and drastically cut emissions of both sulphur dioxide and nitrogen oxide (key components of acid rain), in large part by reducing coal burning (Parry, 2018).

Indoor Air Pollution

Because Canadians spend a large majority of their days indoors (upwards of 90% of the time), indoor air quality, usually defined as the quality of air in and around buildings and other common structures, is a significant determinant of health. Indoor pollutants are usually classified as either biological (things such as moulds, *legionella,* dust mites, and allergens), chemical (VOCs, carbon monoxide, and other pollutants that are also found indoors), or radiological (e.g., radon, described earlier). The most frequent pollutants include tobacco smoke (described earlier) and VOCs.

Volatile organic compounds refer to a range of different chemicals that have a high vapour pressure, meaning they are emitted from objects in gas form at room temperature (i.e., they vapourize easily). They are omnipresent in the environment, and in the indoor environment, they are usually emitted by building materials, furniture, and consumer products such as household cleaners (Health Canada, 2018). Examples of VOCs include acetone, chloroform, isopropyl alcohol, and tetrachloroethylene, among others (Health Canada, 2018). The degree of ventilation and entry rate of fresh air, as well as the reaction rate between chemicals, determines the concentration of indoor pollutants such as VOCs.

Health effects of poor indoor air quality depend on the specific causal agent but typically include allergic-type diseases, respiratory infections, and other respiratory symptoms, as well as irritative and nonspecific symptoms (e.g., fatigue, nausea, eye and upper respiratory tract irritation) (Tham, 2016). Chronic, noncommunicable diseases such as asthma and cancer (linked specifically with tobacco smoke exposure and radon, for example) are also implicated (Tham, 2016).

Two concepts that have been written about extensively in recent years are sick building syndrome and building-related illness. **Building-related illnesses** refer to any illness for which a specific cause can be identified and is related to the indoor environment. For example, Legionnaire's disease (caused by the bacteria *Legionella pneumonia*) causes pneumonia, fever, and other respiratory symptoms in susceptible people who are exposed to things such as showers and decorative water fountains found in indoor environments. **Sick building syndrome**, on the other hand, refers to nonspecific signs and symptoms that cannot to be linked back to a specific etiology. It has been hypothesized that elements of the indoor air environment, such as the presence of VOCs, for example, are associated with sick building syndrome (Tham, 2016).

In terms of control measures, adequate ventilation, measuring and tracking various indoor air pollutants, the development of Residential Indoor Air Quality Guidelines that set out reference or "safe" levels, and implementing building codes and other regulations have all been used to address this issue.

Water Quality

Ensuring a safe potable water supply has long been a prerequisite for good health. In Canada, this issue was brought to the forefront in 2000, when the municipal drinking water supply in Walkerton, Ontario, became contaminated with *Escherichia coli* 0157:H7. Seven people died, and more than 2 300 became ill. The contamination resulted from a combination of the spreading of manure near a town well and improper disinfection of the water supply through inadequate chlorination. The problem was compounded by a lack of monitoring of water quality (Walkerton Inquiry, 2002).

Contamination of the drinking water supply by microorganisms is not the only factor of concern. Protecting the water supply from chemical contamination (e.g., lead) as well as radiological contaminants is also important (see Table 11.1 for a list of common contaminants).

In terms of the regulation of drinking water in Canada, the federal government sets out the guidelines for Canadian drinking water quality. Provinces and territories, however, are responsible for setting out regulation related to potable water (e.g., requiring various agencies to monitor, inspect and report on adverse water quality results, mandating that drinking water operators follow specific rules and guidelines and be licensed). Municipal governments are the purveyors of potable water and are typically responsible for maintaining and funding water treatment and waste water treatment plants, as well as distribution systems. In some areas, such as Indigenous communities and military bases, the federal government is more directly involved in ensuring availability of safe water. (The In the News box provides a more detailed explanation of water safety on Indigenous reserves.) Last, through the *Food and Drugs Act,* the federal government regulates the production and safety of bottled water.

⊕ IN THE NEWS

Access to Safe Drinking Water in Indigenous Communities

In recent years, the issue of safe drinking water on Indigenous reserve communities has gained a lot of media attention. As of 2015, there were approximately 136 drinking water advisories posted in 91 Indigenous communities across the country (Dyck, Plummer, & Armitage, 2015). Reasons for this are wide ranging and context specific. Some cited reasons include a lack of regulatory protection of drinking water sources, a lack of funding and infrastructure related to water treatment, troubles with monitoring and reporting adverse water quality results for private water systems (e.g., wells that are separate from large distribution networks and more common in rural areas), jurisdictional complexities when it comes to responding to adverse water quality results, and colonialism and a lack of involvement of Indigenous people when addressing issues such as access to safe drinking water (Dyck et al., 2015).

A multibarrier approach to protecting the water supply, from source to tap, is often defined as a set of policies, procedures, and tools that prevent or reduce water contamination. The three most commonly described elements of a multibarrier approach are (1) protecting source water from contamination (which can be surface water from lakes and rivers or ground water), (2) protecting the distribution system (which delivers water from the treatment plant to individual homes), and (3) drinking water treatment (e.g., ensuring that drinking water is treated with disinfectants like chlorine) (Dyck et al., 2015). A fourth element, namely, monitoring and responding to adverse events or reports of water quality, is often added to this approach.

> **EXERCISE 11.5:** List one example of each of the three elements of the multibarrier approach to protecting the water supply.

In many parts of Canada, fluoride is added to drinking water to prevent tooth decay. The recommended level of fluoride in drinking water is 0.7 mg/L (Government of Canada, 2017). Community water fluoridation (CWF) is endorsed by many public health agencies (including the WHO, CDC, Public Health Agency of Canada [PHAC], and a number of professional bodies) as a policy measure that is both safe and effective, particularly in preventing tooth decay and its results in children. It has been estimated that CWF can reduce tooth decay by up to 30% in children and adults, and the CDC has named CWF as one of public health's 10 greatest achievements. In addition to its effectiveness, CWF is cited by many as having a high return on investment. Recent estimates suggest that for every dollar invested, between $6 and $90 is gained in health benefits (PHAC, 2017). CWF is thought to be a policy measure that also improves health equity because most people have access to safe drinking water in Canada, including low-income Canadians who may not be able to afford preventive dental care or curative dental care for things such as cavities.

Despite its benefits, however, CWF remains hugely controversial. In fact, as of 2017, only 39% of Canadians reside in places where the water is fluoridated. Many municipalities have actually discontinued the practice of CWF. Reasons for this include concerns about safety (and the risk of fluorosis and recent concerns regarding the effect of fluoride on IQ at high levels), cost, questions regarding the magnitude of the efficacy of CWF interventions, and occupational health risks associated with fluoridating the water. Safety concerns, however, have been largely discredited because of the fact that most studies examining adverse effects do so in areas where fluoride is naturally occurring in the water at very high levels, greater than the recommended 1.5 mg/L maximum acceptable concentration (Health Canada, 2017c). In Canada, however, the average fluoride levels to which Canadians are exposed as a result of CWF are closely monitored at an optimal level of 0.7 mg/L, below which adverse effects are not expected to occur (Health Canada, 2010; Safe Drinking Water Foundation, 2017).

Although contamination of drinking water is very directly linked to human health, safety of beach water and other recreational water sources (e.g., pools, hot tubs, splashpads) must not be forgotten. More and more attention is being paid to keeping these supplies safe, after recent outbreaks of gastrointestinal illnesses, such as *Salmonella* and *Cryptosporidium* spp., have been linked back to exposure to water parks and splash pads (Clayton et al., 2017). In addition to guidelines for drinking water, Health Canada has also published *Guidelines for Canadian Recreational Water Quality*.

Blue-green algae is a phenomenon that is increasing across the country (Pick, 2016). It is caused by bacteria called cyanobacteria that multiply in the late summer and early fall to cause a large mass in the water, called an "algae bloom." This bloom usually looks like pea soup but can be a variety of colours and in its later stages may emit a foul smell. The danger of cyanobacteria is that they form toxins, known as cyanotoxins, that are toxic to the skin, liver, and nervous system and in very high amounts can even be fatal to both humans and animals. Humans can be exposed by drinking water with algae blooms or by swimming in contaminated waters. Eating fish from contaminated waters is another route of exposure. Short-term exposure to the toxins can cause vomiting, diarrhea, rash, and numbness in addition to paralysis. Chronic exposure can lead to cancer over a long period of time.

Blue-green algae blooms occur in waters that are warmer in temperature and water that is high in nutrients (e.g., phosphorous and nitrogen because of run-off from agricultural operations). Climate change is expected to increase blue-green algae blooms because of the warmer water temperatures (Hamilton, Salmaso, & Paerl, 2016), and this may become an increasing cause of morbidity in the future.

Food Quality

Although Canada's food supplies are considered to be among the safest in the world, environmental contamination of food continues to be a concern. Whereas food contamination accounts for up to 95% of our daily intake of persistent toxic chemicals, air contributes approximately 15%, and drinking water contributes very little. Common concerns about the quality of food are the use of pesticides and chemicals during food production and handling, use of drugs such as antibiotics and hormones to treat livestock, use of food additives and preservatives, quality of sport-caught fish, genetically modified foods, and food irradiation. Major sources of food contamination in Canada are microbial contamination, environmental contamination, naturally occurring contaminants, pesticide residues and chemicals in meat and milk products, and food additives and preservatives. The common microbial contamination in raw foods are *Salmonella* spp., *Campylobacter* spp., and *Escherichia coli*.

Most foodborne illnesses in Canada result from consumers not storing, handling, or cooking food properly; therefore, education on safe handling and cooking practices can significantly reduce foodborne illness (Canadian Public Health Association [CPHA], n.d.). However, with the globalization of the food supply and the manufacturing and processing of foods in large industrial operations, outbreaks from commercial foods (e.g., bagged lettuce, processed and packaged meats) are expected, and regulations, inspections, and strict food handling protocols and training for those involved need to be in place.

Persistent chemicals such as polychlorinated biphenyls (PCBs), dioxins, and some pesticides (as well as heavy metals such as mercury and lead) are of concern because of their tendency to accumulate in the fat or organs of fish and wildlife. Fish and small insects absorb these chemicals directly from contaminated water and concentrate them in target tissues, such as fat. Larger predators consume these small organisms, and the concentration of the contaminants increases up the food chain, which is known as **biomagnification**.

Just like with drinking and recreational water, all levels of government have a role to play in ensuring food safety. At the federal level, Health Canada sets out safety standards and guidelines and performs risk assessments on specific products, and the Canadian Food Inspection Agency enforces regulations, conducts inspections to ensure the food industry is compliant with various standards and regulations, and initiates recalls of contaminated food products. Local public health agencies typically inspect food establishments that fall under their jurisdiction and regional boundaries, as well as investigate and manage outbreaks that may be related to food products, at the local level (CPHA, n.d.). The Real-World Example box provides an introduction to public health inspectors who play a key role in the public health workforce and are responsible for enforcing various environmental health regulations, including those relating to food safety.

 REAL-WORLD EXAMPLE

Public Health Inspectors

Key to the public health workforce are public health inspectors (PHIs), also sometimes known as Environmental Health officers, who often work in multidisciplinary teams along with public health nurses, physicians, dietitians, and others at various local, provincial or territorial, and federal public health agencies. PHIs are specifically trained in environmental public health and hold certification in public health inspection, a designation that is recognized across the country. Six Canadian postsecondary institutions currently offer this specific training, and training ranges in length from 2 to 4 years (Canadian Institute of Public Health Inspectors, n.d.).

The role of a PHI is to reduce the incidence of food- and water-borne diseases and ensure compliance with infection prevention and control practices. At the local level, they are typically involved in inspecting premises such as restaurants, daycares, public pools, spas, long-term care facilities, tattoo parlours, and other businesses to ensure compliance with legislation and regulation.

Toxic Chemicals

Canadians are exposed to a wide array of chemicals throughout the course of the day, through food, water, air, household products, cosmetics, and so on. Although most of these chemicals are not thought to be harmful

to human health, they are widespread, and only a small number of chemicals in use today have had adequate toxicological testing before their introduction. A detailed review of the adverse health outcomes of the differing classes of chemicals is beyond the scope of this chapter. Instead, this section examines a small number of the most prominent chemical classes in relation to environmental health.

A few key terms related to classification of chemicals are worth noting to frame the rest of the discussion. **Persistent organic pollutants (POPs)** are a category of substances that are able to persist in the environment for a very long period of time, can biomagnify in the ecosystem, and can be carried very long distances away from the source of their release (and thus represent a global concern). POPs typically affect human health by altering the immune system, nervous system, reproductive system, and endocrine system (WHO, n.d.b). Examples of POPs include some pesticides, PCBs, and dioxins (discussed later).

Another class of substances commonly reported on in the mainstream media these days are **endocrine-disrupting chemicals (EDCs)**. These chemicals are typically human made and are known to affect the body's endocrine system by mimicking the body's naturally made hormones, thereby disrupting processes such as reproduction, metabolism, growth and development, and immune system function. Examples of EDCs include some pesticides, some heavy metals, PCBs, dioxins, and bisphenol A. As you can see, some chemicals are both EDCs and POPs, some are one or the other, and some do not fall into either category (Ribeiro, Ladeira, & Viegas, 2017; Gore, 2016).

Heavy Metals

Heavy metals are a group of chemicals that are high in density and are typically released into the environment through both natural sources (because they are present in the Earth's crust) and human activity (e.g., mining, smelting, industrial operations, and application of some metal-containing pesticides). Heavy metals are typically toxic even at low doses and tend to persist in the environment for a long time without degrading. They impact the health of the environment and of humans. Some heavy metals are also essential human micronutrients; these include copper, nickel, iron, and zinc (Gall, Boyd, & Rajakaruna, 2015). Examples of the five most common metals of environmental public health significance are lead, mercury, cadmium, chromium, and arsenic. Lead and mercury, in particular, are discussed later in more detail.

Lead

Source and exposure. Lead is a naturally occurring metal that has been used since prehistoric times. Lead exposure occurs chiefly through ingestion, although inhalation is the exposure pathway for those who are occupationally exposed. Drinking water and food are sources of environmental exposures to lead. Automobile emissions were a significant source of exposure until 1975, when unleaded gasoline was introduced in Canada. Industrial emissions of lead now exceed automobile emissions. Lead paint is an important source of exposure for children. The older the home, the more likely it is to have lead-based paint, which is an important potential source of lead exposure for people who renovate homes. Domestic drinking water may be contaminated through the leaching of lead from water pipes and lead solder. Hobbies that put people at increased risk of lead exposure include pottery, artistic painting, stained-glass making, glass or metal soldering, target shooting, electronic soldering, and construction of bullets, slugs, and fishing sinkers.

Health effects and control. Lead is absorbed into the bloodstream and deposited in bone and other tissues. The toxicity of lead is multisystemic. Acute exposure to large amounts of lead may cause abdominal pain, anemia, kidney problems and brain problems. Chronic exposure can result in central nervous system (CNS) effects ranging from impaired concentration to encephalopathy, anemia, kidney problems, and adverse reproductive outcomes, including miscarriage, low birth weight, and impaired neurological development. In the general population, two groups—the unborn child and children up to 6 years of age—are at a greater risk of the adverse health effects of lead. During pregnancy, lead can cross the placenta and reach the unborn child. Neurological development may be compromised. Young children are a high-risk group for several reasons: they take in more lead per unit of body weight than adults, develop at a rapid rate, and are more susceptible to the adverse effects of lead. Children also absorb a higher proportion of ingested lead (50% compared with 10% in adults). Over the past decade, some researchers have found that exposure to even low levels of lead before birth or during infancy and early childhood can cause impaired intellectual development, behavioural disturbances, decreased physical growth, and hearing impairment. High levels of lead exposure have been linked to increased spontaneous abortion and stillbirth rates in pregnant women (Amadi, Igweze, & Orisakwe, 2017). Elevated lead levels can be detected by a simple blood test.

Canadians have some of the lowest levels of blood lead in the world, and levels have declined substantially since the introduction of unleaded gasoline. However, some groups still remain at risk, particularly people who have a low income and live in older houses and people who were born outside of Canada (Statistics Canada, 2015).

Lead levels over a certain level warrant interventions such as identification of the source of exposure, control of the source, or removal of individuals to prevent further exposure. Municipal water treatment removes lead effectively, and the alkalization of water can reduce leaching from corroded pipes. To avoid posttreatment exposure, if water is left standing for more than a few hours, taps should be flushed until the water is as cold as it will get; if lead levels at point-of-use exceed recommended levels, then replacement of lead pipes and lead solder by municipalities and homeowners may be necessary.

Mercury

Source and exposure. Mercury is a naturally occurring metal that is found in cinnabar ore. It is used in the manufacture of chlorine and caustic soda, in electrical equipment, and in thermometers and other instruments. It is released into the environment through natural degassing of the Earth's crust as well as through industrial releases. Organic mercury (predominantly methyl mercury) is the form that is most toxic to humans, and it is formed by the conversion of inorganic mercury by microorganisms that live in water.

Thus, most exposure to mercury today occurs through the eating of fish (Pirkle, Muckle, & Lemire, 2016). Fish bioconcentrate mercury in their muscle tissue by a factor of 10 to 100 000. Canadians who rely on subsistence fishing and do not heed consumption guidelines are at particular risk of exposure to mercury. Pregnant women who consume large quantities of mercury-contaminated fish are at risk of exposing their unborn children to mercury (Pirkle et al., 2016).

Although Health Canada encourages fish consumption because of its positive effects on heart health, it also advises Canadians to limit their consumption of shark, swordfish, and fresh and frozen tuna (fish that are near the top of the food chain and thus have higher levels of mercury compared with other commercial fish), especially for pregnant women and young children (Health Canada, 2017b).

People who live in northern communities in Canada, including Indigenous communities, are a particularly vulnerable group when it comes to mercury exposure. The greater accumulation of mercury at higher latitudes, increased consumption of fish high in mercury, industrial activities, and local ecosystems high in mercury are some of the factors that contribute to why northern communities may have higher blood mercury levels compared with the general population (Pirkle et al., 2016). In 2016, for example, a large controversy unfolded over the construction of a hydroelectric dam in Muskrat Falls, Labrador, that was located close to Inuit communities. Inuit people were concerned about the risk of methylmercury contamination in a nearby lake, which could result from the flooding of a reservoir required for the dam. The local Inuit people protested, with some engaging in hunger strikes to advocate for appropriate risk-management strategies to protect the lake, which the Inuit people rely on heavily for fishing, from mercury poisoning. Eventually, these community-led advocacy efforts resulted in government officials creating a special committee to mitigate the risk of methylmercury contamination and prevent the harmful health effects of mercury in these nearby communities (CBC News, 2017). Another example of a catastrophic event in Canadian history involving Indigenous communities is discussed in the Case Study Box.

Health effects and control. Unlike elemental and inorganic mercury, organic mercury is rapidly absorbed from the gut. Acute exposure can cause balance issues, numbness, impaired vision and hearing, psychosis, and kidney damage. Chronic low-dose poisoning can cause liver and kidney damage as well as damage to the CNS. The brains of developing fetuses are particularly at risk if exposed to high levels of circulating maternal organic mercury. Possible effects include impaired physical growth and coordination; cerebral palsy; and more subtle effects on coordination, behaviour, and intelligence quotient (Pirkle et al., 2016).

CASE STUDY

Mercury Poisoning Among Indigenous People in Northern Ontario

During the 1960s and 1970s, the Dryden Chemical Company discharged nearly 10 tonnes of mercury waste into the English–Wabigoon river system, causing extensive mercury exposure for residents of Grassy Narrows and Wabaseemoong Indigenous reserves for generations. Many people suffered the health effects of mercury poisoning, including Minamata's disease (which causes neurological symptoms such as weakness, numbness, and vision and hearing changes, among others). Animals such as cats and turkeys were also affected and were found by residents to be acting strangely. Other than the purely physiological effects to both humans and animals, this incident resulted in widespread community harm because the Asubpeecho-Seewagong people not only relied on that river for their drinking water, but also for fishing and for their livelihood (Mosa & Duffin, 2017). In addition to community members losing their livelihoods (because they could no longer fish), they also lost a healthy dietary staple, which was replaced by foods much lower in nutritional quality, thereby contributing to risks of developing chronic disease.

This catastrophe continues to adversely affect these communities today and is still resulting in disruptions to economic activities and to physical and mental health. Shockingly, there continues to be ongoing evidence of high mercury levels in the local ecosystem. Trust in government authorities has undoubtedly also been affected by this crisis (Mosa & Duffin, 2017). Last, the impact on future generations is immense, given the association of mercury poisoning in childhood with cognition, memory, attention, and language later in life (US EPA, 2018c).

Polychlorinated Biphenyls and Dioxins

Polychlorinated biphenyls

Source and exposure. Polychlorinated biphenyls are a class of highly stable, noncorroding, and relatively nonflammable chemicals first manufactured on a commercial scale in 1929. For several decades, they were used extensively in a wide range of industrial applications, especially the manufacture of electrical and heat exchange equipment. In the past, PCBs have also been used in such products as inks, oil, sealants, caulking compounds, and carbonless copy paper. In the 1970s, concerns over health and the environmental impact of PCBs led to their substitution by other compounds and eventually to a North American ban in 1977 on the manufacture, importation, and most nonelectrical uses of PCBs. Electrical uses of PCBs are now being phased out, with stringent requirements for their handling and disposal.

Studies have found trace levels of PCBs everywhere in the environment even though they are no longer being manufactured. This is because PCBs do not readily break down (they are a type of POP). This persistence, coupled with their tendency to accumulate in the fat of living organisms, means that they are often present and biomagnified in the food chain. Humans are regularly exposed to minute amounts of PCBs in food, air, and water (Loganathan & Masunaga, 2015; Enault et al., 2015). Ingestion is the most common route of entry. As a result, all humans have a low level of PCBs in their body fat and blood.

Health effects and Control. Sustained, high-level exposure to PCBs has been associated with adverse health effects. These include a severe form of acne (chloracne), eye discharge, swelling of the upper eyelids, darkening of the nails and skin, numbness, weakness, muscle spasms, chronic bronchitis, and decreased birth weight and head circumference in newborns. Scientists generally agree that short-term, low-level exposure to PCBs is unlikely to have a significant health impact on adults. However, there is potential cause for concern about long-term exposure to low concentrations (Faroon & Ruiz, 2015; Office of Response and Restoration, National Oceanic and Atmospheric Administration, 2014).

Long-term, high-level PCB exposure has been linked to an increased incidence of cancer, particularly liver cancer, and it is now considered a group 1 agent, according to IARC (Zani et al., 2017).

Like other POPs, PCBs affect the immune system, reproductive system, nervous system, and endocrine (or hormonal) system (US EPA, 2018b). As mentioned previously, PCBs are being phased out because of legislation banning their production. However, transport and storage of existing wastes containing PCBs pending destruction are also heavily regulated to prevent further exposure.

Dioxins and Furans

Source and exposure. Dioxins are a family of toxic substances called polychlorinated dibenzo-para-dioxins. A second family of closely related toxic substances known as polychlorinated dibenzofurans is very often present with dioxins. Dioxins and furans, which have never been purposely manufactured, are byproducts of the production of certain chemicals (e.g., some pesticides and wood preservatives) of the chlorine-bleaching process used in some pulp and paper mills, and of the incomplete combustion of materials that contain both chlorine atoms and organic matter. Although they are most often human made, some natural occurrences, such as forest fires, are believed to contribute to the presence of dioxins and furans in the environment.

People living in industrialized nations are constantly exposed to minute amounts of dioxins and furans in food, air, water, soil, and some consumer products. Scientists have shown that food is the major source of dioxins and furans for humans.

Health effects and control. Just like PCBs, dioxins and furans are present in nearly all humans at low levels, and this low-level background exposure isn't thought to cause significant harm. However, these agents have the potential at higher doses to be very toxic and cause cancer and immune system, nervous system, endocrine system, and reproductive system issues in the longer term.

As a result, the government of Canada recognizes that these compounds are undesirable environmental contaminants and that, when possible, their unintentional production should be limited. To date, the government has produced guidance to minimize the release of these compounds from waste incinerators, have eliminated dioxins and furans from pesticides, and have regulated release from industries such as pulp mills—all of which have contributed to a more than 60% decline in the release of dioxins and furans in Canada.

Pesticides

Pesticides are unique as a class of environmental agents because they are deliberately added to the environment for the express purpose of killing some form of life. They have been categorized as economic poisons because they have some important beneficial effects on food supply and on health. For example, the use of insecticides has eliminated or controlled vector-borne disease in many parts of the world.

Both acute and chronic human health effects related to pesticide exposure have been identified. Acute health effects include things such as skin and eye irritation, headaches, dizziness, and nausea and typically are occupational in origin. Chronic health effects include asthma, cancer, diabetes, allergies, hormone disruption, and birth defects (Kim, Kabir, & Jahan, 2017). Pesticide residues contaminate food products and can concentrate in the ecological food chain. Almost every human body is born with measurable organochlorine pesticide levels related to widespread use of pesticides. Most people are exposed through eating foods or drinking liquids that are contaminated with pesticides.

The delayed effects of pesticide exposure are difficult to investigate because exposures are universal and not easily measured; it takes years and years before the health effects (e.g., cancer) are seen, and there are no unexposed control groups. Several municipalities and provinces in Canada have used their powers to limit the use as lawn and garden pesticides (which are used purely for cosmetic reasons) in their jurisdictions. Two provinces that have banned the cosmetic use of pesticides are Manitoba and Ontario. The federal government has also created the Pest Management Regulatory Agency to monitor the impact of pesticides on food supply and their effects on human health and administering the *Pest Control Products Act* and regulations, which regulates all pesticides imported into, sold, or used in Canada. More and more emphasis is now being placed on integrated pest management strategies (which focus on anticipating and preventing pests before they are established) and eco-friendly pesticides (Kim et al., 2017).

CRITICAL THINKING QUESTIONS 11.2: In their efforts to educate and raise awareness among their clients, health care providers often give people mixed health promotion messages and health advice. For example, we warn clients with pre-existing lung disease not to go outdoors or do strenuous activities on days when air pollution is bad. Yet at the same time, we tell people with chronic diseases to stay active, exercise, and get enough vitamin D.

Reflect on your own practices. What other examples of contradictory health messaging can you think of? How might you address the issue of "mixed messages" with your practice or client group?

CREATING A HEALTHY ENVIRONMENT

With increasing recognition of the importance of the ecosystem has come respect for the maintenance of the integrity of the environment for its intrinsic value, as well as for its purpose in meeting human needs. Because of the cross-cutting nature of environmental health issues (affecting human health, infrastructure, ecosystems),

ensuring a healthy environment is the responsibility of citizen groups, individual households, all levels of governments, and all sectors of society. Control strategies that have been described throughout this chapter include educating individual consumers (e.g., fish consumption guidelines to reduce mercury exposure), improved technologies (e.g., fuel-efficient vehicles), better land use planning (e.g., to encourage active transport and reduce air pollution), improving the resiliency of buildings and infrastructure (e.g., improved ventilation, soundproofing walls), and developing evidence-based guidelines for exposure (e.g., Canadian safe drinking water guidelines). Often in environmental public health, policies and other regulatory measures are considered to be the best ways to reduce or limit exposure to various environmental agents. As mentioned in Part 1 of this book, a cornerstone of the Ottawa Charter for Health Promotion is building healthy public policy and creating environments that support health. This is also a key focus of community nursing—moving beyond the level of the individual to impact societies and influencing policies affecting whole communities. Regulatory approaches are examples of both of these elements and, because of their influence on the whole population, they can be very significant in terms of changing the environment for the better compared with interventions that target individual people (e.g., promoting education and awareness).

The following section discusses landmark regulatory policy approaches in more detail. Regulatory approaches often intend to restrict or ban the production, use, and release of various toxicants. See Box 11.1 for a description of a key approach that has been used to regulate environmental health agents.

EXERCISE 11.6: If in the example given in Box 11.1, it was unknown whether the infertility caused by a new chemical was temporary or permanent, what would be the risks and benefits (both ethical and practical) of using the precautionary principle to institute a full ban on its use?

Regulatory Approaches
Global

Many of the current initiatives to deal with environmental issues are undertaken at an international level. For example, the Paris Agreement—signed by 195 countries at the Paris Climate Conference in 2015—is a legally binding deal with the stated goal of limiting global warming to less than 2°C (compared with pre-industrial temperatures). It commits countries to reducing global emissions of greenhouse gases, strengthening their abilities to adapt to climate change, and helping low-income countries achieve these goals, among others.

Another key international agreement was the Stockholm Convention, adopted in 2001. This convention is a global treaty that prohibits and restricts the production, use, and release of various persistent organic pollutants. Other key agreements include the Rotterdam Convention (which aims to reduce the harmful effects of pesticides) and the Minamata Declaration (which protects humans and the environment from harmful mercury exposure).

Federal

Jurisdictional responsibility for environmental issues is shared between the federal and provincial or territorial governments, and areas of overlap are usually resolved through close cooperation. The Canadian *Environmental Protection Act* is the cornerstone of federal environmental legislation. It provides the framework for protection from hazardous substances, enforcement tools, and powers to reduce pollution and to eliminate and regulate emissions of toxic substances. It ensures that substances not specifically covered under other legislation meet Canadian standards in the areas of human health and safety and environmental protection. Environment Canada enforces the Act, and Health Canada contributes to the development of regulations and guidelines.

Other pieces of federal legislation relevant to environment and health include the *Food and Drugs Act* and the *Pest Control Products Act*. The environmental assessment and review process is formalized in the *Canadian Environmental Assessment Act*. This process is used to identify and review the implications to multiple sectors, including health, of all projects, with both public and professional input being obtained. For example, the location of dams, nuclear facilities, or pipelines to carry crude oil or natural gas are major issues in Canada, and environmental assessments are a means of identifying implications for the whole ecosystem as well as for human health. Provinces have also developed environmental assessment processes and regulations.

Provincial and Territorial

The provinces and territories have primary responsibility for the quality of local air and water, the quantity and types of emissions allowed by industries, the disposal of toxic waste products, and the identification and management of environmental health hazards. For example, the regulation of drinking water is primarily the responsibility of the provinces and territories.

Municipal

Local municipalities also have an important role to play when it comes to regulation. Examples of regulatory policies enacted at the local level include restricting where people can smoke tobacco and waterpipes, banning the use of tanning salons by minors, and making policy decisions when it comes to community water fluoridation.

Role of Local Public Health Agencies

Public health departments usually have municipal and provincial mandates for the enforcement of regulations regarding safe food and water, sanitation, and other environmental hazards, with public health inspectors playing a significant role in this work. Public health agencies also work with municipalities to support healthy built environments (e.g., addition of bike lanes and transport infrastructure for people to take public transportation). The role of public health departments is described in more detail in Chapter 14.

CRITICAL THINKING QUESTIONS 11.3: We have discussed the role of local public health agencies and various levels of government in creating healthy environments. What can individual health care providers do in their personal lives, professional lives within their teams in specific practice settings (e.g., within their hospitals or clinics), across sectors (beyond the walls of their practice setting), and with their communities to drive action on improving the environment? What concrete actions might one take?

(HINT: Consider using the Ottawa Charter for Health Promotion, as well as the CMA and CNA's *Joint Position Statement on Environmentally Responsible Activity in the Health Care Sector*, to help support your answer.)

SUSTAINABLE DEVELOPMENT

Sustainable development is defined as development that meets the needs of the present without compromising the ability of future generations to meet their own needs. It refers to use of resources, direction of investments, the orientation of technological development, and institutional development in ways which ensure that the current development and use of resources do not compromise the health and well-being of future generations (IISD, n.d.). Certain widely held human values and practices, such as support for population growth, increased production of goods and services, increasing material expectations, and the belief in technology have caused specific ecological phenomena that threaten human health. The major issues are climate change, with possible consequent food shortages and change in distribution of vector-borne diseases, ozone pollution, ecosystem contamination, and resource depletion. Sustainable development is a conceptual model that incorporates a number of approaches to reverse the deterioration of the earth, to prevent pollution beyond the point where natural systems cannot cope, to conserve natural resources by sparing or reducing use or by recycling and reuse (with municipal recycling programs

being a positive indication of action in this area), and to sustain yield, whereby renewable resources are used at a rate that does not exceed their continued replenishment.

In 2015, the global community agreed to 17 **sustainable development goals (SDGs)** as part of the *2030 Agenda for Sustainable Development*. Fundamental aspirations of the 2030 agenda include poverty eradication as well as environmental protection. Of the 17 SDGs (which replaced the earlier Millennium Development Goals), those most relevant to environmental public health include sustainable cities and communities, affordable and clean energy, climate action, reduced inequalities, clean water and sanitation, good health and well-being, responsible consumption and production, and protecting the land and oceans (United Nations Development Programme, 2016).

CRITICAL THINKING QUESTIONS 11.4: Look into the concept of "complete streets." Describe what this notion entails and analyze what impacts designing complete streets could have on environmental health. What environmental exposures could be reduced by embracing a complete streets approach? What health outcomes (e.g., disease states, like cancer) might this impact?

WASTE MANAGEMENT

Waste management involves the disposal, destruction, or storage of solid waste and sewage (and industrial discharges and nuclear waste). On average, Canadians produce around 720 kg of waste per capita and spend just over $3 billion a year on waste management (Conference Board of Canada, 2016).

There are three main approaches to solid waste disposal in Canada: burial, ideally in modern sanitary landfills that satisfy criteria relating to aesthetics, health, and the monitoring and prevention of leaching (which is the diffusion of substances into groundwater from the landfill site); incineration (in which controlled combustion is used to stabilize and eliminate hazardous material, convert organic into inorganic matter, and kill pathogens); and transformation (e.g., digestion by microorganisms or chemicals). Liquid waste, or sewage, is treated in Canada in municipal sewage treatment plants (except from areas where septic tanks are used).

The best way to manage waste is for society—including government, industry, and individuals—to produce less of it, by following the "4 Rs": reduce, reuse, recycle, and recover. Reducing the consumption of goods is the most effective waste management strategy because it results in less waste and consumes less energy. Reusing products is the next best option. Examples of this strategy include returnable beverage bottles, garage sales, and used furniture and clothing outlets. Recycling involves using material from old products to make new products; commonly recycled materials include newspapers, aluminum cans, glass containers, plastics, cardboard, and auto parts. Recovery involves harvesting energy or economically worthwhile components from waste materials. Industrial-scale examples include heat energy generated from the incineration of solid wastes and methane gas recovered from composting organic wastes. It is estimated that after recycling plastic, glass and metal containers, and paper products, backyard composting could reduce the volume of remaining residential waste in Canada by up to 60%.

An issue that has received much global attention is that of inappropriately disposed-of plastics ending up in the world's oceans. It is estimated that globally, more than 8 million metric tons of plastic are thrown into the ocean every year, and according to recent projections, by 2050, there will be more kilograms of plastic in the ocean than there are fish. This causes significant problems in marine environments because it negatively affects coral; as well, many marine creatures ingest the plastic, causing damage to their digestive systems (Earth Day Network, 2018). Because the fish that we consume ingest plastic and the harmful chemicals associated with it, this issue also affects fish-consuming humans. It is estimated that Canadians generate about 3.25 million tonnes of plastic waste annually—which translates into a 140 000 garbage trucks' worth.

Some strategies that individual people can take to address this issue include reusing and recycling plastic as well as decreasing their consumption of single-use, disposable products such as plastic bags and plastic bottles. Communities and institutions can also take action by eliminating plastic straws (A&W announced in 2018 that it would be doing so, for example) and single-use plastics (IKEA also has plans to phase these out by 2020) (Chin, 2018).

Governments and policy makers at various levels (municipal, provincial, and federal) also have very important roles to play and can introduce legislation to support this initiative. In the regional municipality of Wood Buffalo in Alberta, a bylaw was passed in 2010 that banned retailers from using single-use plastic bags (Chin, 2018). Health care providers can adopt similar measures in their own practices and institutions and can be part of movements that advocate to government to pass laws and bylaws such as these.

SUMMARY

Environmental health may be defined as the study of conditions in the natural and human-made environment that can influence health and well-being. The focus of study in environmental health is the impact of environmental or hazardous agents on the health of the population, and it can be divided into workplace and nonworkplace categories. The workplace environment (occupational health) is often associated with high-level exposure, with the exposed population being predominantly of adult age and in good health. In contrast, nonworkplace environmental exposures are generally low level and often chronic. The population at risk contains the extremes of age, developing fetuses, and ill or immunocompromised persons.

The study of environmental health relies heavily on the fields of epidemiology and toxicology. Toxicology, the science of poisons, identifies adverse effects and predicts harmful dosages. One of the fundamental tenets of toxicology is that any substance can be a poison if given in a large enough dose. Canadians are exposed to toxic substances through a variety of sources, including food, water, air, soil, and consumer products. Risk assessment, management, and communication are strategies for dealing with health risks posed by the environmental contaminants. There are four major steps in the risk assessment of any environmental contaminant. These are hazard identification, exposure assessment, dose response determination, and risk characterization. Risk management follows risk assessment and involves making decisions and implementing options for managing the identified risk. Environmental health issues focus on the outdoor and indoor environment, water quality, food quality, and toxic chemicals. Factors in the outdoor and indoor environments that affect health consist of electromagnetic radiation (ionizing and nonionizing), noise pollution, light pollution, and air pollution (both indoor and outdoor). Climate change is a growing concern and is a known threat to human health, adversely affecting humans through a variety of mechanisms.

Common categories of toxic chemicals include heavy metals, POPs, endocrine disrupters, and pesticides. A number of strategies have been proposed to create a safer environment, including those undertaken at the global, national, provincial or territorial, and local levels. These strategies consist of education or awareness raising among the general public, the development of evidence-based guidelines and exposure limits, technological improvements, adaptation strategies, and regulatory policy approaches.

KEY WEBSITES

Agency for Toxic Substances and Disease Registry (ATSDR): https://www.atsdr.cdc.gov
The ATSDR is a federal public health agency (part of the US Department of Health and Human Services) that responds to environmental health emergencies, investigates environmental health threats, conducts research on hazardous waste sites and their health impact, and provides actionable guidance to health partners. Visit the link to access ATSDR's publications, press releases, education and training resources, and more.

Canadian Environmental Law Association (CELA): http://www.cela.ca
CELA is a nonprofit public interest organization that advocates for human health and the environment by tackling policies to increase environmental protection and safeguard communities. Since 1970, CELA has been using legal tools and research evidence to focus on environmental justice and influence policies. Currently, CELA's work is focused on access to environmental justice, water sustainability, pollution and health, green energy, planning and sustainability, green energy, planning and sustainability, and acting globally. Visit the CELA's website to learn more about these focus areas.

Canadian Institute of Public Health Inspectors (CIPHI) http://www.ciphi.ca
The CIPHI aims to protect the health of all Canadians by advancing the profession and field of environmental public health. The organization represents and unites environmental public health professionals across Canada by offering certification and competency development resources as well as events and education opportunities. Follow the link to learn more about these resources and opportunities.

Intergovernmental Panel on Climate Change (IPCC): https://www.ipcc.ch
Established in 1988 by the World Meteorological Organization and the United Nations Environment Program, the IPCC provides policymakers with scientific, technical, and socioeconomic assessments of climate change. These assessments written by leading scientists are policy-relevant but not policy-prescriptive assessments, providing balanced, evidence-based scientific information to decision makers. Access the link to access the assessment reports and learn more about the IPCC's rigorous review process.

International Agency for Research on Cancer (IARC): https://www.iarc.fr
The IARC specializes in cancer research for cancer prevention by promoting international collaboration in cancer research. The independent role as an international organization facilitates its expertise in coordinating interdisciplinary research across countries and organizations, bringing together skills in epidemiology, laboratory sciences, and biostatistics. Working with the World Health Organization, the IARC produces evidence-based resources for cancer control policies. Visit the link to access research information and publications from the IARC.

International Dark-Sky Association (IDA): http://darksky.org
Since 1988, the IDA has aimed to combat light pollution. Specifically, the IDA aims to preserve and protect the nighttime environment by advocating for protection of the night sky, educating the public and policymakers about night sky conservation, promoting environmentally responsible outdoor lighting, and empowering the public with relevant resources and tools.

International Institute for Sustainable Development (IISD): https://www.iisd.org
The IISD was established in 1990 and impacts economies, communities, ecosystems, and lives in nearly 100 countries by conducting research, reporting international negotiations, and engaging citizens, businesses, and policy makers. This independent think tank tackles challenges that include ecological destruction, social exclusion, unfair laws and economic rules, and climate change. The IISD's work for promoting sustainable development is organized around programs for economic law and policy, energy, water, resilience, knowledge on sustainable development goals, and reporting services. Follow the link to access the IISD's resources and e-library.

United Nations Environment Programme (UN Environment): https://www.unenvironment.org

UN Environment strives to inspire, inform, and enable nations and peoples to improve their quality of life while encouraging sustainability for future generations. As a leading global environmental authority, UN Environment sets the global environmental agenda, promotes coherent implementation of sustainable development, and acts an authoritative advocate for the global environment. Access the link to find out more and find out how to get involved.

United States Environmental Protection Agency (EPA): https://www.epa.gov/iris

The EPA aims to protect human health and the environment. As a national organization, the EPA develops and enforces environmental regulations, gives grants to support environmental programs, conducts research, sponsors partnerships, provides educational resources, and publishes evidence to inform the public. Visit the link to access information and resources from the EPA.

REFERENCES

Amadi, C. N., Igweze, Z. N., & Orisakwe, O. E. (2017). Heavy metals in miscarriages and stillbirths in developing nations. *Middle East Fertility Society Journal*, 22(2), 91–100. https://doi.org/10.1016/j.mefs.2017.03.003.

Australian Radiation Protection and Nuclear Safety Agency. (n.d.). *Radiofrequency radiation*. Retrieved from https://www.arpansa.gov.au/understanding-radiation/what-is-radiation/non-ionising-radiation/radiofrequency-radiation.

Braun, J. M., Gennings, C., Hauser, R., et al. (2016). What can epidemiological studies tell us about the impact of chemical mixtures on human health? *Environmental Health Perspectives*, 124(1), A6–A9. https://doi.org/10.1289/ehp.1510569.

Canadian Centre for Occupational Health and Safety. (2018). *OSH answers fact sheets: Synergism*. Retrieved from https://www.ccohs.ca/oshanswers/chemicals/synergism.html.

Canadian Institute of Public Health Inspectors. (n.d.). *Start your career*. Retrieved from http://www.ciphi.on.ca/career.

Canadian Nurses Association & Canadian Medical Association. (2009). *Joint position statement: Environmentally responsible activity in the health-care sector*. Retrieved from https://www.cna-aiic.ca/-/media/cna/page-content/pdf-en/jps99_environmental_e.pdf?la=en&hash=5919DEC0BF2C282E71BFBCE1DC-649672562164CF.

Canadian Public Health Association. (n.d.). *Who is responsible for food safety in Canada?* Retrieved from https://www.cpha.ca/who-responsible-food-safety-canada.

Cancer Care Ontario. (2017). *Risk of residential radon exposure varies geographically (June 2017)*. Retrieved from https://archive.cancercare.on.ca/cms/One.aspx?portalId=1377&pageId=380327.

Carex Canada. (2017). *Radon in schools: A summary of testing efforts across Canada*. Retrieved from https://www.carexcanada.ca/en/announcements/radon_in_schools/.

Carlberg, M., & Hardell, L. (2017). Evaluation of mobile phone and cordless phone use and glioma risk using the Bradford Hill viewpoints from 1965 on association or causation. *BioMed Research International*. https://doi.org/10.1155/2017/9218486.

CBC News. (2017). *Battle over Muskrat Falls: What you need to know*. October 27. Retrieved from https://www.cbc.ca/news/indigenous/muskrat-falls-what-you-need-to-know-1.3822898.

Centers for Disease Control and Prevention. (2011). *Impact of the built environment on health*. Retrieved from https://www.cdc.gov/nceh/publications/factsheets/impactofthebuiltenvironmentonhealth.pdf.

Chin, J. (2018). Single-use plastics in Canada: Here are the businesses and governments tackling the problem. *Huffington Post*. Retrieved from https://www.huffingtonpost.ca/2018/06/11/single-use-plastics-canada_a_23456208/.

Clayton, J. L., Miller, S., Shepherd, C., et al. (2017). Water quality survey of splash pads after a waterborne Salmonellosis outbreak—Tennessee, 2014. *Journal of Environmental Health*, 79(10).

Conference Board of Canada. (2016). *Provincial and territorial ranking, waste generation*. Retrieved from https://www.conferenceboard.ca/hcp/provincial/environment/waste.aspx.

Cousins, I. T., Vestergren, R., Wang, Z., et al. (2016). The precautionary principle and chemicals management: The example of perfluoroalkyl acids in groundwater. *Environment International*, 94, 331–340. https://doi.org/10.1016/j.envint.2016.04.044.

Craig, S., Earnshaw, C. H., & Virós, A. (2018). Ultraviolet light and melanoma. *The Journal of Pathology*, 244(5), 578–585. https://doi.org/10.1002/path.5039.

Dyck, T., Plummer, R., & Armitage, D. (2015). Examining First Nations' approach to protecting water resources using a multi-barrier approach to safe drinking water in Southern Ontario, Canada. *Canadian Water Resources Journal/Revue Canadienne Des Resources Hydriques*, 40(2), 204–223. https://doi.org/10.1080/07011784.2015.1033759.

Earth Day Network. (2018). *Fact sheet: Plastics in the ocean.* Retrieved from https://www.earthday.org/2018/04/05/fact-sheet-plastics-in-the-ocean/.

Emanuele, E., Spencer, J. M., & Braun, M. (2014). From DNA repair to proteome protection: New molecular insights for preventing non-melanoma skin cancers and skin aging. *Journal of Drugs in Dermatology, 13*(3), 274–281.

Enault, J., Robert, S., Schlosser, O., et al. (2015). Drinking water, diet, indoor air: Comparison of the contribution to environmental micropollutants exposure. *International Journal of Hygiene and Environmental Health, 218*(8), 723–730. https://doi.org/10.1016/j.ijheh.2015.06.001.

Environment and Climate Change Canada. (2017). *Air pollution: Drivers and impacts.* Ottawa: Government of Canada. Retrieved from http://www.ec.gc.ca/indicateurs-indicators/default.asp?lang=En&n=D189C09D-1.

Falchi, F., Cinzano, P., Duriscoe, D., et al. (2016). The new world atlas of artificial night sky brightness. *Science Advances, 2*(6), e1600377. https://doi.org/10.1126/sciadv.1600377.

Faroon, O., & Ruiz, P. (2015). Polychlorinated biphenyls: New evidence from the last decade. *Toxicology and Industrial Health.* https://doi.org/10.1177/0748233715587849. 0748233715587849.

Gall, J. E., Boyd, R. S., & Rajakaruna, N. (2015). Transfer of heavy metals through terrestrial food webs: A review. *Environmental Monitoring and Assessment, 187*(4), 201. https://doi.org/10.1007/s10661-015-4436-3.

Gore, A. C. (2016). Endocrine-disrupting chemicals. *JAMA Internal Medicine, 176*(11), 1705–1706. https://doi.org/10.1001/jamainternmed.2016.5766.

Government of Canada. (2006). *Community noise annoyance.* Retrieved from https://www.canada.ca/en/health-canada/services/healthy-living/your-health/lifestyles/community-noise-annoyance.html.

Government of Canada. (2017). *Fluoride and oral health.* Retrieved from https://www.canada.ca/en/health-canada/services/healthy-living/your-health/environment/fluorides-human-health.html.

Government of Canada. (2018). *Acid rain: Causes and effects.* Retrieved from https://www.canada.ca/en/environment-climate-change/services/air-pollution/issues/acid-rain-causes-effects.html.

Habeeb, D., Vargo, J., & Stone, B. (2015). Rising heat wave trends in large US cities. *Natural Hazards, 76*(3), 1651–1665. https://doi.org/10.1007/s11069-014-1563-z.

Hamilton, D. P., Salmaso, N., & Paerl, H. W. (2016). Mitigating harmful cyanobacterial blooms: Strategies for control of nitrogen and phosphorus loads. *Aquatic Ecology, 50*(3), 351–366. https://doi.org/10.1007/s10452-016-9594-z.

Hammer, M. S., Swinburn, T. K., & Neitzel, R. L. (2014). Environmental noise pollution in the United States: Developing an effective public health response. *Environmental Health Perspectives, 122*(2), 115–119. https://doi.org/10.1289/ehp.1307272.

Harvard Health Publishing. (2018). *Radiation risk from medical imaging.* Retrieved from https://www.health.harvard.edu/cancer/radiation-risk-from-medical-imaging.

Health Canada. (2010). *Guidelines for Canadian drinking water quality: Guideline technical document—Fluoride.* Retrieved from https://www.canada.ca/en/health-canada/services/publications/healthy-living/guidelines-canadian-drinking-water-quality-guideline-technical-document-fluoride.html.

Health Canada. (2014). *Radon—Reduction guide for Canadians.* Retrieved from https://www.canada.ca/content/dam/hc-sc/migration/hc-sc/ewh-semt/alt_formats/pdf/pubs/radiation/radon_canadians-canadiens/radon_canadians-canadien-eng.pdf.

Health Canada. (2015). *Safety Code 6: Health Canada's Radiofrequency Exposure Guidelines.* Ottawa: Government of Canada. Retrieved from https://www.canada.ca/en/health-canada/services/environmental-workplace-health/reports-publications/radiation/safety-code-6-health-canada-radiofrequency-exposure-guidelines-environmental-workplace-health-health-canada.html.

Health Canada. (2017a). *Guidelines for Canadian drinking water quality—summary table.* Ottawa: Government of Canada. Retrieved from https://www.canada.ca/en/health-canada/services/environmental-workplace-health/reports-publications/water-quality/guidelines-canadian-drinking-water-quality-summary-table.html.

Health Canada. (2017b). *Mercury in fish.* Ottawa: Government of Canada. Retrieved from https://www.canada.ca/en/health-canada/services/food-nutrition/food-safety/chemical-contaminants/environmental-contaminants/mercury/mercury-fish.html.

Health Canada. (2017c). *Fluoride and oral health.* Ottawa: Government of Canada. Retrieved from https://www.canada.ca/en/health-canada/services/healthy-living/your-health/environment/fluorides-human-health.html#s4.

Health Canada. (2018). *Indoor air reference levels for chronic exposure to volatile organic compounds.* Ottawa: Government of Canada. Retrieved from https://www.canada.ca/en/health-canada/services/publications/healthy-living/indoor-air-reference-levels-chronic-exposure-volatile-organic-compounds.html.

International Dark-Sky Association. (n.d.). *Light pollution.* Retrieved from http://darksky.org/light-pollution/.

International Dark-Sky Association. (2018). *Kanab, Utah preserves view of the stars with outdoor lighting ordinance.* Retrieved from http://darksky.org/10099-2/.

International Institute for Sustainable Development. (n.d.). *Sustainable development.* Retrieved from https://www.iisd.org/topic/sustainable-development.

International Institute for Sustainable Development. (2017). *Costs of pollution in Canada, Measuring the impacts on families, businesses and governments.* Retrieved from https://www.iisd.org/sites/default/files/publications/costs-of-pollution-in-canada.pdf.

Kim, J. (2015). *Case Study: Health effects of traffic-related air pollution in a small community.* Toronto: Ontario Agency for Health Protection and Promotion (Public Health Ontario). Retrieved from https://www.publichealthontario.ca/en/eRepository/Traffic_Pollution_Small_Community_2015.pdf.

Kim, K. H., Kabir, E., & Jahan, S. A. (2017). Exposure to pesticides and the associated human health effects. *Science of The Total Environment, 575,* 525–535. https://doi.org/10.1016/j.scitotenv.2016.09.009.

Landis, M. S., Edgerton, E. S., White, E. M., et al. (2018). The impact of the 2016 Fort McMurray Horse River Wildfire on ambient air pollution levels in the Athabasca Oil Sands Region, Alberta, Canada. *Science of the Total Environment, 618,* 1665–1676. https://doi.org/10.1016/j.scitotenv.2017.10.008.

Loganathan, B. G., & Masunaga, S. (2015). PCBs, dioxins and furans: Human exposure and health effects. In *Handbook of toxicology of chemical warfare agents* (2nd ed., pp. 239–247). https://doi.org/10.1016/B978-0-12-800159-2.00019-1.

McKitrick, R., & Aliakbari, E. (2017). *Canada's air quality is much improved—no need for more costly regulation.* Vancouver: Fraser Institute. Retrieved from https://www.fraserinstitute.org/article/canadas-air-quality-is-much-improved-no-need-for-more-costly-regulation.

Moan, J., Grigalavicius, M., Baturaite, Z., et al. (2015). The relationship between UV exposure and incidence of skin cancer. *Photodermatology, Photoimmunology & Photomedicine, 31*(1), 26–35. https://doi.org/10.1111/phpp.12139.

Momoli, F., Siemiatycki, J., McBride, M. L., et al. (2017). Probabilistic multiple-bias modeling applied to the Canadian data from the Interphone Study of mobile phone use and risk of glioma, meningioma, acoustic neuroma, and parotid gland tumors. *American Journal of Epidemiology, 186*(7), 885–893. https://doi.org/10.1093/aje/kwx157.

Mosa, A., & Duffin, J. (2017). The interwoven history of mercury poisoning in Ontario and Japan. *Canadian Medical Association Journal, 189*(5), E213–E215. https://doi.org/10.1503/cmaj.160943.

Munnangi, S., & Boktor, S. W. (2017). *Epidemiology, study design.* StatPearls Publishing. Retrieved from https://www.ncbi.nlm.nih.gov/books/NBK470342/.

Natural Resources Canada. (2017). *About renewable energy.* Ottawa: Government of Canada. Retrieved from https://www.nrcan.gc.ca/energy/renewable-electricity/7295.

Office of Response and Restoration, National Oceanic and Atmospheric Administration. (2014). *PCBs: Why are banned chemicals still hurting the environment today?* Retrieved from https://response.restoration.noaa.gov/about/media/pcbs-why-are-banned-chemicals-still-hurting-environment-today.html.

Olive, A. (2016). What is the fracking story in Canada? *The Canadian Geographer/Le Géographe Canadien, 60*(1), 32–45. https://doi.org/10.1111/cag.12257.

Parry, T. (2018). Years ago, Canada and the U.S. came together to end the acid rain threat. What changed? *CBC News ,* December 6. Retrieved from https://www.cbc.ca/news/politics/acid-rain-bush-climate-change-mulroney-1.4934402.

Pick, F. R. (2016). Blooming algae: A Canadian perspective on the rise of toxic cyanobacteria. *Canadian Journal of Fisheries and Aquatic Sciences, 73*(7), 1149–1158. https://doi.org/10.1139/cjfas-2015-0470.

Pirkle, C. M., Muckle, G., & Lemire, M. (2016). Managing mercury exposure in northern Canadian communities. *Canadian Medical Association Journal, 188*(14), 1015–1023. https://doi.org/10.1503/cmaj.151138.

Public Health Agency of Canada. (2017). *The state of community water fluoridation across Canada.* Ottawa: Government of Canada. Retrieved from https://www.canada.ca/en/services/health/publications/healthy-living/community-water-fluoridation-across-canada-2017.html.

Ribeiro, E., Ladeira, C., & Viegas, S. (2017). EDCs mixtures: A stealthy hazard for human health? *Toxics, 5*(1), 5. https://doi.org/10.3390/toxics5010005.

Safe Drinking Water Foundation. (2017). *Water fluoridation in Canada.* Retrieved from https://www.safewater.org/fact-sheets-1/2017/1/23/water-fluoridation-in-canada.

Sagar, S., Dongus, S., Schoeni, A., et al. (2018). Radiofrequency electromagnetic field exposure in everyday microenvironments in Europe: A systematic literature review. *Journal of Exposure Science and Environmental Epidemiology, 28*(2), 147. https://doi.org/10.1038/jes.2017.13.

Sifakis, S., Androutsopoulos, V. P., Tsatsakis, A. M., et al. (2017). Human exposure to endocrine disrupting chemicals: Effects on the male and female reproductive systems. *Environmental Toxicology and Pharmacology, 51*, 56–70. https://doi.org/10.1016/j.etap.2017.02.024.

Statistics Canada. (2015). *Blood lead concentrations in Canadians, 2009 to 2011.* Retrieved from https://www150.statcan.gc.ca/n1/pub/82-625-x/2013001/article/11779-eng.htm.

Statistics Canada. (2016). *Environment fact sheets: Radon awareness in Canada.* Retrieved from https://www150.statcan.gc.ca/n1/pub/16-508-x/16-508-x2016002-eng.htm.

Tham, K. W. (2016). Indoor air quality and its effects on humans—a review of challenges and developments in the last 30 years. *Energy and Buildings, 130*, 637–650. https://doi.org/10.1016/j.enbuild.2016.08.071.

United Nations Development Programme. (2016). *Sustainable development goals.* Retrieved from http://www.undp.org/content/undp/en/home/sustainable-development-goals.html.

United States Environmental Protection Agency. (2017). *Risk assessment, conducting a human health risk assessment.* Retrieved from https://www.epa.gov/risk/conducting-human-health-risk-assessment#tab-5.

United States Environmental Protection Agency. (2018a). *Environmental justice.* Retrieved from https://www.epa.gov/environmentaljustice.

United States Environmental Protection Agency. (2018b). *Learn about polychlorinated biphenyls (PCBs).* Retrieved from https://www.epa.gov/pcbs/learn-about-polychlorinated-biphenyls-pcbs.

US Environmental Protection Agency. (2018c). *Health effects of exposure to mercury.* Retrieved from https://www.epa.gov/mercury/health-effects-exposures-mercury.

US National Library of Medicine & National Institutes of Health. (n.d). *What is environmental health?* Retrieved from https://kidsenvirohealth.nlm.nih.gov/generic/11/what-is-environmental-health.

Walkerton Inquiry. (2002). *Report of the Walkerton Inquiry: Parts I and II.* Toronto: Publications Ontario/Government of Ontario.

World Health Organization (n.d.a.). *Radiation (non-ionizing).* Retrieved from http://www.who.int/topics/radiation_non_ionizing/en/.

World Health Organization (n.d.b). *Persistent organic pollutants (POPs).* Retrieved from http://www.who.int/foodsafety/areas_work/chemical-risks/pops/en/.

World Health Organization. (2001). *Climate change and human health—risks and responses. Summary, international consensus on the science of climate and health: The IPCC Third Assessment Report.* Retrieved from http://www.who.int/globalchange/summary/en/index-2.html.

World Health Organization. (2009). *WHO night noise guidelines for Europe.* Retrieved from http://www.euro.who.int/en/health-topics/environment-and-health/noise/policy/who-night-noise-guidelines-for-europe.

World Health Organization. (2018). *Climate change and health.* Retrieved from http://www.who.int/news-room/fact-sheets/detail/climate-change-and-health.

Zani, C., Ceretti, E., Covolo, L., & Donato, F. (2017). Do polychlorinated biphenyls cause cancer? A systematic review and meta-analysis of epidemiological studies on risk of cutaneous melanoma and non-Hodgkin lymphoma. *Chemosphere, 183*, 97–106. https://doi.org/10.1016/j.chemosphere.2017.05.053.

Zuo, F., Li, Y., Johnson, S., et al. (2014). Temporal and spatial variability of traffic-related noise in the City of Toronto, Canada. *Science of The Total Environment, 472*, 1100–1107.

Occupational Health and Diseases

LEARNING OBJECTIVES

- Define *occupational health* and list examples of chemical, biological, physical, mechanical or ergonomic, and psychosocial exposures in the workplace.
- Describe the major shifts that have occurred in the Canadian labour market over the past several decades.
- Name and describe the principles of legislation that are relevant to occupational health, including

workplace health and safety and workplace compensation acts.
- Describe the hierarchy of controls for occupational health exposures and list an example of each type of control measure.
- Be familiar with the scope of workplace health promotion interventions.
- Describe the key features of specific workplace hazards that are of public health significance in Canada.

CHAPTER OUTLINE

KEY TERMS

administrative controls
asbestosis
barotrauma
carpal tunnel syndrome (CTS)
coal workers' pneumoconiosis (CWP)
contact dermatitis
decompression sickness
due diligence
hazard identification
internal responsibility system

elimination
engineering controls
Job Strain Model
hand-arm vibration syndrome (HAVS)
Meredith principles
mesothelioma
occupational health
personal protective equipment (PPE)
primary prevention

precarious employment
Raynaud's phenomenon
risk assessment
risk control
silicosis
substitution
vulnerable workers
Workplace Hazardous Materials Information System (WHMIS)
workplace wellness programs

INTRODUCTION

Chapter 5 discusses the importance of employment and the work environment on health and its distribution. Most adults spend a considerable amount of time at their workplace (8 hours on average) and are exposed to a variety of work-related situations. Some of these situations are pleasant, but others expose workers to stressful situations and to physical, chemical, mechanical, ergonomic, and biological hazards. The effects of these hazards are not always immediate, because some have a long latency period. This chapter deals with the impact of employment (including employment policies) and the workplace environment as it relates to Canadians.

For this chapter, it is important to keep in mind the differences between the terms *hazard*, *exposure*, and *risk* (also discussed in Chapter 11). Whereas *hazard* refers to any type of agent (e.g., biological, psychological) that can cause harm, *risk* refers to the actual probability or chance that the hazard will result in harm. Hazards do not pose harm unless one is exposed to them. So, risk (or probability of harm) is really the product of a specific hazard and a person or group's *exposure* to it (through ingestion, inhalation, skin absorption, and so on).

OCCUPATIONAL HEALTH

Occupational health is defined as the maintenance and promotion of health in the work environment. The delivery of occupational health services involves, nurses, physicians, occupational hygienists, engineers and safety officers, ergonomists, chiropractors, physicists, and technicians. The jurisdiction for enforcement of occupational health legislation lies with the provinces and territories. Exceptions to this are the federally regulated industries covered under the *Canada Labour Code,* which include those within the federal government and those within industries operating across provincial/territorial or international borders (listed in Box 12.1). In total, workers who are covered under the *Canada Labour Code* make up about 6% of the Canadian workforce; the remaining 94% are covered under their provincial or territorial health and safety acts (described later). Because of this provincial jurisdiction, there are variations in legislation and regulations governing occupational health across Canada. However, the principles of occupational safety underlying most occupational health acts are constant. For example, the internal responsibility system is the main philosophy that underlies occupational health and

---

> ## BOX 12.1 Sectors Covered by the *Canada Labour Code*
>
> - Airports and airlines
> - Banks
> - Canals
> - Exploration and development of petroleum on lands subject to federal jurisdiction
> - Ferries, port services, tunnels, and bridges
> - Grain elevators licensed by the Canadian Grain Commission, and certain feed mills and feed warehouses, flour mills and grain seed-cleaning plants;
> - Highway transport
> - Many Indigenous activities
> - Pipelines
> - Radio and television broadcasting and cable systems
> - Railways
> - Shipping and shipping services
> - Telephone and telegraph systems
> - Uranium mining and processing

safety laws across Canada. The **internal responsibility system** posits that everyone is responsible for their safety and the safety of co-workers. It helps to promote a culture of safety and self-reliance and holds everyone in the workplace accountable for safety (Canadian Centre for Occupational Health & Safety [CCOHS], 2019a). Additionally, the rights of workers are the same across Canada; they include the worker's right to (1) know workplace hazards, (2) refuse dangerous work, and (3) participate in workplace health and safety initiatives.

The work environment contains a wide range of hazards grouped as chemical (e.g., solvents, heavy metals), physical (e.g., radiation, noise), biological (e.g., blood-borne pathogens, viruses), ergonomic (e.g., work processes involving repetitive movements or an awkward posture), and psychosocial (e.g., workplace violence, harassment, stress, isolation). Protecting the worker from exposure to these factors requires a commitment on the part of management to ensure that activities are carried out in the areas of health promotion (work design and worker education), health protection and disease prevention (implementing controls to decrease exposure to hazards and monitoring the health of the worker), and rehabilitation (returning the worker to safe, meaningful, productive work).

The Canadian Workforce

Although most of Canada's wealth has traditionally come from natural resources, today most Canadian workers are employed in the service sector. In 2017, there were just over

18 million people over the age of 15 years in the workforce across the country, 9.6 million of whom were male and 8.7 million of whom were female (Statistics Canada, 2018).

The most recent estimates of the unemployment rate in Canada suggest that it ranges between 5% and 6% federally, although important geographic differences in unemployment exist. For example, the unemployment rate in Newfoundland and Labrador in January 2019 was much higher, at 11.4%, than the national average, whereas in Quebec, the unemployment rate was slightly lower than the national average, at 5.4% (Statistics Canada, 2019).

Employment status is an important determinant of health. High rates of unemployment undoubtedly affect population health because employment provides income (another critical health determinant), can be important in feeling a sense of purpose and accomplishment (important to mental health), and can often act as a place for social connection as well.

Aside from the presence or absence of employment, type of work and the age and composition of the workforce also impact population health outcomes. Other notable trends in the Canadian workforce include more Canadians working past the age of 65 years; fewer people aged 24 to 54 years working full time, all year; more recent immigrants participating in the labour force; and declining employment rates among youth and some Indigenous groups (Statistics Canada, 2017a) (for more details, refer to Chapter 5). Box 12.2 presents a detailed description of vulnerable workers and the effects of precarious employment on population health in Canada.

EXERCISE 12.1: What factors might account for the higher unemployment rate in Newfoundland and Labrador compared with Quebec?

Statistics Canada defines the goods-producing industry as including manufacturing, construction, utilities, agriculture, and the other primary industries (fishing, trapping, logging, mining, quarrying). All other sectors of industry, including government, are considered to be services. In general, growth in employment has been the greatest among service sectors, with almost four of five workers working in the service industry. Notably, roughly 12% of Canadian workers are employed in health care and social service industries. In health care, specifically, women outnumber men by a ratio of nearly four to one. Nowadays, women also make up half of the physician workforce (Statistics Canada, 2017b).

BOX 12.2   Vulnerable Workers and the Health Effects of Precarious Employment

Precarious employment is a complex concept that encompasses characteristics such as having insecure employment (including temporary or part-time work), low wages, and limited ability to access workplace rights and protections. The number of people who experience precarious employment is thought to be growing in Europe and North America. These changes are thought to have come about because of the decreased influence of unions, automization of the workforce, and globalization.

Precarious employment is increasingly being viewed as an important determinant of health and has been shown to influence things such as perceived mental and physical health, quality of life, and exposure to hazardous working environments (Benach et al., 2016). In Canada, certain groups of people are more likely to end up in precarious employment situations, including youth, older adults, women, racialized groups, Indigenous people, and people with disabilities (Fleury, 2016).

An important concept related to precarious employment is that of the vulnerable worker. **Vulnerable workers** are at an increased risk of work-related injury or illness because of a combination of increased exposure to hazardous work and decreased ability or power to alter these conditions. Such vulnerability frequently arises from the lack of access to information about one's health and safety rights and from being unable to exercise these rights or raise health and safety concerns for fear of losing one's job or being deported. Examples of vulnerable workers include young workers, recent immigrants, workers who are new to their job, and foreign workers hired to address temporary or seasonal labour shortages (CCOHS, 2019b).

Discrimination against some groups (women, Indigenous peoples, visible minorities, and people living with disabilities) is prevalent in the Canadian workforce. For example, although women are participating more in the workforce than they did 50 years ago, they are still overrepresented in traditionally female occupations such as teaching, nursing, and social work; more often work part time (because of caregiving responsibilities); are underrepresented in leadership positions in the private sector; and continue to experience wage inequities (women earn $0.87 for every dollar earned by a male counterpart) (Statistics Canada, 2017b).

EXERCISE 12.2: Brainstorm some reasons to explain the wage gap that we see between men and women.

Racism also continues to exist in the workplace and tends to work on several levels: by excluding individuals from entering the workforce and hindering their promotion; by not providing suitable work for level of training (underemployment), which is particularly common among recent immigrants with professional qualifications; and by both overt and systemic racism in the workplace. For example, a recent study examining trends in employment between 2011 and 2017 in the Greater Toronto and Hamilton areas reported that, on average, more people with university degrees found stable employment over the reported time period, although this gain did not hold true to the same degree for all groups. White workers with university degrees did better than racialized workers with the same qualifications in terms of rates of stable employment, and men did better than women. Furthermore, racialized women with a university degree were the only ones who did not see an increase in stable employment over the study time period (Poverty and Employment Precarity in Southern Ontario, 2018).

Discrimination increases the general level of stress in the workplace, and causes considerable demoralization and financial strain, which in turn, affects health. The issue of racism and employment is discussed again in Chapter 6.

> **CRITICAL THINKING QUESTION 12.1:** Many global nongovernmental organizations dedicate their work to increasing women's participation in the labour force, arguing that this is key to development and achieving health and well-being for all.
>
> Why might greater female labour force participation rates translate into improved population health outcomes?

Health Indicators Among Canadian Workers

The Association of Workers' Compensation Boards of Canada (AWCBC) collects information from the provincial and territorial workers' compensation boards (WCBs). According to the most recent AWCBC data, in 2016, just over 900 workplace deaths were recorded, and about 240 000 claims were accepted to compensate people for lost time because of work-related injuries or illnesses across the country. Overall, workplace-related injuries and fatalities have declined over the years (Tucker & Keefe, 2018). Based on the most recent statistics from the AWCBC, contacts with objects and equipment, falls, bodily reaction and exertion, exposure

to harmful substances and environments, and transportation-related accidents made up the highest proportion of claims for lost time in Canada. Traumatic injuries made up the bulk of claims and far exceeded claims for communicable or noncommunicable diseases (NCDs). Most fatalities occurred in the construction industry, and most injuries (nonfatal) for people who claimed lost time occurred in the health and social services, manufacturing, and retail industries (AWCBC, 2016).

Workplace musculoskeletal (MSK) disorders—painful conditions affecting one or more nerves, tendons, or muscles—are some of the most common health issues experienced by workers today. These MSK disorders include tendinitis (inflammation of a tendon), carpal tunnel syndrome, neck and back pain as a result of repetitive motions, and awkward postures (CCOHS, 2014). Skin diseases also make up a bulk of occupational health issues. Contact dermatitis, for example, is prevalent among health care workers and some other occupations, such as food handlers who engage in frequent handwashing.

> **EXERCISE 12.3:** Can you think of occupations that might make workers more prone to MSK disorders?

Increasing attention is being paid to the impact of workplaces on mental health and vice versa. The Mental Health Commission of Canada estimates that nearly 500 000 people do not go to work every week because of an issue related to mental health. Given the fact that many people spend 25 to 40 hours every week at work, attention must be paid to ensuring that the workplace is fostering positive mental health. Currently, nearly 47% of Canadians consider work to be the most stressful part of their day. Workers who come to work with less than optimal psychological health perform less well, take more time off, and are less engaged while at work. This reduced productivity while at work is called *presenteeism*, and it is estimated to cost more than absenteeism (being away or off work because of illness or injury). Thus, much incentive exists to address the root causes of poor mental health in the workplace. In fact, according to some estimates, up to 14% of new cases of common mental health issues (e.g., depression and anxiety) are preventable through the elimination of work-related psychosocial hazards (Brooks, 2018).

An issue that is gaining much public and media attention is that of post-traumatic stress disorder (PTSD), particularly among people in the military, as well as first responders (e.g., police, paramedics, fire services). With constant exposure to violence, trauma, and death (particularly during a time of rising opioid deaths across the country), many of these workers are at risk of PTSD, which may go unrecognized and untreated. Some Canadian estimates suggest that nearly 70 000 first responders across the country have experienced PTSD at some point in their lifetime (Wilson, Guliani, & Boichev, 2016). See the Research Perspective box for a discussion of PTSD among military personnel in Canada.

RESEARCH PERSPECTIVE

Post-traumatic Stress Disorder in the Canadian Military

Widespread attention is being paid to the issue of PTSD among current and past Canadian Armed Forces personnel. PTSD has significant societal consequences, including disability, risk of suicide, family violence, and substance use disorders, among others, and as such, researchers across the nation have aimed to describe the burden of PTSD in this population.

In 2010, Veterans Affairs Canada, the Department of National Defence, and Statistics Canada launched the Life After Service Studies (LASS). This series of surveys helps to elicit how people cope with the transition from military life to civilian life. Of note, LASS 2016 found that 14% of veterans reported having PTSD (Veterans Affairs Canada, 2018). Statistics Canada also surveys active members of the Canadian Armed Forces. In 2013, their survey revealed that nearly 11% of regular force members experienced symptoms of PTSD in their lifetime. In fact, it was the third most common disorder reported among those surveyed (Pearson, 2015). These studies reveal the vulnerability of members of the military to PTSD for reasons including being far away from friends and family, living through harsh physical conditions, experiencing loss and grief, stigma around mental health, and the culture and norms around seeking help for mental health challenges.

Exercise

Changing the culture of a workplace or professional group can be quite challenging. Imagine that you are a health care provider at a Canadian Armed Forces base, where speaking about feelings and emotions is ridiculed and stigma for people living with mental health issues is prevalent. How might you promote talking about and seeking help for mental health challenges among your clients and begin to change the culture?

Issues Related to Occupational Health Data

Injury and illness prevention are among the most important issues in occupational health. The lack of coordinated data collection in Canada has long been recognized as a major hindrance to the prevention of occupational injury and illness. One of the problems is deciding who should be responsible for collecting this information—which is difficult because occupational health falls under federal, provincial, and territorial jurisdictions. At the provincial/territorial level, occupational injury and illness are mostly the responsibility of labour departments rather than health departments. Although illness data are collected from hospitals, primary care physicians, emergency department visits, medical examiner reports, health surveys, cancer registries, and death certificates, these sources often fall short in terms of providing information about work exposures and work attribution. There is no systematic data collection from occupational medicine specialists, industry, and health insurance firms. WCBs provide the bulk of the information about work-related injuries and illnesses. However, WCB data tend to be imperfect; the data focus mostly on the illness of the worker, with little information on substances to which all workers were exposed in the same work situation. WCB data is also inherently biased because only claims that are accepted are counted.

Epidemiological studies are also fraught with challenges because they require unique patient-identifying data, accurate medical diagnosis, and standardized ways of coding exposures and occupational diseases. An additional problem exists with the interpretation of epidemiological data, even if data collection is satisfactory, because there is the confounding effect of nonoccupational disease. For example, when researchers try to determine the causation between coal mining and lung cancer, smoking becomes an extremely powerful confounding factor. This makes for challenging study design, as well as problematic WCB compensation claims in miners who smoke.

In addition to lifestyle, there is also the issue of genetic, or inherent, disease. For instance, not all asthma or cancer cases in workers are caused by chemical exposures. A segment of these cases would have developed even without exposures in the workplace. The multifactorial causation of most chronic conditions complicates how confidently we can attribute a person's illness to the workplace, and affects workers' compensation claim acceptance. Finally, underreporting is a significant challenge. Workers and employers don't always fill out claims or report injuries, accidents, or illnesses, particularly if they are perceived to be minor.

CRITICAL THINKING QUESTION 12.2: How might big data analytics (discussed in Chapter 2) change how occupational health data are captured and analyzed?

OCCUPATIONAL HEALTH RESOURCES

Occupational health resources are based in government, industry, educational institutions, union-based centres, and hospitals. The federal government's jurisdictional responsibility in occupational health is mainly for federal employees and a few special sectors, such as banks, nuclear power, and transportation (listed in Box 12.1). The federal government relies on both Employment and Social Development Canada and Health Canada to set standards and provide appropriate occupational health services. The provinces and territories have the most responsibility for occupational health. At the provincial/territorial level, regulatory responsibility lies with one or more departments or ministries. (The Ministry of Labour is usually the lead agency; others with responsibility are the Ministry of Mining and the Ministry of Health.) Major industries have corporate occupational health departments where company-hired health care professionals are responsible for the surveillance and monitoring of workers as prescribed by law and corporate policy. The range of health care professionals hired depends on the size and complexity of the industry or corporation and may include occupational health nurses, ergonomists, occupational hygienists, physicians, psychologists, chiropractors, and physiotherapists or kinesiologists. For a description of occupational health nursing and the role of an occupational health nurse in the interprofessional care team, refer to the Interprofessional Practice box.

Educational institutions, hospitals, union-based centres, and consultants provide some, if not all, occupational health services on a fee-for-service basis or through other payment mechanisms. The occupational health services provide health promotion and health protection (primary prevention), management of injury and illness (secondary prevention), and rehabilitation services (tertiary prevention). Unfortunately, however, there is a trend for many corporate occupational health departments to focus on disability management (i.e., tertiary prevention) and pay only minimal attention to health promotion (primary prevention).

INTERPROFESSIONAL PRACTICE

Occupational Health Nurses and their Role in the Broader Interprofessional Occupational Care Team

The Canadian Nurses Association (CNA) offers an RN certification in the field of occupational health. RNs who have taken this certification are officially certified in Occupational Health Nursing (designation: COHN(C)). They often work in a range of organizations to protect and promote employee health in a broad sense. They are members of a multi-disciplinary team providing advice to managers, supervisors, and employees of a given institution. Examples of their day-to-day work include disability management; finding strategies to reduce absenteeism; and designing health promotion programs to improve the health of workers, occupational health, and safety.

Occupational health nurses typically work in collaboration with a range of other health care professionals, including other nurses (e.g., public health nurses), physicians, occupational therapists, physiotherapists, pharmacists, and ergonomists. As such, occupational health—like many other health care disciplines—requires a focus on collaboration and team dynamics, including active listening, understanding each other's roles and responsibilities, and frequent and clear communication between team members.

Exercise
Research, compare, and contrast the role of an occupational therapist with that of an occupational health nurse. What are areas of similarities, and what are the key differences in the role when it comes to the area of occupational health—improving, maintaining, and restoring health of workers?

In terms of legislation that supports occupational health, federally, part two of the *Canada Labour Code* and provincial and territorial occupational health and safety legislation remain the strongest tools. Although the specifics of the provisions may differ among federal, provincial, and territorial occupational health and safety acts, there are three aspects that are universal across the country. The first is the concept of **due diligence**. That is, the employer must demonstrate that reasonable steps were taken to become familiar with the inherent dangers in the workplace and that action was taken to ensure that the workplace was safe. Ignorance is no excuse for an unsafe workplace if it can be demonstrated that no effort was made to understand the hazards of the workplace.

Second, the federally legislated **Workplace Hazardous Materials Information System (WHMIS)** applies across Canada. WHMIS is intended to ensure that workers are protected from hazards in the workplace by labelling all chemical substances in the workplace according to a globally recognized classification system (refer to Fig. 12.1 for common WHMIS symbols), educating all workers at the work site with respect to the WHMIS program, and keeping a centralized record of all hazards in the workplace on Safety Data Sheets (SDSs), which detail important information on handling hazardous substances and cleaning up spills properly.

Third, provincial occupational health and safety acts mandate the existence of *joint health and safety committees* or health and safety representatives, depending on the size of a company. Joint health and safety committees are composed of representatives drawn from both management and workers. Their purpose is to identify workplace health and safety hazards and to communicate their concerns to management in writing. Workers must be granted time, with pay, to prepare for and attend committee meetings and to participate in inspections of the workplace.

Additionally, most occupational health and safety legislation outlines specific rights and duties of the employee and employer—a key one being that of reporting. Employees must report hazards and accidents or incidents to their employers, and employers must report accidents or incidents to the appropriate authorities (a ministry of labour [or an equivalent organization] at the provincial/territorial level or the Labour Program, which falls under Employment and Social Development Canada at the federal level). See Table 12.1 for a more detailed description of the rights and duties of both employees and employers under the Canada Labour Code and most provincial and territorial occupational health and safety laws.

> **CRITICAL THINKING QUESTION 12.3:** Review Table 12.1, particularly the asterisked note at the bottom of the table. As is mentioned in the note, some workers (e.g., health care workers) have some limitations in their right to refuse work, particularly if it endangers the life, health, or safety of another person.
>
> Research the severe acute respiratory syndrome (SARS) crisis of 2003. If you were a health care worker at that time, how might you have responded to the need to treat ill clients but also protect yourself? Is this type of risk a "normal part of your work"? Is refusing work in this type of situation endangering health or safety of others? What professional standards and ethical principles apply (depending on your profession)? What protections should be in place for those continuing to work in risky situations?

PREVENTION AND CONTROL STRATEGIES

As already explained, the prevention of injury and illness is very important for maintaining the physical, mental, and social well-being of employees in the workplace. The goal of **primary prevention** is to take action in the workplace so that the worker is protected from injury and illness occurring in the first place. Ideally, of course, this is the preferred level of prevention and includes ongoing **risk assessment**, including identifying hazards in the workplace (**hazard identification**), assessing the actual level of exposure of workers to these hazards (exposure assessment), and reducing these exposures (through risk control and risk communication), similar to those described in Chapter 11. **Risk control** can be achieved in many ways, and a common occupational health framework, developed by the Centers for Disease Control and Prevention (CDC) (2018), is used to classify and prioritize different control strategies (see Fig. 12.2 for a visual depiction).

According to the CDC, the best method of control is **elimination**—or getting rid of the hazard. For example, the removal of lead from aviation fuel for large airplanes has eliminated the source of lead toxicity for aircraft mechanics. If elimination cannot be achieved, **substitution**—the replacement of a hazardous substance with one that is less hazardous—is the next best option (e.g., replacing a very dangerous pesticide in the agricultural sector with another, less harmful, one).

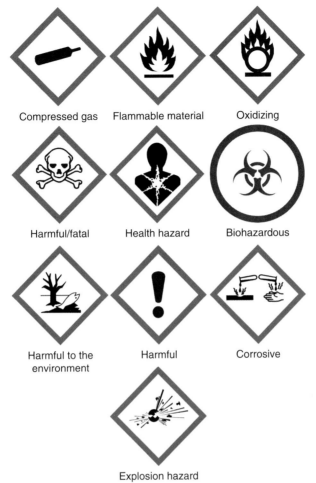

Fig 12.1 Workplace Hazardous Materials Information System symbols (from top left to bottom): Compressed Gas, Flammable and Combustible Materials, Oxidizing Materials, Materials Causing Immediate and Serious Toxic Effects, Materials Posing a Health Hazard, Materials Posing a Biohazard, Materials Posing an Environmental Hazard, Materials Posing an Irritation Hazard, Materials Posing a Corrosion Hazard, and Explosive Hazard). Source: Canadian Centre for Occupational Health and Safety. (2015). *WHMIS 2015 pictograms kit.* Retrieved from https://www.ccohs.ca/WHMISpictograms.html.

TABLE 12.1	Rights and Duties of the Employee and the Employer under the *Canada Labour Code*
Employee	**Employer**
Rights • Right to know about hazards • Right to refuse dangerous work[a] • Right to participate in ensuring a safe workplace **Duties** • Use protective materials, equipment and devices given by employer to protect employee • Report all work-related accidents to employer • Report hazards to employer	**Duties** • Ensure workers have the needed training, information, and supervision to be safe at work • Ensure that complaints, accidents, and injuries are thoroughly investigated • Ensure health and safety committees are formed and carry out their functions (including inspections)

[a]Workers with the responsibility to protect public safety, such as many health care workers, have limitations to the right to refuse work. They cannot refuse work if the danger is a normal part of their job or if the refusal will endanger the life, health, or safety of another person. From Statistics Canada. (2017). *Workplace safety.* Retrieved from https://www.canada.ca/en/employment-social-development/services/health-safety/workplace-safety.html.

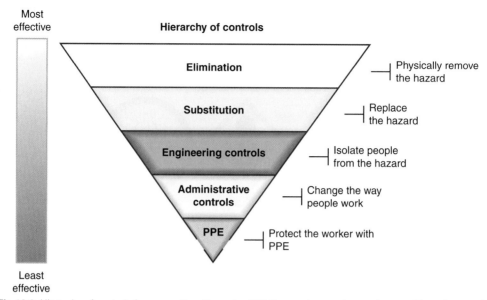

Fig 12.2 Hierarchy of controls for occupational hazards. *PPE,* Personal protective equipment. (From Centers for Disease Control and Prevention. [2018]. *Hierarchy of controls: overview.* Retrieved from https://www.cdc.gov/ niosh/topics/hierarchy/default.html.)

Engineering controls, although more costly than administrative ones, are the next most effective control strategies. **Engineering controls** reduce the exposure to the hazard by affecting the path between the source and the person. An example is designing a negative-pressure isolation room whereby ventilatory and air circulation systems prevent airborne pathogens such as tuberculosis (TB) from spreading outside the isolation room to nearby environments.

Administrative controls tend to be less expensive and complex than engineering controls. They include job rotation, whereby employees rotate through jobs that have exposure to hazardous materials and minimize exposure to certain repetitive tasks. Refer to the Case Study box for a more detailed description of a well-known Canadian disaster and some of the hazard control measures put into place after this tragedy.

Lastly, personal protective equipment (PPE) (e.g., wearing masks, gloves) is the control strategy of last resort because it is often expensive to purchase and maintain, requires training, and often must be individually fitted. However, the major problem with PPE is that its effectiveness depends solely on workers' compliance. Similar to other strategies in public health, strategies targeting individual behaviours are the least effective. Noncompliance is frequently a problem in the workplace because PPE is often uncomfortable to wear, and the long-term benefits of

improved health are often not perceived as being as desirable as the relief afforded by removing the equipment.

EXERCISE 12.4: At one time, asbestos fibres were commonly used in building materials and for insulation in Canada, and they are still used internationally because the fibres are fire resistant and very stable in the environment. Currently, most exposures in Canada occur during the renovation of old buildings. When inhaled, asbestos fibres can cause lung disease (called asbestosis) and cancers (specifically, mesotheliomas and lung cancers).

Applying the CDC's hierarchy of controls framework, brainstorm one strategy under each type of control that could minimize the harm of asbestos exposure to construction workers when working with disturbed asbestos fibres.

CASE STUDY

Lessons Learned About Hazard Control from the Ocean Ranger Tragedy

The *Ocean Ranger* was a large drilling rig used to drill for oil off the shores of Newfoundland. On February 14, 1982, a large storm hit and toppled the drilling rig, tragically killing all 84 crew members aboard. As a result, this incited outrage and questions regarding the safety of workers involved in such risky operations (Kelly, 2012). About a month after the incident, a Royal Commission on the Ocean Ranger Marine Disaster was formed to explore what happened and to find solutions to ensure that a similar incident didn't happen again. The findings of the two reports written by the commission pointed towards the failure of the physical infrastructure (e.g., the design of the rig and its components), a lack of survival equipment kits, and a lack of training for worker safety, to name a few factors contributing to the deaths. Thus, engineering controls, protective equipment, and administrative controls were put into place on all oil rigs. The engineering controls included creating standards for rig design. More protective equipment was mandated so that each drilling unit had to carry enough survival suits and lifeboards for every crew member to have at least two. Last, but perhaps most important, is that a key administrative control—training—was emphasized. Training standards (related both to how to do the job as well as safety training) were developed by both the provincial and federal governments (Higgins, 2018). These standard competencies are now updated on a regular basis and are delivered to all workers without fail.

This emphasis on training and fostering a culture of safety among all staff should not be understated. In certain lines of work, the control measures of substitution and elimination may not consistently be able to be used (though they are always the "gold standard"). In these situations, in particular, fostering a culture of safety with training and administrative measures—such as policies, rules, and regulations in place that are routinely audited and practised—can go a long way. In fact, even when substitution and elimination are in place, using administrative controls to enhance and promote a culture of safety is of utmost importance.

Workplace Health Promotion

Health promotion in the workplace has emerged as an effective approach, enabling access to the substantial number of people in the workplace, not only for prevention of work-associated health problems but also for general wellness programs that incorporate attention to lifestyle and other health determinants. Making workplaces into supportive health-promoting environments was the call to action declared in the *Third International Conference on Health Promotion: Supporting*

Environments for Health—the Sudsvall Conference in 1991. Promoting health in the workplace can include interventions that aim to change individual and organizational practices, as well improve the overall workplace environment.

The shift towards more service-sector jobs is associated with greater levels of sedentary work environments (e.g., desk jobs). Given the significant amount of time that Canadians spend at work, the impact of work on stress (as described earlier) and the rise in NCDs resulting from the four most significant risk factors (described in Chapter 8, namely, smoking, alcohol consumption, low levels of physical activity, and poor diets), the need for broad-based workplace health-promotion strategies has never been more important.

Workplace wellness programs, defined as organizational-level programs that aim to improve people's health while at work, are becoming increasingly popular in North America. They often include multiple strategies such as health education and awareness raising (e.g., seminars on nutritional diets), weight management and fitness (e.g., providing employees with discounted gym memberships or in-house gyms, policies regarding the types of foods sold in the cafeteria), stress management (described further below), employee assistance programs (described later), screening and immunizations (e.g., routinely offering the influenza vaccine to employees every fall), and physical space design (e.g., designing appealing and well-lit stairwells and walking paths around an office building). These types of programs have a significant benefit to employers because they have been shown to result in improved productivity, worker satisfaction, and reduced absenteeism. Additionally, because they improve health, employers save money spent on employee health benefits (Jacobs et al., 2017).

One example of an innovative and gender-sensitive workplace mental health promotion intervention is the POWERPLAY program, which aimed to increase physical activity and fruit and vegetable consumption among male workers in Northern British Columbia. This program consisted of promoting healthy competition related to progressively increasing physical activity and healthy eating among four male-dominated worksites that included trucking companies and a shipping terminal. Resources, weekly tips, and log-books (targeting the attitudes and beliefs of males who work and live in rural environments) were given to participants to support their progress, and two 6-week challenges were held over a 6-month period. Kick-off events at which blood pressure, heart rate, and so on were measured helped with engaging and motivating participants. This initiative resulted in increases in the average level of physical activity the men were engaging in on a weekly basis over the 6-month study period (Johnson et al., 2016).

EXERCISE 12.5: What other interventions (e.g., tackling the environment and root causes) can a workplace take to ensure that these initiatives are sustainable and that the changes workers make are maintained in the long run after the program has been completed?

Other types of workplace wellness initiatives also include things such as smoking cessation programs, stress management programs, and employee assistance programs.

Smoking cessation programs have been extensively studied and are one of the few lifestyle programs that are justifiable to employers based on cost-effectiveness alone because the investment in the program costs less than the savings achieved through a reduction in absenteeism from smoking-related illnesses.

Stress management programs help to both reduce and manage stress at the workplace. They may include offering meditation, yoga, or mindfulness classes, instituting strategies that encourage work–life balance (e.g., flexible work schedules, opportunities to work from home), providing opportunities for social interaction while at work, and being mindful of the design of physical workspace (e.g., ensuring access to windows and sunlight).

Employee assistance programs are often a component of stress management programs and are designed to help employees deal with stress. They provide a third party to be available for counselling services to help employees deal with workplace and home or personal problems (which may include the stress of relationships, financial issues, or drug or alcohol abuse).

The extensive focus on stress reduction and management in workplace wellness programs is warranted, given the impact of work on stress. Additionally, as described in Chapters 8 and 9, stress has been shown to contribute to a number of different physical and mental health disease states, including anxiety, depression, and cardiovascular disease, among others.

Workplace stress is a result of the interplay between a complex array of factors. One of the most validated and cited models relating to stress in the workplace is called the **Job Strain Model**. This model posits that workplace stress is influenced by three main domains: demand (i.e., more stress results from work that is too hard or is unmanageable), decision latitude (more strain is associated with having no control over decisions in the workplace), and social support (i.e., having more stress relates to being poorly supported by colleagues and supervisors) (Niedhammer et al., 2018). Thus, institution-level strategies that are aimed at ensuring manageable workloads, training and support for people to accomplish their workplace goals, engaging employees in decision making, and fostering positive organizational cultures and relationships can also go a long way towards reducing and managing workplace stress.

Lastly, healthy public policy options related to working conditions are instrumental in improving health because they address the broad, systemic, and social conditions or environments that influence employee health. For example, provision of a daycare centre onsite, flexible work hours, and adequate parental leave facilitate the health of employees of childrearing age and help reduce inequities in employment across genders.

Much research has focused on the benefits of parental leave—both for parents and children. Studies have shown that parental leave policies help improve employment continuity, labour force participation (particularly among women), and physical and mental health among children (through the promotion of breastfeeding and promoting more time and bonding between parent and child) and reduce school drop out rates in children (Ruhm, 2017). The Case Study box provides an example of a healthy public policy initiative that was instituted by the federal government to help address employment inequities among certain groups.

CASE STUDY

Federal Government Interventions to Improve Equity, Diversity, and Inclusion

A few strategies have been introduced at the federal government level to assess their potential in addressing inequities in the labour market, including gender inequities and racism. The *Canadian Employment Equity Act* was introduced in 1995 and applies to industries under federal jurisdiction (listed in Box 12.1), as well as federal public sector employees. Under the Act, employers must identify and eliminate barriers to employment and institute positive practices to encourage equitable employment for four designated groups: women, Indigenous people, people with disabilities, and visible minorities (Treasury Board of Canada Secretariat, 2003). Under this Act, employers must assess how representative their workforce is (compared with the general Canadian population), review their policy and practices with an equity lens to eliminate barriers for certain groups, correct underrepresentation of these four groups, and do their best to accommodate differences and diversity. A key principle highlighted in the Act is the notion that "employment equity means more than treating persons in the same way but also requires special measures and the accommodation of differences" (Treasury Board of Canada Secretariat, 2003).

Another initiative taken by the federal government is the Federal Contractors Program, which applies to organizations that do business with the Canadian government. This program stipulates that eligible contractors maintain a representative workforce and include members of the four designated groups (Employment and Social Development Canada, 2018).

Other interventions that have been piloted are ones that address issues with hiring (e.g., résumé blinding—a practice that has mixed results), promotion and retention (e.g., mentorship programs), and fostering an inclusive work space (e.g., explicitly stating equity, inclusion, and diversity as key organizational values), among others.

These initiatives can be very influential in promoting health among groups experiencing health inequities because employment is one way in which people feel they are contributing meaningfully in society, people derive fulfillment through work, and work can provide social interaction and in some cases reduce sedentary time and boredom. Being respected and valued and in a positive workplace that supports health can also have immense mental and physical health benefits (in addition to simply providing work opportunities). As discussed earlier, sometimes exercise and diet initiatives work better when done in a group setting (e.g., in the workplace) or in an environment that fosters fun and healthy competition because there are others to support you in a behaviour change, and there is a group to whom you are accountable. Having positive social support networks at work can influence physical and psychological health status and health behaviours.

EXERCISE 12.6: Referring to the Case Study box about government interventions, brainstorm three other interventions that a workplace might implement to address inequities in hiring, retention, and promotion.

CRITICAL THINKING QUESTION 12.4: Reflect on your current (or future) role as a member of an interdisciplinary care team in the health sector. What might you be able to do as an individual to reduce stress in the workplace?

Secondary Prevention

The goal of secondary disease prevention is to monitor workers' health in order to prevent the development of disease. Secondary prevention in occupational health involves the use of preplacement and periodic examinations. The preplacement examination findings help in establishing an individual's baseline characteristics. Periodic examinations facilitate early, and often presymptomatic, diagnosis.

It must be emphasized that the periodic exams are not the regular check-ups performed by the family physician but are highly selective examinations that focus on the organ systems at risk because of specific hazards in the work environment. This includes directed history taking (with emphasis on specific symptoms), directed physical examinations, and appropriate tests, including biomonitoring specific to certain hazard exposures (e.g., measuring annual blood lead levels in workers exposed to lead). For example, a worker who has been exposed to lead will have a physical examination that places a greater focus on the function of the nervous system and blood pressure. In addition, ordering blood lead level tests and other tests to assess kidney function might be indicated.

Another aspect of secondary prevention in the workplace is the issue of employee screening for substance abuse. Mandatory pre-employment and random testing have been introduced in many industries in the United States. The Canadian Medical Association (CMA) is opposed to routine pre-employment drug testing and recommends that random drug testing among employees be restricted to safety-sensitive positions and be undertaken only when measures of performance and effective peer or supervisory observation are unavailable (CMA, 2001). This position mirrors the sentiment of Canadian Human Rights Commission's position on alcohol and drug testing because alcohol and substance use disorders are classified as disabilities. People with these specific types of disabilities cannot be discriminated against under human rights laws (and random screening for alcohol and drugs would be considered discrimination) unless one is dealing with a safety-sensitive job (Canadian Human Rights Commission, 2009), defined as a job in which impairment may result in a direct and significant risk of injury to the employee, the public, or the environment (Martin, 2010). An additional consideration when thinking through the implications of screening for substance use is that although many drugs can be detected in urine, the tests do not indicate when the substance was used because levels may persist for weeks. There is also individual variation between levels detected and extent of impairment of work performance.

The legalization of recreational cannabis in Canada has resurfaced this debate. Like some other substances, marijuana can remain present in the urine well past the time when a person may experience its effects, and there is no clear detectable level at which a person is considered "impaired." As such, employee drug testing for cannabis can be tricky. Additionally, it is unclear whether legalization of marijuana will result in an increase in use among workers who do jobs for which marijuana consumption could be dangerous, calling into question the utility of conducting drug screens. The issue of drug testing for safety-sensitive jobs generates much concern with regard to the topic of civil liberties and represents an interesting ethical dilemma.

If substance misuse is detected, whether it is by organized screening or by observation of impaired performance (such as may occur with alcoholism) an organizational response is warranted. This includes provision of counselling and cessation programs, and many employers also offer employee assistance programs for those with alcohol problems.

Tertiary Prevention

Tertiary prevention in occupational health refers to the treatment of injury or illness with the safe return of an employee to the workforce in the most timely and appropriate manner. A rapid return to the workplace reflects the employer's desire to reduce costs associated with a worker's absence and the employee's desire to be a functioning and productive member of society. The cornerstones of a successful early return-to-work philosophy include the prompt initiation of treatment and rehabilitation and the return to the workplace as soon as possible, using a modified program when appropriate. A modified program is work that has been selected to accommodate any limitations (i.e., what a worker is not able to do) and restrictions (i.e., what a clinician has prescribed to do or not do to reduce the risk of worsening the condition) that the worker may have while recovering. The CMA has published guidelines for the physician's role in helping the worker safely return to meaningful work after injury or illness. These focus on the physician's role in diagnosing and treating injury or illness, advising the worker, communicating, and working with the worker and the employer to facilitate the return to productive employment (CMA, 2013).

After a work-related injury or illness, the individual may be temporarily or permanently disabled. If these individuals are covered under their provincial workers' compensation act, financial awards might be available to cover medical expenses, rehabilitation services, and loss of earnings, as well as compensation for permanent loss of function and survivor's benefits.

Workers' Compensation Boards

The injury and disease related to work are compensable in all provinces and territories. The agency that deals with compensation in most provinces is the WCB. Workers' compensation mostly falls within the jurisdiction of provincial/territorial statutes, although the general principles are uniform across Canada. The main principles that workplace compensation systems across Canada follow are known as the **Meredith principles** and include:

1. **No-fault compensation:** No matter which party is at fault (i.e., employee or employer), benefits are paid out to the injured employee. Both the employee and the employer waive their right to sue, and thus no debate occurs regarding who is at fault.

2. **Security of benefits:** Funds must be established to make sure an employee can be paid when she or he sustains an injury at work.

3. **Collective liability:** All employers in a province or territory must contribute to the cost of the compensation system.

4. **Independent administration:** The administrator for a workplace compensation system must be separate from a government entity.

5. **Exclusive jurisdiction:** Only insurers that are designated as workplace compensation organizations can provide worker's compensation insurance (Workers' Safety and Compensation Commission of the Northwest Territories and Nunavut, n.d.).

Also contained under most workplace compensation laws are provisions that the employer notify the WCB within a specified time of an employee's becoming injured and is responsible for first aid to the worker and transport to hospital. The treating physician should submit a report to the WCB (in Quebec, reporting is mandatory), and physicians are typically reimbursed for their services through WCB, not through their provincial health insurance plan. In addition to treatment, the WCB offers rehabilitation consisting of physiotherapy, occupational therapy, counselling, social work, and chiropractic services for those injured, delivered either through a WCB clinic or through an independent clinic paid by the WCB.

CRITICAL THINKING QUESTIONS 12.5: Look up your current (or future) professional regulatory body's position and relevant process or recommendation when it comes to screening for substance use at work (e.g., college of nurses, college of pharmacists at the provincial/territorial level). Remember that screening can be through a questionnaire asking people to self-report or by random urine screens (it is not limited just to a biochemical test). Does the regulatory body you most associate with have a policy whereby they ask members to declare whether they have a substance use problem as they renew their membership, for example? Do you agree with the policies and processes in place? Why or why not?

COMMON OCCUPATIONAL EXPOSURES

The balance of this chapter provides a brief overview of certain occupational exposures and diseases relevant to public health that have not been discussed in previous chapters. Many occupational health issues overlap with environmental health issues, and thus, only those that have not been covered in Chapter 11 are discussed here.

Similar to an environmental health history, the occupational health history must be a routine component of any health history. When occupational disease is suspected, the history should be suitably detailed, as disease can manifest many years after the exposure. Generally speaking, there are two main parts: a work history, which includes exposure and controls, and a health history, which reviews the symptoms to determine any relationship to work. While this history is being elicited, other significant environmental exposures (e.g., hobbies or travel history) should also be ascertained. Although occupational diseases have their origin in the working environment, it should be noted that similar diseases can also be caused by nonoccupational exposures, the distinction being the location of the exposure. (Refer to the Clinical Example box and exercise that follows it to apply these learnings.)

 CLINICAL EXAMPLE

Mr. Gonzales

Mr. Gonzales is a 53-year-old man who works in a mine. For the past several years, he has been coughing, producing sputum, and experiencing sharp chest pains on and off. He has also lost around 6.8 kg (15 lb) over the past 1.5 years, although he does not exercise or eat what he considers to be a "healthy diet."

Exercise

As a nurse working in an occupational health clinic, you are eliciting an initial history from this client. What questions might you ask to gather more information to assess if this worker has an occupational disease?

The agents (hazards) that cause occupational disease may be divided into five broad groups: chemical, physical, biological, mechanical and ergonomic, and psychosocial. Table 12.2 provides some examples of different categories of occupational health hazards, several of which are discussed towards the end of this chapter. At the time of diagnosis, certain conditions must be fulfilled before attributing causality to the workplace (criteria for causality are described further in Chapter 2). These conditions, when applicable, include presence of a work hazard known to be associated with the condition in question, sufficient duration of exposure to the hazard, appropriate dose (based on concentration of the hazard, duration of

TABLE 12.2   Categories and Examples of Occupational Hazards

Category	Example of Hazards
Chemical agents	Organic dust
	Mineral dust
	Asbestos
	Lead
	Mercury
	Nickel
	Cadmium
	Volatile organic solvents
	Methyl alcohol
	Carbon monoxide
	Second-hand tobacco smoke
Biological agents	Hepatitis B
	Hepatitis C
	HIV
	Anthrax
	Brucellosis
Physical	Noise
	Heat
	Cold
	Changes in air pressure
	Ionizing radiation
	Nonionizing radiation
Mechanical or ergonomic	Repetitive movements
	Vibration
	Undue force
	Awkward posturing
Psychosocial	Workplace bullying
	Workplace harassment
	Lack of organizational support
	Stress
	Isolation
	Frequent travel
	Precarious work

exposure, absorption by the body), appropriate temporal sequence, and consistency of ill-health effects with the putative exposure. The list of occupational diseases may be endless. However, this chapter focuses on those deemed significant because of their frequency of occurrence in Canada or the severity of the disability produced.

Chemical Agents and Resulting Health Conditions

Crystalline Silica Dust

Crystalline silica is a ubiquitous mineral that is commonly found in sand, soil, glass, and granite. When inhaled by workers who work in industries such as coal and metal mining; stone crushing; quarrying; construction; and manufacturing of building materials, glass, and clay and those involved in ceramic and pottery and brick industries, it can be harmful to human health. In particular, exposure to silica dust is linked to lung disease, TB, autoimmune disease, and possibly, cardiovascular disease (Poinen-Rughooputh et al., 2016). Perhaps the most commonly cited condition linked to inhaling silica dust is known as silicosis. **Silicosis** is a progressive lung disease that is, generally speaking, irreversible. It causes lung scarring (known as fibrosis), which can eventually lead to respiratory failure and death (Agency for Toxic Substances and Disease Registry, 2017). Crystalline silica dust is also a group 1 carcinogen according to the International Agency for Research on Cancer, meaning there is sufficient evidence from human studies of a causal association between the exposure to crystalline silica and cancer. In particular, crystalline silica is thought to increase the risk of lung cancer (Agency for Toxic Substances and Disease Registry, 2017), although this has been controversial in the research literature.

According to CAREX (CARcinogen EXposure) Canada, an organization dedicated to the surveillance of workplace and community carcinogens, nearly 380 000 Canadian workers are exposed to crystalline silica in the workplace. Most often, these are workers involved in construction, plastering, drywalling, and operating heavy equipment (CAREX, 2018a).

Asbestos

Asbestos has been the subject of much media attention for decades in Canada. Asbestos refers to a group of fibrous, naturally occurring minerals, including chrysotile, amosite, crocidolite, actinolite, tremolite, and anthophyllite (CAREX, 2018b). Before 1990, asbestos was used very widely for insulating and fire-proofing buildings, including homes, because it is fire resistant and does not break down easily in the environment (Health Canada, 2018). Today it is still used in some materials, including tiles, brake pads, and clutches (Health Canada, 2018.

Historically, Canada was one of the principal asbestos-producing countries in the world, producing about 6% of all global asbestos between 2008 and 2010 (CAREX, 2018b). However, in 2012, the two remaining asbestos mines closed in Quebec (as a result of a loss of funding and political support by the government of the day and significant advocacy by the public health sector), and in December 2016, the Canadian government announced it would ban asbestos by 2018 (Ruff, 2017). This move was welcomed by scientists and public health professionals who recognized the adverse health impacts of asbestos exposure.

In particular, exposure to asbestos, primarily through inhalation, is linked to three adverse health effects:

1. **Lung cancer:** Like silica dust, the International Agency for Research on Cancer has classified asbestos as a group 1 carcinogen.
2. **Mesothelioma:** a rare but aggressive type of cancer affecting the lining of the lung, heart, or abdomen
3. **Asbestosis:** a chronic lung disease that results in scarring of the lung and, eventually, difficulty breathing and respiratory failure.

CAREX Canada estimates that more than 150 000 Canadian workers are exposed to asbestos. Workers who are more at risk include carpenters, cabinetmakers, construction workers, electricians, plumbers, plaster and drywall installers, and auto mechanics. Generally speaking, people who work in building construction, automotive repair, and shipbuilding industries are more commonly exposed (CAREX, 2018b).

When it comes to mesothelioma specifically, in 2013, 595 people were diagnosed with this aggressive cancer, and 485 Canadians died from it (Canadian Cancer Society, n.d.). Rates of mesothelioma have risen over the years and tend to be more concentrated in Quebec, where most asbestos mines were located. Globally, Canada has one of the highest incidence rates of mesothelioma because of asbestos exposure in the workplace, highlighting the importance of the workplace on health.

Coal Dust

Coal miners are exposed to coal dust, which, if inhaled over long periods of time, causes a number of different chronic health issues, including chronic bronchitis, chronic obstructive pulmonary disease (COPD), silicosis, and **coal workers' pneumoconiosis** (CWP). CWP, also known as "black lung," was first described in 1831 and is characterized by chronic, irreversible inflammation and scarring in the lungs. Symptoms often include cough, shortness of breath, wheeze, and in the later stages, coughing up black-coloured phlegm (Zosky et al., 2016).

Coal dust comes in many different forms and is usually a complex mixture of carbon (the main constituent in coal dust) mixed with contaminants such as silica, iron, cadmium, and lead, for example.

Globally, in 2013, CWP was responsible for around 25 000 deaths (Zosky et al., 2016). Interestingly, there has been a shift away from coal mining both because of the environmental effects of coal burning (e.g., the contribution of coal burning to global warming) and because of the very real occupational health effects of coal mining on human health.

Occupational Skin Diseases that Result from Occupational Chemical Exposures

Skin disease also makes up a large proportion of occupational health issues. More specifically, **contact dermatitis** (chronic inflammation of the skin because of contact with either an irritating compound or an allergen that often causes pain, redness, itching, cracking, and sometimes infection) is commonly reported among workers, particularly those who work often with their hands, with chemicals or cleaners, or even in health care (because of frequent handwashing and hand sanitation requirements, as well as prolonged glove wearing). Interestingly, some studies have reported the prevalence of contact dermatitis to be nearly 30% in the health care sector among nurses, doctors, personal support workers, and others who frequently handwash and engage in patient care (Nichol et al., 2018).

> **EXERCISE 12.7:** If you are in charge of occupational health and safety in a health care setting, what steps might you take to reduce contact dermatitis as a result of frequent handwashing?

Physical Agents
Abnormalities of Air Pressure

Exposure to abnormally high atmospheric pressures occurs in diving operations and in occupations in which compressed air shafts and caissons are used, as in construction of tunnels, bridge piers, and building foundations. Workers are exposed to air pressures exceeding the hydrostatic pressure of water at the depths in which they work. Rapid gain in altitude can also cause adverse health effects as a result of the body's difficulty in adjusting to reduced oxygen availability at high altitudes. Acute mountain sickness may present as headache, fatigue, loss of appetite, nausea, vomiting, difficulty sleeping, or confusion at altitudes above 2500 m. In severe cases, it may progress to fluid accumulation in the brain and, eventually, death.

Decompression sickness. Most frequently encountered by divers, **decompression sickness**, also known as "the bends," occurs when a person moves too quickly from an area of high pressure (e.g., being underwater) to low pressure (e.g., being at the surface). Under higher pressure, nitrogen gets dissolved in tissues. During a rapid decompression, tissues cannot unload nitrogen rapidly enough and become supersaturated, and nitrogen comes out of solution and forms bubbles. This may cause severe body pains (the name "the bends" comes from the observation that people acquire a stooped posture from the pain), mottling of skin, shortness of breath, strokes, and other interruptions of blood flow (Badesh, 2018).

Barotrauma. **Barotrauma** refers to the actual physical damage that can occur when there is a significant pressure difference between certain closed compartments in the body and the environment. Most commonly, barotrauma occurs in the middle ear and the sinuses. It can occur during activities and work that involve diving, flying, or mountain climbing and usually happens if a person ascends or descends too quickly.

A sudden increase in pressure, for example, can cause the tympanic membrane (also known as the eardrum) to rupture. A sudden decrease in pressure, particularly if a person has blocked nasal sinuses, can cause sinus barotrauma, which can be extremely painful (Battisti & Murphy-Lavoie, 2018).

Biological Agents

These include bacteria, viruses, fungi, and parasites. Diseases caused by such agents may be regarded as occupational in origin when the nature of the work involves exposure to the organism. Thus, TB may be accepted as an occupational disease when it occurs in health care professionals whose daily work has caused them to be exposed to *Mycobacterium tuberculosis*. Most occupational diseases of infectious origin result from exposure to patients and other infected people in a health care setting. Other occupations at risk include those that expose people to animals or birds (e.g., abattoirs, veterinary occupations, and pet shops), laboratory workers, food handlers, travelling workers, and flight attendants.

Blood-Borne Occupational Diseases

Exposure to human blood is associated with a risk of blood-borne infection (e.g., HIV, hepatitis B and C). At-risk workers include health care workers, police, and other first responders. Some studies have reported that health care workers experience high rates of needlestick injuries (a common way to be exposed to blood-borne pathogens among health care providers). A German study, for example, found that nearly 30% of respondents had sustained a needlestick injury at least once in the past year (Brewer et al., 2017).

The occurrence of occupationally acquired blood-borne infection depends on the frequency and types of hazardous exposures, the risk associated with each type of discrete exposure, and the prevalence of infection in the patient population. The prevalence of potentially infectious individuals within the Canadian general population varies depending on the virus involved: hepatitis B (<0.5%; Public Health Agency of Canada [PHAC], 2016), hepatitis C (~1%; Challacombe, 2017), and HIV (~0.15%; Challacombe, 2018). Their prevalence in population subgroups, such as intravenous drug users, people who are incarcerated, and certain new Canadians, can be substantially higher. In general, the risk of acquiring hepatitis B from occupational exposure to blood is higher than the risk of acquiring hepatitis C, which is higher than the risk of acquiring HIV. The estimated transmission rate of HIV via a needlestick injury is around 0.3%, which is much lower than the transmission rate of hepatitis C (estimated as being around 1.8%–3%) or hepatitis B (estimated as being between 1% and 30%, depending on the infectivity of the index case; Brewer et al., 2017). See the Case Study box for an example of legislation in Ontario that helps ensure workers are made aware of the blood-borne infection status of the clients they engage with if an exposure occurs.

CASE STUDY

Ontario's Mandatory Blood Testing Act

In 2006, Ontario passed the *Mandatory Blood Testing Act (MBTA)*. Under the *MBTA*, members of certain occupational groups (in particular, police officers, firefighters, nurses, nursing students, doctors, medical students, paramedics, correctional institution workers) and some members of the public can make an application to the Medical Officer of Health in their area to analyze the blood of a person they have had an exposure to during the course of their duties. After the application is made, the Medical Officer of Health will request that the respondent (i.e., the person whose blood came into contact with a worker or member of the public) voluntarily provides a blood sample to be tested for HIV, hepatitis C, and hepatitis B. If the person declines, the application can be referred to the Consent and Capacity Board, which will make a decision regarding issuing a mandatory order for the person to have his or her blood analyzed and results shared with the applicant (or exposed worker; Ministry of Community Safety & Correctional Services, 2018; College of Physicians and Surgeons of Ontario, 2011).

CASE STUDY—Cont'd

Exercise

In your opinion, what are the ethical arguments for and against this type of a law? Do you feel that workers at high risk of exposure (e.g., health care professionals and first responders) should have the right to this type of protection? Can the same argument be made for recipients of their care? For example, should nurses or doctors who are HIV positive have to disclose this to a patient on whom they may be performing a significant procedure?

EXERCISE 12.8: What are some control strategies that may be used to prevent exposure to blood-borne pathogens among health care professionals?

Anthrax

Anthrax is an infectious disease caused by the bacterium *Bacillus anthracis*. The spores produced by these bacteria are very infective, and humans could be exposed through inhaling or ingesting the spores. When inhaled, the infection can be very serious and even life threatening. Animals can be infected with anthrax and, as a result, workers who work closely with animals or with contaminated animal products—such as farmers, veterinarians, or anyone who handles livestock—are at increased risk. Cases of anthrax have also developed in people who process animal hides or wool, for example, people who make drums out of animal hides (CDC, 2015). Luckily, in Canada, cases of human anthrax are quite rare, with the last reported case occurring in 1990 (CCOHS, 2016).

Mechanical and Ergonomic Agents
Tenosynovitis and Bursitis

Tenosynovitis (inflammation of the membrane surrounding a tendon) and bursitis (inflammation of tissues near joints) occur as a result of chronic repetitive movements, exertions, impacts, pressure, or the resumption of aggressive work after an extended break (e.g., winter layoff for bricklayers). The resulting inflammation often manifests as pain and swelling in the tendons, joints, or muscles

Hand-Arm Vibration Syndrome

The clinical effects resulting from prolonged use of handheld vibrating tools (e.g., drills, jackhammers) have been recognized for some years. In Canada, it is estimated that there are around 70 000 to 144 000 cases, most often among workers in the construction, mining, forestry, foundry work, automobile assembly, and metal-working industries.

Hand-arm vibration syndrome (HAVS) usually takes several years to develop, depending on the intensity of the exposure to vibrations. One of the most common symptoms of HAVS is something known as **Raynaud's phenomenon**, which affects the blood vessels of the fingers. In people who have Raynaud's phenomenon, exposure to the cold or stress causes the blood vessels to contract, resulting in discolouration, numbness, and pain, most often in the fingers and toes. Other symptoms that a person with HAVS might experience include numbness and tingling and reduced grip strength (Shen & House, 2017).

Carpal Tunnel Syndrome

Carpal tunnel syndrome (CTS) results from damage to the median nerve as it passes through the wrist from the arm, into the hand. CTS causes symptoms such as pain, numbness and tingling, and reduced grip strength. Workers who perform repetitive hand movements, maintain their wrists in prolonged awkward postures, are exposed to ongoing arm vibration, or sustain repetitive force to the wrist are most commonly affected. CTS is quite common in Canada. In one prospective study of working adults, the annual incidence of CTS was found to be 103 per 100 000 people. Workers in trades involving repetitive wrist movements, such a seafood packers and carpenters, are at increased risk (Squissato & Brown, 2014).

Occupational Back Pain

Back pain is said to be the leading cause of absenteeism and lost workplace productivity. More specifically, work-related back pain accounts for just over one third of all disability-adjusted life years lost because of occupational health issues globally (Fan & Straube, 2016). Ergonomic factors most often underlie occupational low back pain.

Low back pain disorders are associated with work-related lifting, forceful movements, and whole-body vibration, as well as working in awkward positions. Psychosocial factors, such as job satisfaction, personality traits, perception of intensified workload, and job control are also associated with low back pain (Yilmaz & Dedeli, 2014; Urquhart et al., 2013; Esquirol et al., 2017).

CRITICAL THINKING QUESTION 12.6: Refer to Table 12.2. Using the table format shown below, categorize the hazards mentioned in the Table 12.2 that are relevant to the health care setting.

High Probability of Occurring; High Impact if it Occurs	High Probability of Occurring; Low Impact if it Occurs
Low Probability of Occurring; High Impact if it Occurs	Low Probability of Occurring; Low Impact if it Occurs

Based on the results of this categorization, which hazards might you prioritize when it comes to taking action to reduce the risk? Other than probability of occurrence and likely impact, what other factors would you consider if you were trying to choose one hazard to address in your institution over the next year? Are there health promotion strategies that can be implemented at the workplace to create a supportive, health-enhancing environment when it comes to tackling this hazard?

■ SUMMARY

Occupational health may be defined as the maintenance and promotion of health in the working environment. Most Canadians today are employed in service industries. Although the national unemployment rate ranges between 5% and 6%, inequities, including safe and secure employment, continue to exist, particularly among certain groups, such as women, Indigenous peoples, people with disabilities, and racialized groups.

Overall, workplace-related injuries and fatalities have declined over the years, with certain types of injuries (namely, falls, transport-related events, exposure to harmful substances and environments, and contacts with objects and equipment) making up the bulk of disability claims. Trauma, MSK problems, and skin conditions are also responsible for a significant proportion of occupational diseases.

The specifics of corporate responsibility to workers' safety are determined to a large part by provincial/territorial legislation, more specifically, occupational health and safety acts that outline the rights and duties of both employees and employers. Primary prevention in occupational health first involves substitution of the hazardous material with something safer, and if this is not possible, then segregation is attempted, including ventilation. Personal hygiene and protective equipment are used if the other measures outlined in this chapter are not feasible. Secondary prevention in occupational health involves the use of preplacement and periodic examinations that are usually directed to a specific exposure or workplace substance (e.g., blood lead levels for lead exposure). Tertiary prevention involves treatment, rehabilitation, and retraining under the auspices of workers' compensation. The injury and disease related to work are compensable in all provinces and territories by workers, compensation boards.

Because of the shift in the type of work that Canadians are engaging in, chronic diseases including mental health problems remain a challenge with respect to lost productivity. As such, workplace wellness initiatives, which address risk factors for poor mental and physical health, are becoming more popular.

Lastly, healthy public policy options to improve employment conditions and employment inequities are of critical importance. Examples include parental leave policies and laws to ensure equitable employment for certain groups. The agents causing occupational disease may be divided into five broad groups: chemical, physical, biological, mechanical or ergonomic, and psychosocial. Examples of exposures and some resulting conditions of note include dust, asbestos, coal, abnormalities in air pressure, HAVS, low-back pain, tenosynovitis and bursitis, chronic dermatitis, blood-borne pathogens (including hepatitis B and C and HIV), anthrax, and stress (or job strain).

KEY WEBSITES

Association of Workers' Compensation Boards of Canada (AWCBC): http://awcbc.org

The AWCBC is a nonprofit organization that facilitate information exchange between workers' boards and commissions. The site offers information for contacting provincial or territorial boards and commissions, as well as summaries of prevention campaigns, workers' benefits, and statistics on time claims (see http://awcbc.org/?page_id=14).

Canadian Centre for Occupational Health and Safety (CCOHS): https://www.ccohs.ca

The CCOHS is a resource from the Government of Canada. It offers information about occupational standards and legislation as well as workers' wellness and occupational hazards.

Canadian Occupational Health Nurses Association (COHNA): https://cohna-aciist.ca

COHNA aims to promote occupational health practices in nursing. The organization and its members work to develop standards and guidelines, foster regional relationships, influence legislation and regulations, and promote the role of occupational health nurses. The COHNA site provides additional information on membership, regional networks, awards and bursaries.

CAREX (CARcinogen EXposure) Canada: https://www.carexcanada.ca/en/about

As a multi-institutional research project, CAREX is a Canadian evidence-based carcinogen surveillance program. It is based on a Finnish model for estimating the burden of occupational cancer in Europe and has been hosted at Simon Fraser University in British Columbia since 2013. Visit the site for CAREX tools, news, and publications.

Occupational Medicine Specialists of Canada (OMSOC): http://www.omsoc.org

OMSOC is composed of occupational specialists and physicians devoted to promoting health policy and encouraging discussion in occupational medicine. OMSOC members also interact with employers, labour groups, and other allied health professionals to advance practice of occupational medicine. The weblink provides access to OMSOC resources.

Ontario Occupational Health Nurse Association (OOHNA): http://oohna.on.ca

OOHNA represents a broad network of Ontario occupational health nurses, providing its members with educational programs and peer networks. Visit the link to learn more about occupational health nursing, OOHNA membership, education, and events.

REFERENCES

Agency for Toxic Substances and Disease Registry. (2017). *Toxicological profile for silica.* [Draft for Public Comment]. U.S. Department of Health and Human Services. Retrieved from https://www.atsdr.cdc.gov/toxprofiles/tp211.pdf.

Association of Workers' Compensation Boards of Canada. (2016). *2016 Lost time claims in Canada.* Retrieved from http://awcbc.org/?page_id=14.

Badesh, M. (2018). Decompression sickness. Retrieved from https://www.cancercarewny.com/content.aspx?chunkid=11914.

Battisti, A. S., & Murphy-Lavoie, H. M. (2018). Trauma, barotrauma. *StatPearls* [Internet]. Retrieved from https://www.ncbi.nlm.nih.gov/books/NBK482348/.

Benach, J., Vives, A., Tarafa, G., et al. (2016). What should we know about precarious employment and health in 2025? Framing the agenda for the next decade of research. *International Journal of Epidemiology, 45*(1), 232–238. https://doi.org/10.1093/ije/dyv342.

Brewer, J. D., Elston, D. M., Vidimos, A. T., et al. (2017). Managing sharps injuries and other occupational exposures to HIV, HBV, and HCV in the dermatology office. *Journal of the American Academy of Dermatology, 77*(5), 946–951.e6. https://doi.org/10.1016/j.jaad.2017.06.040.

Brooks, M. (2018). Job stress may be a "substantial contributor" to mental illness. *Medscape.* May 18. Retrieved from https://www.medscape.com/viewarticle/896891?src=wnl_tp10n_180607_mscpedit&uac=231814MR&impID=1650872&faf=1.

Canadian Cancer Society. (n.d.). *Mesothelioma statistics.* Retrieved from http://www.cancer.ca/en/cancer-information/cancer-type/mesothelioma/statistics/?region=sk.

Canadian Centre for Occupational Health and Safety. (2019a). *What is the internal responsibility system?* Retrieved from https://www.ccohs.ca/oshanswers/legisl/irs.html.

Canadian Centre for Occupational Health and Safety. (2019b). *Precarious employment and vulnerable workers.* Retrieved from https://www.ccohs.ca/oshanswers/legisl/vulnerable.html.

Canadian Centre for Occupational Health & Safety. (2014). *Work-related musculoskeletal disorders (WMSDs).* Retrieved from https://www.ccohs.ca/oshanswers/diseases/rmirsi.html.

Canadian Centre for Occupational Health & Safety. (2016). *Anthrax.* Retrieved from https://www.ccohs.ca/oshanswers/diseases/anthrax.html.

Canadian Human Rights Commission. (2009). *Canadian human rights commission's policy on alcohol and drug testing.* Retrieved from https://www.healthunit.com/uploads/padt_pdda_eng_1.pdf.

Canadian Medical Association. (2001). *Drug testing in the workplace (Update 2001).* Retrieved from https://www.cma.ca/Assets/assets-library/document/en/advocacy/policy-research/CMA_Policy_Drug_testing_in_the_workplace_Update_2001_PD01-14-e.pdf.

Canadian Medical Association. (2013). *The treating physician's role in helping patients return to work after an illness or injury (update 2013)*. Retrieved from http://policybase.cma.ca/dbtw-wpd/Policypdf/PD13-05.pdf.

CAREX. (2018a). *Silica (crystalline)*. Retrieved from https://www.carexcanada.ca/en/silica_(crystalline)/.

CAREX. (2018b). *Asbestos*. Retrieved from https://www.carexcanada.ca/en/asbestos/.

Centers for Disease Control and Prevention. (2015). *Exposure to hides/drums*. Retrieved from https://www.cdc.gov/anthrax/specificgroups/animal-workers/hides-drums.html.

Centers for Disease Control and Prevention. (2018). *Hierarchy of controls: Overview*. Retrieved from https://www.cdc.gov/niosh/topics/hierarchy/default.html.

Challacombe, L. (2017). *The epidemiology of hepatitis C in Canada*. Retrieved from http://www.catie.ca/en/fact-sheets/epidemiology/epidemiology-hepatitis-c-canada.

Challacombe, L. (2018). *The epidemiology of HIV in Canada*. Retrieved from https://www.catie.ca/en/fact-sheets/epidemiology/epidemiology-hiv-canada.

College of Physicians and Surgeons of Ontario. (2011). *Physicians with blood borne pathogens mandatory questions for registration renewal: Frequently asked questions 2011*. Retrieved from http://www.cpso.on.ca/cpso/media/uploadedfiles/members/membership/bbp-faq(1).pdf.

Employment and Social Development Canada. (2018). *Federal contractors program*. Retrieved from https://www.canada.ca/en/employment-social-development/programs/employment-equity/federal-contractor-program.html.

Esquirol, Y., Niezborala, M., Visentin, M., et al. (2017). Contribution of occupational factors to the incidence and persistence of chronic low back pain among workers: Results from the longitudinal VISAT study. *Occupational and Environmental Medicine, 74*(4), 243–251. https://doi.org/10.1136/oemed-2015-103443.

Fan, X., & Straube, S. (2016). Reporting on work-related low back pain: Data sources, discrepancies and the art of discovering truths. *Pain Management, 6*(6), 553–559. https://doi.org/10.2217/pmt.16.8. Retrieved from https://www.futuremedicine.com/doi/pdf/10.2217/pmt.16.8.

Fleury, D. (2016). *Precarious employment in Canada: An overview of the situation. HillNotes: Research and Analysis From Canada's Library of Parliament*. Retrieved from https://hillnotes.ca/2016/01/27/precarious-employment-in-canada-an-overview-of-the-situation/.

Health Canada. (2018). *Health risks of asbestos*. Retrieved from https://www.canada.ca/en/health-canada/services/air-quality/indoor-air-contaminants/health-risks-asbestos.html.

Higgins, J. (2018). *Response to the Ocean Ranger Disaster. Heritage Newfoundland and Labrador*. Retrieved from https://www.heritage.nf.ca/articles/politics/ocean-ranger-disaster-response.php.

Jacobs, J. C., Yaquian, E., Burke, S. M., et al. (2017). The economic impact of workplace wellness programmes in Canada. *Occupational Medicine, 67*(6), 429–434. https://doi.org/10.1093/occmed/kqx075.

Johnson, S. T., Stolp, S., Seaton, C., et al. (2016). A men's workplace health intervention: Results of the POWERPLAY program pilot study. *Journal of Occupational and Environmental Medicine, 58*(8), 765–769.

Kelly, S. (2012). PR lessons from the Ocean Ranger tragedy. *Journal of Professional Communication, 2*(1), 13–18.

Martin, S. (2010). Determining fitness to work at safety sensitive jobs. *British Columbia Medical Journal, 52*(1), 48.

Ministry of Community Safety & Correctional Services. (2018). *Mandatory blood testing*. Retrieved from https://www.mcscs.jus.gov.on.ca/english/MandatoryBloodTesting.html.

Nichol, K., McKay, S. M., Ruco, A., et al. (2018). Testing the hand dermatitis screening tool in the home health care sector. *Home Health Care Management & Practice*. https://doi.org/10.1177/1084822318780012.

Niedhammer, I., Milner, A., LaMontagne, A. D., et al. (2018). Study of the validity of a job–exposure matrix for the job strain model factors: An update and a study of changes over time. *International Archives of Occupational and Environmental Health, 1–14*. https://doi.org/10.1007/s00420-018-1299-2.

Pearson, C. (2015). *Mental health of the Canadian Armed Forces*. Ottawa: Statistics Canada. Retrieved from https://www150.statcan.gc.ca/n1/pub/82-624-x/2014001/article/14121-eng.htm.

Poinen-Rughooputh, S., Rughooputh, M. S., Guo, Y., et al. (2016). Occupational exposure to silica dust and risk of lung cancer: An updated meta-analysis of epidemiological studies. *BioMed Central Public Health, 16*(1), 1137. https://doi.org/10.1186/s12889-016-3791-5.

Poverty and Employment Precarity in Southern Ontario. (2018). *Getting left behind*. Retrieved from https://pepso.ca/documents/pepso-glb-final-lores_2018-06-18_r4-for-website.pdf.

Public Health Agency of Canada. (2016). *Report on hepatitis B and C in Canada: 2013*. Retrieved from https://www.canada.ca/en/public-health/services/publications/diseases-conditions/report-hepatitis-b-c-canada-2013.html.

Ruff, K. (2017). How Canada changed from exporting asbestos to banning asbestos: The challenges that had to be overcome. *International Journal of Environmental Research and Public Health, 14*(10), 1135. https://doi.org/10.3390/ijerph14101135.

Ruhm, C. J. (2017). *A national paid parental leave policy for the United States. Driving growth through women's economic participation* (107). Retrieved from https://www.brookings.edu/wp-content/uploads/2017/10/es_121917_the-51percent_ebook.pdf#page=112.

Shen, S. C., & House, R. A. (2017). Hand-arm vibration syndrome: What family physicians should know. *Canadian Family Physician, 63*(3), 206–210. Retrieved from http://www.cfp.ca/content/63/3/206.

Squissato, V., & Brown, G. (2014). Carpal tunnel syndrome. *Canadian Medical Association Journal, 186*(11), 853. https://doi.org/10.1503/cmaj.131177.

Statistics Canada. (2017a). *Labour in Canada: Key results from the 2016 Census.* Retrieved from https://www150.statcan.gc.ca/n1/daily-quotidien/171129/dq171129b-eng.htm.

Statistics Canada. (2017b). *Women and paid work.* Retrieved from https://www150.statcan.gc.ca/n1/pub/89-503-x/2015001/article/14694-eng.htm.

Statistics Canada. (2018). *Table 14-10-0018-01 Labour force characteristics by sex and detailed age group, annual (x 1,000).* Retrieved from https://www150.statcan.gc.ca/t1/tbl1/en/tv.action?pid=1410001801.

Statistics Canada. (2019). *Labour force characteristics by province, monthly, seasonally adjusted.* Retrieved from https://www150.statcan.gc.ca/t1/tbl1/en/tv.action?pid=1410028703.

Treasury Board of Canada Secretariat. (2003). *Overview of the Employment Equity Act (1996) from a public service perspective.* Retrieved from http://www.tbs-sct.gc.ca/pubs_pol/hrpubs/tb_852/overpr-eng.asp.

Tucker, S., & Keefe, A. (2018). *2018 report on work fatality and injury rates in Canada.* Regina: University of Regina Business Faculty. Retrieved from https://www.uregina.ca/business/faculty-staff/faculty/file_download/2018-Report-on-Workplace-Fatalities-and-Injuries.pdf

Urquhart, D. M., Kelsall, H. L., Hoe, V. C., et al. (2013). Are psychosocial factors associated with low back pain and work absence for low back pain in an occupational cohort? *Clinical Journal of Pain, 29*(12), 1015–1020. https://doi.org/10.1097/AJP.0b013e31827ff0c0.

Veterans Affairs Canada. (2018). *Life After Service survey 2016.* Retrieved from https://www.veterans.gc.ca/eng/about-us/research-directorate/publications/reports/lass-2016.

Wilson, S., Guliani, H., & Boichev, G. (2016). On the economics of post-traumatic stress disorder among first responders in Canada. *Journal of Community Safety and Well-Being, 1*(2), 26–31. Retrieved from https://www.journalcswb.ca/index.php/cswb/article/view/6.

Workers' Safety and Compensation Commission of the Northwest Territories and Nunavut. (n.d.). *The Meredith Principles.* Retrieved from http://www.wscc.nt.ca/about-wscc/meredith-principles.

Yilmaz, E., & Dedeli, O. (2014). *Effect of physical and psychosocial factors on occupational low back pain.* Retrieved from http://www.hsj.gr/medicine/effect-of-physical-and-psychosocial-factors-on-occupational-low-back-pain.pdf.

Zosky, G. R., Hoy, R. F., Silverstone, E. J., et al. (2016). Coal workers' pneumoconiosis: An Australian perspective. *The Medical Journal of Australia, 204*(11), 414–418. https://doi.org/10.5694/mja16.00357.

The Health Care System

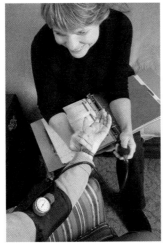

iofoto/Canstockphoto.com

Health systems are essential platforms for accessible quality health services and population health improvements. According to the World Health Organization (2010), a well-functioning health system responds in a balanced way to a population's needs and expectations in the following ways:
- Improving the health status of individuals, families, and communities
- Defending the population against what threatens its health
- Protecting people against the financial consequences of ill health and providing equitable access to people-centred care
- Making it possible for people to participate in decisions affecting their health and health system

A health system requires staff, funds, information, supplies, transport, communications, and overall guidance and direction to function. Thus, strengthening health systems means addressing key constraints in each of these areas.

The Canadian Institute for Health Information (CIHI)'s *Health System Performance Measurement Framework [HSPMF]* (see introductory chapter) contributes to the strengthening of health systems in different ways (CIHI, n.d.). In Part III of the text, CIHI's HSPMF will be applied with a focus on the governance and leadership, the health system inputs and characteristics, and health system outputs.

Part III provides an overview of the health system and the constant turmoil it faces because of jurisdictional disputes between federal and provincial governments. It begins with the evolution and history of health care in Canada and describes the federal, provincial, and local delivery structures for funding, resource allocation, and accountability. It also discusses health care professionals and their role in the system. For several years, Canada has been voted as among the top countries to live in, thanks in no small part to our health system. The traditional Canadian values of social justice and equity that are reflected in our political system have shaped the health system.

The Evolution of National Health Insurance

LEARNING OBJECTIVES

- Understand the history of the Canadian health care system.
- Describe four main models of health care systems.
- Describe the various Canadian government legislative acts that have informed our current health care system.

- Understand how the Canadian health care system is financed from the federal government to the provincial government.
- Outline the five criteria for federal health care funding.
- Understand how Canada's health care compares with that of other countries.

CHAPTER OUTLINE

KEY TERMS

accessibility
British North America (BNA) Act
Canada Health & Social Transfer (CHST) Act of 1996
Canada Health Act (CHA) of 1984
Canada Health Transfer (CHT)
Canada Social Transfer (CST)
Canada Assistance Plan (CAP)

Canadian health care system
comprehensiveness
equalization program
gross national product (GNP)
Hospital Insurance and Diagnostic Service Act of 1957
medicare
Medical Care Act
National Health Grants Act

portability
privately funded health care
public administration
publicly funded health care
social union
territorial formula financing
universality

INTRODUCTION

The terms *health care system* and *health system* are used interchangeably in this book. In 2000, the World Health Organization (WHO) defined a health system as "all the activities whose primary purpose is to promote, restore or maintain health" (WHO, 2009). It is important to keep in mind that although health care providers may have a tendency to equate the health system with service delivery, the health care system is far more than that. In addition to the delivery of services, it also includes population and public health activities, research, health promotion intended for the population at large, policy work to promote health, financing, technology, and many other components.

This chapter provides an overview of the organization of the delivery and financing of the Canadian health care system; offers a review of its historical evolution, and finally; and, for comparison purposes, describes the organization of the delivery and financing of health care systems in the United Kingdom and the United States. The historical review provides insights into the governance and leadership that were required to create our current health care system and how federal, provincial, and territorial governments have worked together to ensure the system has been responsive to the health needs of Canadians. These insights align with CIHI's Health System Performance Measurement Framework (HSPMF) regarding governance and leadership capacities in the system. Ensuring that strategic policy frameworks exist and are combined with effective oversight plays a role in the governance of Canada's health care system. Additionally, supporting the provision of appropriate regulations and incentives and paying attention to system design and accountability are examples of leadership roles in Canada's health care system.

The choice that each country makes with respect to health policy reflects the extent to which it is a just and caring society (Simpson & McDonald, 2017). For example, in countries where individual choices are valued above the societal goods and government involvement is considered an infringement on personal rights, as in the United States, the health care system is to a large extent private. However, in countries where liberal socialism exists and where health care is viewed as an individual right and social good, the health care system is mainly financed and delivered by the public sector, such as in the United Kingdom. In Canada, where a large majority of people hold dear the values of social justice and equity but still believe to some degree in individualism, certain important or expensive components of the health care system are in the public sector, and others are in the private domain (Romanow, 2002).

Political leaders and health ministries of every country are faced with a series of decisions about how best to meet the health care needs of their populations. Conceptually, the organization of a health care system can be divided into two parts: (1) how health services are *delivered* to those in need (i.e., the institutions and organizations like hospitals and clinics that provide services) and (2) how payments for the provision of these services are *financed*.

The terms *public* and *private* often come up in discussions regarding the health care system. These terms are not precise, but in general, *public* refers to being under the guise of the state or government, and *private* refers to anything beyond government boundaries (e.g., individual citizens or families, and the private market). The term "public" can be used to describe either the financing or delivery of health care. "Public" health care is often confused with public health (although these two terms mean different things). Whereas public health care implies that there is some sort of government involvement in either the delivery or financing of health care, public health (defined in Chapter 1) is much broader and refers to all of society's efforts to keep people healthy.

Other terms you may see to describe various health care delivery models are *for profit* and *not for profit*. Just like the term *public*, *for profit* and *not for profit* can be used both to describe how institutions that *deliver* health care do their finances or accounting or how health insurers (i.e., those responsible for the *financing* of health care) do their business. Although the terms may make you think that for-profit agencies make a profit and not-for-profit agencies do not, this is not entirely accurate. The main difference between for-profit and not-for-profit organizations is that whereas for-profit organizations issue shares (i.e., they have shareholders that are considered owners in the corporation), not-for-profit organizations do not have shareholders, and their intent is not solely to make profit but also to improve things such as social welfare and recreation. They *can* make a profit; however, doing so is not the primary reason for their existence. Nonprofit organizations (also known as registered charities) are a specific type of not-for-profit organization that benefits the community. As a special class of not-for-profit agency, nonprofit organizations have special rules when it comes to paying taxes (Government of Canada, 2017).

Applying these terms to health care organizations, there are four main models for health care system organization, which are described below (Chung, 2017):

1. *The Beveridge model* was developed in the 1940s in the United Kingdom and forms the basis of the United Kingdom's National Health System (NHS). Under this model, the government is the primary payer for health care services, which means that people do not pay out of pocket for the services covered under the NHS. The government raises funds to be able to pay for these services by taxing the public. The health care providers that deliver services are typically government employees, and the government owns many hospitals and clinics, so delivery is "public" because it is provided by the government and is not for profit. The purpose behind this model is to ensure universal coverage so all people have access to funded health care services.

2. *The Bismarck model* was created near the end of the 19th century. This model of health care organization includes private delivery models (i.e., health care providers do not work for the government as they do in the Beveridge model). When it comes to financing, however, the Bismarck model does not necessarily have one single government funder; instead it has government-controlled, tightly regulated rules for health insurance that can be provided by one or more insurers that are usually not for profit. Most commonly, this model provides coverage to people in the workforce only because employers have to contribute to a "sickness fund" (i.e., a health insurance plan), as do the employees. However, under this model, not every citizen is covered (e.g., those who do not work are not covered). Examples of countries that have adopted variant(s) of this model include Germany, Belgium, Japan, and Switzerland.

3. The *national health insurance model* is the model that Canada has adopted. Under this model, the government is the sole payer (funder) of health care services, so people do not pay out of pocket for essential services such as hospital and physician services (essential services are described later in this chapter). However, providers (deliverers of health care services) are private. Examples of other countries that have adopted version(s) of this model include South Korea and Taiwan.

4. In the *out-of-pocket model*, the health care system payers are private individuals and families who pay for services out of pocket. Delivery systems and providers are also private and independent from government. The United States is an example of a country that has adopted this model.

EXERCISE 13.1: List one advantage and disadvantage of each of the four health care organization models discussed in this chapter.

Although these models provide a rough idea of the types of systems that exist, it is rare to find a system that fits purely into one model or another. Almost every country uses a mix of financing and delivery models, relying on various public–private combinations in various sectors of the health care system or for various groups of the nation's population (Deber, 2017). So although we have described the Canadian system as an example of the national health insurance model, provinces and territories only finance what they consider to be "essential," "medically necessary," or "medically required" physician and hospital services, as will be described further later in the chapter.

When it comes to financing the health care system, the government is the sole payer and offers insurance (financial coverage) to every Canadian to access many physician and hospital services in a not-for-profit manner. However, in many provinces and territories, some of the types of services that provinces and territories consider nonessential, or elective, (e.g., some elective dermatological procedures or vision care) actually fall under the Bismarck model (with an employer and employee providing the funds to access it) or out-of-pocket model for those without benefits and health insurance. Furthermore, although the national health insurance model describes a private delivery system, this holds true mostly for outpatient clinical settings (e.g., nurse practitioner- or physician-based practices), which are largely independent from government oversight when it comes to how they deliver care. However, most Canadian hospitals, although they are privately run and are usually not-for-profit institutions (with respect to their delivery of services), do receive financial support and oversight by government (e.g., the government may set a global hospital budget) and so are more like semiprivate delivery institutions because they are still held to government rules and regulations. Indeed, the combination of varying delivery and financing models makes each individual health system unique.

Additionally, because of the division of federal–provincial responsibilities at the time of Confederation, Canada does not have a single health system but rather 10 provincial and 3 territorial health systems with uniform federal guidelines. The current legal foundation of Canada's health system is based on three statutes: the *Constitution Act* of 1867, which deals primarily with the jurisdictional power between federal and provincial governments; the **Canada Health Act (CHA) of 1984**; and the *Federal-Provincial Fiscal Arrangements Act* of 1985. The CHA outlines the national terms and conditions, and the *Federal-Provincial Fiscal Arrangements Act* sets the conditions for fiscal transfers from the federal government to the provinces and territories. To understand these particular Canadian features and how they evolved from a free-enterprise system of medicine, one first must examine the historical development of health care in Canada and how collective Canadian values have shaped and continue to shape the health care system.

CRITICAL THINKING QUESTION 13.1: If everyone's basic needs were met in the public system but some people could get more timely treatment by paying for it privately, would this constitute a serious inequality? Would you be prepared to accept this inequality in order to allow those with means the freedom to spend their money as they wished?

Adapted from Government of Canada. [2004] *Canada Health Action: Building on the Legacy—Volume II, Synthesis Reports and Issues Papers (Scenario 2)*. Retrieved from https://www.canada.ca/en/health-canada/services/health-care-system/reports-publications/health-care-renewal/canada-health-action-building-legacy-volume2.html#p1a13_1.

CRITICAL THINKING QUESTION 13.2: How might interprofessional practice and interdisciplinary team dynamics be affected if a health care institution (e.g., a clinic or hospital) was for profit versus not for profit? Might this have an impact on how team members behave? If so, how?

HEALTH CARE BEFORE 1950

Health and the *British North America Act*

In 1867, Canada's Confederation was proclaimed in the **British North America (BNA) Act** (now known as the *Constitution Act* of 1867), our most fundamental constitutional document. At that time, the government's role in the health care system was minimal. Most Canadians had to rely on their own resources for medical care, and hospital services were provided only by charitable trusts and religious organizations. Naturally, those who drafted the *BNA Act*, and even the Fathers of Confederation, could not predict the volume of industrial and technological growth or the health care needs for the coming years.

Although the constitution makes minimal mention of health, specifically, it does outline the differences between what the federal government is responsible for versus what the provincial and territorial governments are responsible for. In general, the federal government gets involved in matters of the federal economic role, including the regulation of trade, taxation, external affairs, defence, quarantine, immigration, criminal law, and the powers of reservation and disallowance. Provincial responsibility, on the other hand, includes social welfare, education, civil law, and agriculture. The *Constitutional Act*, and subsequent interpretations of it, gave the provinces jurisdiction over most health services (in keeping with its role for social welfare and such). The federal government was given jurisdiction only for the specific populations mentioned in the *Constitutional Act* These include Indigenous peoples with whom the federal government has signed treaties, the armed forces, the RCMP, immigrants or refugees at certain stages in the immigration process, those living in the territories, and a few other small groups. Table 13.1 outlines the historical evolution of the role of federal government involvement in personal health care in Canada.

Since the establishment of the first federal health department, the role of the federal government has expanded. This increased role is discussed in the next chapter.

1867 to 1948

The origin of publicly financed medical care and hospital care can be traced to Saskatchewan. In 1914, the rural municipality of Sarnia, Saskatchewan, experimented with a form of medical care insurance that offered physicians a retainer to practise in the area, because the population was sparsely distributed and physicians were unwilling to settle. This plan guaranteed the physician certain remuneration based on the number of health care services (e.g., number of client visits, assessments,

TABLE 13.1	**Historical Evolution of Federal Government Involvement in Personal Health Care**
1867 Confederation	*British North America Act* (now *Constitution Act,* 1867); no involvement
1935-45	Proposed national health care and security legislation; the idea of legislation rejected by provinces
1944	Veterans Affairs Health Care Programs which provides veterans and dependents with health and social programs
1947	Saskatchewan Hospital Services Plan introduced the first universal insurance plan for hospital services in North America
1948	National Health Grants; beginnings of infrastructure for national health insurance
1957	Equalization Program, which addresses horizontal imbalances between provinces and territories
1957	*Hospital Insurance and Diagnostic Services Act;* universal hospitalization for acute care
1961	Saskatchewan extended public health insurance to cover physicians services outside hospital
1966	Canada Assistance Plan (CAP) introduced by the federal government, a cost-sharing plan for comprehensive welfare programs; the plan also covered certain health services
1966	*Medical Care Act;* universal coverage for physicians' services
1977	*Established Programs Financing Act* and Extended Health Care Services; revised financial arrangements and coverage for additional services
1979	Medical Services Branch
1984	*Canada Health Act;* consolidation of previous two acts with some revisions
1985-86	Territorial Formula Financing introduced to replace a system of annual grants negotiated by federal and territorial governments
1996	*Canada Health and Social Transfer Act;* consolidation of finances under previous arrangement of *Established Programs Financing Act,* Canada Assistance Plan, and postsecondary education
1997	Report of National Forum on Health
1997	Health Transition Fund
1999	Social Union Framework Agreement signed by the Prime Minister and all premiers and territorial leaders except Quebec
1999	Announcement in the Federal Budget of a new five-year funding arrangement for Canada Health and Social Transfer
1999	1999 Federal Budget announced key steps to strengthen health care in Canada, improve the health of Canadians and enhance health research
2000	Primary Health Care Transition Fund
2002	Reports by Kirby Commission and Romanow Commission
2003	Health Care Renewal Accord; federal government commits new funding for health care renewal and reform
2004	CHST is split into the Canadian Health Transfer and the Canadian Social Transfer First Ministers' Accord on Health Care Renewal (2004–2014)
2016	Negotiations for a new Health Accord began; all provinces signed the Accord individually by 2018

vaccines) performed. This is known as fee-for-service payment. The physicians would be paid on this basis by government funds. The experiment was so successful that 2 years later, the provincial government passed the *Rural Municipality Act,* which permitted any rural municipality in Saskatchewan to levy property taxes to retain doctors who provided primary medical care and public health services in that area. This legislation encouraged doctors to settle in the province. Eventually, the same type of system was used to finance hospitals.

The first attempt to develop a national health insurance program was in 1935, when the conservative federal government of Prime Minister R.B. Bennett proposed the *Employment and Social Insurance Act* to collect taxes to provide certain social security benefits, including health benefits. However, the provinces challenged the Act because it encroached on their jurisdiction (because according to the interpretation of the constitution, health was considered to be primarily a provincial or territorial responsibility, not federal). The provincial governments were so concerned with Bennett's proposals that they took the matter to the British Privy Council for a constitutional determination. The program was ruled *ultra vires* in 1937, meaning it was outside of the federal government's area of responsibility. This was the first formal determination that health was a provincial responsibility. The federal government's attempts to introduce a national insurance program (to deal with the rising costs of health care and new technologies) failed because the issue became entangled with jurisdictional dispute between the federal and provincial governments.

Meanwhile, under the leadership of Tommy Douglas (Box 13.1), Saskatchewan decided to proceed on its own. In 1947, it became the first province to introduce a hospitalization plan for all residents, financed by a combination of premiums and general taxes. This meant the provincial government would to pay for the delivery of hospital services so people wouldn't have to pay out of pocket for this. Other provinces followed. British Columbia introduced its universal hospital insurance program in 1949, and Alberta initiated a limited plan in 1950. Newfoundland and Labrador joined Confederation in 1949, and one of the conditions of joining was the maintenance of its Cottage Hospital Plan (discussed further in Chapter 16).

THE HEALTH CARE SYSTEM BETWEEN 1948 AND 1977

National Health Grants

Recognizing constitutionally that the federal government could not unilaterally move forward with a national health system, federal politicians and bureaucrats decided they could advance their agenda by means of providing cash incentives to the provinces. Because provinces had primary jurisdiction over health, the role of the federal government was restricted to assistance in paying the bills. However, the federal government could steer the health care system by imposing conditions whenever it shared the cost of programs, and this is what it did.

In 1948 the ***National Health Grants Act*** was enacted. This act marked the entry of the federal government into the health field. Under it, grants-in-aid were provided to the provinces for a variety of health services, such as hospital construction, laboratory services, and professional training for public health. The federal government viewed these grants as the fundamental prerequisites of a nationwide system of health insurance. Later, other grants were added, but except for professional training grants and public health research grants, they were all gradually abolished after the introduction of Canadian medicare and the contemporary provincial health insurance programs.

The Equalization Program

Initiated in 1957, the Equalization Program is renewed every 5 years by legislation. Its purpose is to address the horizontal imbalances among provinces and territories when it comes to money the federal government passes on to them. This program enables provincial and territorial governments to provide their residents with reasonably comparable levels of public services at reasonably comparable levels of taxation. The equalization payments are calculated according to a formula set out in federal legislation. Equalization payments are unconditional in that the receiving provinces are free to spend them on public services according to their own priorities. Unlike the other federal transfers, the Equalization Program is entrenched in the Canadian Constitution and is one of the few federal programs exempted from restraint measures over the past few years.

The *Hospital Insurance and Diagnostic Services Act* of 1957

There have been several federal acts related to health and hospitals passed since 1950; one of the first was the *Hospital Insurance and Diagnostic Services (HIDS) Act,* passed by Parliament in 1957 and enacted in 1958. HIDS provided for federal cost sharing of all services delivered in hospital except for those provided by physicians in provinces with a universal hospital insurance plan. Five provinces immediately agreed to the terms of the HIDS. By 1961, it was operating in all provinces and territories and covered 99% of the population of Canada. Although all residents of Canada were eligible for hospital insurance coverage, the federal law excluded services for those already eligible for similar benefits under other federal or provincial legislation, such as workers covered by workers' compensation legislation or veterans covered by the *Pensions Act*.

One basic principle influenced the development of hospital insurance legislation: the belief that existing traditions should be maintained as far as possible. Therefore, provincial autonomy in health care was not affected. The policy of provincial autonomy allowed each province to decide on its own administrative methods while ensuring a basic uniformity of coverage throughout the country.

Terms and Conditions

HIDS stipulated that the following must be insured services provided to inpatients for the provinces and territories to receive financial assistance from the federal government:

- Accommodation and meals
- Necessary nursing service
- Laboratory, radiology, and other diagnostic procedures
- Drugs, biological products, and related preparations
- Use of operating room, case room, and anaesthetic facilities, including necessary equipment and supplies

- Routine surgical supplies
- Use of radiotherapy facilities, where available
- Use of physiotherapy facilities, where available
- Such other services as specified in the agreement

At the option of each province, any of the above could also be provided as insured outpatient services. Provinces may include additional benefits in their plans without affecting the federal–provincial agreements. The Act also made hospital insurance portable for residents who temporarily left their home province, although coverage was subject to provincially regulated limits. HIDS was replaced by the CHA in 1984, which has similar provisions.

The *Medical Care Act* of 1966

Events Leading to the *Medical Care Act* of 1966

Hospital insurance paved the way for medical care insurance. Saskatchewan again was the first province to experiment with a compulsory, government-sponsored medical care insurance program. The program's principles were prepayment, universal coverage, and acceptability both to providers and receivers of services. The legislation received royal assent in November 1961, and despite a strike by physicians (see In the News box), the program was implemented on July 1, 1962. British Columbia, Alberta, and Ontario adopted their own medical insurance programs between 1963 and 1966.

🌐 IN THE NEWS

Saskatchewan Physician Strike

Many physicians in Saskatchewan were very unhappy with the *Medical Care Act* when it was first enacted in 1961. Some of the doctors thought that the Act would result in the government dictating how practitioners practised medicine and that the province was heading down a "slippery socialist slope" (CBC, 2001). As a result, the day the Act took effect, Saskatchewan physicians went on strike for a full 23 days and eventually returned to work after the Act was amended (to allow physicians to work outside the model and have more independence).

Although the public was initially supportive of the physicians (and even campaigned against the government in the name of keeping the doctors), public support eventually waned, and the length of the strike left many members of the public concerned about the lack of access to medical care. The province brought in physicians from the United Kingdom, United States, and some other Canadian provinces to help out in the meantime.

After the strike ended, it had lasting effects on clients' trust of their health care providers, and some resented the fact that the doctors had gone on strike. Interestingly however, by 1965, many physicians actually supported the program (Larmour, 2015).

Critical Thinking Question

As a health care provider of any type, research your rights in the province or territory where you are training or currently practice when it comes to striking. What are the ethical and societal implications for health care providers who decide to strike? What about the implications societally when providers are not allowed by law to strike?

In the scenario presented, do you think that the providers were justified in their decision to strike? Why or why not? What is a providers' responsibility when it comes to advocating for policies that make health care more affordable or accessible when it compromises your own practice philosophy?

In 1965, the federal government's Royal Commission on Health Services completed the most comprehensive assessment of health services undertaken to that date. It found that nearly 60% of Canadians had some form of insurance against the costs of medical care, but for approximately 30% of those insured, this coverage was inadequate. The commission recommended strong federal government leadership and financial support for medical care. However, it also recommended that the operating controls of the program be decentralized under the provincial governments. General standards and guidelines were suggested as part of the federal government's conditions, but the commission recommended that each province should be permitted wide latitude in its program. In the summer of 1965, a new federal proposal based on the recommendations of the Hall Commission was introduced (i.e., the future *Medical Care Act*). (Marchildon, 2014).

Enactment of the *Medical Care Act* of 1966

The *Medical Care Act* was implemented in 1968. By 1971, all provinces had set up programs that complied with the Act. Under the *Medical Care Act*, each province received a federal government contribution to health care. Following the intent of the equalization program, a larger proportion of payments were given to provinces with fewer resources. Hence, the federal contribution as a proportion of the total cost for medical care varied among provinces. In 1975 to 1976, the proportion ranged from 40.8% in British Columbia and 49.2% in Ontario to 67.7% in Prince Edward Island and 75.6% in Newfoundland. All physicians' services and some additional services provided by dentists and chiropractors were covered. To be eligible for federal contributions, the provincial Medicare plan was required to meet criteria very similar to those in HIDS, which were called the "Four Points": medical insurance must be comprehensive, universal, portable, and publicly administered. These terms are explained and discussed further next.

Terms and Conditions

Comprehensive Coverage. At a minimum, the plan was to provide coverage for all services rendered by medical practitioners, without dollar limit or exclusions, provided there was medical need, unless coverage was available under other legislation. The plan was to be administered so that no financial limitation prevented an insured person from receiving necessary medical care. Certain surgical-dental procedures by dental surgeons (when rendered in hospital) were included from the beginning, and other professional services were added as the provincial government considered fit. Each province could provide additional insured benefits but without federal cost sharing.

Universality. The plan was to be uniformly available to all eligible residents (no fewer than 95% of the population must be covered). Each province determined whether its residents should be insured on a voluntary or compulsory basis. Provinces were allowed to charge premiums to the enrollees in the program. No discrimination according to previous health, race, age, or nonmembership in a group was permitted, but partial or complete premium subsidization for low-income groups or older adults was allowed if all qualifying residents were treated equally. Similarly, utilization charges at the time of service were not precluded by the federal legislation if they did not impede, either by their amount or by the way they were applied, reasonable access to necessary medical care, particularly for low-income groups.

Portability. Under the *Medical Care Act*, benefits were portable when the insured person was temporarily absent from the province, whether travelling anywhere in the world or changing jobs, retiring, or moving from one province to another, provided the individual remained enrolled in the program and paid premiums in those provinces that charged premiums. When an insured resident moved to another province, the province of origin would provide medical care benefits during any waiting period imposed by the medical insurance plan of the destinations. No province could impose a waiting period longer than 3 months before a new resident was entitled to obtain coverage. Some provinces required that people obtain approval before having elective (i.e., nonemergency) care outside their province. In general, provinces limited the amount payable for medical services received out of province to the amount payable for similar services in the person's province.

Public Administration. The plan was nonprofit and administered by a public agency accountable to the provincial government for its financial transactions. The criteria gave each province substantial flexibility in determining the administrative arrangements for the operation of its medical care insurance plan and in choosing its financing plan (through premiums, sales tax, other provincial revenues, or a combination thereof). Federal contributions to the provinces under this program totalled $1.7 billion by the fiscal year 1975 to 1976. Like HIDS, this act was replaced by the CHA in 1984, which has similar provisions.

> **CRITICAL THINKING QUESTION 13.3:** Before 1948, what economic event occurred that had an influence on the development of the *HIDS Act* and eventually the CHA in 1984?

1977 TO 1984: NEW FINANCING OF HEALTH CARE PROGRAMS AND THE *CANADA HEALTH ACT*

By the middle of the 1970s, the shared-cost health programs had become a critical problem for both the federal and provincial governments. The chief point of contention between the two levels of government was increasing health care costs as the cost was transferred from the private sector to the public sector. In 1976, total health expenditures in Canada exceeded $13 billion. Because these programs were open-ended (i.e., the federal government paid the provinces about half of the cost for insured hospital and medical care costs), they impeded federal governmental program planning in other fields. The provincial governments were also dissatisfied because although the most expensive costs of health care were shared, other important and innovative aspects (e.g., the development of community-based services instead of general hospital care) were not shared. To alleviate this, a new agreement on financing arrangements was reached at the Conference of First Ministers in December 1976. The legislation was enacted on March 31, 1977, as the Federal-Provincial Fiscal Arrangements and *Established Programs Financing Act (EPF), 1977*, and included extended health care services.

Established Programs Financing Act of 1977
Description of Financing Arrangements
As of April 1, 1977, federal contributions to the provinces and territories for the established programs of hospital insurance, medical care, and postsecondary education changed. In the new model, about 70% of all the EPF transfers were designated for the health component, and the remaining 30% went to education. This breakdown was arbitrary because EPF was a "block" funding mechanism. In other words, unlike the shared-cost programs, EPF transfers were not determined

based on the province's expenditures on health care and education. Each province was free to allocate the EPF transfers according to its own priorities.

These financing arrangements initially provided each province with more money than it might have received with the previous cost-sharing formula, but the increase was tied to the **gross national product** (**GNP**) (a measure of the levels of production of all the citizens or corporations from a particular country working or producing in any country) and population growth. There was greater equality among the provinces in what they received from the federal government per capita, and they had greater flexibility in the use of their own funds and federal contributions.

The federal government had attached broad conditions to its cash payments to guarantee adequate standards of health care across the country. The conditions were the same as those used for hospital and medical care insurance since the beginning: comprehensiveness, universal coverage, portability of benefits, and nonprofit administration by a public agency.

Extended Health Care Services
Under the EPF, the federal government made a financial contribution for extended health care services. The Extended Health Care Services Program allowed the federal government to make block-funded contributions (one payment to cover all services) to the provinces to assist them in providing nursing homes (intermediate care), adult residential care, converted mental hospitals, health-related aspects of home care, and ambulatory health care. These types of care were all referred to as "extended" because they were outside of the physician and hospital essential types of services that were covered under the *HIDS Act* and the *Medical Care Act*.

This program had three purposes:
- To provide the provinces with financial assistance for providing less costly forms of health care in conjunction with the insured services of the *HIDS Act* and the *Medical Care Act*
- To encompass most of health and institutional health services within a similar block-funding financial arrangement
- To provide the provinces with greater flexibility

Because this program was viewed as complementary to basic hospital insurance (covered by the *HIDS Act*) and medical care insurance (covered under the *Medical Care Act*), the only condition of payment was that the provinces furnish the federal minister of health with information required by the federal government for its international obligations, national planning and standards, and information exchanges with the provinces.

In 1995 to 1996, the last year of the EPF, provinces and territories received a total of $22 billion in EPF entitlements (cash and tax), 71.2% of which was intended for health care and the rest for postsecondary education. This arrangement was replaced by the Canada Health and Social Transfer (CHST) in 1996, which has similar provisions.

Territorial Formula Financing. Territorial Formula Financing (TFF) was introduced in 1985 to 1986 to replace a system of annual grants negotiated by federal and territorial governments. The TFF enables the territories to provide a range of public services comparable to those offered by provincial governments. TFF is an unconditional cash transfer based on the difference between the expenditures needs and revenue means of the territorial governments, a formula designed to fill gaps.

In 2001 to 2002, the federal government transferred almost $1.5 billion to the three territorial governments: $510 million to the Northwest Territories, $611 million to Nunavut, and $346 million to the Yukon (Department of Finance Canada, 2016).

The *Canada Health Act*

The EPF no longer tied federal payments to particular forms of health services, which reduced the effect of imposed federal steering. During the late 1970s, health care costs increased faster than the GNP, leading the provinces to bear greater costs because of an increase in demand for health care and relatively lower contributions by the federal government. As a result, the provinces introduced measures of cost containment such as restraints on raising physicians' fees. An increasing number of physicians responded to this by extra-billing their patients, that is, billing patients above the fee schedules, which were negotiated with their provincial health insurance plans. These factors led to charges from the public and interest groups that medicare was being eroded (because people had to pay out of pocket, which could limit access to services for the poor, meaning that the criteria of universality wasn't being met). The federal government established another commission to review the Canadian health care system, led again by the Honourable E.M. Hall, who had reviewed the health care system in early 1960s.

In 1980, Mr. Justice Hall published the results of this health services review, which emphasized the issue of accessibility of services (Hall, 1980). He concluded that extra-billing threatened to violate the principle of uniform terms and conditions and would prevent access to services for some people. He therefore recommended that this practice be banned and that fair compensation for physicians' services to be determined through negotiation between physicians and governments, with binding arbitration if negotiations failed. Physicians unwilling to accept the plan as payment in full would be required to practise entirely outside the plan, as was already the case in Quebec. They would bill their patients directly, and patients would be responsible for the full cost of the service.

Separate from the commission's report, in 1981, the Parliamentary Task Force on Federal-Provincial Fiscal Arrangements, an all-party task force of members of Parliament, published a review of the EPF, titled *Fiscal Federalism in Canada* (Parliamentary Task Force, 1981). This report included a review of the problems in delivering health care and fulfilling various program conditions outlined in the original hospital and medical care insurance acts. As well, it addressed the question of whether health care in Canada was underfunded and recommended, as had Mr. Justice Hall, that a national health council be formed that would be independent of government and of health care providers. This council would act as a coordinating body for defining, planning, and implementing health policy for Canada. Such a council could monitor whether the conditions of the various health care programs were being met. The Health Council of Canada was eventually established for this purpose (discussed later in the chapter).

Enactment of the *Canada Health Act* of 1984

Following these two major reports, the federal government introduced proposals for a new CHA in May 1982, which was enacted on April 1, 1984, with support from all political parties.

Criteria, Provisions, and Conditions of the *Canada Health Act*

The CHA combined and updated the 1957 *HIDS Act* and the 1966 *Medical Care Act*. It reaffirmed national principles but added specific restrictions to discourage any form of direct patient charges and to provide citizens of all provinces and territories access to health care, regardless of their ability to pay.

The CHA sets out nine requirements that provincial and territorial governments must meet through their public health care insurance plan to qualify for federal funding under the 1977 EPF. These nine requirements consist of five criteria, two provisions, and two conditions. The five criteria are as follows:

- **Public administration:** The program must be administered on a not-for-profit basis by a public authority accountable to the provincial government.
- **Comprehensiveness:** The program must cover all medically necessary hospital and medical services and surgical-dental services rendered in hospitals.
- **Universality:** 100% of the eligible residents must have access to public health care insurance and insured services on uniform terms and conditions.
- **Portability:** Provinces and territories must cover insured health services for their citizens while they are temporarily absent from their province of residence or Canada; the home province must pay for out-of-province services at the host province rates and must pay for out-of-country services at the home province rates.
- **Accessibility:** Reasonable access to insured health services must be neither obstructed, either directly or indirectly, by financial charges nor discriminated against on the basis of such factors as income, age, or health status.

EXERCISE 13.2: Violations of the *Canada Health Act*

Public administration and portability are essentially administrative and do not place substantive restrictions on the terms by which public health insurance is provided to citizens. The remaining three criteria—universality, comprehensiveness, and accessibility—embody the overarching policy goal of facilitating reasonable access to health services without financial or other barriers.

For the criteria of universality, comprehensiveness, and accessibility, provide examples of practice that may violate the *Canadian Health Act*.

The two provisions of the Act specifically discouraged financial contributions by patients, either through user charges or extra-billing for services covered under the provincial health care insurance plans. However, the Act makes a distinction between insured health services (i.e., those that have been deemed medically necessary) and extended health care services. Medically necessary services are defined only in the broad sense of the term in the Act. Section 2 states that *insured health services,* which must be fully insured by provincial health care insurance plans, comprise:

- Hospital services that are medically necessary for the purpose of maintaining health; preventing disease; or diagnosing or treating an injury, illness, or disability, including accommodation and meals, physician and nursing services, drugs, and all medical and surgical equipment and supplies
- Any medically required services rendered by medical practitioners
- Any medically required surgical-dental procedures that can only be properly carried out in a hospital

Essentially, the terms "medically required," "medically necessary," or "essential services" are left to interpretation and debate.

Section 2 of the Act also stipulates that *extended health care services* include intermediate care in nursing homes, adult residential care service, homecare service, and ambulatory health care services. Because these services are not subject to the two provisions relating to user charges and extra-billing, they can be charged at either partial or full private rates. In addition, provincial health care insurance plans may cover other health services, such as optometric services, dental care, assistive devices, and prescription drugs, which are not subject to the Act and for which provinces may demand payment from patients. The range of such additional health benefits that are provided under provincial government plans, the rate of coverage, and the categories of beneficiaries vary greatly from one province to another, and there is always controversy when considering and debating what is a medically necessary service and what isn't. See the Case Study box for an example of one type of service that is covered under some provincial and territorial plans but not others.

Furthermore, not all health disciplines and health care professional services are covered. Whereas physician services are specified under the CHA and in-hospital nursing services and so on are often covered, services by other disciplines, including opticians, chiropractors, physiotherapists, and naturopaths, among others, are not covered to a great extent in most provinces and territories. This impacts service-delivery models and the ability of practitioners to seamlessly work together.

Health Care Coverage for Sex-Reassignment Surgery Across Canada

Gender identity disorder, according to the *Diagnostic and Statistical Manual*, 5th edition (*DSM-5*, a diagnostic tool published by the American Psychiatric Association that is described further in Chapter 9) is the term ascribed to people who present with a "persistent and compulsive desire to become a member of the opposite sex," who many refer to as transgendered individuals. This disorder is recognized by health care practitioners, and although its listing in the *DSM-5* may help provide awareness to people, as well as greater understanding and less stigma, many people advocate that it should not be designated as a medical condition because this may imply pathology.

Transgender people often experience a range of inequities and challenges when it comes to interfacing with the health system, including discrimination from health care providers and other societal inequities (such as discrimination related to employment, for example, as described more in Chapter 6).

Some but not all transgender people find sex-reassignment surgery (SRS, which refers to a range of surgical procedures aimed at transforming one's body to match the physical attributes of the opposite sex) to be an effective and beneficial treatment. However, this range of treatment options is not fully covered as a medically necessary service under provincial health plans in all provinces and territories. Although some provinces and territories are silent on the matter, others cover only some types of SRS and not other types. Additionally, expertise with SRS only exists in some places, so many who need the treatment cannot easily access it, have to travel great distances, and often have to go through many processes (e.g., extensive psychological testing) to be able to access it when the surgery is covered, which further restricts access (Egale, 2019).

Critical Thinking Questions

For a treatment such as SRS, which has been shown to be beneficial in a group that is already experiencing high levels of health inequity, what are the implications of not considering it "medically necessary"? What are implications of making it a medically necessary procedure, and how can one go about prioritizing the list of what is considered medically necessary and what isn't? What criteria do you feel should be used to make these decisions about what is covered under the single-payer health insurance and what isn't? How might interprofessional collaboration and practice be impacted when some health care professional services are covered and others are not?

Penalties for defaults under the CHA are linked to federal transfers to the provinces. The financial penalties stipulated in the Act vary, depending on whether a default is directly related to extra-billing and user charges or involves failure to satisfy any of the five criteria. The federal Department of Finance has been responsible for making payments to the provinces and territories since the enactment of the CHST on April 1, 1996 (which replaced the EFP). However, the Minister of Health is responsible for determining the amounts of any deductions or withholdings pursuant under the CHA.

As indicated earlier, one of the conditions of the CHA was a partial withholding of funds from provinces that allowed extra-billing and user charges. Ontario, Alberta, Manitoba, Saskatchewan, and New Brunswick allowed extra-billing. With the introduction of the CHA, these provincial governments had to enact legislation to ban extra-billing or they would lose revenue from the federal government. This stipulation strained relations between the two levels of governments and also between provincial governments and their respective medical associations. For example, in 1986, when Ontario introduced legislation banning extra-billing, some physicians in that province went on strike. However, by 1987, all provinces had banned extra-billing. The Canadian health care system was moving toward an increased federal role, especially in the areas of formulation, monitoring, and enforcement of program conditions.

> **EXERCISE 13.3:** Which services are not covered by the CHA?

FROM THE *CANADA HEALTH ACT* TO THE SOCIAL UNION

The Canada Health and Social Transfer Act of 1996

Health and social transfer payments have developed over the years from cost-sharing programs to block-funding transfers. Fig. 13.1 shows the evolution of these transfers.

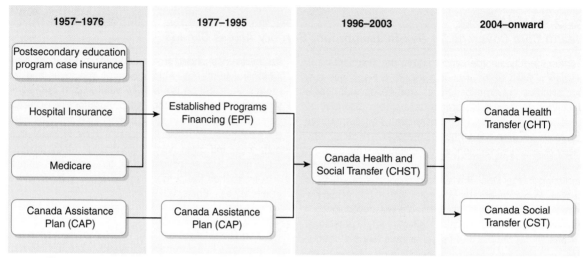

Fig 13.1 History of social and health funding in Canada. (From Government of Canada. [2014]. *History of health and social transfers.* Retrieved from https://www.fin.gc.ca/fedprov/his-eng.asp.)

As described earlier, the CHST (which replaced the EFP) was a block fund designed to give provinces enhanced flexibility in designing and administering efficient health care and social programs while upholding basic principles of medicare and safeguarding social programs. In 2004, the CHST was split into the **Canada Health Transfer (CHT)** and the **Canadian Social Transfer (CST)** with the aim of providing greater accountability and transparency for federal health funding.

Social Union: New Prescription for Canadian Health Care

The **social union** framework forms the basis of a new partnership between the federal government and the provinces and territories. On February 4, 1999, the Prime Minister and all premiers and territorial leaders, except Quebec, signed the agreement on the Social Union Framework Agreement (SUFA). The SUFA clearly laid out roles in health care, social services, postsecondary education, and social assistance.

The first ministers declared that Canadians will have publicly funded health services that provide quality health care and that promote the health and well-being of Canadians in a cost-effective and fair manner. To achieve this, they made the following commitments. Their governments will:

- Support the principles of universality, accessibility, comprehensiveness, portability, and public administration for insured hospital and medical services.

- Continue to renew health care services by working with other governments, communities, service providers, and Canadians.

- Promote those public services, programs, and policies that extend beyond care and treatment and that make a critical contribution to the health and wellness of Canadians.

- Further address key priorities for health care renewal and support innovations to meet the current and emerging needs of Canadians.

- Expand the sharing of information on best practices and thereby contribute to continuing improvements in the quality and efficiency of health care services.

- Report regularly to Canadians on health status, health outcomes, and the performance of publicly funded health services and the actions taken to improve these services.

- Work in collaboration with Indigenous people, their organizations, and their governments to improve their health and well-being.

The progress in the health care system in Canada has been incremental because of jurisdictional disputes and divided federal–provincial responsibility. For the past half century, Canadians have witnessed acrimonious stands taken by both levels of government on how to reform the health care system, and the changes have been slow. In the beginning of this century, the federal government and a number of provinces had appointed commissions and committees to review their health care systems and recommend blueprints for reform in health care; these are described in Chapter 18.

In late 2002, the Commission on the Future of Health Care (the Romanow Commission) and the Senate Committee Report on the Health of Canadians (the Kirby Commission) recommended the need for specific reforms in the Canadian health care system and an infusion of new funds (Romanow, 2002; Kirby & LeBreton, 2002). When the First Ministers met in February 2003, they agreed on an action plan to improve access to quality care for all Canadians. The First Ministers' Meetings led to a First Ministers' Accord on Health Care Renewal, which set out plans for change. One of the changes was the establishment of the Health Council of Canada, which reported regularly to Canadians on the quality of their health care. However, in 2014, the federal government ended the funding to the Health Council after more than 60 reports were drafted regarding Indigenous health, access and wait times, health promotion, health system performance, home and community care, pharmaceuticals management, and primary health care (see In the News box for more discussion regarding the dissolution of funding for the Heath Council).

🌐 IN THE NEWS

The Demise of the Health Council of Canada

A great uproar occurred when the federal government announced the end of the funding for the Health Council of Canada—the group that was charged with monitoring the 2004 health accord between the federal and provincial or territorial governments and collecting information to monitor how well the health care system was working for Canadians. Groups such as the Canadian Medical Association, Canadian Doctors for Medicare, and Council of Canadians criticized the Conservative government's decision to stop the funding, saying the federal government was removing itself from its responsibility as the guardians and champions of our publicly funded health care system, leaving it to the provinces and territories to do on their own, without much coordination. The Conservative government, on the other hand, defended their decision by citing that other bodies were taking on that work of the council and that money should instead be going to front line services instead of bodies like the health council (CBC News, 2013). Much political tension arose between the political left and right who often have differing opinions on how strongly provinces and territories should adhere to the principles of the CHA.

Discussion Question

Often decisions such as the one mentioned result from political beliefs, and different political parties have different stances on our health care system's future. In your province and territory, how supportive is your governing political party when it comes to championing and maintaining a single-payer national health insurance system? What can you do as a health care provider to influence the future of our health system?

One year after the First Ministers' meeting that focused on access to health care in 2003, a more detailed 10-Year Plan to Strengthen Health Care was established. The Government of Canada provided $41.3 billion from 2004 to 2014 for the following: to relieve immediate pressure on the health care system; for a new Health Reform Fund for primary care, home care, and catastrophic drug coverage; for the purchase of diagnostic and medical equipment and investment in information technology; and to increase funding to address the health of Indigenous people to reduce health inequity.

In 2016, Canada began renegotiating a new Health Accord (i.e., new agreement when it comes to the health sector between the federal government and the provincial or territorial government). However, the First Ministers' discussions were difficult and failed to produce a consensus agreement. Instead, separate agreements were secured with each province and territory except Quebec. The federal, provincial, and territorial governments (FPT) did agree, however, on endorsing a *Common Statement of Principles on Shared Health Priorities* (Collaboration, Innovation, and Accountability) to work together to ensure health care systems continue to respond to the needs of Canadians. The Government of Québec will continue to report to Quebecers on the use of all health funding and will continue to collaborate with other FPT governments by sharing information and best practices.

Guided by the Shared Health Priority principles, all governments recognize the following:

- Mental illness and addictions are serious issues for Canadians.
- There is a need to improve access to appropriate services and supports in home and community, including palliative and end-of-life care.
- Collection and public reporting of outcomes is key to enabling Canadians to assess progress on health system priorities.
- Working with Indigenous populations to improve their access to health services and health outcomes is a priority.
- FPT governments will continue to work on areas of mutual interest, specifically supporting health

innovation and improving the affordability, accessibility, and appropriate use of prescription drugs, including taking steps toward harmonization of drug plan formularies.

As negotiated in the bilateral deals, new money for home care and mental health was allocated in the 2017 federal government budget, totalling $11 billion. The $6 billion for home care over 10 years includes support for home and community care, palliative care, and informal care providers, as per the Liberal mandate. Unlike the CHT, funds for home care and mental health are to come with an accountability framework that includes a detailed plan outlining how the funds will be spent, performance indicators, and mechanisms for annual public reporting.

CRITICAL THINKING QUESTION 13.4: Some people claim that our health care system is vitally important to our national identity. Do you agree? What is it about our health care system that makes you most proud as a Canadian?

- Its high level of quality?
- Its efficiency?
- Its success in meeting the needs of the sick and vulnerable?
- Its equality?

EXERCISE 13.4: Where are we now? Review the Canadian Nurses Association document *Review of the 10-Year Plan to Strengthen Health Care* (2011) (https://www.cna-aiic.ca/-/media/cna/page-content/pdf-en/brief_10_year_plan_e.pdf?la=en&hash=D6B333AD9AA01C7ADD3F054A0C5E10449FCDC3D3). Seven priority areas for action are outlined in the document. Re-

view the priorities and assess where we are now with progress on each one. Compare and contrast the CNA document with the *Health Council of Canada Review of the 10-year Plan to Strengthen Health Care* (2011) (https://healthcouncilcanada.ca/files/3.6.10_HeatlhCouncilReview.pdf).

EXERCISE 13.5: Canada's Health Care Timeline Project

Working in a group or by yourself, after reading the chapter, create a digital timeline (using TimelineJS, Tiki-Toki, or Prezi) that includes major Canadian historical considerations. The aim of the online project is to explore the historical, political, and socioeconomic evolution of Canada's current health care system. The chapter will provide some details; however, you will also need to review a variety of sources (grey or research literature) to answer the following questions that will help you create your timeline.

- What was the economic climate?
- What was the political climate?
- Media of the time—how was information conveyed?
- What major events were happening (domestic, global)?

- What changes were taking place?
  - Health care reform
  - Research
  - Notable inventions or medical breakthroughs
- What key documents were shaping the health care system?
  - Government reports
  - Critical reports
  - Legislation
- What issues or controversies were being discussed?
  - Areas of social justice
- How does each of the above questions organize the way individuals are able to function within the health care system? For example, the outbreak of severe acute respiratory syndrome (SARS) had a number of

impacts on the function of various types of individuals. Training is now required in personal protective
equipment for all health care workers; annual mask-fit
testing has also become a requirement by employers
in health care settings. SARS changed the way health
care workers and visitors are able to enter and leave a
room or a health care facility when they are seeing a
patient or client, and it also changed the work of health
care workers requiring a systematic screening of respiratory symptoms.

Analyze how certain situations, events, government reports, and so on in your time period changed the function
of these groups of individuals:

- Health care professionals
- Patients
- Caregivers
- "The public"
- Indigenous peoples
- Vulnerable populations

You can divide your timeline into decades (10-year span
each) to explore these questions.

In Reflection

What knowledge have you gained by contextualizing the
past that helps you as current or future health leaders to
make change in the health care system?

Source: Adapted with permission from Dr. Nicola Waters course assignment for HLTH 5200 at Thompson Rivers University, British Columbia.

DESCRIPTION OF THE FINANCING AND DELIVERY OF HEALTH CARE IN SELECTED COUNTRIES

The first sections of this chapter traced the evolution of Canada's medicare system from Confederation in 1867 to the present. What started as a minimal state role in a privately financed and mostly privately delivered system has evolved into a largely publicly funded system referred to by many as Canada's public policy success story. The evolution of the Canadian health care system as it faces its many current challenges, however, is not yet over. Some of the main issues currently facing the system are described in subsequent chapters in this book.

The 1990s were a decade of restructuring of health care systems, both in North America and abroad. Triggered largely by fiscal considerations and concerns about increases in costs, virtually every government in the industrialized world sought to reform its health care system.

Reform measures were introduced to contain costs and enable health care resources to be used more efficiently. In general, these changes have meant reduced public coverage, decreased publicly funded services, and increased out-of-pocket payments (Box 13.2). The private sector is now more involved in health care. Increasingly, the public and private sectors are working conjointly to fund and deliver health care.

BOX 13.2 Out-of-Pocket Spending on Health Care in Canada

Since 2000, the split between what is publicly financed (through the federal, provincial or territorial, or municipal governments) and what is privately financed in Canada has been at a 70% (public), 30% split (private). Private financing can occur either by people participating in private insurance (e.g., through their employers to cover extended health benefits mostly) or through families or individuals paying out of pocket (literally with their own individual funds).

In 2017, it was estimated that nearly 15% of health services were paid for out of pocket and, in general, out-of-pocket expenditures for health have been increasing since the 1980s. For example, in 1988, the average out-of-pocket health expenditure was $278 per person, and in 2015, it was $902 per person (CIHI, 2017). Examples of what people may pay for out of their own pockets include services that are not fully covered by provincial or territorial plans (because they are not deemed to be medically necessary where they live, including extended health benefits such as long-term care), prescription drugs (because Canada does not have universal drug coverage), and medical devices (e.g., wheelchairs, walkers), among others. In fact, a recent report drew attention to the extent of out-of-pocket expenditures that Canadian seniors may face in the future. According to this 2014 Bank of Montreal Wealth Institute report, without private insurance, Canadian seniors may pay up to $5 000 a year on out-of-pocket health costs (Sharratt, 2015). For many seniors, particularly those who live on low incomes, this could present a barrier to accessing care and may therefore impact equity in health status.

continued

OECD, Organisation for Economic Co-operation and Development.

The United Kingdom (A Public–Public Model)

The United Kingdom has the same parliamentary system as Canada. However, unlike Canada, the United Kingdom is a unitary state comprising England, Scotland, Wales, and Northern Ireland. Each nation is responsible for managing its own health care system. The principles upon which the health care systems function are basically the same. The British NHS has existed since 1948 as a publicly financed and centralized system providing free universal access to health care. It was the first publicly funded and publicly owned health system to appear in Western Europe. With $4 192 per capita USD spent on health in 2016 (Organisation for Economic Co-operation and Development, 2017, p. 32; see Table 13.2), the United Kingdom consistently spends less on health care than most of its European or North American neighbours.

Financing

The NHS is a universal system of national health insurance financed mainly through central government general taxation. The NHS funds 80% of health care spending, which is a higher proportion than in Canada, where the public sector funds 70% (CIHI, 2016; NHS Confederation, 2016).

> **EXERCISE 13.6:** In Canada, the public sector funds 70% of health care spending. To recap earlier chapter discussion, how is the other 30% of health care spending financed in Canada?

The NHS is financed mainly through central government general taxation, together with an element of national insurance contributions made by employers and employees. It provides comprehensive coverage, not only for professional services but also for hospitalization and preventive services. Preventive services are comprehensive and include screening, immunization, and vaccination programs; inpatient and outpatient hospital care; physician services; inpatient and outpatient drugs; clinically necessary dental care; some eye care; mental health care, including some care for those with learning disabilities; palliative care; some long-term care; rehabilitation, including physiotherapy (e.g., after-stroke care); and home visits by community-based nurses. Eligibility for medical benefits is universal based only on citizenship, and care is provided free of charge at time of delivery. There are no user charges for physician services, specialist services, and hospital services. User charges do apply to prescription drugs and to dental and optical services. User charges account for only 3% of the total NHS financing. Unlike in Canada, the United Kingdom allows individuals to purchase private health insurance(usually for elective services), and providers can offer services in both the public and private systems. In 2015, an estimated 10.5% of the UK population had private voluntary health insurance (LaingBuisson, 2015), mostly offered through their employers.

> **EXERCISE 13.7:** How might having a parallel system, in which people can purchase private health insurance and providers can work in both the NHS and the "private system," affect the publicly funded, publicly financed model of health care?

Delivery

Until 1989, the United Kingdom's health care system was almost entirely public delivery, with the NHS owning and operating most health facilities. However, in the

TABLE 13.2 A Comparison of Health Care Spending, Mortality Rate, and Human Resources per Capita for Selected Countries in 2016–2017

Country	Health Care Expenditures (Total Spending per Capita USD PPP)	MORTALITY RATE FROM ALL CAUSES (STANDARD-IZED DEATH RATES PER 100 000 POPULATION)		Infant Mortality Rate (Deaths per 1 000 Live Births)	LIFE EXPECTANCY (IN YEARS)		Nurses per Capita (Number of Practicing Nurses per 1 000 Population)	Doctors per Capita (Number of Practicing Physicians per 1 000 Population)
		Male	Female		Male	Female		
Canada	4 753	755[a]	719[a]	4.8	79.6	83.8	9.9	2.7
United Kingdom	4 192	1,124[b]	836.8[b]	3.9	79.2	82.8	7.9	2.8
United States	9 892	616[c]	616[c]	6.8	76.3	81.2	11.3	2.6

[a]2016: from https://www150.statcan.gc.ca/t1/tbl1/en/tv.action?pid=1310039201&pickMembers%5B0%5D=2.1&pickMembers%5B1%5D=3.3.

[b]2017:   from   https://www.ons.gov.uk/peoplepopulationandcommunity/birthsdeathsandmarriages/deaths/bulletins/deathsregistrationsummarytables-/2017#age-standardised-mortality-rates-continued-to-decrease-in-2017.

[c]2016: from https://www.cdc.gov/nchs/data-visualization/mortality-leading-causes/index.htm.

All other nonannotated figures come from https://read.oecd-ilibrary.org/social-issues-migration-health/health-at-a-glance-2017_health_glance-2017-en#page32.

PPP, Purchasing power parity (allows one to estimate what the exchange rate between two currencies would have to be for the exchange to be at par with the purchasing power of the two countries' currencies).

early 1990s, reforms were put into place that maintained the public financing role, but providers of specialist services were to compete in a quasi or internal market for secondary health care.

In the past decade, the NHS has been undergoing a period of unprecedented structural change. The 2012 *Health and Social Care Act* (HSCA12) significantly altered the NHS architecture. It removed responsibility for the health of citizens from the Secretary of State for Health, which the post had carried since the inception of the NHS in 1948. The then Minister for Health, Andrew Lansley, said the Act had three key principles: patients were to be at the centre of the NHS; a change in the emphasis of measurement to clinical outcomes; and the empowering of health professionals, in particular general practitioners (GPs). Critics of the HSCA12 argued that the Act was ideologically motivated and intended to undermine professional dominance and to force private providers (to the exclusion of public providers) into the NHS model (Speed & Gabe, 2013).

In 2013, the Better Care Fund (BCF) was launched as a collaborative partnership between local government and the NHS. The partners work closely together to help local areas plan and implement integrated health and social care services across England. In theory, the BCF was meant to begin to align health and social care budgets by sharing money across the divide of Local Government and the NHS. However, in reality, with shrinking budgets, there was not enough money in either pot to achieve significant change to benefit communities. As a result, an extensive "privatization" of social care provision has occurred. In 2017, the National Audit Office produced a report suggesting that the money spent in 2015 to 2016 had not delivered value for money (National Audit Office, 2016).

Primary care is delivered mainly through GPs, who act as gatekeepers for secondary care, and most primary care providers are private delivers of health care. In 2015, there were 34 592 general practitioners (full-time equivalents) in 7 674 practices, with an average of 7 450 patients per practice and 1 530 patients per GP (Health and Social Care Information Centre, 2015). Specialists are mostly salaried government employees of the NHS and work in NHS-run hospitals. An estimated 548 private hospitals (meaning they are not government owned) and between 500 and 600 private specialist clinics in the United Kingdom offer a range of services, including treatments either unavailable in the NHS or

subject to long waiting times, such as bariatric surgery and fertility treatment, but generally do not have emergency, trauma, or intensive-care facilities (Competition and Markets Authority, 2014). Just like Canada, then, the United Kingdom's health system does not entirely fit into one of the four main types of health care models described in the chapter introduction but represents more of a mixed model in some areas.

The United States (A Private–Private Model)

The United States has a federalist system of government consisting of a national government and 50 state governments. Each level of government plays some role in the financing or delivery of health care services. As in Canada, the national government provides health services to specific groups of the population, including military personnel, veterans with service-related disabilities, Indigenous people, and inmates of federal prisons. The US government has the authority to raise taxes and appropriate funds for the purpose of the general welfare of the population, including health care. The Health Care Financing Administration in the Department of Health and Human Services is responsible for administering the health care insurance programs Medicare and Medicaid and the Children's Health Insurance Program (CHIP). The US government is also responsible for regulating the health care insurance provided by employers and managed care organizations participating in federally subsidized health care.

The responsibilities of state governments with respect to health care include the licensing of hospitals and health care personnel, the provision of public health services (sanitation, water quality, and so on), and the provision of mental health services. States can raise their own revenue by various types of taxes, and there is no federal limit on their taxing powers. State governments must conform to federal regulations in order to receive funds from the national government under Medicaid and CHIP. They are also responsible for regulating private health care insurance. Although the federal and state governments provide public coverage for health care, the US. health care system remains unique around the world because it strongly relies on the private sector to provide health care coverage as well as deliver health services.

In 2016, the Commonwealth Fund found that although the US health care system is the most expensive in the world, it ranks last on most dimensions of

TABLE 13.3 Major Provisions of the US *Affordable Care Act*

Provision	Explanation
Guaranteed issue	Prohibits insurers from denying coverage to individuals with pre-existing conditions
Continued coverage	Allows financially dependent children to remain on their parents' health insurance until age 26 years
Actuarial rating adjustments	Obliges insurers to offer the same premium price paid by other insurees of the same age and geographical location regardless of gender
Health insurance exchanges	Operate as the primary pathway for individuals and small businesses to compare and purchase insurance policies in an "open" market
Individual mandate	Requires all citizens not covered by an employer-sponsored or public insurance program to purchase an approved policy or pay a penalty
Employer mandate	Requires businesses with 50 or more employees to offer health insurance to their full-time employees or pay a penalty
Federal subsidies	Provide several types of aid to ensure implementation of other provisions; for example, low-income individuals receive subsidies to purchase insurance policies they could not afford otherwise, and states are entitled to billions of dollars in subsidies to expand Medicaid eligibility for their low-income citizens

performance when compared with Canada, France, and the United Kingdom. Although several publicly funded and delivered health care programs exist in the United States, 55% of health care is financed and delivered privately. The United States provides an interesting case study regarding how political systems (i.e., governing parties) play a major role in the financing and delivery of health care. The *Affordable Care Act (ACA)* was passed in 2010 during a period in which the Democratic Party controlled the presidency and both houses of Congress. Major provisions of the ACA can be found in Table 13.3. Before the time of the ACA, health insurance coverage was always voluntary. About 30% of the population was covered through the two major public programs, Medicare for seniors (later extended to the disabled) and Medicaid for low-income Americans (Kaiser Commission on Medicaid and the Uninsured, 2013). Most others received coverage through their employment, either as employees or dependents, but such coverage was always voluntary: employers did not have to provide it, and individuals were not required to buy it. Fewer than 10% purchased coverage on their own (Medicaid.gov, 2018). Those with pre-existing illnesses generally found individual insurance policies to be unaffordable because insurers could charge higher premiums to those with a history of illness. The ACA increased individual coverage by prohibiting insurance companies from excluding people or charging more for pre-existing conditions, mandating that all individuals obtain insurance, and

helping individuals pay for this through income-based premium subsidies (Obama, 2017). Also before the ACA, only about half of low-income adults were covered by Medicaid, and almost 30% of low-income individuals younger than 65 years of age lacked coverage (Medicaid.gov, 2018).

In 2017, when the Republican Party controlled the presidency and both houses of Congress, an unsuccessful attempt was made to repeal the ACA. However, the Republicans were able to make a major legislative dent by repealing the individual mandate. In 2018, the Medicaid expansion remains in place in 31 states; those eligible will continue to receive coverage, which typically has a broad benefit package and little or no premiums or patient cost sharing. However, because many physicians do not accept Medicaid patients, largely because of low fees, access is often not the same as for those with private insurance and Medicare.

Financing

There are multiple methods of financing health services in the United States, including both private funds and public funds. The majority of health care funding comes from private sources, including private health insurance and out-of-pocket payment. The private health insurance industry covers three quarters of the population (e.g., Blue Cross/Blue Shield, private insurance companies, corporate self-insurance, managed care plans). Insurance coverage is largely employment based and entirely voluntary. Small employers generally cannot afford to offer their employees insurance coverage, and even large companies do not cover most part-time and contractual workers.

Both the national and state governments provide public funds for health care. The three publicly funded government plans are Medicare, Medicaid, and CHIP. Medicare is a federally subsidized program for those older than age 65 years, some people with disabilities, and people with chronic renal diseases. Benefits that are not generally transferable outside Medicare fall into two parts: Part A, a hospital insurance program for the populations mentioned and generally requiring contributions by participants for a minimal period of their working lives, and Part B, an optional social security arrangement for medical care insurance that covers some of the costs of services provided by medical practitioners and certain other benefits.

Medicaid is a series of state programs with federal cost sharing. Eligibility for Medicaid benefits is based on income- and means-tested criteria and is determined by county welfare boards. Basic benefits cover inpatient and outpatient hospital services, laboratory and radiology, basic physician medical services, and skilled nursing facility coverage for people older than 21 years of age. Each state is responsible for the administration, establishment of eligibility standards, type and scope of services, and reimbursement for services. As a result, Medicaid programs vary from state to state.

The federal government initiated CHIP to expand health care coverage to otherwise uninsured children. This program allows for the coverage of children from working families with incomes too high to qualify for Medicaid and too low to afford private health insurance. A growing proportion of the population is uninsured. It is currently estimated that 10.4% of the population younger than 65 years of age in the United States have no health insurance (Centers for Disease Control and Prevention, 2017). In addition, a significant proportion of the US population are underinsured, meaning that they have some insurance coverage but there is no limit on out-of-pocket costs.

Delivery

In the United States, the dominant system of health services delivery is private and usually for profit. Government-owned (i.e., public) services are usually limited to providing care to special groups such as veterans, mentally ill individuals, and people with low socioeconomic status. Some jurisdictions (cities or counties) operate public hospitals and community health centres as a social safety net, although many such institutions are now under fiscal pressure and are being downsized or closed.

EXERCISE 13.8: Compare and Contrast Health Care Systems

Compare and contrast the health care system of France with Canada's health care system. Use Table 13.2 as a guide and then explain how the financing and delivery are different in both countries.

Although different models of health system organization and delivery exist across the globe, many health system policymakers are now exploring interventions to improve interprofessional collaboration—defined as the process by which different health and social care professional groups work together to positively impact care. Researchers in both the United States and the United Kingdom have been exploring what tools exist to bring various professionals together in collaborative relationships for the purposes of improving patient safety and quality of care (see the Interprofessional Collaboration box).

INTERPROFESSIONAL COLLABORATION

Tools for all Health Care Systems

An area of focus over the past 10 years for health system researchers has been that of interprofessional collaboration. Whether one is operating within an out-of-pocket system, a Beveridge model, or some other type of health system, interprofessional collaboration and the constant bringing together of various health care and social care providers in practice (often around individual client care) can be hugely beneficial, given the complexities of clients and the holistic needs that need to be addressed to restore people back to good health and well-being.

Some tools that have been evaluated across various health systems in the published literature when it comes

INTERPROFESSIONAL COLLABORATION—cont'd

Tools for all Health Care Systems

to fostering better interprofessional collaboration include the following:

- Interdisciplinary hospital rounds in which all members of the team get together to discuss various clients
- Interdisciplinary meetings in which all members of the team can discuss organizational and client-based issues
- Interprofessional checklists to guide who needs to be involved when and for what, for things such as surgeries and other complex interventions (Reeves et al., 2017)

Thus, although we must be aware of the larger laws and agreements shaping the health system in the province and country where we practice, equally important is gaining an understanding of how these laws, agreements, and delivery systems affect our ability to work together as a diverse team of practitioners. As we saw in Part II of this book, Canada's health needs are diverse, requiring skill sets from many different disciplines. We know that health is holistic in nature and encompasses well-being, social health, emotional health, spiritual health, and mental health; thus, the more we work in systems that foster collaboration, the better and more comprehensively we can serve our communities.

SUMMARY

Conceptually, the organization of health care systems can be divided into how health services are delivered to those in need and how payments for the provision of these services are financed. The terms *public* and *private* are not precise but are often used to describe health care systems, both in terms of their delivery and in terms of their financing. In general, whereas the terms *public sector* refers to government involvement, *private sector* is generally thought of as what lies beyond the boundaries of government. *Private* is generally thought of as what lies beyond the boundaries of government to include both the family and the market.

Four main models of health care system organization prevail: the Beveridge model, the Bismarck model, the national health insurance model, and the out-of-pocket model, but in reality, most countries have a health care system with elements of multiple models and a mix of private and public service and delivery.

The *Constitution Act* of 1867 gave the federal government a minimal role in the health care system. Section 91 defines the primacy of the federal economic role, including the regulation of trade, taxation, external affairs, defence, quarantine, immigration, criminal law, and the powers of reservation and disallowance. Section 92 defines the provincial role in social welfare, including health, education, civil law, and agriculture. However, the federal government has become involved in health care by sharing the cost of programs and thus steering the health care system. Since 1950, a number of federal acts have been passed, most significantly the *HIDS Act* of 1957 (which provided universal hospitalization) and the *Medical Care Act* of 1966 (which provided universal

coverage of necessary medical services). The federal government shared 50% of the cost of these programs with the participating provinces, provided the provinces and territories met four criteria: universality, portability, comprehensiveness, and public administration. All provinces and territories participated in these programs. In the 1970s, the shared cost of health programs became a critical problem for the federal and provincial governments alike and this led to the legislation of the EPF of 1977. In this act, the federal government agreed to pay the provinces by the transfer of income tax points and cash contribution linked to an increase in the GNP instead of the previous 50% cost sharing. The EPF no longer tied federal payments to a particular form of health services, thus reducing the extent to which the federal government could dictate how money could be spent.

During the early 1980s, critical reviews of national health insurance programs and financing arrangements led to the 1984 enactment of the CHA. This act amalgamated the HIDS Act and the Medical Care Act. It also established five criteria that provincial health programs must meet in order to be eligible for the full cash portion of the federal government contribution, namely, public administration, comprehensiveness, universality, portability, and accessibility. The Act also banned extra-billing, and by 1987, all the provinces had complied. It appeared that the Canadian health care system was moving towards an increased federal role, especially in the areas of formulation, monitoring, and enforcing of program conditions. However, as a result of budgetary deficits, the federal government was forced to reduce transfer payments for health care and postsecondary education to the provinces. In an attempt to stabilize the amount of federal health and social transfers to the provinces and maintain a role in health, the federal government passed the *Canada Health and Social Transfer Act* in 1996—a block grant to the provinces covering health care, higher education, and social programs. Since 1999, the federal government has increased its financial contribution to sustain and reform the health care system. In 2016, Canada began renegotiating a new Health Accord—the agreement under which health system transfer payments would occur from the federal to the provincial and territorial governments. Although widespread consensus could not be reached and each province and territory negotiated with the federal government separately, key principles were agreed to in order to best ensure that the health care system continues to meet the needs of Canadians. These principles included a commitment to enhancing Indigenous health, focusing on mental health, and enhancing care that can be accessed at home and in the community (versus a hospital or institutional setting).

Although it appears that Canada has a national **medicare** program, this is incorrect: health care is actually a provincial responsibility. The involvement of the federal government is through financial contributions, which enables the federal government to establish national standards. As a result, Canada has 10 provincial and 3 territorial health care systems that are structured on federal guidelines and provide mainly sickness care and, to a lesser extent, preventive practices carried out by physicians. However, the jurisdictional dispute between the provinces and the federal government in the health sector has become a source of increasing tension. The primary objective of the social union initiative is to reform and renew Canada's social services and to reassure Canadians that their pan-Canadian social programs are strong and secure.

Both the United Kingdom and the United States have very different health care systems than Canada—both in terms of how health services are financed and how they are delivered. Whereas Canada's health system most closely matches the National Health Insurance model, the UK health care system aligns most closely with the Beveridge model and, for the most part (with the exception of the Medicare, Medicaid, and CHIP program), the US system matches an out-of-pocket model. Although none of these systems exclusively match one model but represent a mix of a few elements, each one has its own set of strengths and weaknesses.

KEY WEBSITES

Canada Health Act (CHA) **Annual Reports:** https://www.canada.ca/en/health-canada/services/health-care-system/reports-publications/canada-health-act-annual-reports.html
This Government of Canada's landing page contains the *CHA* annual reports that provide an overview of how well each provincial and territorial health system is meeting the requirements of the *CHA*.

Canada's History—The Fight for Medicare: http://www.canadashistory.ca/explore/politics-law/the-fight-for-medicare
This site houses a video made by the National Film Board, which showcases the history of Medicare and the role that Tommy Douglas of Saskatchewan played in moving the agenda forward for a single-payer health care system.

Canadian Foundation for Healthcare Improvement: https://www.cfhi-fcass.ca

This not-for-profit, Health Canada–funded organization works to improve innovation in our heath care system. One of their areas of work is in health care system transformation, and they are currently working on developing programs to support both value-based health care and primary care reform.

The European Observatory on Health Systems and Policies: http://www.euro.who.int/en/about-us/partners/observatory/about-us
This observatory organization represents a partnership among institutions such as the World Bank, the London School of Hygiene and Tropical Medicine, and national governments and is hosted by the World Health Organization (Europe). The observatory's work includes analyzing health systems in Europe to help promote evidence-based health policy. The website houses many resources, including policies, briefs, studies, and reviews of various health care system analyses and policy trends.

REFERENCES

Centers for Disease Control and Prevention. (2017). *Health insurance coverage.* Atlanta: Author. Retrieved from https://www.cdc.gov/nchs/fastats/health-insurance.htm.

Canadian Institute for Health Information. (n.d). A performance measurement framework for the Canadian health system. Ottawa: Author. Retrieved from https://secure.cihi.ca/free_products/HSP-Framework-ENweb.pdf

Canadian Institute for Health Information. (2016). *OECD Interactive Tool: International comparisons—Peer countries.* Canada. Ottawa: Author. Retrieved from https://www.cihi.ca/en/oecd-interactive-tool-peer-countries-can.

Canadian Institute for Health Information. (2017). *National health expenditure trends, 1975 to 2017*. Ottawa: Author. Retrieved from https://secure.cihi.ca/free_products/nhex2017-trends-report-en.pdf.

CBC. (2001). The fight for Medicare Saskatchewan faces a bitter doctors' strike over Canada's first universal health care plan. Retrieved from https://www.cbc.ca/history/EPISCONTENTSE1EP15CH2PA4LE.html.

CBC News. (2013). Health Council's demise 'just made sense,' spokesman says. Retrieved from https://www.cbc.ca/news/politics/health-council-s-demise-just-made-sense-spokesman-says-1.1309302.

Chung, M. (2017). *Health care reform: Learning from other major health care systems*. Princeton Public Health Review. Retrieved from https://pphr.princeton.edu/2017/12/02/unhealthy-health-care-a-cursory-overview-of-major-health-care-systems/.

Competition and Markets Authority. (2014). *Private healthcare market investigation*. Retrieved from https://assets.publishing.service.gov.uk/media/533af065e5274a5660000023/Private_healthcare_main_report.pdf.

Deber, R. B. (2017). *Treating health care: How the Canadian system works and how it could work better*. Toronto: University of Toronto Press.

Department of Finance Canada. (2016). *Backgrounder on territorial formula financing*. Retrieved from https://www.fin.gc.ca/n16/data/16-024_1-eng.asp.

Egale Canada Human Rights Trust. (2019). *Sex reassignment surgery (SRS) backgrounder*. Retrieved from https://egale.ca/sex-reassignment-surgery-srs-backgrounder/.

Government of Canada. (2017). *Are all not-for-profit corporations the same?* Retrieved from https://www.ic.gc.ca/eic/site/cd-dgc.nsf/eng/cs07310.html.

Hall, E. M. (1980). *Canada's national-provincial health program for the 1980s: A commitment for renewal*. Ottawa: Health and Welfare Canada, Special Commissioner.

Health and Social Care Information Centre. (2015). *General and personal medical services, England 2005–2015*. Retrieved from http://webarchive.nationalarchives.gov.uk/20180328140045/http://digital.nhs.uk/catalogue/PUB20503.

Kaiser Commission on Medicaid and the Uninsured. (2013). *Medicaid: A primer*. Retrieved from https://www.kff.org/medicaid/issue-brief/medicaid-a-primer/.

Kirby, M., & LeBreton, M. (2002). *The health of Canadians: the federal role. Interim report, volume 3: Health care systems in other countries*. Standing Senate Committee on Social Affairs, Science and Technology. Retrieved from http://www.parl.gc.ca/37/1/parlbus/commbus/senate/com-e/SOCI-E/rep-e/repjan01vol3-e.htm

LaingBuisson. (2015). *Health cover UK market report* (12th ed.). Retrieved from. http://www.laingbuisson.com/wp-content/uploads/2016/06/Health_Cover_12ed_Bro_WEB.pdf.

Larmour, J. (2015). Saskatchewan doctors' strike. *The Canadian Encyclopedia*. Retrieved from https://www.thecanadianencyclopedia.ca/en/article/saskatchewan-doctors-strike

Marchildon, G. P. (2014). The three dimensions of universal Medicare in Canada. *Canadian Public Administration, 57*(3), 362–382.

Medicaid.gov. (2018). *Program history*. Retrieved from https://www.medicaid.gov/about-us/program-history/index.html.

National Audit Office. (2016). *Departmental overview 2015–2016*. Department of Health. Retrieved from https://www.nao.org.uk/report/departmental-overview-2015-16-department-of-health/.

NHS Confederation. (2016). *Key statistics on the NHS*. Retrieved from http://www.nhsconfed.org/resources/key-statistics-on-the-nhs.

Obama, B. H. (2017). Repealing the ACA without a replacement—the risks to American health care. *New England Journal of Medicine, 376*(4), 297–299.

Organisation for Economic Co-operation and Development. (2017). *Health at a glance 2017: OECD indicators*. Paris: OECD Publishing. Retrieved from.

Parliamentary Task Force on Federal-Provincial Fiscal Arrangements. (1981). *Fiscal federalism in Canada*. Ottawa: Ministry of Supply and Services. [seminal].

Reeves, S., Pelone, F., Harrison, R., et al. (2017). Interprofessional collaboration to improve professional practice and healthcare outcomes. *Cochrane Database of Systematic Reviews* (6).

Romanow, R. (2002). *Building on values: The future of health care in Canada*. Ottawa: Commission on the Future of Health Care in Canada. [seminal].

Sharratt, A. (2015). Hidden health-care costs can be a shock for retirees. *The Globe and Mail*, November 18. Retrieved from https://www.theglobeandmail.com/globe-investor/retirement/retire-health/hidden-health-care-costs-can-be-a-shock-for-retirees/article27324248/

Simpson, C., & McDonald, F. (2017). The big picture: ethics, health policy, health systems and rural health care. In *Rethinking rural health ethics* (pp. 139–160). Switzerland: Springer, Cham.

Speed, E., & Gabe, J. (2013). The Health and Social Care Act for England 2012: The extension of "new professionalism." *Critical Social Policy, 33*(3), 564–574.

World Health Organization. (2009). *WHO Guidelines on hand hygiene in health care: First global patient safety challenge: Clean care is safer care*. Retrieved from https://www.ncbi.nlm.nih.gov/books/NBK144006/.

World Health Organization. (2010). *Key components of a well-functioning health system*. Retrieved from https://www.who.int/healthsystems/EN_HSSkeycomponents.pdf.

14

Federal and Provincial Health Organizations

ⓔ Additional resources are available online at http://evolve.elsevier.com/Canada/Shah/publichealth/

LEARNING OBJECTIVES

- Understand and analyze the pertinent history, structure, and function of the federal health system.
- Understand and analyze the pertinent history, structure, and function of the provincial and territorial health system.
- Describe the following at a basic level:

- Relationships between the federal, provincial, and territorial health systems
- National health strategies
- Provincial and territorial funding models for health care

CHAPTER OUTLINE

KEY TERMS

Centre for Emergency Preparedness and Response (CEPR)
Canada Health Transfer (CHT)
Canadian Strategy for Cancer Control
Canadian Centre for Occupational Health & Safety (CCOHS)
Canadian Institute for Health Information (CIHI)
Canadian Institutes of Health Research (CIHR)
Centre for Health Promotion
Federal Initiative to Address HIV/AIDS in Canada
First Nations and Inuit Health Branch (FNIHB)

Health Canada
Health Products & Food Branch
Healthy Eating Strategy
Healthy Environments and Consumer Safety (HECS) Branch
income security programs
infectious disease prevention and control
National Collaborating Centres (NCCs)
Natural and Non-prescription Health Product Directorate
Office of Border Health Services (OBHS)

INTRODUCTION

The social determinants of health play a major role in the health of Canadians; they focus on living and working conditions and on the inequitable distribution of income and power. However, the structure and function of the ever-evolving and changing federal and provincial or territorial government departments also play a role in determining health as it relates to our access to health care. This chapter focuses on the organization of the federal and provincial or territorial organizations; as you read through the transformations of organization, you will also see how the shuffling, renaming, devolution, and creation of departments has an impact on the health of Canadians.

Under the *Constitution Act* of 1867, the federal government had almost no power in personal health care. However, through a number of financial arrangements as seen in Chapter 15, the government influenced two major areas: medical care and hospital care. Whereas provinces and territories in Canada have primary responsibility for organizing and delivering health services and supervising health care providers, the federal government transfers health funding to provinces and territories. Cash funding to the provinces and territories is on a per capita basis through the **Canada Health Transfer (CHT)**. The estimated CHT in 2016 to 2017 was CAD $36 billion, accounting for an estimated 24% of total provincial and territorial health expenditures (Canadian Institute for Health Information [CIHI], 2015a). This chapter deals with the major functions of federal and provincial governments as they relate to health care. (Fig. 14.1 provides an overview of the Canadian health care system.) The chapter also relates to CIHI's Health System Performance Measurement Framework (see introductory chapter) regarding the role of federal, provincial, and territorial leadership and governance and as manager of health system resources in Canada. To have a high-performing health care system, leadership and governance must play a major role.

HEALTH CANADA: FEDERAL HEALTH ORGANIZATION

As seen in Chapter 13, under the terms of Confederation, the federal government had relatively little jurisdiction over health care. In 1872, the Department of Agriculture had primary responsibility for federal health activities, which were gradually dispersed among several departments: Agriculture, Inland Revenue, and Marine and Fisheries. In 1919, the Department of Health was established by an act stating that its duties, powers, and functions "extend to and include all matters relating to the promotion or preservation of the health, social security and social welfare of the people of Canada over which the Parliament of Canada has jurisdiction." In 1929, the Department of Soldiers' Civil Re-establishment was discontinued, and the Department of National Health became the Department of Pensions and National Health. In 1945, it was split into Health and Welfare Canada and the Department of Veterans' Affairs. At that time, the task of Health and Welfare Canada was twofold: (1) to promote, preserve, and restore the health of Canadians and (2) to provide social security and social welfare to Canadians.

Over the past two decades, the department has undergone a number of reorganizations. As of 2015, there are two departments—one responsible for employment, workforce and labour, and the other responsible for health, now known as Health Canada.

Health Canada is responsible for helping the people of Canada maintain and improve their health. In partnership with provincial and territorial governments, Health Canada provides national leadership to develop health policy, enforce health regulations, promote disease prevention, and enhance healthy living for all Canadians. Health Canada ensures that health services are available and accessible to Indigenous communities. It also works closely with other federal departments, agencies, and health stakeholders to reduce health and safety risks to Canadians.

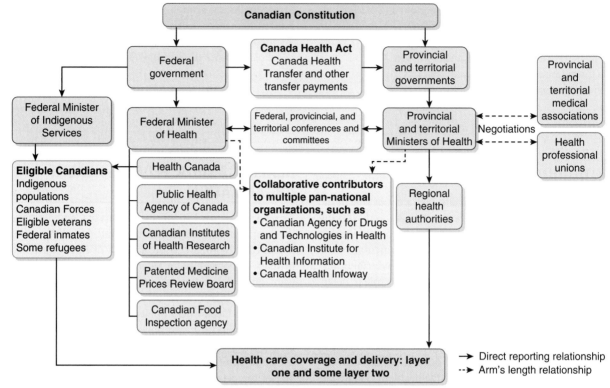

Fig. 14.1 Overview of the Canadian health care system. (Reprinted with permission from Elsevier (Martin, D., Miller, A.P., Quesnel-Vallée, A., et al. (2018). Canada's universal health-care system: achieving its potential. *Lancet, 391*(10131), 1718–1735.))

Although Health Canada branches, divisions, and units are frequently reorganized in an effort to streamline operations and reduce waste, the basic priorities have remained fairly stable over the past several years (Fig. 14.2). Health Canada publishes the most up-to-date and accurate information regarding its organizational structure on its website (Health Canada, 2018a). The following section outlines some of the functions and activities carried out by each branch and its sub-divisions.

The federal Minister of Health is responsible to parliament for maintaining and improving the health of Canadians (Health Canada, 2018b). The Deputy Minister and Associate Deputy Minister of Health, working with the Departmental Secretariat, support the Minister and manage departmental operations. The offices and branches are under the jurisdiction of the Deputy Minister and Associate Deputy Minister of Health. The Health Portfolio managed by the Ministers comprises Health Canada, the Public Health Agency of Canada,

the Canadian Institutes of Health Research (CIHR), the Patented Medicine Prices Review Board, and the Canadian Food Inspection Agency.

Branches, Offices, and Bureaus of Health Canada

Only Health Canada offices that are directly related to health activity are included in this chapter; they are the First Nations and Inuit Health Branch (FNIHB), Strategic Policy Branch, Health Products & Food Branch, Public Health Agency of Canada (PHAC), Healthy Environments & Consumer Safety Branch, and Pest Management Regulatory Agency. Offices not listed have mainly administrative and management functions.

Because provinces and territories have the primary responsibility for health matters, the federal government is restricted to acting as a clearinghouse for information in many instances and developing a national consensus or guidelines. The federal government develops and implements policies whenever there is a joint

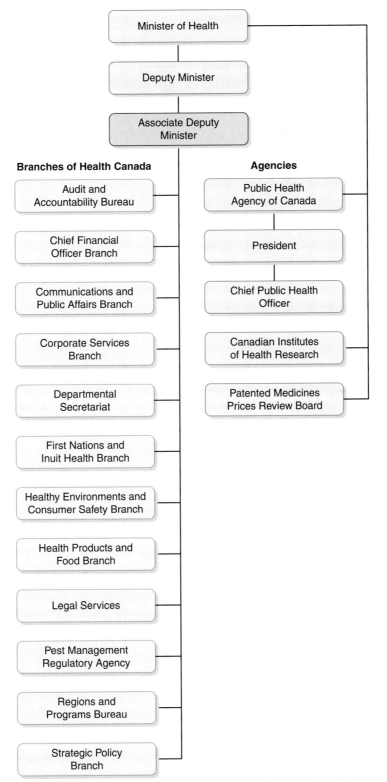

Fig. 14.2 Organization of Health Canada. (From Government of Canada. [2017]. Branches and agencies. Retrieved from https://www.canada.ca/en/health-canada/corporate/about-health-canada/branches-agencies.html. © All rights reserved. Organization of Health Canada: Branches and Agencies. Health Canada, 2017. Adapted and reproduced with permission from the Minister of Health, 2019.)

federal–provincial or –territorial initiative, when both parties have signed agreements or accords, or when there are constitutional amendments. Most of the time, the federal government exerts its influence through financial incentives or disincentives.

First Nations and Inuit Health Branch

The **First Nations and Inuit Health Branch (FNIHB)** is responsible for providing health services to Indigenous peoples with whom the government of Canada had signed treaties and who are living on reserves, which does not include services to Métis. However, in 2017, the department of Indigenous and Northern Affairs Canada (INAC) was dissolved, and two new departments were created: Indigenous Services Canada (ISC) and Crown-Indigenous Relations and Northern Affairs Canada (CIRNAC). ISC's focus includes high-quality services for Indigenous populations that support and empower Indigenous peoples to independently deliver services and address the socioeconomic conditions in their communities. The move to include Métis peoples, a broader view of the determinants of health, and self-determination positions these new departments on a path towards reconciliation as set out in the Truth and Reconciliation Commission (TRC) of Canada's *Calls to Action* report (TRC, 2015). The health status of Indigenous peoples is described in Chapter 7, which provides contextual framework for this section. The mandate of FNIHB is to assist Indigenous communities and people to address health inequalities and disease threats through health surveillance and population health interventions; to ensure the availability of, or access to, health services for Indigenous people; and to devolve the control and management of community-based health services to Indigenous communities and organizations (Health Canada, 2018c).

There are three main programs. The Non-Insured Health Benefits (NIHB) Program is a national program that provides coverage to registered First Nations and recognized Inuit for a specified range of medically necessary items and services that are not covered by other plans and programs. NIHB include drugs, dental care, vision care, medical supplies and equipment, short-term mental health services, and transportation to access medical services. The Community Programs Directorate (CPD) works in partnership with First Nations and Inuit peoples to deliver a wide range of programs in key community health sectors. All CPD activities have the goal of maintaining and improving the health of First Nations and Inuit and facilitating First Nations and Inuit control of health programs and resources. CPD is organized as follows: Children and Youth Division, Mental Health and Addiction Division, and Chronic Disease Prevention Division (Health Canada, 2018d). The Primary Health Care and Public Health Directorate (PHCPH) of the FNIHB is responsible for primary health care delivery in partnership with First Nations and Inuit health authorities. All PHCPH activities are directed towards supporting knowledge and capacity building among First Nations and Inuit and facilitating First Nations and Inuit control of health programs and resources. The PHCPH has the following divisions: the Primary Health Care Division, the Infectious Disease Control Division, the Environmental Health Division, and the Dental and Pharmacy Programs Division (Health Canada, 2018e).

Community health nurses, nurse practitioners, or physicians provide primary care in remote and isolated communities. In certain provinces and territories, several universities provide medical personnel and students on rotation. Because Indigenous peoples live all over Canada, there is a network of specially designed health facilities that operate in all provinces and territories, including nursing stations, health stations, health offices, health centres, and hospitals. Provincial departments of public health do not provide services on reserves, which creates gaps in services (e.g., when FNIHB and the province do not offer the same services). Unlike in the provincial and territorial health care systems, public health programs for reserve residents are not mandated by legislation. A comprehensive public health program attempts to provide dental care for children, immunization, school health services, health education, and prenatal, postnatal, and healthy baby clinics, and it provides care on reserves that other residents of Canada would receive from provincial and territorial governments, such as home care. Because of a chronic shortage of qualified staff, however, many services are either not delivered or are inadequate.

As residents of a province or territory, Indigenous people are entitled to the benefits of the cost-shared provincially operated plans for medical and hospital insurance on the same terms and conditions as other Canadians. Because many of the Indigenous communities are small and often located in remote and isolated areas, these insured benefits are supplemented by the FNIHB, which assists Indigenous bands to arrange transportation and to obtain drugs and prostheses. The FNIHB is in the process of transferring control of health services to Indigenous communities and, with the creation of Indigenous Services Canada and the inclusion of Métis peoples, changes are occurring in how services will be offered. This involves the development of policies, health-funding arrangements, planning strategies and activities leading to the negotiation and conclusion of self-government agreements with Indigenous people.

Strategic Policy Branch

The **Strategic Policy Branch (SPB)** plays a lead role in health policy, communications, and consultations, which are described below.

The Canada Health Act Division administers the *Canada Health Act,* provides policy advice related to the Act, and monitors a broad range of sources to assess provincial and territorial compliance with its criteria and conditions. It also informs the minister of possible noncompliance with the Act and recommends appropriate action. The division develops interpretations under the Act, provides support to legal counsel in court cases involving the Act, and maintains a centre of expertise on the Canadian health insurance system. As required by section 23 of the Act, the division produces an annual report for each fiscal year on the extent to which provincial and territorial health care insurance plans have satisfied the criteria and conditions for payment. These reports are excellent sources of detailed and up-to-date information on each provincial and territorial health insurance program. The branch's other major departments include Applied Research and Analysis Directorate (ARAD), Canada Health Act Division (CHAD), Federal/Provincial Relations Division (FPRD), Health Care Policy Directorate (HCPD), Office of Nursing Policy (ONP), Official Language Community Development Bureau, Policy Coordination and Planning Directorate (PCPD), and Science Policy Directorate (SPD).

Health Products and Food Branch

The two main goals of the **Health Products and Food Branch (HPFB)** are to promote good nutrition and informed use of drugs, food, and natural health products and to maximize the safety and efficacy of drugs, food, natural health products, medical devices, and biologics and related biotechnology products in the Canadian marketplace and health care system. Its three major programs are described next.

The Therapeutic Products Directorate (TPD) is responsible for the regulation of pharmaceutical drugs, medical devices, and other therapeutic products available to Canadians. This includes evaluating and monitoring their safety, effectiveness, and quality (Health Canada, 2018f). By definition, Canada's *Food and Drugs Act* encompasses a range of products:

- Therapeutic products, including pharmaceuticals, prescription drugs, and over-the-counter drugs
- Homeopathics, herbal remedies, and nutraceuticals
- Biological products, such as vaccines, blood and blood products, certain hormones and enzymes, tissues, and organs
- Xenografts
- Medical devices, such as medical and dental implants, medical equipment and instruments, test kits for diagnosis, and contraceptive devices
- Disinfectants
- Low-risk products, such as sunscreens, antiperspirants, and toothpaste
- Narcotic, controlled, and restricted drugs

The TPD regulates both the manufacture and distribution of pharmaceutical drugs in Canada. Facilities that manufacture biological products to be sold in Canada, such as serums and vaccines, must be licensed according to the specifications of the *Food and Drugs Act* and Regulations, whether they are located in Canada or abroad.

Another major activity of HPFB is the Quality Assessment of Drugs Program, which includes inspection of manufacturing facilities, assessment of claims and clinical equivalency of competing brands, and provision of information to professionals and to the general public.

The Marketed Health Products Directorate (MHPD) is responsible for maintaining consistency in postapproval surveillance and assessment of signals and safety trends concerning all marketed health products. The MHPD works closely with other directorates in the HPFB and other branches.

The HPFB's Food Directorate is responsible for establishing policies and standards for the safety and nutritional quality of food sold in Canada, as well as the administration of those provisions of the *Food and Drugs Act* that relate to public health, safety, and nutrition. It is also responsible for assessing the effectiveness of the Canadian Food Inspection Agency's activities related to food safety (Health Canada, 2017). In 2018, the government introduced new changes to nutrition labelling found on food items. Products will now be labelled according to the amount of sugar, sodium, or saturated fat per serving. Any product that includes more than 15% of the daily recommended intake of each ingredient will get a label. This label is intended to make choosing the healthier option easier for consumers (Health Canada, 2018g).

The **Natural and Non-prescription Health Products Directorate** ensures that Canadians have ready access to safe, effective, high-quality natural health and nonprescription products by maintaining proper labelling and implementing a regulatory framework that supports freedom of choice and cultural diversity. It was established in March 2002 and is based on the 53 recommendations contained in the Standing Committee on Health's report titled *Natural Health Products: A New Vision* (Health Canada, 2003).

The Biologics and Genetic Therapies Directorate (BGTD) is responsible for the regulation of biological and radiopharmaceutical drugs, including blood and blood products, viral and bacterial vaccines, genetic therapeutic products, tissues, organs, and xenografts. This includes evaluating and monitoring their safety, effectiveness, and quality.

Public Health Agency of Canada

The **Public Health Agency of Canada (PHAC)** was created from a response to the aftermath of a number of public health emergencies. In 2000, an *Escherichia coli* outbreak killed seven people in Walkerton, Ontario, and affected thousands of others. Then, in 2001, approximately 6 000 people in North Battleford, Saskatchewan, contracted cryptosporidiosis because of problems with the water supply. In 2002 and 2003, severe acute respiratory syndrome (SARS), a previously unknown disease, reached near-pandemic levels, causing more than 8 000 cases in 16 countries, and killed 44 Canadians. At the same time, experts in public health were warning of an impending influenza pandemic.

A number of reports examined how the outbreaks were handled, including *Learning from SARS—A Renewal of Public Health in Canada, A Report of the National Advisory Committee on SARS and Public Health* (frequently referred to as the Naylor Report, after Dr. David Naylor, Chair of the Committee), and *Reforming Health Protection and Promotion in Canada:*

Time to Act, a report of the Standing Senate Committee on Social Affairs, Science and Technology. Born out of these reports was Bill C-5—the *Public Health Agency of Canada Act,* which established the Public Health Agency of Canada and amended certain other Acts (the *Public Health Agency of Canada Act*). The control and supervision of the Population and Public Health Branch of Health Canada was transferred to the Public Health Agency of Canada by Order in Council pursuant to the *Public Service Rearrangement and Transfer of Duties Act,* effective 24 September 2004.

The PHAC is primarily responsible for policies, programs, and systems relating to prevention, health promotion, disease surveillance, community action, and disease control. There are three main programs and several subprograms within the PHAC. The three main programs are health promotion and chronic disease preventions, infectious disease prevention and control, and health security. There are also several centres attached to the various programs, which are described next (Health Canada, 2018h).

A number of programs fall under the health promotion and chronic disease prevention area of PHAC, for example:

- Aboriginal Head Start in Urban and Northern Communities (AHSUNC) program
- Canada Prenatal Nutrition Program (CPNP)
- Community Action Program for Children (CAPC)
- Innovation Strategy
- Nutrition North Canada
- Preventing Gender-Based Violence: The Health Perspective
- Canadian Diabetes Strategy (CDS)
- Healthy Living Fund, Canadian Breast Cancer Initiative
- Federal Tobacco Control Strategy
- Integrated Strategy for Healthy Living and Chronic Disease—Cancer
- Integrated Strategy for Healthy Living and Chronic Disease—Cardiovascular Disease Program
- International Health Grants Program
- Men's Health
- Economic Action Plan 2015 Initiative
- Fetal Alcohol Spectrum Disorder (FASD) —National Strategic Projects Fund
- Integrated Strategy for Healthy Living and Chronic Disease—Enhanced Surveillance for Chronic Disease

- Integrated Strategy for Healthy Living and Chronic Disease—Joint Consortium for School Health
- Integrated Strategy for Healthy Living and Chronic Disease—Observatory of Best Practices

The **National Collaborating Centres (NCCs)** are funded through the Public Health Agency of Canada and include six National Collaborating Centres (NCCs) for Public Health that are located across Canada; each focuses on a different public health priority. The NCCs work together to promote the use of scientific research and other knowledge to strengthen public health practices, programs, and policies in Canada. The NCCs identify knowledge gaps, foster networks, and provide the public health system with an array of evidence-based resources, multimedia products, and knowledge translation services. These six centres are:

- NCC for Indigenous Health at the University of Northern British Columbia in Prince George
- NCC for Determinants of Health at St. Francis Xavier University in Antigonish, Nova Scotia
- NCC for Healthy Public Policy at L'Institut national de santé publique du Québec in Montreal
- NCC for Environmental Health at the BC Centre for Disease Control in Vancouver
- NCC for Infectious Diseases at the University of Manitoba in Winnipeg
- NCC for Methods and Tools at McMaster University in Hamilton, Ontario

The **Centre for Health Promotion** is responsible for implementing policies and programs that enhance the conditions within which healthy development takes place through life stages. The CHP was founded on the principles of population and public health and uses a determinants of health approach in its programs, policies, and research.

Infectious disease prevention and control includes the following:

- Laboratory science leadership and services
- Communicable diseases and infection control
  - HIV and Hepatitis C Community Action Fund (CAF)
  - Strengthening the Canadian Drugs and Substances Strategy (Harm Reduction Fund)
  - Blood Safety
  - International Health Grants Program

The National Microbiology Laboratory, located in Winnipeg, Manitoba, consists of external national reference centres across Canada. The laboratory houses the only Containment Level 4 (also known as Biosafety Level 4) facility in Canada, allowing scientists to work safely with the most serious of pathogens, including Ebola, Marburg fever, and Lassa fever. The Laboratory for Foodborne Zoonoses, a science-based organization in Guelph, Ontario, provides and integrates scientific information for the development, implementation, and evaluation of policies and programs that reduce risks to health associated with food-borne microorganisms across the food chain. It includes:

- Immunization
  - Immunization Partnership Fund
- Foodborne and zoonotic diseases
  - National Collaborating Centres for Public Health (NCCPH)
  - Infectious Diseases and Climate Change Fund—Adapting to the Impacts of Climate Change
- Health security
  - Emergency preparedness and response
  - Biosecurity
  - Border and travel health

The **Centre for Emergency Preparedness and Response (CEPR)** aims to strengthen Health Canada's capacity to respond to global and domestic public health threats, including natural disasters, accidental and deliberate emergencies, and international public health risks. The CEPR acts as the coordinating point for dealing with public health emergencies. Active 24 hours a day, 7 days a week, it also works closely with other internal experts in areas such as infectious disease, food, blood, nuclear emergencies, and chemicals.

The PHAC is also responsible for the National Emergency Stockpile System, Emergency Social Services, and Health Canada is responsible for the Federal Nuclear Emergency Plan, as well as providing emergency health care for Indigenous communities, the health of travellers to Canada, and occupational health for federal government employees and providing expert health advice when assessing potential threats.

The **Office of Border Health Services (OBHS)** includes the Quarantine Program and the Travelling Public Program (TPP). Together, these programs are responsible for protecting Canada from the importation of dangerous communicable diseases that might pose a threat to the public's health. OBHS is responsible for the *Quarantine Act* and Regulations, which control the importation of infectious diseases into Canada through the international movement of people, conveyances, and goods. As well, OBHS plays the lead role in coordinating Canada's response to outbreaks of international disease, which may involve implementing contingency plans and other measures. Under the umbrella of the TPP, environmental health conditions on board conveyances entering Canada, including goods and cargo, is monitored.

Healthy Environments and Consumer Safety Branch

The **Healthy Environments and Consumer Safety (HECS) Branch** is responsible for promoting safe living, working, and recreational environments. It emphasizes health in the work environment and delivering occupational health and safety services, assessing and reducing health risks posed by environmental factors, promoting initiatives to reduce and prevent the harm caused by tobacco and the abuse of alcohol and other controlled substances, and regulating tobacco and controlled substances. It also provides drug analytical services, regulates the safety of industrial and consumer products in the Canadian marketplace, and promotes their safe use (Health Canada, 2014).

The Drug Strategy and Controlled Substances program regulates controlled substances, such as opiates, opiates derivatives, and hallucinogenic substances, and promotes initiatives that reduce or prevent the harm associated with these substances and alcohol. It also provides expert advice and drug analysis services to law enforcement agencies across the country.

The **Canadian Centre for Occupational Health & Safety (CCOHS)** program establishes workplace health and safety policies and provides services to protect the health of the public sector, the travelling public, and dignitaries visiting Canada.

The Product Safety program regulates the safety of commercial and consumer chemicals and products and promotes their safe use. The Safe Environments program promotes healthy and safe living, working, and recreational environments. It also assesses and reduces health risks posed by environmental factors. The Tobacco Control program regulates tobacco and promotes initiatives that reduce or prevent the harm associated with tobacco use (see later).

Pest Management Regulatory Agency Branch

The **Pest Management Regulatory Agency (PMRA)** is responsible for protecting human health and the environment by minimizing the risks associated with pest control products. All products that are used, sold, or imported into Canada to manage, destroy, attract, or repel pests are regulated by the PMRA. These pesticides include chemicals, devices, and even organisms. The use of pesticides is regulated by the *Pest Control Products Act,* as well as provincial and territorial legislation. The agency's health activities are linked to those of other branches, with emphasis on monitoring disease trends to provide a signal of potential health effects from pesticide exposure, assessing the impact of pesticide use on the quality of the Canadian food supply, and regulating pesticides that are no longer registered but find their way into the environment as contaminants. The PMRA collaborates with Environment Canada, Agriculture and Agri-Food Canada, the Canadian Food Inspection Agency, and other organizations in environmental and pesticide research and monitoring, including sustainable pest management (Pest Management Regulatory Agency, 2009).

Independent Agencies of Health Canada

These agencies report to the Minister of Health at arm's length.

Canadian Institutes of Health Research

Canadian Institutes of Health Research (CIHR) constitute Canada's federal agency for health research, established in 2000 to replace the former Medical Research Council. CIHR's objective is to excel, according to internationally accepted standards of scientific excellence, in the creation of new knowledge and its translation into improved health for Canadians, more effective health services and products, and a strengthened health care system. This involves a multidisciplinary approach, organized through a framework of "virtual" institutes, each dedicated to a specific area, and linking and supporting researchers located in universities, hospitals, and other research centres across Canada. The institutes embrace four pillars of research: biomedical research, clinical science, health systems and services, and the social, cultural, and other factors that affect the health of populations. CIHR's 13 institutes are Indigenous Peoples' Health; Aging; Cancer Research; Circulatory and Respiratory Health; Gender and Health; Genetics, Health Services, and Policy Research; Human Development, Child, and Young Health; Infection and Immunity; Musculoskeletal Health and Arthritis; Neurosciences, Mental Health, and Addiction; Nutrition, Metabolism, and Diabetes; and Population and Public Health (CIHR, 2018). The CIHR invests approximately $1 billion each year to support health research. This funding is divided into two types of research: investigator-driven and priority-driven, out of which it funded 1 431 grants, 1 486 awards, 14 Career Awards, and approximately 898 trainees in 2017.

Patented Medicine Prices Review Board

The **Patented Medicine Prices Review Board (PMPRB)** is an independent quasi-judicial body, created in 1987 under the *Patent Act* to protect consumer interests in light of increased patent protection for pharmaceuticals. Its mandate is to ensure that the prices charged by manufacturers of patented medicines in Canada are not excessive, to report annually to Parliament on the price trends of all medicines in Canada, and on the ratio of research and development expenditures to sales by patentees. The PMPRB does not review the prices of nonpatented medicines, but it does oversee the selection and utilization process of any medicines, patented or not, including which drug the doctor prescribes, the amount prescribed, how the product is used, and the coverage provided by third-party and provincial and territorial drug plans (Patented Medicine Prices Review Board, 2018).

Canadian Centre for Occupational Health and Safety

The Canadian Centre for Occupational Health and Safety (CCOHS) is an independent departmental corporation under Schedule II of the *Financial Administration Act* and is accountable to Parliament through the Minister of Labour. CCOHS is responsible for the advancement of safe and healthy workplaces and preventing work-related injuries, illnesses, and deaths. CCOHS was created in 1978 by an Act of Parliament—the *Canadian Centre for Occupational Health and Safety Act* (S.C., 1977-78, c. 29). This act was based on the belief that all Canadians had ". . . a fundamental right to a healthy and safe working environment." The CCOHS promotes the total well-being—physical, psychosocial, and mental health—of working Canadians by providing information, training, education, management systems, and solutions. It makes credible information about workplace hazards and conditions easily and widely accessible to all Canadians, promoting safe and healthy workplaces.

Women's Health Bureau

Health Canada is also responsible for the **Women's Health Bureau**, which is guided by Health Canada's Women's Health Strategy (Canadian Women's Health Network, 2018). It has four main objectives: (1) to ensure that Health Canada's policies and programs are responsive to gender differences and to women's health needs, (2) to increase knowledge and understanding of women's health and women's health needs, (3) to support the provision of effective health services to women, and (4) to promote good health through preventive measures and the reduction of risk factors that imperil the health of women.

One of the major activities of the Women's Health Bureau is the Centres of Excellence for Women's Health Program. Based in Halifax, Montreal, Toronto, Winnipeg, and Vancouver, these multidisciplinary centres operate as partnerships among academics, community-based organizations, and policy makers. The Canadian Women's Health Network is responsible for disseminating the research findings of the centres and other information on women's health.

Workplace Hazardous Materials Information System

Health Canada is the government body responsible for making the required changes to the overall federal **Workplace Hazardous Materials Information System (WHMIS)**–related laws. The *Hazardous Products Act* and the new Hazardous Products Regulations (HPR) guide WHMIS regulations. The Hazardous Materials Information Review Commission (HMIRC) is charged with providing the protection mechanism for trade secrets within the WHMIS.

The WHMIS requires that manufacturers and suppliers provide employers with information on the hazards of materials produced, sold, or used in Canadian workplaces (Canadian Centre for Occupational Health & Safety, 2018). Employers, in turn, provide that information to employees through product labels, worker education programs, and material safety data sheets (MSDS). A product's MSDS must fully disclose all hazardous ingredients in the product, its toxicological properties, and any safety precautions workers need to take when using the product and treatment required in the case of exposure. The WHMIS is a nation-wide system that contributes to the reduction of illness and injury caused by using hazardous materials in the Canadian workplace (see Chapter 12).

CRITICAL THINKING QUESTION 14.1: In the past 2 decades, major structural changes have been made to federal government departments in health. Why do you think these major changes have occurred?

RELEVANT SOCIAL PROGRAMS

The federal social programs described briefly below promote and strengthen the income security of Canadians; share the cost of provincial and territorial social assistance, welfare services, and rehabilitation programs; and assist in the development of social services to meet changing social needs.

Income Security Programs

The **income security programs** promote and preserve the social security and social welfare of Canadians through the administration of a number of programs, including Guaranteed Income Supplement; Home Adaptations for Seniors Independence; Canada Pension Plan Disability Benefits; Employability Assistance for People with Disabilities; Veteran Disability Pension; Canada Child Tax Benefit; and Maternity, Parental, and Sickness Benefits (Government of Canada, 2017). Through a network of regional offices and client service centres, these programs provide financial assistance to people with disabilities, older adults, single-parent families, orphans, unemployed, and low-income individuals. The programs complement existing social welfare, provincial and territorial, and local programs.

Social Service Programs

Social service programs consist of major federal–provincial cost-sharing programs that provide basic assistance for those whose budgetary needs exceed available resources (for whatever reason). They also provide consultation on social and welfare-related issues, including employability and vocational rehabilitation; alcohol and drug treatment and rehabilitation; services to people with physical and mental impairment; child welfare, child abuse, and family violence; family and community services; and voluntary action. Contributions are provided to help seniors maintain and improve their quality of life and independence and to encourage seniors to use their skills, talents, and experience within the community.

OTHER RELEVANT PROGRAMS

Health Canada is involved in a number of other interdepartmental activities related to health. The tasks of these relevant advisory councils are given next.

Canadian Institute for Health Information

The **Canadian Institute for Health Information (CIHI)** grew out of a report by the National Task Force on Health Information, released in June 1991. This task force highlighted the need for a nationally coordinated approach to Canada's health information system. In September 1992, federal, provincial, and territorial ministers of health approved the creation of CIHI, which was launched in 1994 after the amalgamation of the Hospital Medical Records Institute and the Management and Information Systems Group. The following year, specific health information programs from Health Canada and activities from Statistics Canada joined. CIHI is a not-for-profit organization funded primarily through bilateral funding agreements with federal and provincial and territorial ministries of health and individual health care institutions (CIHI, 2018).

The CIHI is governed by a board of 16 directors who are chosen from health sectors and regions of Canada to create a balance. The board provides strategic guidance to CIHI, as well as to Statistics Canada's Health Statistics Division. In addition, it maintains strong links with the Conference of Deputy Ministers of Health, advising them on health information matters. CIHI has one of the best websites for data on Canadian health and health care system (CIHI, 2018).

The Federal Initiative to Address HIV/AIDS in Canada

Canada's response to the HIV/AIDS epidemic has evolved significantly over the past 2 decades. In 1990, the federal government established the National AIDS Strategy (NAS) to help organize the various players, which then included professional associations, the medical community, researchers, and the private sector, into a more formal, interconnected approach. In 1993, the NAS was renewed for 5 years, with annual funding increased from $37.3 million to $42.2 million.

After extensive stakeholder consultations in the summer of 1997, the Canadian Strategy on HIV/AIDS (CSHA) was launched in 1998, now known as the **Federal Initiative to Address HIV/AIDS in Canada**. It receives permanent funding for an ongoing, coordinated national response and represents a shift from a disease-oriented approach under NAS to one that looks at the root causes, determinants of health, and other dimensions of the HIV epidemic (Health Canada, 2015). People living with HIV/AIDS and those at risk of

HIV infection are the focus and centre of CSHA efforts. The Canadian HIV Vaccine Initiative (CHVI) is a partnership between the government of Canada and the Bill & Melinda Gates Foundation. The CHVI is a key element in the Government of Canada's commitment to a comprehensive, long-term approach to addressing HIV/AIDS, both domestically and internationally.

Tobacco Control Strategy

Initiated in 2018 and building on the success of the National Strategy to Decrease Tobacco Use in Canada, Canada's **Federal Tobacco Control Strategy's** goal is to drive down the smoking rates in Canada to less than 5% by 2035 (Health Canada, 2018i). The government has committed $330 million dollars over 5 years to do the following:

- Help Canadians who smoke to quit or reduce the harms of their addiction to nicotine.
- Protect the health of young people and non-smokers from the dangers of tobacco use.

This new strategy notes that tobacco use is not equally spread across the population. It is often linked to other health and social inequities. LGBTQ+, young people, and Indigenous populations who have higher rates of tobacco use are a focus of the new strategy. Additionally, the *Tobacco and Vaping Products Act,* passed on May 23, 2018, makes it legal for adults to buy vaping products that contain nicotine, as a less harmful option than smoking. This is part of the Tobacco Control Strategy for dealing with tobacco use.

Health Canada's Healthy Eating Strategy

The **Healthy Eating Strategy** aims to improve the food environment in Canada to make it easier for Canadians to make healthier choices. Health Canada has taken a number of actions to improve the food environment:

- Improving healthy eating information
- Improving nutrition quality of foods
- Protecting vulnerable populations
- Supporting increased access to and availability of nutritious foods

Improving healthy eating information includes updating regulations about food labels and their nutrition facts table, list of ingredients, and updating Canada's Food Guide. In 2019, Canada's Food Guide was updated, based on broad consultation, and released to the public with mixed reviews. The revised guide focuses on plant-based proteins, drinking water, and avoidance of processed foods. However, the amount to eat each meal or each day is unclear because portion sizes are pictured rather than described, and recommendations state that we should "have plenty of vegetables and fruit," leaving Canadians with fuzzy advice. Additionally, two separate consultations on front-of-package (FOP) nutrition labelling occurred: Toward Front-of-Package Labels for Canadians (in 2016) and Proposed Front-of-Package Labelling in 2018 (Health Canada, 2018j). Consultations with consumers provided valuable feedback regarding how to improve food labelling because some consumers found the information provided on food labels too complex to understand and use. As a result of these consultations, FOP labelling requirements on prepackaged foods are now required to note when that food is high in sodium, sugars, and saturated fat.

Improving nutrition quality of foods includes regulations to ban industrially produced trans fat in foods. Additionally, sodium reduction is a priority for the Government of Canada, and efforts are currently underway to ensure that the food industry is meeting the voluntary sodium reduction targets that were established in 2012 and working with restaurants and food services to develop goals for reducing sodium in their foods.

Protecting vulnerable populations involves restricting marketing of unhealthy foods and beverages to children. Public consultations were held in 2017 and pending Royal Assent of Bill S-228, the *Child Health Protection Act,* Health Canada will publish proposed regulations in the Canada Gazette for consultation.

Supporting increased access to and availability of nutritious foods targets Canada's Northern population, for whom extremely high prices for food and decreased accessibility to nutritious food are issues. The Nutrition North Canada program supports increased access and availability to nutritious foods by providing a retail subsidy through Crown-Indigenous Relations and Northern Affairs, to make perishable nutritious foods more accessible and affordable to residents of isolated northern communities. After the 2014 Auditor General's report demonstrating a lack of government monitoring of the Nutrition North program, a number of changes were implemented, including increasing subsidies and adding more foods to the subsidy list. However, it is still unclear how the government plans to ensure there is a rigorous monitoring process to ensure that the full subsidy is being passed on to Northerners.

Mental Health Strategy for Canada

The Mental Health Commission of Canada (MHCC) is leading the way in developing and disseminating innovative programs and tools to support the mental health and wellness of Canadians. Through its unique mandate from the Government of Canada, the MHCC supports federal, provincial, and territorial governments, as well as organizations in the implementation of sound public policy. The MHCC's current mandate aims to deliver on priority areas identified in the Mental Health Strategy for Canada. *Advancing the Mental Health Strategy for Canada: A Framework for Action (2017–2022)* has identified the need for improved access to services that cross the continuum of care, with an emphasis on improving the experiences of transitions across life stages (MHCC, 2018). In its 2017 budget, the Government of Canada confirmed $11 billion in funding over 10 years for provinces and territories, starting in 2017 to 2018, targeted specifically to improve access to mental health services and home care.

Canadian Cancer Control Strategy

The Canadian Partnership Against Cancer (CPAC) is an independent organization funded by the federal government to accelerate action on cancer control for all Canadians (Canadian Partnership Against Cancer, 2018). The CPAC was founded in 2007 as the steward of the **Canadian Strategy for Cancer Control**. The CPAC has outlined three main goals that it aims to reach within 30 years:

- Fewer Canadians develop cancer.
- Fewer Canadians die from cancer.
- Canadians affected by cancer have a better quality of life.

> **CRITICAL THINKING QUESTION 14.2:** Over the past decade, several federal government health strategies have come and gone. Can you think of two reasons why this has occurred? Brainstorm possible new federal government strategies to come.

PROVINCIAL AND TERRITORIAL HEALTH SYSTEMS

Constitutionally, the provincial and territorial governments have primary responsibility for all personal health matters, such as disease prevention, treatment, and maintenance of health—a right that provinces and territories increasingly cite to exercise greater freedom in health system restructuring and reform without perceived federal interference. This has become an increasingly contentious issue, although there appears to be a conciliatory gesture on parts of the federal government and all provinces and territories except Quebec, by being signatory to the Social Union Agreement in 1999 and by committing to reform the health care system in 2000. Additionally, the 2017 Shared Health Priorities Health Accord was signed individually by each province, indicating a desire to work in partnership to meet the health needs of Canadians (see Chapter 13).

The financing of services such as preventive health services, medical services, hospital services, and treatment services for tuberculosis and other chronic diseases and rehabilitation and care for people who are chronically ill and disabled depends chiefly on provincial and municipal governments. Provincial and territorial administrations fund and regulate hospitals and some functions of voluntary community health associations, a number of health care professions, and teaching and research institutions. Methods of organizing, financing, and administering health ministries vary from province to province and information from the ministry of health in each province is accessible through the website of the provincial or territorial ministry of health. For instance, programs such as hospital insurance, medical care insurance, tuberculosis control, cancer control, and mental health and addictions may be administered directly by the province or territory. Alternatively, the same programs may be the responsibility of separate public agencies directly accountable to a provincial or territorial minister of health. Other ministries can also finance some of the health-related services. This diversity stems from traditional and financial considerations because health consumes the largest percentage of provincial budgets, in a range of 38% to 45% (CIHI, 2016). There are two likely explanations for these diversities. First, provincial governments differ in their views of health—that is, what is to be included in health, such as services for children with special needs or health surveillance in the workplace. Second, to reduce the power of a single ministry with such a large budget, the functions of the health ministries are distributed across different ministries; however, this results in the fragmentation and duplication of services. More recently, fiscal constraints and political and ideological shifts have also encouraged the implementation of private sector tools, such as lean management and Six Sigma, which focus on reducing waste and improving efficiency and effectiveness (Dunn, 2016).

Local and Regional Health Authorities

Beginning in the early 1990s, many provincial ministries of health have held extensive public consultations and reviews in an effort to improve the functioning of their health systems. A key component of these recent reforms are the devolution and decentralization of decision making for health to the regional and local levels. Based on the premise of increased community and consumer empowerment through increased participation in health and on the belief that the health sector needed greater flexibility and responsiveness to local needs, regionalization has proceeded swiftly in every province except Ontario. However, within the health community, there is a growing suspicion that regionalization has been created to cut health care costs and to shift "blame" from the provincial government to the local level.

In the 1990s, most provinces and territories in Canada partially devolved their responsibility to subprovincial regions. This resulted in the establishment of regional health authorities (RHAs) across Canada. One objective was to streamline the delivery system, making it less fragmented and more responsive to local needs. Some provinces and territories set additional goals to increase community-based services, improve public participation in health care, and encourage policies and programs to promote health.

Regionalization has taken different forms across the country. Typically, however, there is a provincially appointed (sometimes locally elected) board responsible for the delivery of health care services and programs to the region. The implications of regionalization for improving health effectiveness and efficiency and its broader social implications for community participation and understanding of health have yet to be fully documented and evaluated; nonetheless, recent reports indicate that regionalization has been beneficial in many ways, such as in better integration of service delivery, reduced administrative costs, increased focus on illness prevention and public health, and greater flexibility in reallocating and consolidating clinical services between health care providers and institutions (Barker & Church, 2017).

Regional Health Authorities

Regional health authorities (RHAs) across Canada differ in size, structure, scope of responsibility, and number per province. RHAs are autonomous health care organizations that are responsible for health administration within a defined geographic region within a province or territory (Statistics Canada, 2016). They have appointed or elected boards of governance and manage the funding and delivering of community and institutional health services within their regions.

Many changes have taken place over the past 2 decades concerning RHAs. Although in the 1990s nearly every province and territory (except Ontario) had created RHAs, many have now evolved back into one health authority (e.g., Prince Edward Island [2005], Alberta [2008], Nova Scotia [2015], Northwest Territories [2016], and Saskatchewan [2017]). The remaining provinces and territories are divided into RHAs (regions), ranging from 5 in British Columbia to 18 in Quebec, based partly on population size and natural geographic and administrative boundaries. Each region's health needs are managed by a regional or district health board composed of roughly 10 to 15 members. In Alberta, one health authority exists that is organized into five zones (Calgary, Edmonton, North, South, and Central). Saskatchewan has recently transitioned from 12 RHAs to a single health authority to plan and deliver health care services that will break down geographic boundaries and service silos and to provide more consistent and coordinated health care services across the province. Additionally, Saskatchewan has two ministers of health, with one minister being dedicated to rural and remote health. Ontario opted for creating 14 Local Health Integration Networks (LHINs), which are mandated to plan, fund, and integrate hospital, home, and community services. However, at the time of writing, the current government in Ontario is discussing reducing the number of LHINs to five. In British Columbia, the First Nations Health Authority (FNHA) was created in 2013 and is Canada's first province-wide health authority focusing on Indigenous health (see Case Study box: The First Nations Health Authority of British Columbia).

The process of choosing board members varies from province to province, but generally a board includes both elected and appointed officials who represent a wide variety of constituencies and interests. They are usually drawn from consumer or special needs groups, hospitals and health services centres, professional groups, voluntary agencies, and elected officials. This mix of membership increases the board's accountability before its community and simultaneously ensures the inclusion of particular areas of expertise or the representation of particular cultural backgrounds that may not already be represented. Several provinces, such as British Columbia and Ontario, have provided for direct links between regional boards and organizations of physicians to ensure that physicians have a voice in regional planning and resource allocation decisions.

CASE STUDY

The First Nations Health Authority of British Columbia

The FNHA is responsible for planning, management, service delivery, and funding of health programs, in partnership with Indigenous communities in British Columbia. Guided by the vision of embedding cultural safety and humility into health service delivery, the FNHA works to reform the way health care is delivered to British Columbia's Indigenous communities through direct services, provincial partnership collaboration, and health systems innovation. Services are largely focused on health promotion and disease prevention.

The work of the FNHA does not replace the role of the Ministry of Health and Regional Health Authorities but strengthens their work through collaboration, coordination, and integration of their respective health programs and services.

CASE STUDY

Regional Health Authorities

After waiting three weeks for an appointment, Mr. S., a 55-year-old independent truck driver, met with a heart specialist, who advised him that he needed coronary bypass surgery. Unfortunately, it would take up to 10 weeks before he could have the surgery.

Mr. S. was told that his angina was stable and not immediately life threatening, but serious all the same. For his safety and the safety of others, the specialist said he should not return to work and that she would review his fitness to work after the surgery.

Mr. S. complained that being laid up would bring him financial ruin and that it would be maddening to live under the shadow of the operation for that long. The doctor listened carefully and sympathetically but responded that there was nothing she could do.

Dejected by this news, Mr. S. pulled some strings with an old friend and got a meeting with a specialist in another major city. The specialist said he could get him in for surgery in about 2 weeks.

Mr. S. was pleased about this but curious about the reason for the difference in waiting lists between the two cities. He investigated and discovered that 5 years earlier,

the regional board for the city where he lives had decided to spend more money on prevention, and consequently, to spend less on acute care.

The regional board in the other city, however, considered and rejected this option and decided instead to ensure that programs such as the coronary bypass program were well funded.

According to a recent newspaper article, the prevention program has been very successful. The incidence of heart disease in Mr. S.'s region has decreased by 5% and is a full 10% lower than in the region to which he travelled for the bypass. "Maybe the board in my region made the right decision," he remarked to his wife, "but I'm sure glad I won't have to suffer its negative consequences."

Discussion Questions
1. Given the information above, which board do you think made the right decision, and why?
2. Is it consistent with the "equal access" stipulation in the *Canada Health Act* that there should be such great variation in waiting lists between different regions in the same province?

Source: Government of Canada. (2004). *Canada Health Action: Building on the Legacy. Volume II: Synthesis Reports and Issues Papers* (Appendix A, Scenario 2). Retrieved from https://www.canada.ca/en/health-canada/services/health-care-system/reports-publications/health-care-renewal/canada-health-action-building-legacy-volume2.html. © All rights reserved. Organization of Health Canada: Branches and Agencies. Health Canada, 2017. Adapted and reproduced with permission from the Minister of Health, 2019.

Functions of Regional Health Authorities. The exact functions of RHAs across provinces and territories vary but in general include the following:

- Assessing health needs of the population in its region
- Developing policy and program priorities within the region and related allocation of resources
- Administering funding, including allocating funds to community and nongovernmental organizations for primary care
- Planning and coordinating service delivery, including planning of capital projects
- Guaranteeing reasonable access to high-quality health services in a coordinated and integrated system of care
- Maintaining liaisons with community agencies and with the provincial and territorial ministry of health
- Managing and operating service delivery and financing of institutions, including hospitals, long-term care, and other health services centres
- Evaluating health system outputs and outcomes
- Promoting public participation in the decision-making process (Martin et al., 2018)

EXERCISE 14.1 *ONLINE RESEARCH:* Do a quick on-line search to see if the RHAs in your province have changed. What has happened and why? If the RHAs in your province have not changed, how are they functioning compared with the list of functions (see Functions of Regional Health Authorities) of RHAs? Do you think there is change coming? Why or why not?

Core Health Services. The following are core services that are administered and funded by provincial and territorial RHAs:

- Public health
- Home care and community-based services
- Mental health services
- Long-term care institutions
- Substance use programs (Barker & Church, 2017)

Hospitals are governed or funded by RHAs in all Canadian jurisdictions with regional structures and are considered private and not for profit. In Quebec, the *Act to Modify the Organization and Governance of the Health and Social Services Network* came into force in 2015. This Act abolished the regional agencies and now includes the following:

- Twenty-two integrated health and social services centres, 9 of which named university health and social services integrated centres. Only integrated centres located in a health region where a university offers a complete undergraduate medical program or operates a university institute in the social field are entitled to use the wording "university health and social services integrated centre" in their title.
- Seven institutions that were not amalgamated with an integrated centre, of which 4 are university hospital centres (CHU) and three are university institutes (IU)
- Five institutions not covered by the Act that offer services to an Indigenous and northern population.
- Hospitals in Manitoba and Ontario have the option of maintaining individual boards.

There are some key services that continue to be administered and funded centrally by provincial and territorial governments, and the most significant services are physicians services, with the exception of salaried physicians; prescription drugs except for the Northwest Territories; and cancer services (Government of Northwest Territories, n.d.).

Funding Formulas. To increase the effectiveness of RHAs, which were usually only advisory in nature, most provinces and territories have passed legislation to restructure their ministries of health and devolve financial decision making and planning and prioritizing activities. With cuts at all level of government, one potential reason for restructuring was to transfer difficult funding decisions to the regional level during a time of downsizing, so the provincial government does not have to bear the blame for unpopular decisions.

In general, provincial legislation has changed funding formulas to allow for the devolution of decision making. Whereas the provincial and territorial ministries collect taxes to finance the health care system and develop regional funding envelopes, regional health boards allocate funds to service organizations based on their own needs assessments and policy priorities. RHAs are accountable to the provincial or territorial governments for the money they spend and for the decisions they make. A **population needs-based funding formula (PNBF)** for the provision of health services is how many RHAs and governments are determining how and where to spend health care dollars. The PNBF is based on the characteristics and need of a population (i.e., the number of chronic versus acutely ill individuals, the number and type of accidents and injuries). For example, in Quebec, government funding to regions is based on needs assessments and population counts. Each district can borrow the money but is not allowed to tax local communities. Alberta, Saskatchewan, and Newfoundland and Labrador have adopted a population needs-based funding model. Other provinces and territories are also moving toward funding formulas based on population needs. Funding for physician remuneration through provincial health insurance plans is, as a rule, maintained as a separate budget category within ministry (not regional board) budgets (see Chapter 15); consequently, physicians have not been integrated into any regionalization within Canada (Marchildon, 2016).

Different concerns about regionalization have been expressed from different perspectives. Concerns about regionalization generally include the notions that regional boards create more government bureaucracy instead of increasing responsiveness to local needs and that appointed rather than elected board members may cause the positive aspects of accountability to be lost. There are also concerns about regional boundaries and the maintenance of freedom of consumers to choose their health care provider regardless of region and about funding envelopes and resource allocation mechanisms, especially with regard to specialized tertiary and quaternary care centres (e.g., does a region with highly specialized hospitals pay for the services of those hospitals that serve multiple regions?). In addition, in an era of fiscal restraint, many public health activists fear that public health and community services will lose in the funding allocation struggle as each board identifies which services it can and will fund.

Functional Organization of Provincial Ministries of Health

The role of the provincial and territorial ministries of health, in most cases, has been revised to meet the increased role of regional and local boards. In most cases, ministries have devolved service delivery responsibilities to regional boards while maintaining responsibility for overall health sector planning, corporate services, financing and the administration of funding envelopes, the administration of provincial and territorial insurance plans covering physician remuneration, evaluation and monitoring, and the management of computerized information systems. The main exception to this trend is the Ontario Ministry of Health and Long-Term Care, in which the organizational structure remains more or less unchanged and oriented toward financing individual hospitals and agencies rather than regional boards.

Because the administrative structures of provincial and territorial health ministries are constantly changing, no organizational chart of the ministries is included here; for up-to-date information, readers are advised to visit the websites of each provincial and territorial ministry of health. However, the functional organization remains stable. Provincial and territorial health responsibilities fall into three areas: service delivery, financing of health services, and administrative services (Table 14.1).

Service Delivery

Service delivery involves services that, in most provinces and territories, fall under the jurisdiction of the ministry of health with regard to budget, policies, and control. For the most part, the actual delivery of health services

---

TABLE 14.1   Functions of Provincial and Territorial Health Systems

Service Delivery	Service Financing (Direct or via Regional Health Board)	Administrative Services
Services for tuberculosis and cancer patients	Public health services[a]	Health services planning
Health services in remote areas	Homecare programs	Health human resources planning, training, and regulation
Ambulance services	Mental health services	Standard setting for health institutions and public places
Public health laboratories	Hospital and medical care	Health research
	Dental care	Health surveillance (communicable disease control)
	Prescription drugs	Emergency health services
	Services for allied health professionals	Vital statistics
	Other services, e.g., health appliances and equipment	
	Services for welfare recipients	

[a]Most provinces, except Ontario.

is now the responsibility of regional health boards, with the function of the ministry of health at the provincial and territorial level limited to financing health services, administration, and planning (see later). Thus, regionalization represents the centralization of most services to regional levels from local bodies and decentralization from the ministries of health.

Public Health Laboratories

Public health laboratories assist with the identification and control of epidemic and endemic diseases. All provinces and territories maintain a central public health laboratory, and most have branch laboratories to assist local health departments and the medical profession in the protection of community health and the control of infectious diseases.

Occupational Health

Services designed to prevent accidents and occupational diseases and to maintain the health of employees are the common concern of provincial and territorial health departments, labour departments, workers' compensation boards, industrial management, and unions (see Chapter 12).

Emergency Health Services

All provinces and territories have emergency health services that deal with the transportation of patients from their homes or institutions to service-providing institutions, either in their community or farther away. This is accomplished by land, air, or water ambulance systems. In Manitoba, Quebec, and New Brunswick, RHAs are responsible for these services; in other provinces and territories, the municipalities or provincial and territorial departments are responsible for service provision and the provinces and territories set standards. All provinces and territories have emergency or disaster plans for such situations as ice storms, floods, forest fires, chemical spills, rail derailment, or threats of biological or nuclear warfare.

In most emergency situations, Health Canada works closely with the provinces and territories and local health officials. Cooperation can include working together on emergency preparedness, intelligence gathering, disease surveillance, detection, and diagnosis, as well as on keeping the public informed during emergency situations, training first-responders (ambulance, fire, police, and emergency room staff), providing on-site field hospitals and pharmaceutical and medical supplies, protecting assets, decontaminating affected sites, and maintaining emergency equipment.

Health Canada also leads a provincial and territorial emergency response team that convenes during times of crisis. On the morning of September 11, 2001, for example, Health Canada's Centre for Emergency Preparedness and Response activated its Emergency Response Centre on a round-the-clock basis. Early links were established with provincial emergency response coordinators, the Office of Critical Infrastructure Protection and Emergency Response (OCIPEP), and the United States Department of Health and Human Services Office of Emergency Preparedness.

Service Financing

As indicated, all of the services listed in Table 14.1 are financed totally or partially by the provincial and territorial governments. As a result, provinces and territories exert pressure on professionals and institutions for setting standards for the services and controlling costs. Provinces and territories try to manage the system through their financial clout.

Health Insurance Programs

The basic principles of hospital and medical insurance stated by the federal government are described in Chapter 15, so only the relevant features of the provincial programs are described here (see also Box 14.1). In some provinces and territories, the administration of the hospital insurance plan and the medical insurance plan is combined, but in others, the two plans have separate administrative structures.

Health insurance coverage is automatic and compulsory across Canada, requiring only some form of registration. All provinces and territories, except Alberta and British Columbia, fund their health care only through general revenues or a levy on payrolls, or both. Alberta and British Columbia also have a component of premiums based on income. Coverage for insured services is available to all Canadian residents on equal terms and conditions and cannot be denied on grounds of age, income, or pre-existing conditions.

EXERCISE 14.2: What nonphysician services are available outside the hospital in your area?

Map out on a geographical city/area map where these services and programs are located. What do you notice about their location? Who are they serving? Who are they not serving?

The federal government has established a Health Insurance Supplementary Fund (administered by the Canada Health Act Division) with provincial and territorial contributions to provide for payment of claims for hospital or medical services for residents of Canada who have lost coverage through no fault of their own. This might occur, for example, if someone changing residence was not recognized as eligible under the rules of any province. It would not apply if coverage was lost through the individual's own fault, as in nonpayment of premiums. Contributions to the fund are made by all provinces and territories in proportion to population and are matched by the federal government. Those that charge premiums make some provision to cover those unable to pay (e.g., welfare recipients and those whose incomes are slightly above the poverty level) through full and partial subsidies. All provinces and territories also provide additional services for recipients of public assistance and for those older than 65 years of age. These commonly include prescription drugs and may also include dental services, eyeglasses, prostheses, home-care services, and nursing home care, depending on the province. Additionally, provinces and territories such as Ontario, Manitoba, Saskatchewan, and British Columbia provide limited insurance coverage for the services of chiropractors, podiatrists, and optometrists, often for specific populations only. Usually there is a dollar limit on these services covered.

The Alberta Health Care Insurance Plan offers additional health insurance to residents who cannot obtain Alberta Blue Cross coverage through an employer on an individual basis at special rates. Two government-sponsored supplementary health programs are available from Alberta Blue Cross (Alberta Health Services, 2018): (1) nongroup coverage for Alberta residents younger than 65 years of age whose Alberta Health Care Plan premiums are paid and who are not eligible to receive the Alberta Widows' Pension and (2) coverage for seniors for Albertans 65 years of age and older and their spouses and dependants and all recipients of the Alberta Widows' Pension and their dependants. Benefits of each program include maximum amounts per year, depending on the benefit. For example, diabetic supplies are covered up to a maximum of $600 per eligible person each benefit year. Diabetic supplies include needles, syringes, lancets, and both blood glucose and urine testing strips. Coverage for clinical psychological services are up to $60 per visit, to a maximum of $300 per family each benefit year, for treatment of mental or emotional illness by a registered chartered psychologist.

Drug Plans

All countries with universal health insurance systems also provide universal coverage of prescription drugs, with the exception of Canada. However, in 2018, talks between the provincial leaders and the federal government were underway, with online public consultations taking place. Eric Hoskins, the former Ontario health minister was appointed as head of the federal advisory council on how to implement a national pharmacare program, and he has been working with the provincial premiers on a strategy.

The greatest concern regarding implementing a national pharmacare program is the cost. A study by Morgan et al. (2015) estimated that by implementing a universal public drug program, Canada would reduce total spending on prescription medications by $7.3 billion per year, or 32%. The private sector (employers and unions) would save $8.2 billion, but costs to government could increase by about $1.0 billion, related to the potential of inappropriate use of medications (Morgan et al., 2015). Medications continue to consume an increasing share of Canada's health care dollar and currently account for the second largest category of health expenditure next to hospital services.

In Canada, prescription medications are generally financed through a combination of public funding (provincial–territorial and federal government) and

---

BOX 14.1 Have You Read Lately?

The *Canada Health Act* Annual *Report*, published by Health Canada, accounts the extent to which provincial and territorial health care insurance plans have satisfied the criteria and the conditions for payment under the Act. It is an excellent source of details on the functioning of the health insurance plans in each province. The Minster of Health in the 2016 annual report stated the following:

Canadians should have equitable access to required medical care based on their need and not on their ability, and willingness, to pay. This is why the Prime Minister has charged me with the responsibility to Promote and defend the Canada Health Act *to make absolutely clear that extra-billing and user fees are illegal under Canada's public Medicare system, and develop policies in collaboration with provinces and territories to improve verification and recourse mechanisms when instances of non-compliance arise (Health Canada, 2018k).*

TABLE 14.2 Overview of Characteristics of Publicly Funded Drug Plans Across Canadian Provinces and Territories

Province and Territory	Number of Plans	COMMON TARGET POPULATIONS FOR PUBLICLY FUNDED DRUG PLANS (X) AND WHETHER COVERAGE IS SUBJECT TO A PREMIUM		
		General Population	Seniors[a]	Social
Alberta	10	Premiums	Yes	Yes
British Columbia	10	Yes	Born before 1939	Yes
Saskatchewan	11	Yes	Yes	Yes
Manitoba	5	Yes	Same as general population	Yes
Ontario	7	Yes	Yes	Yes
Quebec[b]	1	Premiums	Premiums	Yes
Newfoundland and Labrador	5	Yes	Yes	Yes
Nova Scotia	5	Yes	Premiums	Yes
New Brunswick	10	Premiums	Low income only	Yes
Prince Edward Island	27	Combination of plans[c]	Yes	Yes
Yukon	3	Chronic disease plan	Yes	No
Northwest Territories	3	Specified disease conditions	Older than 60 yr	No
Nunavut	5	Chronic disease plan	Yes	No

[a]Older 65 years of age unless otherwise denoted.
[b]All persons are mandated to have insurance (private or public).
[c]Prince Edward Island has a variety of disease- and drug-based plans for those under 65 years of age.
Source: Adapted from Clement, F., Soril, L., Emery, H., et al. (2016). *Canadian publicly funded prescription drug plans, expenditures and an overview of patient impacts* (Table 1, p. 9). Retrieved from https://obrieniph.ucalgary.ca/system/files/comparison-of-canadian-publicly-funded-drug-plans-for-alberta-health-feb-1-2016.pdf.

nongovernment sources (third-party private insurance or out of pocket). Currently, most Canadians (95%) are covered by public or private drug plans; however, not all Canadians (only 11.3%) are enrolled for either public or private coverage despite being eligible; the remaining 5% have no coverage at all. Generally, all provinces and territories use a number of plans (range, 1–27) to offer financial assistance for many drug categories across a wide range of populations (e.g., seniors, those on social assistance, and the general population younger than 65 years of age) (Table 14.2). Many programs also target patients who have specific diseases (e.g., cancer), low-income families, and those with a high medication burden.

All provinces and territories have public prescription drug programs for recipients of social assistance, and seniors (except in New Brunswick, where eligibility in the government-sponsored drug plan is based on income). For seniors, Quebec and Nova Scotia offer plans to seniors with premiums, and Alberta, Quebec, and New Brunswick offer plans to the general population with a premium. Of special note: Quebec has mandated that all persons have drug insurance (either public or private) with an out-of-pocket cap no greater than

$1 046 for all residents, whether under employer-sponsored programs or the provincial program. Most provinces and territories provide drugs for the treatment of sexually transmitted infections, tuberculosis, and other infections that pose a public health hazard, and for which treatment costs are very high (e.g., cystic fibrosis, AIDS). The federal government assumes the full cost of providing prescription drugs for some Indigenous populations and certain armed forces veterans. The *Canada Health Act* includes drugs and biological and related preparations administered in the hospital within the definition of hospital services.

It is hoped that the implementation of a national pharmacare program will mean that issues relating to inequities that exist across provinces and within populations will be decreased as Canada moves towards a more equity-oriented health system.

Dental Plans

Good oral health is a key factor in general well-being and quality of life. However, inequities in access to dentistry or oral care exist in Canada, whereby insured people receive subsidized dental services, and people with relatively low incomes and limited public benefits must pay for dental care out of their own pockets. Private health insurance plays a crucial role in the provision of dental care in Canada. Approximately 60% of all private dental care expenditures originate from private insurance sources and 40% directly out of pocket (CIHI, 2015b). Most provinces and territories provide emergency basic dental health services to children, adults, and seniors on social assistance. A few provinces and territories, such as British Columbia, Quebec, Newfoundland, and Labrador, have special provision for children's dental programs, mainly in the area of preventive dentistry. The federal government provides basic dental services to those with recognized Indigenous status, with three delivery options: fee for service, contract session, or salaried staff.

Administrative Services

Administrative services are those operational functions that government undertakes to plan, forecast, and evaluate necessary services.

Planning of Health Services

All provincial and territorial ministries of health have a group of civil servants who, with the help of outside consultants, do short- and long-range planning of health services. These groups may be loosely structured or have a defined status within the ministry, such as the division of strategic health planning within the Ministry of Health and Long-Term Care in Ontario.

Often the minister, recognizing the deficit in services, appoints a special committee composed of selected citizens and professionals who receive support from civil servants. The task of these committees is to recommend mechanisms for delivering health services to the population or sub-groups of the population. Recent reports are listed in references (see also Chapter 18).

The ministry of health in many provinces and territories actively assesses the future needs for health human resources. Most provinces and territories go through the cycle of over and undersupply of their health human resources. At the time of writing, all provinces and territories are faced with undersupply of health professionals (e.g., doctors and nurses), especially in rural and remote areas in Canada. Many provinces have taken active steps to increase the number of students admitted into these professional schools or to facilitate licensing of foreign-trained professionals. When there is a lack of human resources, subsidies or student loan forgiveness have been provided to students entering that profession. Several provincial and territorial governments provide incentives for recruitment and retention of health care practitioners in rural areas.

Regulation of Health Professions

The established health professions, including medicine, nursing, chiropractors, dentistry, and pharmacy, are regulated by their respective licensing bodies, which are mandated by provincial and territorial legislation. Other health professionals and technicians are also usually regulated or certified (for details, see Chapter 17).

Standard Setting for Health Institutions and Public Places

All acute, chronic, rehabilitation, extended care, and mental health hospitals are governed by specific legislation. Standards are set for nursing homes in many provinces and territories as well. There are definite standards and guidelines for public places, such as restaurants, food-handling venues, industries, and factories. Legislation usually emanates from within the civil service or from concerned members of the legislature.

EXERCISE 14.3 *DEBATE A TOPIC OF PROVINCIAL IMPORTANCE RELATED TO HEALTH:* A debate is a particular way to explore opinions and perspectives. It starts with a proposed action. An individual presents reasons and evidence for supporting the action. Then another person presents the opposite viewpoint: reasons and evidence for not supporting the action. The discussion goes back and forth, like a tennis match, as different ideas are brought forward, first on one side and then on the other. (A good source to guide how to structure your debate can be found at https://www.debatingsa.com.au/wp-content/uploads/2017/07/Debating-An-Introduction-For-Beginners.pdf.)

Debate a current event topic you identify from TV, the radio, or in your local newspaper regarding health care organization or design. For example, you could choose to debate that a national drug program will save the province money, and your opponents would debate that a national drug program will cost the province more money.

CRITICAL THINKING QUESTIONS 14.3:
1. How does the structure of health services in your province or territory help you participate in them?
2. Why do you think Saskatchewan and Quebec's organization of health departments looks different than those of many of the remaining provinces?

SUMMARY

This chapter dealt with the types of health services provided by the federal and provincial and territorial governments.

At the time of Confederation, the federal government had relatively little jurisdiction and involvement in the health care of Canadians. In 1919, the Department of Health was established, and its responsibilities included "all matters relating to the promotion or preservation of health, social security and social welfare of the people of Canada over which the Parliament of Canada has jurisdiction." In 1945, Health and Welfare Canada was created, with two primary tasks: (1) to promote, preserve, and restore the health of Canadians and (2) to provide social security and social welfare to Canadians. In 1993, the Welfare Department of the ministry was separated. The federal ministry of health is now known as Health Canada and is composed of six branches: (1) Chief Financial Officer Branch, (2) Communications and Public Affairs Branch, (3) First Nations and Inuit Health Branch, (4) HPFB, (5) Healthy Environments and Consumer Safety Branch, and (6) Strategic Policy Branch. There are also several offices and bureaus that make up Health Canada, including the Audit and Evaluation Bureau, Departmental Secretariat, Legal Services, Pest Management Regulatory Agency, and Regions and Programs Bureau.

Two branches are of particular relevance to public health: the SPB plays a lead role in health policy, communications and consultations. The HECS Branch is responsible for promoting safe living, working, and recreational environments, including occupational health and regulating tobacco and controlled substances, and it provides drug analytical services, regulates the safety of industrial and consumer products in the Canadian marketplace, and promotes their safe use.

The Employment and Social Development Canada (ESDC) programs of the Ministry of Families, Children and Social Development also influence health. They promote and strengthen the income security of Canadians; share in the cost of provincial and territorial social assistance; welfare services, and rehabilitation programs; and assist in the development of social services to meet changing social needs.

As noted in earlier chapters, provincial and territorial governments have primary responsibility for all personal health matters, such as disease prevention, treatment, and maintenance of health. Activities such as preventive health services, hospital services, treatment services for tuberculosis and other chronic diseases, and rehabilitation and care of people who are chronically ill and disabled are all under the jurisdiction of the provincial and territorial governments. The responsibilities of the provincial and territorial governments can be classified as service financing, service delivery, and administrative services.

In the 1990s, most provinces and territories in Canada partially devolved their service delivery responsibility to subprovincial regions, resulting in the establishment of RHAs everywhere except in Ontario. However, a more recent trend is to amalgamate all the RHAs in a province into one health authority. Health, again, is being centralized in many provinces. The objective of RHAs was to streamline the delivery system, making it less fragmented and more responsive to local needs. In some provinces and territories, additional goals were to increase community-based services, improve public participation in health care, and encourage policies and programs to promote health. RHAs and health authorities are autonomous health care organizations responsible for health administration within a defined geographic region within a province or territory. They have appointed or elected boards of governance and are responsible for funding and delivering community and institutional health services within their regions.

Regional health authorities and health authorities fund and administer core services, including public health, home care and community-based services, mental health services and long-term care institutions, alcohol and substance abuse programs, and hospitals. Whereas the provincial and territorial ministries collect taxes to finance the health care system and develop regional funding envelopes, regional health boards allocate funds to service organizations based on their own needs assessments and policy priorities. Health insurance claims covering physician remuneration and prescription drugs covered under the provincial plans remain, for the most part, under the administrative auspices of the province.

Service financing involves services that are paid for either totally or partially by either government-run health insurance programs (e.g., hospital and medical services provided by a physician) or by subsidizing the cost for services, drugs, or appliances.

Health insurance coverage is automatic and compulsory in all provinces and territories, requiring only some form of registration. All, except Alberta and British Columbia, fund their health care only through general revenues, a levy on payrolls, or both. Alberta and British Columbia also have a component of premiums based on income.

Most Canadians (95%) are covered by public or private drug plans. All provinces and territories except New Brunswick and Newfoundland and Labrador have public prescription drug plans for seniors (in these two provinces, seniors' eligibility is based on income), and coverage for the general population differs among the provinces and territories.

Most provinces and territories provide emergency basic dental health services to children, adults, and seniors on social assistance. Medical appliances and equipment comprise devices and equipment necessary or complementary to medical treatment. Provinces and territories differ in the benefits provided.

Administrative services are those operational functions that government undertakes to plan, forecast, and evaluate the necessary services.

KEY WEBSITES

Canada's National Centre for Occupational Health and Safety: https://www.ccohs.ca
This website provides links to Canadian occupational health and safety information that is provided by federal, provincial and territorial government agencies, Workers' Compensation Boards, and the Canadian Centre for Occupational Health and Safety. The site aims to make this information readily and easily accessible to Canadians in the continuing effort to prevent workplace injury and illness and help create healthy workplaces.

Canadian Partnership Against Cancer: https://www.partnershipagainstcancer.ca
This website provides current and relevant evidence-based information and data related to cancer control in Canada.

Mental Health Commission of Canada: https://mentalhealthcommission.ca/English
This website provides information for policy makers, health care providers, employers, and individuals interested in mental health issues.

National Collaborating Centres for Public Health: http://nccph.ca
This website provides information regarding research on public health and makes the information more relevant and understandable for individuals and organizations that could use this information in their day-to-day practices and in policy-making.

The Women's Health Bureau: http://www.cwhn.ca/en/node/39529
This website is bilingual and provides information for women's health, including breaking news, feature articles, webinars and podcasts, an online database, and links to other useful sites.

REFERENCES

Alberta Health Services. (2018). *Non-group coverage benefit.* Retrieved from http://www.health.alberta.ca/services/drugs-non-group.html#Benefits.

Barker, P., & Church, J. (2017). Revisiting health regionalization in Canada: More bark than bite? *International Journal of Health Services, 47*(2), 333–351.

Canadian Centre for Occupational Health & Safety. (2018). *WHMIS 2018 general.* Retrieved from http://www.ccohs.ca/oshanswers/chemicals/whmis_ghs/general.html.

Canadian Institute for Health Information. (2015a). *About CIHI.* Retrieved from https://www.cihi.ca/en/about-cihi.

Canadian Institute for Health Information. (2015b). *Expenditure trends, 1975 to 2015.* Ottawa: CIHI. Retrieved from https://www.cihi.ca/en/spending-and-health-workforce/spending/national-health-expenditure-trends.

Canadian Institute for Health Information. (2016). *Expenditure trends, 1975 to 2016.* Ottawa: CIHI. Retrieved from https://www.cihi.ca/sites/default/files/document/nhex-trends-narrative-report_2016_en.pdf.

Canadian Institute for Health Information. (2018). *National expenditure trends; Government of Canada, federal support to provinces and territories.* Retrieved from https://www.fin.gc.ca/fedprov/mtp-eng.asp.

Canadian Institutes for Health Research. (2018). *CIHR.* Retrieved from http://www.cihr-irsc.gc.ca/e/193.html.

Canadian Partnership Against Cancer. (2018). *Canadian Strategy for Cancer Control: 2017-2022: We see progress.* Toronto: Author. Retrieved from https://www.partnershipagainstcancer.ca/wp-content/uploads/2016/02/canadian-strategy-cancer-control-2017-2022-en.pdf.

Canadian Women's Health Network. (2018). *The Women's Health Bureau.* Retrieved from http://www.cwhn.ca/en/node/39529.

Dunn, C. (Ed.). (2016). *Provinces: Canadian provincial politics.* Toronto: University of Toronto Press.

Government of Canada. (2017). *Benefits.* Retrieved from https://www.canada.ca/en/services/benefits.html.

Government of Northwest Territories. (n.d.). *Supplemental health benefits.* Retrieved from https://www.hss.gov.nt.ca/en/services/supplementary-health-benefits/extended-health-benefits-specified-disease-conditions

Health Canada. (2003). *Natural health products in Canada—a history.* Retrieved from https://www.canada.ca/en/health-canada/services/drugs-health-products/natural-non-prescription/regulation/history.html.

Health Canada. (2014). *Healthy Environments and Consumer Safety Branch.* Retrieved from https://www.canada.ca/en/health-canada/corporate/about-health-canada/branches-agencies/healthy-environments-consumer-safety-branch.html.

Health Canada. (2015). *The federal initiative to address HIV/AIDS in Canada.* Retrieved from http://www.tbs-sct.gc.ca/hidb-bdih/plan-eng.aspx?Org=0&Hi=25&Pl=756.

Health Canada. (2017). *Food Directorate.* Retrieved from https://www.canada.ca/en/health-canada/corporate/about-health-canada/branches-agencies/health-products-food-branch/food-directorate.html.

Health Canada. (2018a). *Health Canada.* Retrieved from https://www.canada.ca/en/health-canada.html.

Health Canada. (2018b). *Health Canada's organizational structure.* Retrieved from https://www.canada.ca/en/health-canada/corporate/organizational-structure.html.

Health Canada. (2018c). *First Nations and Inuit Health.* Retrieved from https://www.canada.ca/en/indigenous-services-canada/services/first-nations-inuit-health.html.

Health Canada. (2018d). *Community Programs Directorate.* Retrieved from https://www.canada.ca/en/indigenous-services-canada/corporate/first-nations-inuit-health-branch/community-programs-directorate.html.

Health Canada. (2018e). *Public Health Care & Public Health Directorate.* Retrieved from https://www.canada.ca/en/indigenous-services-canada/corporate/first-nations-inuit-health-branch/primary-health-care-public-health-directorate.html.

Health Canada. (2018f). *Therapeutic Products Directorate.* Retrieved from https://www.canada.ca/en/health-canada/corporate/about-health-canada/branches-agencies/health-products-food-branch/therapeutic-products-directorate.html.

Health Canada. (2018g). *Regulations and compliance—nutrition labelling.* Retrieved from https://www.canada.ca/en/health-canada/services/food-nutrition/food-labelling/nutrition-labelling/regulations-compliance.html.

Health Canada. (2018h). *Programs and Policy Development PHAC.* Retrieved from https://www.canada.ca/en/public-health/programs.html.

Health Canada. (2018i). *Canada's tobacco strategy.* Retrieved from https://www.canada.ca/en/health-canada/services/publications/healthy-living/canada-tobacco-strategy.html.

Health Canada. (2018j). *Canada's healthy eating strategy.* Retrieved from https://www.canada.ca/en/services/health/campaigns/vision-healthy-canada/healthy-eating.html.

Health Canada. (2018k). *Canada Health Act Annual Report 2016-2017.* Retrieved from https://www.canada.ca/en/health-canada/services/publications/health-system-services/canada-health-act-annual-report-2016-2017.html.

Marchildon, G. P. (2016). *Regionalization: what have we learned?* Retrieved from https://www.ihf-fih.org/resources/pdf/Regionalization-HealthcareCan_June_8th.pdf.

Martin, D., Miller, A. P., Quesnel-Vallée, A., et al. (2018). Canada's universal health-care system: achieving its potential. *The Lancet, 391,* 1718–1735. https://doi.org/10.1016/S0140-6736(18)30181-8.

Mental Health Commission of Canada. (2018). *The mental health strategy for Canada: A framework for action (2017–2022).* Retrieved from https://www.mentalhealthcommission.ca/English/who-we-are/annual-report/framework-action-2017-2022.

Morgan, S. G., Law, M., Daw, J. R., et al. (2015). Estimated cost of universal public coverage of prescription drugs in Canada. *Canadian Medical Association Journal, 187*(7), 491–497. https://doi.org/10.1503/cmaj.141564.

Patented Medicine Prices Review Board. (2018). *About the PMPRB.* Ottawa. Retrieved from http://pmprb-cepmb.gc.ca/home.

Pest Management Regulatory Agency. (2009). *About PMRA.* Retrieved from https://www.canada.ca/en/health-canada/corporate/about-health-canada/branches-agencies/pest-management-regulatory-agency.html.

Statistics Canada. (2016). *Health regions. What are health regions?* Retrieved from http://www12.statcan.gc.ca/health-sante/82-228/help-aide/Q01.cfm?Lang=E.

Truth & Reconciliation Commission of Canada. (2015). *Truth and Reconciliation Commission of Canada: Calls to Action.* Winnipeg: Author. Retrieved from http://nctr.ca/assets/reports/Calls_to_Action_English2.pdf.

15

Funding, Expenditures, and Resources

ⓔ Additional resources are available online at http://evolve.elsevier.com/Canada/Shah/publichealth/

LEARNING OBJECTIVES

- Understand the funding and allocation of health resources.
- Describe strategies used by different levels of government to ensure that the principles of the *Canada Health Act* are being upheld.

- Explain the difference between public sector and private sector financing and expenditure.
- Understand health system performance and the associated indicators.
- Understand the concept of rationing in health care.

CHAPTER OUTLINE

KEY TERMS

alternate level of care (ALC)
Canadian Agency for Drugs and Technologies in
  Health (CADTH)
capitation system
design thinking
fee for service
health technology
home care
integrated delivery systems (IDS)

Lean
medical savings accounts (MSAs)
plan–do–study–act (PDSA)
quality assurance (QA)
rationalization of health services
sessional payments
total quality management (TQM)
Technology Assessment Iterative Loop (TAIL)

INTRODUCTION

The health care industry is the fifth largest industry in Canada and hires about 10% of the workforce. In 2017, total health care expenditures were forecast to be $242 billion CAD, or $6 604 per person (Canadian Institute Health Information [CIHI], 2017). Since the inception of national health insurance programs, constant concerns have been expressed about the financing and delivery of health care.

This chapter describes the financing of health care and the allocation of health resources in Canada. It also provides international comparisons, describes the strategies used by different levels of governments to ensure sustainability, accessibility, and availability of quality health services, and presents indicators that evaluate health system performance, using CIHI's Health System Performance Measurement Framework (HSPMF) (see Introduction).

A goal of the health care system is to provide value for money. *Value* is defined here as the ability of the health care system to balance the allocation of resources to obtain the best outcomes (health status, health system responsiveness and equity) for the resources used (CIHI, 2017).

THE FINANCING OF HEALTH CARE

One of the most basic series of questions about the organization of any health care system relates to the financing of health services: Where does the money for health care come from? Where should it come from? How is it collected? What services and what groups of people are covered?

As discussed in the previous two chapters, Canada does not have a single national health care system but rather has 10 provincial, 3 territorial, and federal systems, all operating under the same founding principles and guidelines. Thus, although every province autonomously makes its own health finance decisions, there are certain generalities that apply to all.

Sources of Health Care Financing

Both the public and private sectors finance Canada's health care systems, with a mix of both private and public funding. As noted in Table 15.1, these sectors are referred to as having various layers—public, public–private, and private.

- Layer one comprises public services (Medicare): medically necessary hospital, diagnostic, and physician services. These services are financed through general tax revenues and are provided free at the point of service, as required by the *Canada Health Act*.
- Layer two services are financed through a mix of public and private insurance coverage and out-of-pocket payments and include outpatient prescription drugs, home care, and institutional long-term care. Provinces and territories each have a diverse mix of public programs in this layer, without any national framework. For example, in some provinces, such as

TABLE 15.1	Funding Structure of the Health System in Canada			
	Services	**Funding**	**Administration**	**Delivery**
Layer one: public services (Medicare): all public funding	Hospitals Physicians Diagnostic	Public taxation	Universal single-payer systems Private self-regulating professions	Private professional for-profit and not-for-profit facilities, and public arm's length facilities
Layer two: mixed services: combination of public and private funding	Prescription drugs Home care Long-term care Mental health care	Public taxation Private insurance Out-of-pocket payments	Public coverage is targeted Public regulation of private services	Private professional for-profit and not-for-profit facilities, and public arm's length facilities
Layer three: private services: almost all private funding	Dental care Vision care Complementary medicine Outpatient physiotherapy	Primarily private insurance, out-of-pocket payments, with some public taxation	Private ownership Private professions Limited public regulation	Private professional for-profit facilities

Source: Reprinted with permission from Elsevier (Martin, D., Miller, A. P., Quesnel-Vallée, A., Caron, N. R., Vissandjée, B., & Marchildon, G. P. (2018). Canada's universal health-care system: achieving its potential. *The Lancet, 391*(10131), 1718–1735).

Ontario, all senior citizens older than 65 years of age have public prescription drug coverage (see Chapter 14), but in other provinces, such as British Columbia, drug coverage is income tested.

- Layer three services are financed almost entirely privately and include dental care, outpatient physiotherapy, and routine vision care for adults when provided by nonphysicians (Marchildon, 2013a).

Layer One: The Public Sector

The annual National Health Expenditure (NHEX) trends for 2017 reported that the public sector will pay for about 70% of total health expenditures (65% from the provincial and territorial governments and 5% from other parts of the public sector) (CIHI, 2017). Since 1997, the public sector share of total health expenditure has remained relatively stable at around 70%.

Public sector revenue includes federal, provincial or territorial, and municipal government revenues that are generated from general taxes and borrowing, as well as from social security funds such as workers' compensation funds and the Quebec Drug Insurance Fund. The individual pays the remainder either directly or through private health insurance (Fig. 15.1).

Federal Financing of Health Care. The federal government has a number of revenue streams, including personal income tax, the goods and services tax (GST), corporate income tax, and employee contributions to social insurance plans (payroll taxes) such

as Employment Insurance and the Canada Pension Plan. The federal government collects more in personal income tax in some provinces, primarily because income levels there are higher (Statistics Canada, 2018). Federal tax rates do not vary from one province to the next; however, the federal government generally collects more revenue in provinces where economic conditions are more favourable. The same holds true for the majority of its revenue sources. There is a redistributive effect to net federal expenditures in Canada: the federal government receives more tax revenues from certain provinces and spends more in others.

National health expenditures are based on the principle of responsibility for payment rather than the source of funds. Federal government transfers are therefore included in the provincial government sector. The federal government contributes to provincial revenue in the form of transfer payments, which are tax credits, and cash as agreed under the Canada Health Transfer (CHT) and the Canadian Social Transfer (CST) (see Chapter 13). Table 15.2 compares federal support to the provinces and territories in 2009 with the projected totals for 2019. Since 2009, there has been an approximate 20% increase in total federal support.

Provincial Financing of Health Care. In 2018 to 2019, provinces and territories received $75.4 billion through major transfers, which accounted for approximately 20% of provincial and territorial revenues. According to the *Canada Health Act,* each provincial health plan must

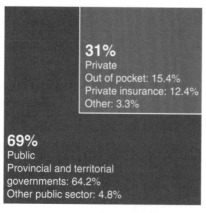
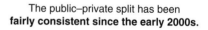
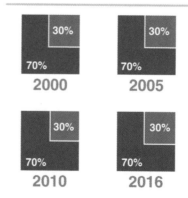

Fig. 15.1 Distribution of public and private sector health care financing. (From Canadian Institute Health Information. [2018]. *National health expenditure trends, 1975–2018* (Figure 5). Ottawa: Canadian Institute for Health Research. Retrieved from https://www.cihi.ca/sites/default/files/document/nhex-trends-narrative-report-2018-en-web.pdf.)

TABLE 15.2 Federal Support to Provinces and Territories, Comparing 2009 with 2019 (in millions of dollars)

Major Transfers	2009–2010	2018–2019[e]
CHT[a]	24 476	38 584
CST[b]	10 857	14 161
Equalization[c]	14 185	18 958
TFF[d]	2 498	3 785
Total federal support	52 736	75 393
Per capita allocation (dollars)	1 570	2 031

[a]Canada Health Transfer (CHT) includes transition protection payments for 2009 to 2010. It includes separate payments to Ontario in respect of the Canada Health Transfer for 2009 to 2010 ($489 million) to ensure Ontario receives the same CHT cash support as other equalization-receiving provinces.
[b]Canada Social Transfer (CST) includes transition protection payments in 2009 to 2010. It excludes $31.9 million from the 2008 budge transition protection payments to Saskatchewan ($31.2 million) and Nunavut ($0.7 million) notionally allocated over 5 and 3 years, respectively, beginning in 2008 to 2009.
[c]Includes payments and additional amounts. Also includes 2009 to 2010 transitional equalization protection to Nova Scotia and Manitoba.
[d]As approved by Parliament, Total Federal Support (TFF) payments include an additional $67 million to Yukon ($16 million), Northwest Territories ($24 million), and Nunavut ($26 million) in 2016 to 2017, stemming from the legislative amendments to enhance the stability and predictability of the program.
[e]CHT and CST amounts for 2018 to 2019 are preliminary. Final amounts for 2018 to 2019 will be determined in September 2019.
Adapted from Department of Finance Canada. (2017). Federal support to provinces and territories. Retrieved from https://www.fin.gc.ca/fedprov/mtp-eng.asp. Reproduced with the permission of the Department of Finance, 2019 (https://www.fin.gc.ca/fedprov/mtp-eng.asp).

cover all "medically necessary" health services delivered in hospital and by physicians. Provinces can choose to provide additional services, as described in Chapter 13.

In Canada, the bulk of total health care expenditures is financed from general revenue by provincial governments. Provincial government expenditure as a proportion of total expenditure gradually fell from 71.4% in 1995 to 64.9% in 1999 and 70% in 2017. The provinces generate their share of the revenue for the health expenditures as follows (CIHI, 2017).

- British Columbia, Ontario, and Quebec charge individual premiums to those who request medicare benefits. Ontario's and Quebec's premiums are remitted through personal income tax; British Columbia collects individual monthly premiums.

- British Columbia, Ontario, Manitoba, Newfoundland and Labrador, and Quebec levy payroll taxes on employers. Payroll taxes tend to be controversial because they do not spread the net as wide, and self-employed individuals escape the tax altogether. Overall, however, payroll taxes do not generate a significant portion of health revenues.

Premiums and payroll taxes do not cover health care spending. General revenue is the predominant funding resource available for health care.

Layer Two: Mixed Public–Private Sector

Provinces and territories each have a range of public programs in this layer, without any national framework. For example, in some provinces, such as Ontario, all senior citizens older than 65 years of age have public prescription drug coverage, but in others, such as British Columbia, drug coverage is income tested (CIHI, 2016a).

Layer Three: The Private Sector

Private sector spending accounted for the other 30% of total health expenditure in 2017. The private sector has three components, the largest of which is out-of-pocket spending (15%), followed by private health insurance (12%) and nonconsumption (3%). Out-of-pocket expenditures include dental and other services, such as those delivered by alternative health care providers not covered by government insurance, and payments for extra services such as private hospital rooms. Some provinces have recently also shifted costs to the private sector for rehabilitative care as a result of motor vehicle collisions by charging personal automobile insurance policies for these fees.

CRITICAL THINKING QUESTION 15.1: What are the benefits and drawbacks of having the federal government transfer money to the provinces versus having a federal system that is fully responsible for the health-care needs of Canadians?

HEALTH EXPENDITURES

Overall Expenditures

In Canada, the ever-increasing growth of health care expenditure has become a great concern for both governments and the public. One concern is the aging population. By 2030, the growing number of seniors is projected to cost the Canadian health care system $24 billion more annually (50% more than today) (Ontario Seniors' Secretariat, 2013). Addressing the delivery of health care services to reduce expenditures and optimally meet the needs of this population are key priorities. See the Critical Thinking Question box for ethical questions related to health expenditures.

It was anticipated that, overall, health expenditure would represent 11.5% of Canada's gross domestic product (GDP) in 2017. The trend over the past 40+ years shows that when there is more economic growth, more is spent on health care (CIHI, 2017). The total health expenditures per capita varies per province and territory because of variety of different factors, including age distribution, population density, geography, population health needs, the organization and financing of health care delivery, and differences in the remuneration of health care workers across the country. The health expenditure per capita is highest in the territories because of their large geographical area and low population density. In the provinces in 2017, total health expenditure per capita was forecast to range from $7 378 in Newfoundland and Labrador and $7 329 in Alberta to $6 367 in Ontario and $6 321 in British Columbia

(CIHI, 2017). Table 15.3 summarizes the three greatest health care expenditures—hospitals, drugs, and physician services throughout Canada.

Health System Sustainability

For several decades now, concerns keep being raised that publicly funded health care is unsustainable. Arguments regarding sustainability have centred around overspending, underfunding, poorly distributed and misdirected spending, and ineffectively managed resources (Deber, 2017). The debates have often focused on the relative importance of provincial revenues and federal transfers in funding the health care system (CIHI, 2017). Projected cost increases combined with pressures health care providers experience addressing health care needs with the resources available supports the argument of unsustainability. Access issues, quality and safety concerns, increasing wait times, increasing prevalence of chronic diseases, the aging population, expensive treatments, and new technologies are all impacting health care costs.

However, not everyone holds the view that the health care system is unsustainable. In his historic report on health care in Canada, Roy Romanow concluded that our health care system was "as sustainable as we want

TABLE 15.3   Provincial and Territorial Health Expenditures on Hospital, Drugs, and Physician Services in 2018

Province or Territory	HOSPITALS		DRUGS		PHYSICIANS	
	Per capita Expenditure ($)	Annual Growth Rate (%)	Per capita Expenditure ($)	Annual Growth Rate (%)	Per capita Expenditure ($)	Annual Growth Rate (%)
Newfoundland & Labrador	2 622	1.3	1 040	2.6	929	0.3
Prince Edward Island	2 211	0.6	927	1.1	958	2.3
Nova Scotia	2 295	0.7	1 192	3.4	937	3.8
New Brunswick	2 283	3.2	1 198	2.0	900	2.0
Quebec	1 618	5.6	1 186	2.1	994	2.1
Ontario	1 766	3.5	1 119	4.3	1 024	2.1
Manitoba	2 275	1.1	841	1.1	1 077	1.8
Saskatchewan	1 929	0.9	937	2.0	992	1.3
Alberta	2 483	0.5	1 054	3.4	1 238	1.7
British Columbia	2 100	3.1	838	2.4	982	2.9
Yukon Territory	2 719	-2.7	870	1.6	1 270	4.7
Northwest Territories	6 428	4.5	855	3.5	479	3.3
Nunavut	5 390	3.4	737	0.0	1 721	-3.7
Canada	**1 933**	**3.0**	**1 074**	**3.2**	**1 032**	**2.2**

Source: Canadian Institute for Health Information. (2018). *National health expenditures trends, 1975 to 2018* (p. 16). Retrieved from https://www.cihi.ca/sites/default/files/document/nhex-trends-narrative-report-2018-en-web.pdf.

it to be" (Romanow, 2002, p. xv). Concerns about unsustainability have provided an impetus for proposed reforms, resulting in a number of commissions, reports, and changes to Canada's health care system (see Chapters 14 and 18). A targeted reform is the payment of physicians on a fee-for-service basis, with Romanow affirming that "Paying physicians for each separate service they provide can create a perverse incentive to focus on the quantity of services provided rather than on the quality of services, in order to maximize physician's income" (p. 124). Other payment models discussed later in the chapter also have drawbacks. Alternative models need to consider incentives for providing care that is focused on prevention, within a primary health care philosophy that uses interprofessional team-based health care providers to address population needs (see Chapter 16). Moving the health care system from a sickness care system to addressing the social determinants of health, where health is conceptualized not only as the absence of disease but also as a resource for everyday life, requires a major transformation in politicians' and decision-makers' thinking.

Trends in Health Care Expenditures

Figure 15.2 shows that after many years of steady increases, the percent of GDP spent on health care in Canada declined in the mid 1990s and is now slowly increasing to its previous level. In 1999, Canada spent 9.2% of its GDP on health care, an increase from the 1996 level of 8.9% but lower than the 1992 level of 9.9%. The first significant rise was in the late 1960s, following the introduction of universal health insurance. By the early 1970s, the federal and provincial governments became alarmed by this rapid rise and set up a task force on the cost of health services, which delivered its report in 1970. Attempts to control the level of health expenditure met with temporary success during the 1970s. The proportion of GDP declined initially and then levelled off to 6.8% in 1979, although both the actual dollars and per capita dollars spent had risen. Since 1980, it has been rising again. (See Box 15.1 for information about GDP.)

International Comparisons

Among 35 Organisation for Economic Co-operation and Development (OECD) countries in 2015 (the latest year for which comparable data was available),

> **BOX 15.1 Gross Domestic Product as an Indicator of Progress**
>
> Gross domestic product (GDP) is considered the "world's most powerful statistical indicator of national development and progress" (Lepenies, 2016). However, it is not without its critics. Noble Laureate Amartya Sen suggests that an increase in a country's GDP or in GDP growth does not necessarily lead to a higher standard of living, particularly in areas such as health care and education (Drèze and Sen, 2013).

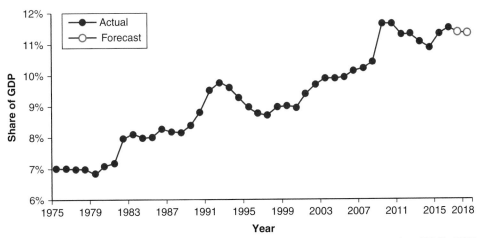

Fig. 15.2 Trends in health expenditures in Canada, percentage of gross domestic product (GDP), 1975 to 2018. (From Canadian Institute Health Information. [2018]. *National health expenditure trends, 1975–2018 (Figure 2)*. Ottawa: Canadian Institute for Health Information. Retrieved from https://www.cihi.ca/sites/default/files/document/nhex-trends-narrative-report-2018-en-web.pdf.)

spending per person on health care remained highest in the United States (CAD $12 865) (CIHI, 2018). Caution should be taken when making cross-country comparisons, however, because countries include different types of expenditures when calculating total health expenditures. For example, Germany excludes expenditures for health research, military health, and prison health, as well as private household expenditures on patient transport and patient care when calculating its total health expenditure, but these expenditures are included in the Canadian determination.

Canada's per capita spending on health care was fifth among the OECD countries, at CAD $6 082 (Fig. 15.3). However, public sector funding in Canada is lower than some other developed nations, where the average is 75%. Figures indicate that the public sector funding for health

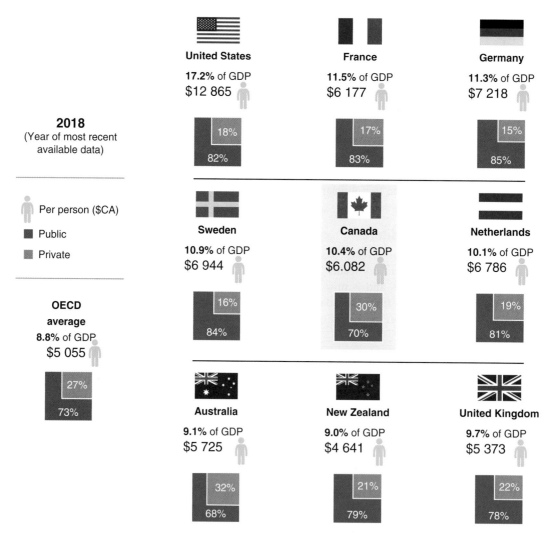

NOTES:

Total current expenditure (capital excluded).

Expenditure data is based on the System of Health Accounts.

Fig. 15.3 Health care expenditures in Organisation for Economic Co-operation and Development countries in Canadian dollars. (From Canadian Institute Health Information. [2018]. *National health expenditure trends, 1975–2018* (p. 10, Figure 4). Retrieved from https://www.cihi.ca/sites/default/files/document/nhex-trends-narrative-report-2018-en-web.pdf.)

care in Canada has declined since 1983, when the total public sector share of health expenditures was 76.6%. The private share of health care expenditure has increased from 23.4% in 1983 to 30% in 2018 (CIHI, 2018).

Many other factors contribute to these international variations in health care expenditures. As described in Chapter 13, health care systems differ widely in their sources of funding, including the balance of private and public funding. They also vary in the degree and form of state planning, the remuneration of health care professionals (particularly physicians), and the nature of services provided. Thus, international comparisons are of questionable significance: they tell us *what* nations spent but little, if anything, about *how* they spent it—the mix of services, possible duplication of facilities, physician-to-population ratios, health care needs, or system inefficiencies. There is no evidence that Americans, for example, are healthier because their country spends a higher share of its GDP on health care.

One significant difference between the health care system in the United States and Canada is the administrative cost (see Chapter 13). In the United States, which has voluntary medical and hospital insurance systems, 12% to 18% of spending goes to administrative overhead, but Canadian administrative costs are less than 2.5%. Furthermore, there are savings in Canadian hospital administrative costs because there is no need to list the price of every service, bandage, and pill on the patient's bill. The savings in accounting, nurses' time, and paperwork are large.

Moreover, there are savings in the more rational distribution of high technology such as magnetic resonance imaging scanners, which US hospitals acquire for competitive reasons and then frequently underuse. The Canadian single-payer system—the provincial government—pays for hospitals and physicians. Provincial governments are directly responsible for the overall allocation and coordination of resources to the health services sector. This avoids the fragmentation of decision making and wasteful competition for resources that can occur when independent nonprofit or fee-for-service providers seek financing from a variety of private and public sources.

Although Canadians are faced with their own set of health system challenges, the single-payer financing system, together with universal coverage for all Canadians, has proven to be more effective than the US market system of health for controlling overall health expenditures, but less effective than the systems of some European countries (Deber, 2017).

Public Sector Expenditures

Table 15.4 summarizes the percentage distribution of total health expenditures by category of expenditure for 2018. The largest category of spending is hospitals, at 28.3%, followed by prescription and nonprescription drugs at 15.4% and physicians at 15.1%, which accounts for a total of 58.8% of the total health expenditure (CIHI, 2018).

Hospital Spending. For two decades, Canada's inpatient hospital sector has been shrinking. In the mid-1970s, hospital spending made up 45% of total health expenditure compared with 28.3% in 2017. Spending on hospitals in 2017 was estimated to grow by 2.9%. Fewer patients are hospitalized overnight each year, and those who are admitted stay, on average, for shorter periods. On average, the per diem cost in acute care hospitals is usually two to three times higher than that in long-term care hospitals.

TABLE 15.4 **Distribution of Health Expenditures by Category of Expenditures, 2018**		
Use of Funds	**Per Capita Health Expenditure ($)**	**Share of Health Expenditure (%)**
Hospitals	1 871	28.3
Drugs: prescribed	909	13.3
Drugs: nonprescribed	166	2.4
Physicians	1 032	15.1
Other institutions	768	11.2
Other professionals: dental services	461	6.7
Other professionals: vision care services	140	2.0
Other professionals: other health professionals	157	2.3
Other health spending (OHS)	369	5.4
OHS: health research	112	1.6
Public health	383	5.6
Capital	225	3.3
Administration	186	2.7

OHS: Other Health Spending.
Source: Canadian Institute Health Information. (2018). *National health expenditure trends, 1975–2018* (pp. 18 & 37, Figure 10). Ottawa: Canadian Institute for Health Information. Retrieved from https://www.cihi.ca/sites/default/files/document/nhex-trends-narrative-report-2018-en-web.pdf.

Almost all the funding for Canada's hospitals comes from provincial governments (89.9% public funds and 10.1% private funds), and hospitals are considered not-for-profit organizations. Wages, salaries, and benefits account for almost three quarters of the operating budgets of public hospitals, with 45% of this budgetary portion paying nurses. Hospitals employ approximately 58.6% of the registered nurses (CIHI, 2016b).

Institutional Resources

Institutional resources consist of acute care hospitals with an ED, medical, surgical, and obstetric services; special allied (e.g., cancer care) services; rehabilitation; mental health; and chronic care (see Chapter 16 for details). As already stated, the most expensive health resources are health-related institutions because they rely heavily on technology and human resources.

Utilization of Institutional Resources

In 2016 to 2017, there were 3 million acute inpatient hospitalizations in Canada. After adjusting for differences in age, sex, and population growth, the hospitalization rate was 7 980 per 100 000 in 2016 to 2017, down from 8 203 per 100 000 in 2012 to 2013. The age-adjusted average length of stay in hospital has been relatively stable over the same time period and was 7.0 days in 2016 to 2017. Although provincial variations continue to exist, because of increasing pressures to use hospital resources more efficiently, the length of stay for inpatient care continues to decrease. For example, in 1995, Ontario reached an average length of stay of 9.7 days for all types of care, with an average of 3.1 days if acute care cases only are considered. In 2016 to 2017, the average length of stay in hospitals in Ontario was 5.8 days, demonstrating that there has been an increase in the past 20 years. Reasons for this are complex and include the aging population and addition of other population groups that have more chronic and complex medical needs.

A growing trend that impacts the utilization of institutional resources is individuals who no longer require acute care, complex continuing care, mental health, and rehabilitation services but must wait in a bed at a facility for placement in a more appropriate setting, such as home or residential care (CIHI, 2012a). This population, referred to as **alternate level of care (ALC)**, is expected to grow as the Canadian population ages. For example, in Ontario, the number of ALC patients—the

majority of whom are older than 75 years—is expected to increase by 32% over the next 10 years (CIHI, 2012b). Persons discharged from acute care to residential care accounted for more than 5 million ALC days in total (CIHI, 2012b). Seniors admitted to residential care with ALC days waited an average of 26 days before being discharged, compared with an average of 7 days among those admitted to home care. Reducing ALC days and transfers to residential care has become a pressing issue.

CASE STUDY

Alternate Level of Care

Meet Robert, aged 70 years. A few days after his back surgery, Robert no longer needed to be in the hospital but still required care while he regained his mobility and the ability to care for himself. On the same day that he was discharged from acute care, Robert found a temporary home at the Jackson Creek Retirement Residence. Not only did the residence have the staff and equipment to support his recovery needs, but it also met his care preferences, including being close to his daughter so she could visit.

Robert's quick match was made possible by the Resource Matching and Referral Program (https://resourcematchingandreferral.com/) which helps facilitate transfers between acute and rehabilitation hospitals and alternate care settings in the community. It is a powerful tool to reduce ALC days and contribute to lower emergency department (ED) wait times.

Patients who are waiting to be transferred from the hospital to a more appropriate care setting are a significant problem for the Canadian health system: in 2009, it was estimated that 1.7 million hospital days were for patients who no longer required acute care services. Nearly half of these patients were waiting for a transfer to a long-term care facility.

Facilitating discharge of patients to a suitable setting increases integration of care and makes sure patients have access to appropriate supports after discharge. This, in turn, ensures high-quality care and reduces readmission rates. Facilitating discharge also liberates costly acute care beds for other patients.

By reusing data collected from patients such as Robert (in the Case Study box, above), health system planning and resource allocation can be better supported. For example, health system managers can better project which services are and will be most in demand. It is also possible to identify where bottlenecks are preventing patients from successfully reintegrating into the community and where local innovations are leading to successful outcomes that could be replicated across the system.

Optimizing the Use of Institutional Resources

In recent years, a number of strategies have been employed to optimize the use of institutional resources that consume the largest proportion of health care dollars.

Rationalization of Health Services. To address growing financial concerns, many provincial governments have adopted rationalization. The **rationalization of health services** may involve restructuring, realignment, downsizing, decentralization, and some institutional closures. These attempt to minimize the duplication of services, provide appropriate levels and types of care, consolidate strengths, and create innovative structures and functional arrangements that make better use of resources and contain costs. Many analysts maintain that the central problem of health services in Canada is that hospitals and other medical institutions have acted in the interests of health care providers instead of the communities they serve. Physicians are now being asked by provincial health ministries to adopt and implement clinical guidelines. There is a constant explosion of scientific and clinical information; thus, clinical guidelines are designed so that the evidence-based approaches to clinical decision making are used. Guidelines have the potential to enhance quality of care, cost containment, and more appropriate use of resources, thus enhancing rationalization. Today there is an ever-increasing public interest in the outcome of health care, the need for cost containment, and the suspicion that some medical care may be unnecessary or inappropriate are all likely to result in a shift toward the supervision of quality of care and the identification of optimal practice patterns.

Rationalization usually involves major transformations of the health care system to contain costs that ensure accessibility and comprehensiveness. The challenge of controlling costs and putting the health care system on more sustainable financial footing is compounded by social and technological changes that are increasing the need for and cost of health services. Rationalization has occurred in every province. Quebec provides a good historical example for rationalization in the health care system. In the early 1970s, Quebec started down the path of regionalization, with Regional Health and Social Service Councils that subdivided the province into 12 regions. However, in 1987, the Rochon Commission recommended a further transformation of the health and social system that required resources be decentralized toward regional authorities that would be governed by a board of directors elected by and accountable to the population (Martin, 2003, as cited in Martin, Pomey, & Forest, 2006). The adoption of Bill 25 in December 2003 moved the management of health care services from the regional to the local level. Regional Boards were transformed into Local Agencies (Local Health and Social Networks) that were responsible for establishing local health and social services networks. Regional health authorities (RHAs) were established in Alberta in the following year, with the goal of ensuring a wellness-based, integrated, accessible, appropriate, and affordable health system.

Home Care. **Home care** is an array of services provided in home and community settings that encompass health promotion and teaching, curative intervention, rehabilitation, support and maintenance, social adaptation and palliative end-of-life care, and integration and support for the family caregiver (Canadian Home Care Association [CHCA], 2013). Publicly funded home care programs exist in every province and territory in Canada. Nationally, home care accounts for 3.3% of total public health care expenditures. Because home care is not included in the *Canada Health Act*, its services are not insured in the same way as hospital and physician services are. Home care policies and their delivery vary across the country (CHCA, 2013).

Home care makes institutional beds available for acute care and costs considerably less than hospital care. Home care clients are better able to adapt to a disability in their own homes, and they tend to adhere more readily with treatment requirements. Home care reduces the chance of hospital-acquired infections and results in psychological benefits experienced by the patient and his or her family. Furthermore, patients who are treated in hospitals often experience confusion, disorientation, anxiety, and personality conflicts, all of which can hinder healing. A home care program can also be tailored to an individual's particular needs and home (see Chapter 16).

Home care remains an uninsured service under the *Canada Health Act* and is listed only as an extended service to which the five principles of the Act do not apply. Therefore, it has no protection under the Act. Although governments are obliged to provide some services through public funds, there are no uniform standards to ensure the quantity or type of home care services to be provided. With the downsizing, closure, and merger of acute hospitals, patients are discharged home much earlier. This has created pressure on home care and has shifted health care costs to consumers.

At present, spending on home care programs accounts for approximately 3.3% of total public spending in the Canadian health care system. Most provincial home care programs are funded by the government, but some provinces charge user fees, often based on the ability to pay (CHCA, 2013). For example, in British Columbia, all public home care programs are fully or partially funded by the Home and Community Branch of the Ministry of Health Services. Whereas home care services such as case management, home nursing care, and community rehabilitation are provided to those who qualify at no charge, the homemaker services charge people according to income testing.

Home care reformers are faced with two opposing trends. On the one hand, with decreasing lengths of stay in hospitals and increasing pressure to push care into the community and home, away from institutional care, ever-increasing numbers of patients require care in the home. On the other hand, as fiscal constraints tighten, provinces may continue to de-list services such as home care that are not strictly required by the *Canada Health Act*. Recent federal reports have recommended postacute home care and palliative home care to be covered under the *Canada Health Act* (Romanow, 2002). The 2003 Health Care Renewal Accord recognized home care as one of the priority areas to receive substantial funding (Health Canada, 2003). In the 2017 federal budget, $6 billion was allocated to improve and support additional home care services over the following 10 years.

Most home care, including palliative care in Canada, is provided informally by unpaid family, friends, and neighbours. The Conference Board of Canada estimates that unpaid caregivers provided 10 times more hours of home care than paid workers in 2007—around 1.5 billion hours from nearly 3.1 million people (Conference Board of Canada, 2015).

Exercise 15.1 A Health Tapestry Sample Client Case:

Watch the video on an innovative home care program called Tapestry by searching for "A Health TAPESTRY Sample Client Case" on the Internet to find the YouTube clip. (The URL can be found at the end of this chapter.)

After watching the video, consider the following questions:

1. With an aging population, how does Tapestry support cost-effectiveness within the health care system?
2. Which principles of primary health care does Tapestry address?
3. Regarding issues of sustainability of Canada's health care system (discussed in a previous section), how does Tapestry address sustainability?

Human Health Resources Expenditures

The largest components of human health resources are nursing, and the expenditure figures for nurses are subsumed under institutional expenditure, as the majority of this staff are in salaried positions. In 2016, the expenditure for professional services by physicians, dentists, and other specialists amounted to 26% of total spending; this does not include professionals employed by institutions, such as nurses, physiotherapists, occupational therapists, social workers, and some physicians (CIHI, 2016b).

Physician Remuneration

Canadian physicians receive remuneration for their services by different methods, namely on a fee-for-service basis, by sessional payment, or by salary. The majority bill for most of their services through provincial health insurance plans (i.e., **fee for service**). The mix varies across Canada. In Alberta, 98% of physicians in 1998 to 1999 were paid only on a fee-for-service basis, compared with 40% in Manitoba. According to 2000 to 2001 estimates from the CIHI, about 11% of the total clinical payments to physicians in the 10 provinces come from some form of payment other than fee for service. Those who receive **sessional payments** receive a lump sum for the time they make their services available; for example, a psychiatrist working a half-day in a mental health clinic receives a flat rate for this service.

However, there is a lot of variation in physician payment modalities. In 2002, 58% of Canadian physicians received at least 90% of their income from fee for services, 8% received at least 90% from a salary, and the remaining 34% did not receive 90% of their income from any single source (Martin, 2002). Provider organizations, such as health services organizations (HSOs) in Ontario and the managed care organizations in the United States, follow the capitation system used by funding organizations. Under the **capitation system**, an organization receives a fixed amount per patient for all services rendered and, in turn, purchases physicians' services by salary or fee for service. Some consider the capitation or salary system to be conducive to a more holistic approach to health care, so that the physician is more likely to pay attention to all determinants of health and practise disease prevention and health promotion. It is used for primary care physicians in the United Kingdom and usually in health maintenance organizations (HMOs) in the United States, and in Ontario HSOs. Traditionally, salaries and sessional payments are more often used in rural regions or underserved areas of the provinces. However, the capitation system is currently drawing increased interest as part of primary health care reforms and endeavors to control health expenditures on physician services.

Nurse Practitioner Remuneration

The number of licensed nurse practitioners (NPs) in Canada grew by 300% between 2006 and 2014, with an employment rate of more than 95% (CIHI, 2015). The majority of NPs work in the family (all ages) and primary care stream, being deployed across a wide variety of settings and sectors and in various models of care. Remuneration for NPs needs to reflect their scope of practice, responsibility, and accountability, and needs to be standardized to address:

- Salary–benefit discrepancies (within provinces and territories)
- Yearly cost-of-living expenses
- Incentives and supports to recruit NPs to difficult-to-recruit areas
- Additional overhead, operating, and infrastructure expenses (Canadian Nurses Association, 2016)

Currently, funding models for NPs vary across Canada. The majority of provinces and territories pay NPs a salary, with some variance in that NPs may be employed directly by physicians in their solo practices and are therefore paid from the physician's salary or fee-for-service revenue. However, there is momentum building among many NPs to advocate for a fee-for-service

payment model that is similar to how many physicians are being paid. Although remuneration is one of the challenges for NPs, Naylor et al. (2015) bring to light another challenge; NPs are underused, despite clear evidence regarding their benefits to the health system and Canadians.

A growing trend is to adopt an interprofessional team approach to health care, particularly in community health centres and urgent care clinics, with the effective utilization of NPs, dietitians, social workers, and other health care providers. These professionals might provide primary care in their field of expertise or work as part of a more comprehensive approach to health care, particularly in its preventive aspects, than is now provided in many primary care settings. Alternative health care delivery models should explore the use of health care professionals other than physicians, such as using NPs to their full scope of practice.

EXERCISE 15.2: What kind of cost-containment strategies have been used in Canadian health care?

CRITICAL THINKING QUESTIONS 15.2
HEALTH CARE ETHICS:

1. Would it be appropriate to redirect money from hospital care to illness prevention if the money spent on prevention would produce more benefit and perhaps even save money in the long run?
2. Do you think it is more important to ensure that people who are sick and disabled are able to achieve the best level of health possible? Or is it more important to ensure that people who are healthy do not become sick and disabled?
3. If the same amount of money could be used either to save the lives of 10 heart attack victims over a 5-year period or, through preventive measures, reduce the number of people who would suffer heart attacks over the same time period and thereby save 100 lives, which option would you choose? Why?

ENHANCING HEALTH SYSTEM PERFORMANCE

The ultimate aim of health expenditures and resources utilization is to produce good health and quality of life. As seen in Chapter 4, indicators to measure health are a difficult to obtain. The public demands accountability from governments, providers, and institutions. Hence, it is important to assess the performance of the health care system using several indicators to account for accessibility, quality, safety, efficiency, and effectiveness of health care. Accords between federal and provincial governments (see Chapter 14) stipulate that health system reforms be monitored by using sets of comparable indicators and providing annual reports to the public. This section describes a number of performance indicators and some of the proposed solutions within the health care system to enhance the performance.

Selected Health Indicators and Improvement of Delivery

In recent years, CIHI, Statistics Canada, and various professional groups have developed a framework to measure health indicators (see Chapters 1 and 4). The framework takes into consideration the evolving performance information needs of its various users, it is grounded in the current state of scientific knowledge, and it is actionable because it offers an analytical and interpretative framework that can be used to manage and improve health system performance (CIHI, 2013). The framework provides the general public, managers, and policy makers with a set of measures to assess health system performance against intermediate and ultimate goals. It also supports an ability to compare their results with other Canadian jurisdictions and to learn from their peers and the best available evidence in their efforts to improve health system performance.

Health system outputs are dimensions that relate to characteristics of the health services (or outputs) produced by the health system, including both the health care system and public health and health promotion services (World Health Organization, 2009). The health system outputs in the CIHI's (2012b) framework encompass four quality attributes (Fig. 15.4). These health system outputs impact the social determinants of health, health system inputs and characteristics, and health system outcome quadrants. These quality attribute dimensions also encompass equity.

The following section describes the four quality attributes in greater detail. The data presented here are derived from CIHI information, which also provides individual provincial and regional data (CIHI, 2017).

Health System Outputs

Access to comprehensive, high-quality health services that are

- Person centred
- Safe
- Appropriate and effective
- Efficiently delivered

Fig. 15.4 The Canadian Institute Health Information's health system outputs.

Access to Comprehensive, High-Quality Health Services

Access refers to the availability of comprehensive, high-quality health services, as well as their ability to meet the needs of the population or an individual without undue delay or financial, organizational, or geographical obstacles. Health services can include public health, health-promotion, and disease-prevention services, as well as curative, maintenance, and palliative services. Access to comprehensive high-quality health services is influenced jointly by the dimensions in the fourth quadrant: efficient allocation of resources, adjustment to population health needs, and health system innovation and learning capacity.

Person-Centred Services. "High-quality" health services are person centred—they are culturally appropriate, respectful of, and responsive to the needs and values of individuals receiving services. Person-centred services put individuals and their caregivers at the centre of delivery and ensure that their preferences guide all clinical decisions. An example of care that falls into this category is physician follow-up within 30 days after hospitalization and caregiver experience.

Safe Services. "Safe" services avoid harming individuals by the care that is intended to help them. A health care example that falls into this category is adverse inpatient drug events. The Canadian Patient Safety Institute (CPSI), established by Health Canada in 2003, works with governments, health organizations, leaders, and health care providers to inspire extraordinary improvement in patient safety and quality. CPSI has developed a variety of evidence-based tools and resources with the assistance of experts in patient safety to:

- Prevent patient safety incidents by properly designing processes and improving communication.

- Identify when incidents do occur, with robust reporting mechanisms.
- Learn from incidents so that prevention strategies can be improved, through excellent analysis and carefully implemented changes.

Appropriate and Effective Services. Appropriate and effective services are based on scientific knowledge of what will best reduce the incidence, duration, intensity, and consequences of health problems. Some examples of measures that fall into this category are addiction services wait times and 30-day readmission for mental illness. Readmission rates can be influenced by the quality of care a patient receives while hospitalized. Although not all readmissions are avoidable or preventable, higher readmission rates for certain conditions reflect the quality of care. The readmission rates of patients to hospital within 28 days because of acute myocardial infarct and asthma reflects such concerns, and their rates were 7.3% and 6.4%, respectively.

Efficiently Delivered Services. Efficiently delivered services avoid wasting equipment, supplies, ideas, and energy. There were no identified measures that addressed delivery of efficient care in relation to access.

Wait Times. Timely access to the health care system is at the crux of wait times. Canadians are waiting too long for an appointment to see a specialist or to schedule surgery, for diagnostic confirmation and treatment for chronic pain or cancer, for discharge from a hospital to home or to a long-term or continuing care facility, and for transfer from the ED to a hospital bed. Canada has one of the longest wait times in the world for health care services (Fig. 15.5).

Strategies to reduce wait times have been implemented for more than a decade. There is increasing evidence to show that when nurses work to their full scope of practice and their roles are optimized, nurses provide more service and help to reduce wait times (Canadian Nurses Association, 2013a). A promising intervention that has been shown to increase the availability of primary care appointments is open access scheduling, also known as advanced scheduling or same-day scheduling (Ansell et al., 2017). Same-day appointments offer individuals an ability to book their appointment on the day they call regardless of the reason for the visit. Compared with the traditional scheduling method, in which the schedule is already full before the start of the workday, the open-access model allows for more flexibility in scheduling, eliminates delays, and improves patient satisfaction and health outcomes (Abou Malham et al., 2017).

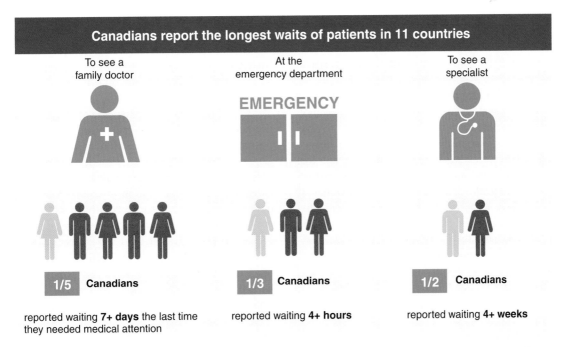

Fig. 15.5 Canadian patient wait times. (From Canadian Institute Health Information. [2016]. *Commonwealth Fund Survey 2016.* Retrieved from https://www.cihi.ca/en/commonwealth-fund-survey-2016-infographic.)

Wait times for surgical procedures such as cataract surgery, knee surgery, hip surgery, and angioplasty have been reduced by creating a central registry system (Damani et al., 2017). It is important to keep in mind that because of a series of health system inefficiencies, solutions require a comprehensive, coordinated response on several fronts—there is no one solution for solving accessibility and wait time issues. See Exercise 15.3 to assess how well your health system is working.

EXERCISE 15.3 HOW WELL IS YOUR HEALTH SYSTEM WORKING?

Access CIHI's website at https://yourhealthsystem.cihi.ca/hsp/indepth?lang=en#.

Look at the big picture for your health system. Check out your province or your territory, your city, or even your local hospital. Explore the five themes that Canadians said were most important to them.

How is your local hospital performing compared with provincial and national standards?

Optimizing Health Care Delivery Systems

There are many entry points into the health care system. With provincial and private health insurance plans (which cover dental, drug, and private nursing), there are relatively few financial barriers at these entry points. The services of psychologists, social workers, dentists, denturists, and NPs in private practice are less commonly covered, however, making these entry points more costly to the consumer, if not to government budgets. Most people, however, receive their primary care through general or family practitioners and use specialized resources upon referral by those practitioners, who play a gatekeeper role.

The current Canadian health care system is heavily oriented towards treating illness. At present in most provinces, RHAs are mandated to coordinate institutional sectors of health services as described in Chapter 14. Nonetheless, services between primary and specialized care are poorly developed in most parts of the country. People have direct access to primary or secondary care, depending upon their proximity to and knowledge of resources and their attitudes towards the system. Many health care planners prefer that there be a linear and seamless progression by the individual from primary care to secondary care to tertiary care, as required (see Chapter 16). However, this progression would be difficult to achieve within the current health care system unless its organization and payment system are drastically restructured. This is why several provinces have been moving towards integrated health systems.

This is one major step toward primary care reform. However, Canada has a long way to go. As reported by the Advisory Panel on Healthcare Innovation in its 2015 final report on integration, "Health care remains disjointed, with poor coordination and alignment within and across the various professions, acute and chronic care institutions and community care" (Advisory Panel on Healthcare Innovation, 2015, p. 58).

Integrated Health Systems

Canada's health system can be viewed as 14 sets of silos (at least from a budgeting perspective) of hospital care, medical services, prescription drug programs, home and community care, mental health and addiction services, cancer care, and long-term care. These services are far from seamless for patients, and there are significant gaps in publicly funded services beyond the hospital and medical care that fall under the *Canada Health Act* (as noted in Chapters 13 and 14). *Integrated health systems (IHS)*, also known as **integrated delivery systems (IDS),** have been promoted as a means to improve access, quality, and continuity of services in a more efficient way, especially for people who have complex needs. Such an integrated system requires interprofessional collaborative teams with a model of primary health care to ensure that patients receive the right provider at the right time, in the right place, and for the right care (Canadian Nurses Association, 2013b).

The continuum of primary and specialized services provided in such arrangements most often includes primary care, health promotion and disease prevention programs, secondary care with links to tertiary care facilities, rehabilitation, palliative care, long-term care, home care, and community support services. IHS or IDS can provide these services or purchase services through contracts with outside care providers—whichever is the most cost-effective use of existing resources. The system of payment for IHS or IDS varies, but most often requires a roster of a particular population group with physician remuneration for services, based on a capitation formula.

As discussed further in Chapter 16, the physical site of service delivery may be the same for primary, specialized, and very specialized care. Certainly, most of these services, as well as their coordination, management, and financing, would occur at a single location. Health Canada has stated that the *Canada Health Act* does not preclude rostering individuals in a plan, as long as the individual can choose to leave the group at a specified time. This interpretation paves the way for reform in primary health care.

Optimizing Quality Assurance and Total Quality Management Programs

Quality assurance (QA) is a management system to assure the quality of health care provided by workers and received by patients. Care should be correctly given, reliable, and empathetic. QA constantly improves standards and the frequency of attaining them. QA has been defined as "all actions taken to establish, protect, promote and improve the quality of health care" (Donabedian, 2003, p. xxiii). Said another way, QA is an effort to find and overcome problems with quality—that is, directing the performance and behaviours of practitioners and institutions toward more appropriate and acceptable health outcomes, expenditures, or both. A number of approaches have been developed specifically for the hospital sector, such as the Medical Audit Committee, which compares care for a specific disease with the standards set for that disease. Another example is the Health Record Committee, which reviews selected patient records for completeness. CIHI also provides large sets of data for comparisons between institutions of similar size. Ontario publishes Measuring Up—a comprehensive report based on the Common Quality Agenda that looks at the health of people living in Ontario and how the provincial health system is performing (Health Quality Ontario, 2018). In 2018, the Canadian Broadcasting Corporation (CBC) also published a report card on hospital ratings across Canada (CBC, 2018).

Although institutions have QA programs, there is rarely an organized review of the community-based practices of health care professionals. Licensing or regulating bodies usually deal with patient complaints; however, recent legislation in a number of provinces now requires quality of care provided by their constituents to be monitored. Increasingly, health care professionals and institutions are required to be accountable to the public and the government for the resources they use and how they practise.

Total quality management (TQM) is a management philosophy for improving quality while controlling costs. In TQM, management focuses on the system rather than the individual, so decisions are made to support quality and remove barriers to quality inherent in the bureaucratic, hierarchical system. Participation and teamwork are vital. Because TQM is based on a continuous feed-forward process called continuous quality improvement (CQI), it differs from QA, which tends to depend on retrospective recognition of exceptions to patterns of care. TQM is slowly being introduced into health care. TQM complements QA by providing a management system for rectifying identified difficulties, an aspect that is frequently missing from QA activities. QA tends to emphasize data collection. QA also focuses on individuals, often in relation to their peers, and is thus less powerful than TQM, which examines issues affecting the performance of the organization as a whole.

Lean is a well-recognized CQI methodology designed to enhance organizational efficiency and effectiveness, which originated as a production line discipline (the "Toyota Production System"). Lean embraces process improvements involving inventory management (Just-In-Time [JIT], and Kanban [a signalling process to support JIT]), waste reduction (5S), and quality improvement techniques (Six Sigma). Lean thinking mainly emphasizes efficiency improvement in speed and waste, in contrast to the Six Sigma focus on effectiveness for process analysis and reduction in variation and errors. The term "Lean Six Sigma" refers to the integration of "Lean" and "Six Sigma." As a more recent option to CQI, Lean and Six Sigma focus on training employees and managers in specific tools and techniques. Health care regions across Canada have been adopting Lean, with 73% of Canadian health regions indicating that Lean was a component of their organizational strategy (Mackenzie & Hall, 2014). Although some health care administrators strongly believe that Lean leads to quality improvements in their organization, the evidence to date does not support this claim (Moraros, Lemstra, & Nwankwo, 2016). Saskatchewan is a case in point (see the Case Study box). Criticisms of Lean in health care organizations include that it fails to take into account patient acuity and complexity and that it has little impact on direct care at the bedside and patient outcomes (Saskatchewan Union of Nurses, 2014).

In 2008, Lean began to be applied to some health care services in Saskatchewan, and by 2010, Lean become a government-wide reform. The provincial ministry of health retained John Black & Associates as consultants on the project to provide an extensive suite of training for health care providers, managers, and staff. According to Marchildon (2013b), it is difficult to find the exact reason for how or why Lean became a government priority; however, Marchildon suggests that there were two key events that may have influenced the adoption. The first was the appointment of Dan Florizone as deputy minister of health; Florizone was a personal proponent of Lean methods. The second was in 2008 when the ministry led a Saskatchewan health system study tour to England, the highlight of which was the NHS Institute for Innovation and Improvement, where the NHS presented results from its Lean initiatives, Releasing Time to CareTM (RTC).

The implementation of Lean in Saskatchewan health, which is underpinned by "goods-dominated" logic systems in health care, frames the relationship of provider as being experienced, knowledgeable, and the source or creator of value; the patient is viewed as being inexperienced, unknowledgeable, passive, and someone who consumes and uses up or destroys value. This relationship is troubling from a Primary Health Care perspective (see Chapter 16), in which patient participation in care is integral to achieving health for all.

An alternative to Lean is design thinking, which is being touted as a bottom-up innovation that is being applied in health care settings across Canada. **Design thinking** is an approach that prioritizes developing empathy for users, working in collaborative multidisciplinary teams, and using "action-oriented rapid prototyping" of solutions. This bottom-up approach distinguishes it from the traditional linear and often top-down approaches to health intervention design, such as the Lean model. Design thinking's five-stage, cyclical approach starts with the designers empathizing with users and then defining the problem, coming up with ideas, prototyping and testing the ideas, and then doing it all over again. However, there are few studies that demonstrate its effectiveness, with interventions being tested primarily in pre and post designs or pilot randomized controlled trials with small samples.

The **plan–do–study–act (PDSA) cycle** is a TQM process that is used for improving a process or for carrying out change (Fig. 15.6). PDSA is a useful model for documenting a test of change by developing a plan to test the change (plan), carrying out the test (do), observing and learning from the consequences (study), and determining what modifications should be made to the test (act). The PDSA cycle is repeated as needed until the desired goal is achieved. The intended output of PDSA is learning and taking informed action for the next PDSA cycle. The PDSA model is used to make and document incremental changes (see Evidence-Informed Practice box).

EVIDENCE-INFORMED PRACTICE

A Plan–Do–Study–Act Example: Improving Emergency Department Flow Through Optimized Bed Utilization

Greater patient volumes in EDs create congestion and can compromise the delivery of high-quality patient care. As the number of patients presenting to an ED outpaces the number of beds available, the increasing patient-to-provider ratio in the waiting room creates an unsafe environment for high-acuity patients and a precarious medicolegal situation for providers. This project was aimed at facilitating the flow of high-acuity patients from the waiting room to a bed in the ED, where comprehensive assessment and close monitoring can be performed by the ED health care team. The transitional care area (TCA) is where ED patients continued to be observed for the duration of their ED visit while not necessitating a bed, thereby freeing up the bed they were previously using for new patients. Several PDSA cycles were performed to test various combinations of locations and processes for the TCA concept. The PDSA served as the framework until the end goal was reached, which was required seven PDSA cycles in all.

Source: Chartier, L. B., Simoes, L., Kuipers, M., & McGovern, B. (2016). Improving emergency department flow through optimized bed utilization. *BMJ Quality Improvement Reports, 5*, u206156.w2532. Retrieved from https://bmjopenquality. bmj.com/content/bmjqir/5/1/u206156.w2532.full.pdf.

Optimizing Technology Assessment

Technology (some of it very expensive) has made tremendous advances in health care in recent times. Technology assessment has been developed to examine the efficacy and safety of a technology, its appropriate clinical use, the relative risks and benefits, and the ethical

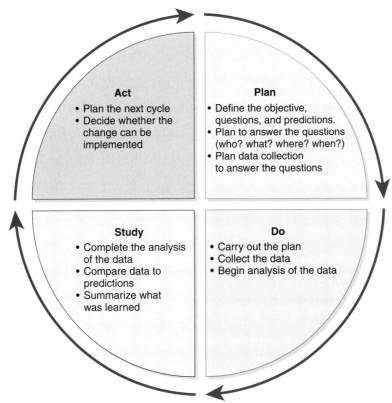

Fig. 15.6 The plan–do–study–act (PDSA) cycle.

and social implications. However, no systematic process for the identification and acquisition of new technology exists in Canada. Interprovincial differences in priorities and disparities in wealth make it difficult to establish uniform approaches to health technology. Health Canada's Health Products and Food Branch administers the *Food and Drugs Act*, which regulates a limited number of medical devices as well as medications. These devices include implantables, condoms, AIDS tests, menstrual tampons, and contact lenses. The Act does not cover devices used externally or most other technology that is introduced independently by the provinces. The **Canadian Agency for Drugs and Technologies in Health (CADTH)** (formerly known as the Canadian Coordinating Office for Health Care Technology Assessment) is a nonprofit organization funded by federal, provincial, and territorial governments. CADTH supports informed decisions about the uptake and use of drugs and other health technologies in Canada. (CADTH, n.d.). **Health technology** or health care technology is the application of organized knowledge and skills in the form of devices, medicines, vaccines, procedures, and systems developed to solve a health problem and improve quality of life (Zisovska, 2016).

Rural and Remote Considerations

Access to health care in rural and remote communities is challenging because of a number of factors, such as geographic distance; limited availability of health care professionals; and logistical, economic, and sociocultural factors that can make medically related travel difficult. Health technology innovation is most promising to address these inequities in health care. Several health technologies are decreasing the barriers to health care access. Three examples of emerging health technologies that are decreasing barriers to health care access in rural and remote communities in Canada are as follows:

1. The Intelligent Retinal Imaging Systems (IRIS) is a platform being used to facilitate the provision of diabetic retinopathy screening in areas that have limited access to eye care professionals.

2. Unmanned aerial vehicles or drones (see Chapter 18) are enabling timely delivery of medical supplies to remote communities.

3. Video directly observed therapy enables patients to record themselves taking their medications at work or at home and send the video to their health care providers, regardless of the time or distances involved to monitor adherence to tuberculosis treatment in remote Canadian communities.

Health Technology Assessment

When a new technology is introduced, people typically question the following:

• Whether it has been adequately tested for safety and efficacy
• How the new technology compares to existing technologies in current practice
• How cost-effective (or costly) the new technology is.

These questions reflect the practical realities of constrained health care spending. Thus, *health technology assessment (HTA)* has become an essential tool for understanding the potential costs, benefits, and side effects that new technologies offer. The International Network of Agencies for Health Technology Assessment (2018) defines HTA as the systematic evaluation of properties, effects, or impacts of health care technology. It may address the direct, intended consequences of technologies, as well as their indirect, unintended consequences. Its main purpose is to inform technology-related policy decisions in health care. HTA is conducted by interdisciplinary groups, using explicit analytical frameworks drawn from a variety of methods.

The World Health Organization (WHO) Collaborating Centre for Health Technology Assessment at the University of Ottawa has developed a tool kit that includes the Technology Assessment Iterative Loop (Feeney, Guyatt, & Tugwell, 1986) framework (Fig. 15.7). The **Technology Assessment Iterative Loop (TAIL)** provides a process for informed decision making as a result of technology assessment. It sets out seven steps: identify technologies with the greatest potential for reducing the burden of illness by primary, secondary, or tertiary prevention or by levels of care; establish efficacy (i.e., therapeutic potential under ideal circumstances); establish procedures for screening and diagnosis (i.e., accurate detection of those in need); determine community effectiveness; assess efficiency (see Chapter 4); develop procedures for synthesis and implementation; and monitor and reassess the process.

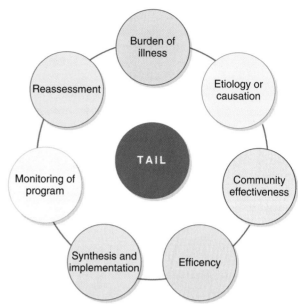

Fig. 15.7 The Technology Assessment Iterative Loop (TAIL). (From Tugwell, P., Bennett, K., Feeny, D., et al. [1986]. A framework for the evaluation of technology: the technology assessment iterative loop [pp. 41–56]. *Health care technology: effectiveness, efficiency, and public policy*. Montreal: Institute for Research on Public Policy.)

An equity-oriented health technology assessment has been developed by the WHO Collaborating Centre for Health Technology Assessment. It emphasizes that technology assessment must be linked to health needs in a systematic manner and that it must also be based on clinical and population health status needs, as opposed to "wants," of the consumers or the vested interests of players such as health care providers, public health specialists, politicians, or industry. Issues of gender equity, social justice, and community participation are key to a needs-based health technology assessment approach. TAIL provides the linkages to these considerations.

> **CRITICAL THINKING QUESTIONS 15.3:**
> 1. What kind of health technologies exist in your local health care system, and how do they facilitate the care of individuals?
> 2. Are there any drawbacks to using health technology?

RATIONING IN HEALTH CARE

When resources for health care and services are finite and limited, rationing is one option that suggests a process of explicit and deliberate decisions about resource allocation. **Medical savings accounts** (MSAs) refer to a family of financing approaches used to pay for specified health care services. Although called by different names, all plans or models have two fundamental features: a personal or household savings account and a high-deductible catastrophic insurance plan (Deber, 2011). Money is put aside either by an employer, an individual, or government in the form of public funds already earmarked for health, in a savings account. Until the high deductible of the catastrophic plan is met, the individual must pay for health services either out of pocket or with money from the savings account. This approach is intended to reduce demand for health services by making individuals financially responsible for their pattern of consumption, with the premise that individuals will buy more efficiently if they have to pay with their own resources rather than having the costs covered by third parties (Deber, 2017).

Supporters of MSAs usually point to Singapore. Measures such as population health, life expectancy, and infant mortality in Singapore are comparable to those of Canada, yet Canada spends a larger percentage of GDP on health care. But as noted earlier, cross-country comparisons can be misleading. The determination of total health expenditure can differ and what gets included in total health expenditure can also differ. A study investigating the effectiveness of MSAs in Manitoba concluded that such a system will not save money but will instead, under most formulations, lead to increased spending on the healthiest members of the population (Forget, Deber, & Roos, 2002). In Deber's (2011) analysis, MSAs "do not appear to be a valuable addition to financing Canadian health care" (p. iii). The WHO concluded that MSAs are neither a panacea nor a catastrophe for the health care system and must be evaluated in the context of the entire health financing system (Hanvoravongchai, 2002).

CASE STUDY

Health Care Funding: Mariella and Pablo

Walking home from the community meeting, Mariella and Pablo continued the discussion about health care funding that had started there.

Mariella: I can't believe you supported the cuts to health care.

Pablo: It's not that I don't think health care is important. But I think we could get better value for our money—more health for our money—by spending this money on other things. That money would do a lot more good if we spent it on job creation and cleaning up the environment.

Mariella: I think it's much more important to look after the people who are sick right now than to improve the health of the general population. And besides, I doubt that the money saved would be spent on making a difference in health. Our health care system is one of the things that makes this country so special, Pablo; I'm very worried about the impact of these cuts.

Pablo: You heard what the experts at the meeting said. There's lots of waste and inefficiency. If we get rid of that, there's plenty of money to fund the system.

Mariella: I'm not so trusting. Maybe there is lots of inefficiency, but do you really believe that quality won't suffer? These cuts will make it very difficult for the provinces to ensure that all Canadians have equal access to high-quality, medically necessary care.

Pablo: That term "medically necessary" is so broad it can mean anything. The health care system has expanded beyond its original intent and beyond what we can afford. Sure, we have to see that no Canadians will lose their houses or burden themselves with debt to meet their medical needs, but maybe the government just can't afford to meet all the lesser needs and wants.

Mariella: Well, who's going to decide what we can and cannot afford, and which and whose needs are greatest? People like the ones at the meeting who supported the cuts? Most of those people were very well dressed and pretty healthy looking. Not very typical of the people I work with every day in the chronic care unit. And not very typical of the people in the neighbourhood where you and I grew up, Pablo. Those are the people I care most about.

Pablo: We agree then, Mariella, because it's these people I care most about, too. I want them to have jobs, and I want their children to have good schools and safe streets. Those things don't come from doctors and hospitals.

Critical Thinking Questions

1. Which one of the two speakers do you most sympathize with, and why?
2. Mariella is concerned about the consequences of funding cuts for poor and needy people. How important is the government's obligation to help these people? Is there anything else that is more important?
3. State whether or not you agree or disagree with the following statement: "We can't afford to pay for everything the public wants; we have to concentrate on what the public really needs." Explain your reasons.
4. In deciding the level of public funding for health care, how much weight should be given to what patients or consumers would like, as opposed to what experts think they need?

SUMMARY

Canada has a predominantly publicly financed health system with universal coverage for all permanent residents, without regard to their ability to pay for care. Most money for health care is raised through provincial and federal taxes and is allocated, for the most part, from general provincial budgets. Both the public and private sectors finance Canada's health systems, with a mix of both private and public funding. Public sector funding accounted for 70% of health expenditures and the remaining 30% came from private sector. As noted in Table 15.1, these sectors are referred to as various levels: level 1, public (Medicare); level 2, public–private; and level 3, private. The largest category of spending is hospitals, followed by prescription and nonprescription drugs and, finally, physicians.

Institutional resources consist of acute care hospitals with an ED, medical, surgical, and obstetric services; special allied health (e.g., cancer care); rehabilitation; mental health; and chronic care. As already stated, institutions are the most expensive element of health care because they rely on both technology and human resources.

A growing trend that impacts the utilization of institutional resources is individuals who no longer require acute care, complex continuing care, mental health, or rehabilitation services but who wait in a bed at a facility for placement in a more appropriate setting, such as home or residential care. This population, referred to as ALC, is expected to grow as the Canadian population ages.

To improve the utilization of institutional resources, the following strategies are considered:

- Rationalization of health care services involving restructuring, realignment, closures, and mergers of institutions

- Increased ambulatory care, day care, and extended care
- Preadmission planning and discharge planning, which shorten hospital stays.

The health system performance measurements include the categories of person-centred, safe, appropriate and effective, and efficiently delivered in high-quality health services. Health services can include public health; health-promotion and disease-prevention services; and curative, maintenance, and palliative services.

Approaches that are suggested to improve health system performance include:

- Technology assessment, a process that examines the efficacy and safety of a technology, its appropriate clinical use, its relative risks and benefits, and its ethical and social implications
- QA, a process for establishing functional goals, implementing procedures to achieve these goals, regularly assessing performance, closing the gap between performance and goal, and documenting and reporting
- Utilization review and management, which involves monitoring the use of services, analyzing variations, assessing interventions to reduce inappropriate use of services, collecting feedback, and providing education based on TQM
- Health care rationing to distribute health care equitably when resources and services are finite and limited. Medical savings accounts have been suggested by some as a possible improvement to Canada's health care funding.

KEY WEBSITES

Accreditation Canada: https://accreditation.ca
Accreditation Canada is a not-for-profit organization that is dedicated to working with patients, policy makers, and the public to improve the quality of health and social services for all.
Canadian Patient Safety Institute (CPSI): https://www.patientsafetyinstitute.ca/en/about/Pages/default.aspx

The CPSI works with governments, health organizations, leaders, and health care providers to inspire extraordinary improvement in patient safety and quality.
Institute for Health Care Improvement PDSA Cycles: http://www.ihi.org/resources/Pages/Tools/PlanDoStudyActWorksheet.aspx
This organization specializes in health and health care improvement globally.

TAPESTRY: A Health TAPESTRY Sample Client Case (YouTube): https://www.youtube.com/watch?annotation_id=annotation_1093172633&feature=iv&src_vid=la1uritj34U&v=zRfYAEdk_U0

The Health TAPESTRY approach is moving primary health care from disease-centred care to person-focused care. Health TAPESTRY is increasing access to health and community-based programs that can help a person stay healthier for longer where they live.

The World Health Organization Collaborating Centre for Health Technology Assessment at the University of Ottawa: http://www.cgh.uottawa.ca/whocc

The Collaborating Centre promotes the concept of technology assessment, the establishment of technology assessment systems, methodological support, training seminars in member countries, and collaborating among institutions with similar intent.

REFERENCES

Abou Malham, S., Touati, N., Maillet, L., et al. (2017). What are the factors influencing implementation of Advanced Access in Family Medicine Units? A cross-case comparison of four early adopters in Quebec. *International Journal of Family Medicine, 2017,* Article ID: 1595406. https://doi.org/10.1155/2017/1595406.

Advisory Panel on Healthcare Innovation. (2015). *Unleashing innovation: Excellent health care for Canada.* Retrieved from http://www.healthycanadians.gc.ca/publications/health-system-systeme-sante/report-healthcare-innovation-rapport-soins/alt/report-healthcare-innovation-rapport-soins-eng.pdf.

Ansell, D., Crispo, J. A., Simard, B., et al. (2017). Interventions to reduce wait times for primary care appointments: A systematic review. *BMC Health Services Research, 17*(1), 295.

Canadian Agency for Drugs and Technologies in Health. (n.d.). Retrieved from http://www.inahta.org/members/cadth/.

Canadian Broadcasting Corporation. (2018). *Canadian hospitals rated by CBC.* Retrieved from https://www.cbc.ca/news2/health/features/ratemyhospital/hospitalratings.html.

Conference Board of Canada. (2015). *Understanding health and social services for seniors in Canada.* Ottawa: Author.

Canadian Home Care Association. (2013). *Portraits of home care in Canada.* Ottawa: Author. Retrieved from http://www.cdnhomecare.ca/content.php?doc=274.

Canadian Institute for Health Information. (2012a). *DAD Abstracting Manual (2011–2012 Edition),* Chapter 10 (pp. 1–7). Ottawa: Author.

Canadian Institute for Health Information. (2012b). *Health care in Canada.* Retrieved from https://secure.cihi.ca/free_products/HCIC_2011_seniors_report_en.pdf.

Canadian Institute for Health Information. (2013). *Better information for improved health: A vision for health system use of data in Canada.* Retrieved from https://www.cihi.ca/en/hsu_vision_report_en.pdf.

Canadian Institute for Health Information. (2015). *Regulated nurses, 2014.* Retrieved from https://secure.cihi.ca/estore/productFamily.htm?locale=en&pf=PFC2898&lang=en.

Canadian Institute for Health Information. (2016a). *Prescribed drug spending in Canada, 2016: A focus on public drug programs.* Retrieved from https://secure.cihi.ca/free_products/Prescribed%20Drug%20Spending%20in%20Canada_2016_EN_web.pdf.

Canadian Institute for Health Information. (2016b). *Regulated nurses.* Retrieved from https://secure.cihi.ca/free_products/regulated-nurses-2016-report-en-web.pdf.

Canadian Institute for Health Information. (2017). *Who is paying for these health services?* Retrieved from https://www.cihi.ca/en/who-is-paying-for-these-health-services-2017.

Canadian Institute for Health Information. (2018). *National health expenditure trends, 1975–2018.* Retrieved from https://www.cihi.ca/sites/default/files/document/nhex-trends-narrative-report-2018-en-web.pdf.

Canadian Nurses Association. (2013a). *Registered nurses on the front lines of wait times—moving forward.* Retrieved from https://www.cna-aiic.ca/-/media/cna/page-content/pdf-en/wait_times_paper_2011_e.pdf?la=en&hash=219FEC089152DC8C52A219448D21EAF12D50D0D9.

Canadian Nurses Association. (2013b). *Integration: A new direction for Canadian health care.* Retrieved from https://www.cna-aiic.ca/-/media/cna/files/en/cna-cma_heal_provider_summit_transformation_to_integrated_care_e.pdf?la=en&hash=094811D-94F0487A196901715B5FE14516ACA194E.

Canadian Nurses Association. (2016). *Canadian Nurse Practitioner initiative: A 10-year retrospective.* Retrieved from https://www.cna-aiic.ca/~/media/cna/page-content/pdf-en/canadian-nurse-practitioner-initiative-a-10-year-retrospective.pdf?la=en.

Damani, Z., Conner-Spady, B., Nash, T., et al. (2017). What is the influence of single-entry models on access to elective surgical procedures? A systematic review. *BMJ Open, 7*(2), e012225.

Deber, R. (2011). Medical savings accounts in financing healthcare. *CHSRF Series of Reports on Financing Models: Paper.* Ottawa: CHSRF.

Deber, R. (2017). *Treating health care: How the Canadian system works and how it could work better.* Toronto: University of Toronto Press.

Donabedian, A. (2003). (1st ed.). *An introduction to quality assurance in health care* (Vol. 1). New York: Oxford University Press.

Drèze, J., & Sen, A. (2013). *An uncertain glory: India and its contradictions.* Princeton, NJ: Princeton University Press.

Feeney, D., Guyatt, G., & Tugwell, P. (1986). *Health care technology: Effectiveness, efficiency, and public policy.* Montreal: Institute for Research on Public Policy. [Seminal Reference].

Forget, E., Deber, R., & Roos, L. (2002). Medical savings accounts: will they reduce costs? *Canadian Medical Association Journal, 167*(2), 143–147. [Seminal Reference].

Hanvoravongchai, P. (2002). *Medical savings accounts: Lessons learned from international experience. EIP/HSF/PHF Discussion Paper No. 52.* Geneva: World Health Organization. [Seminal Reference].

Health Canada. (2003). First ministers' accord on health care renewal. Retrieved from http://www.hc-sc.gc.ca/english/hca2003/accord.html (February 2003). [Seminal Reference].

Health Quality Ontario. (2018). *System performance.* Retrieved from http://www.hqontario.ca/System-Performance/Yearly-Reports.

International Network of Agencies for Health Technology Assessment. (2018). Retrieved from http://www.inahta.org.

Lepenies, P. (2016). *The power of a single number: A political history of GDP.* New York, NY: Columbia University Press.

Mackenzie, J., & Hall, W. (2014). *"Lean" in Canadian health care: Doing less while achieving more (Publication 6262).* Ottawa: The Conference Board of Canada.

Marchildon, G. P. (2013a). *Health systems in transition: Canada (No. 1).* Toronto: University of Toronto Press.

Marchildon, G. P. (2013b). Implementing Lean health reforms in Saskatchewan. *Health Reform Observer–Observatoire des Réformes de Santé, 1*(1).

Martin, S. (2002). More hours, more tired, more to do: Results from the CMA's 2002 Physician Resource Questionnaire. *Canadian Medical Association Journal, 167*(5). Retrieved from http://www.cmaj.ca/content/167/5/521.1.abstract?casa_token=YnDN6qRSNvQAAAAA:turvGCKZI-W_pfWZ1CYZ0e5_GmdXWMbzhkZvKLvGDxJiGjuE-VOO_kqypisYZTbRBf3eH_tpRP8_cB.

Martin, E. (2004).). *La participation publique dans le domaine de la sante au Canada: La regionalisation comme agent de democratisation? (French text).* Bibliogr.: M.A. thesis, Université de Laval, 138–147.

Martin, E., Pomey, M. P., & Forest, P. G. (2006). *A cross provincial comparison of health care policy reform in Canada. The reform of regionalization in Quebec: The introduction of Bill 25 proposing the transformation of regional boards into health and social services agencies and the implementation of local service networks.* Retrieved from https://www.queensu.ca/iigr/sites/webpublish.queensu.ca.iigrwww/files/files/Res/crossprov/QC-Regionalization.pdf.

Moraros, J., Lemstra, M., & Nwankwo, C. (2016). Lean interventions in health care: Do they actually work? A systematic literature review. *International Journal for Quality in Health Care : Journal of the International Society for Quality in Health Care, 28*(2), 150–165.

Naylor, D., Girard, F., Mintz, J. M., et al. (2015). *Unleashing innovation: Excellent healthcare for Canada: Report of the advisory panel on healthcare innovation.* Ottawa: Health Canada.

Ontario Seniors' Secretariat. (2013). *Independence, activity and Good Health Ontario's action plan for seniors.* Retrieved from http://www.oacao.org/images/ontarioseniorsactionplan-en.pdf.

Romanow, R. (2002). *Building on values: The future of health care in Canada.* Ottawa: Commission on the Future of Health Care in Canada; Government of Canada. Retrieved from http://www.hc-sc.gc.ca/english/pdf/romanow/pdfs/HCC_Final_Report.pdf. [Seminal Reference].

Saskatchewan Union of Nurses. (2014). *The real story about Lean.* Retrieved from http://sun-nurses.sk.ca/index/presidents-message/march-2014-the-real-story-about-lean.

Statistics Canada. (2018). *Market income, government transfers, total income, income tax and after-tax income by economic family type (Table 11-10-0190-01: Market income, government transfers, total income, income tax and after-tax income by economic family type).* Ottawa: Author. Retrieved from https://www150.statcan.gc.ca/t1/tbl1/en/tv.action?pid=1110019001.

World Health Organization. (2009). *A WHO framework for health system performance assessment.* Retrieved from https://www.who.int/healthinfo/paper06.pdf.

Zisovska, E. (2016). Few building blocks for evidence-based decision making. *Evrodijalog, Journal for European Issues, 22,* 207–219.

16

Delivery of Health Care Services

Ⓔ Additional resources are available online at http://evolve.elsevier.com/Canada/Shah/publichealth/

OBJECTIVES

- Develop an understanding of the care settings, levels of care, and types of care.
- Explain the difference between primary care and primary health care.
- Develop an understanding of public health services and and the role of public health units.

- Develop an awareness of the various types of home care in Canada.
- Discuss some of the historical milestones in the development of health care and community health services.
- Describe the role of voluntary services in Canada's health care system.

CHAPTER OUTLINE

KEY TERMS

centre
centres locaux des services
  communautaires
divisionally organized hospital
end-of-life care
family health teams (FHTs)

functionally organized hospital
health protection
hospices
hospital boards
hospitalist
institution

mutual aid
palliative care
patient care groups (PCGs)
patient medical homes (PMHs)
primary health care (PHC)
program management

OVERVIEW OF DELIVERY OF HEALTH SERVICES

This chapter discusses the spectrum of health service delivery models for individuals who need preventive and health maintenance care; for those who are acutely or chronically ill needing hospital care, community-based services provided by different health care professionals and support services such as self-help groups and voluntary organizations; and public health services that promote or maintain the health of and prevent diseases in populations. The chapter is divided into two major sections: one discussing hospital or institutional services and the next section discussing community health services.

There are multiple practice settings within the health care system that provide various levels of care to ensure that an individual's health needs are being met. Practice settings that are explored in this chapter are hospitals; walk-in clinics; urgent care; primary care; ambulatory care; and community health, including public health, home care, and mental health. There are four levels of care within the various practice settings. These levels vary in complexity and type of service offered. The four levels discussed are primary, secondary, tertiary, and quaternary care.

Primary Care Services

The role of the primary level of health care is to promote health; prevent disease; and identify diagnostic, curative, rehabilitative, supportive, and palliative services required by the client on a one-on-one basis. Primary care services are usually the first point of contact that people have with the health care system, where their needs and concerns are initially addressed (University of Ottawa, 2017). Examples of primary care facilities that provide these services include family physician offices, primary care nurse practitioner (NP) offices, community health centres (CHCs), and nursing stations. These settings often are multidisciplinary in nature, housing a range of health care professionals, including social workers, nurses, nurse practitioners, dietitians, and family physicians, among others. Primary care providers depend on a stable, long-term, personal relationship (a feature also called "longitudinality") between the individual accessing services and themselves. It is important to note that primary care services are different than the concept of primary health care, which is introduced later in this chapter.

Secondary Health Care

When the primary care provider refers an individual to a specialist, the specialist is part of the secondary care system. **Secondary health care** means that an individual will be taken care of by someone who has more specific expertise than primary care practitioners. Ailments that may require specialized care include serious cardiovascular disorders; unintentional injuries; burns; fractures; cancers; behavioural disorders; and some serious pediatric, medical, and obstetric problems, which usually require care provided by specialists in a community or general hospital. Secondary care services are provided by specialists and other health professionals, who generally do not have first contact with individuals.

Tertiary Health Care

Tertiary health care facilities provide specialized health care, typically for individuals who need hospitalization as inpatients; care is based on referral from a primary or secondary care provider. Tertiary care is provided by an academic teaching facility or large community care hospital with access to specialists and specialized equipment. The services provided by a tertiary care facility can include cancer management, mental health, neurosurgery, cardiac surgery, burn treatment, specialized neonatology services, and other complex medical and surgical interventions

Quaternary Health Care

Quaternary health care provides an advanced level of care that is highly specialized and not widely accessible. This care is usually provided by academic and teaching centres and may include experimental medicine, diagnosis and treatment of rare medical conditions, and uncommon surgical procedures. Examples of quaternary care centres include pediatric facilities (e.g., The Hospital for Sick Children), mental health facilities (e.g., Centre for Addiction and Mental Health [CAMH], described in the Case Study box), and large academic centres (e.g., Montreal General Hospital, Sunnybrook Health Science Centre in Toronto, and The Vancouver General Hospital).

CASE STUDY

The Centre for Addiction and Mental Health in Toronto

Toronto's Centre for Addiction and Mental Health (CAMH) is the country's largest mental health-focused teaching hospital. It is also a well-recognized research centre affiliated with both the University of Toronto and the World Health Organization. CAMH houses a diverse range of staff, including researchers, educators, and clinicians. Some of the work of CAMH includes public policy advocacy, research, health promotion, and clinical services, such as brief interventions, assessments, day hospital services, inpatient programs, outpatient care, and family support for people who have a range of mental health issues (e.g., substance use, dementia, behavioural issues, psychosis, mood disorders, anxiety, trauma).

CRITICAL THINKING QUESTION 16.1 UNDERSTANDING TERMINOLOGY: How are primary, secondary, and tertiary health care different from primary, secondary, and tertiary prevention?

HEALTH CARE SERVICES

The majority of health care services that treat life-threatening illness or injury, surgery, or provide care to those with diseases that require complex diagnostic laboratory or treatment services are provided at institutions such as general and allied special hospitals and chronic care hospitals. In Quebec, the organization and activities of health care institutions is regulated by the *Act Respecting Health Services and Social Services and Amending Various Legislation* (passed in 1991). According to this act, Quebec differentiates

between a centre and an institution. A **centre** is a place where health and social services are dispensed and can include general and specialized hospitals, psychiatric hospitals, local community service centres, residential and long-term care centres, and certain categories of rehabilitative care centres. An **institution** *(établissement)* is an organization responsible for service activities pertaining to the mission of one or more centres and is, in effect, an umbrella organization that ensures the provision of a continuous spectrum of accessible and high-quality health or social services, as well as the reduction of the health and welfare problems of its particular population group. An institution is frequently responsible for the management of several centres with differing missions, thus allowing for better integration and coordination of care, but centres are directly involved in service delivery (Martin, Pomey, & Forest, 2006). Many provinces have adopted similar structures through their regional health authorities (RHAs) (see Chapter 14).

Community Mapping of Health Care Services

One way to get a broad sense of the types of health care services available in your area and to help better integrate and plan, as well as determine community asset and need, is community mapping, an exercise used commonly in the field of community health. Community mapping, or service mapping, means determining what types of services are offered in your community, where, by whom, and what links exist between service providers (Challacombe &Broeckaert, 2016). Community mapping can be much broader than simply mapping out health care and social services, and may also include mapping out and getting a sense of community assets (e.g., social support networks) and gaps or needs (e.g., getting an idea of poverty levels, infrastructure, housing quality in an area). It can be done in a variety of different ways and often involves consultation with service agencies, community organizations, and members of the community. Two prominent ways of undertaking community mapping include *windshield surveys* (in which people observe services, assets, and needs by making observations whilst in a moving vehicle) and *walking surveys* (in which people make these same observations, but on foot) (Community Toolbox, 2018). These two exercises can be immensely valuable in helping figure out what needs exist, how one can go about filling those needs, and initiating discussions about how to better coordinate between community groups or government agencies that are trying to address these needs.

The rest of this section discusses various types of services that one may look out for when engaging in a community health care service mapping exercise.

EXERCISE 16.1 COMMUNITY MAPPING: Investigate in the city or town where you live and find out which kind of health care services are available. Use an existing community map or create your own map to indicate where these services are located in your community.

Notice if there are any clusters of services in a specific geographic area. What can this tell you about the population they serve? Are there accessibility issues? Are you able to infer the type of illnesses or diseases that are prevalent in your community?

Integration of Health Care Services: A Growing Challenge

As may become clear while you read this chapter, Canada's health care system has been described as being "fragmented" and a "hodgepodge patchwork" of acute care facilities, primary care services, public health organizations, and other services—with some facilities being run by the provinces and territories and others by the federal government (Leatt, Pink, & Guerriere, 2000). In other words, the health care system is far from being integrated.

From a client perspective, this often translates into the following types of challenges:

- Having to make multiple phone calls to schedule visit(s)
- Having to repeat one's health history for multiple providers
- Having to undergo multiples of the same test because providers aren't aware of what other providers have already assessed

Enhancing system integration (i.e., better coordination of health services across the continuum of care, as well as better collaboration among service delivery providers) is no easy task. In the early 2000s, a group of researchers proposed a set of strategies for achieving better integration, including really focusing on the actual individual being cared for (taking a client-centred approach to issues), ensuring a strong and accessible primary care system (because this is the first point of contact for people with the broader health care system), and sharing information and exploiting technology (making sure we have electronic systems that talk to each other and that are accessible), among others (Leatt et al., 2000). The concept of achieving better system integration should be kept in mind by readers as they read about the types of health care services provided in Canada.

CRITICAL THINKING QUESTION 16.2: Reflect on your own experiences interacting with our health care system (either as a client yourself or as a trainee or someone in practice). Have you encountered examples of poor integration? How might some of the strategies mentioned above be applied to your example to prevent it from happening in the future?

Acute Care Facilities
The Historical Evolution of Modern Hospitals

The earliest hospitals in Canada were established by religious orders. For example, the first hospital in Canada, Hôtel Dieu de Précieux Sang, was established in Quebec City in 1639 by the Catholic Church. Before 1850, hospitals were perceived as dirty, infested, crowded, and unpleasant places to which people would go only as a last resort. At the time, the overall mortality rate in these institutions generally was high (20%). Florence Nightingale, Joseph Lister, and others revolutionized hospital care by introducing antisepsis, asepsis, good food, and proper nursing; these improvements reduced mortality rates in these settings from 20% to 2%.

By the beginning of the 20th century, people were choosing to go to hospitals to be cured. Canadian hospitals became acceptable places of care and were no longer viewed as "a well of sorrow and charity" but as a workplace for the production of health. The access that private practitioners gained to hospitals, without becoming employees of the hospitals, became one of the distinctive features of medical practice in North America. In Europe and most other areas of the world, when patients enter a hospital, the health care providers that are following them in the community typically relinquish responsibility to the hospital staff. In North America, however, private practitioners (mostly physicians, in this case) often continue to follow their patients into the hospital and continue to attend to them while they are in hospital. This arrangement complicates hospital administration, however, because many of the people making vital decisions are not the institution's employees.

> **CRITICAL THINKING QUESTION 16.3:** Analyze the implications (both positive and negative) of having clinicians who have the authority to admit patients (e.g., nurse practitioners, midwives, and physicians) and be a patient's most responsible provider be actual employees of the hospital institution versus consultants with privileges to provide services to inpatients.

Hospitals' modern role in health care emerged after World War II. A concentration of curative medical technology was developed during the war, primarily because of the advent of modern antibiotics and technology. Until the widespread introduction of antibiotics in the 1940s, hospitals and physicians mainly cared for the ill without being able to cure them. With the introduction of antibiotics, however, providers could in fact cure many diseases and infections. As new technology emerged, health care providers were able to improve their ability to diagnose conditions. The combined impact of these developments in medical science also had its influence on hospitals: hospitals adopted (and often still use) hierarchical organizational structures originally established by the British Army. During the next few decades, the consolidation of hospital dominance occurred through the development of the Canadian health care model, including the Federal Grants-in-Aid (1948), the *Hospital Insurance and Diagnostic Services Act* (1957), the *Medical Care Act* (1966), and the *Canada Health Act* (1984). All these steps resulted in the institutionalization and expansion of the Canadian hospital system. However, in Newfoundland and Labrador, hospitals emerged from a different history. For an interesting example of the cottage hospitals and outpost nursing in Newfoundland and Labrador, refer to Box 16.1.

Hospital Resources

Today hospitals are the major centres for health care activities. Their primary function is to take care of sick people by providing inpatient services, services for many ambulatory patients in outpatient clinics and emergency departments (EDs), and rehabilitation services. In certain cases, they also provide limited public health and home care services. Some large hospitals act as teaching resources for the education of nurses, midwives, physicians, and other allied health

> **BOX 16.1 History of Cottage Hospitals and Outpost Nursing in Newfoundland and Labrador**
>
> The health care system in Newfoundland and Labrador has its roots in the cottage hospital system and the International Grenfell Association facilities. The cottage hospital system, initiated by the Commission government in 1936, was designed to bring a high standard of health care to outpost residents. Small hospitals were constructed in central locations around the Island.
>
> The chronic shortage of physicians in Newfoundland and Labrador and in other remote areas of Canada created a demand for nurses to work in these underserviced areas. According to a national report (Kulig et al., 2003), the first outpost nurses came from England in 1893 as part of the Grenfell Mission. The International Grenfell Association, founded by Sir Wilfred Grenfell in the early 1900s and centred in St. Anthony, provided essential health care services to residents in the north, particularly coastal Labrador, and has now become part of Newfoundland's provincial health care system.

care professionals (e.g., social workers, pharmacists, dieticians, nutritionists, physiotherapists) and are often referred to as academic health science centres (AHSCs). AHSCs conduct research in the form of clinical trials (to test new drugs, devices, and diagnostics), population health studies (to understand diseases at the population level), and translational research (to move basic science to the bedside and back again) (Archer, 2018). In recent years, there has been a trend to decrease the number of hospital beds and move care into the community.

As stated earlier, there are a number of hospital types, including acute care, special allied (e.g., cancer care), rehabilitation, mental health, and chronic care. However, according to Statistics Canada, there has been a marked decline in the number of hospitals and hospital beds that include psychiatric facilities throughout Canada. The deinstitutionalization of mental health patients in 1960 caused a shift to community-based living, which resulted in a decline in bed capacity. In 2017, there were 70 932 hospital beds in Canada (excluding Quebec) (CIHI, 2017a). In 2016, Quebec had more than 21 000 general and specialized care hospital beds in public and private health care institutions (Ministère de la Santé et des Services sociaux du Québec, 2016). Canada has among the lowest ratio of hospital beds in the developed world, about 2.6 per 1 000 population compared with Germany with 8.1 per 1 000 (CIHI, 2017b). A recent trend to address overcrowding (hallway care) in hospitals is adding temporary beds. Ontario announced in 2017 that it would spend $100 million, thereby adding 2 000 temporary beds (Government of Ontario, 2017).

As reported by the Organisation for Economic Co-operation and Development (OECD), the number of hospital beds per 1 000 population in Canada decreased from 3.0 in 2006 to 2.6 in 2016 for publicly owned hospitals in Canada (OECD, 2017) The OECD notes that "the number of hospital beds per capita has decreased over the past decade in most OECD countries. This reduction is part of a voluntary effort in most countries, partly driven by progress in medical technology, which has enabled a move to day surgery for a number of procedures and a reduced need for hospitalisation" (OECD, 2017, p. 172).

Inpatient hospitalization rates have been declining over time. In 2016 to 2017, there were 3 million acute inpatient hospitalizations in Canada, with an average length of stay (LOS) of 7 days (CIHI, 2017b). Giving birth is one of the top reasons for inpatient hospitalization, with an average LOS of 2.3 days. Other major reasons for inpatient hospitalization are chronic obstructive pulmonary disease (COPD) and bronchitis, acute myocardial infarction, pneumonia, and heart failure, respectively.

Organization of Hospitals

A voluntary board of trustees governs hospitals, under legislation such as Ontario's *Public Hospitals Act*. There are various forms of **hospital boards**, which are constantly evolving; some are being phased out. Generally speaking, most board members are not professionals in the health care field and are either elected or appointed to the position. Sometimes health care workers practising in the hospital and other hospital employees, as well members of public representing specific underrepresented population groups, are also represented on hospital boards. In addition, some hospital administrators now sit on hospital boards as nonvoting members. Under provincial legislation, the board is responsible for the governance of the hospital, subject to compliance with the terms of the legislation. The board acts as the agent for the public in assuring proper financial operations and quality of care.

> **CRITICAL THINKING QUESTION 16.4:** Look up the members who sit on the board of your local hospital and try to find out a little bit about their background. Does this group represent the diversity that exists in your community? Does it need to be representative of community diversity? Does having a more diverse board impact the quality and equity of care delivered in the hospital setting? Are there any potential downsides to board diversification?

As the health care system has become regionalized (see Chapter 14), the functions of most hospital boards have been taken over by *regional health boards* (RHBs), and the legislation has been amended accordingly. Nearly all hospitals have a chief executive officer (CEO), president, or administrator in charge of daily operations and executing policies formulated by the regional or hospital board and to whom all personnel report. One or more assistant administrators may support the administrator, each controlling a functional area (e.g., medical director and director of nursing, plant and engineering, finances, and human resources). In Quebec, where health care institutions can oversee the work of several different health centres, the CEO and the senior management staff are responsible for the administration and operation of all of the centres operated by the institution. The CEO and the board are assisted by a management staff (including a director of professional services), a council of physicians, dentists, and pharmacists; a council of nurses; and a multidisciplinary council. Legislation requires that the board establish a *professional advisory committee* (PAC) or a *medical advisory committee* (MAC). In many hospitals, the PAC is responsible for advising on capital purchases of medical equipment, regulation of the professional staff, and similar matters. It is usually chaired by the chief of staff and consists of chiefs of different medical disciplines, chiefs of other health care professional services, and a member from the board.

The work of a hospital is usually organized according to either functions or divisions. A **functionally organized hospital** is divided into different departments, according to the number and type of functions performed, with people who performed similar roles grouped together (e.g., finance department, human resources, clinical services, food and environmental services). This usually involves vertically hierarchical reporting and decision making and is well-suited to small organizations with few goals and uncomplicated environments, such as a small community hospital or a nursing home.

A **divisionally organized hospital** includes smaller, semiautonomous units that are organized according to the type or content area of the work they do (e.g., cardiology, obstetrics and gynecology). Each subunit has its own management team composed of various types of expertise, including medical, nursing, and administrative representatives, and usually has complete authority for the operation of the unit. Although divisional structures are much better at dealing with the multiple tasks required of an academic teaching hospital and usually increase turnaround time for decision making, they run into problems of coordination; competitiveness among units; and, at times, goals that are incompatible with the goals and objectives of the larger corporate structure.

A hospital's size and teaching status determine the complexity of services available. Larger hospitals with multiple stakeholder interactions—frequently teaching hospitals and academic health centres—usually provide the widest range of services and are organized by division or programs.

Organizational measures undertaken to integrate all hospital units (regardless of functional or divisional organization) include *matrix designs* that create dual reporting structures by function and by medical division (e.g., a nurse working in a cardiac unit is responsible to both the director of the cardiac unit and to the director of nursing) and *parallel structures* such as special problem-solving teams or task forces.

In an effort to improve quality of care, responsiveness to patient needs, and accountability, many hospitals across the country have adopted an organizational structure of program management. **Program management** is a management approach, typically arising within a rapidly changing organizational context, that involves the structural regrouping of staff according to patient care "programs" (Hibberd & Smith, 2005). In this structure, the hospital is a portfolio of separate businesses with decision making pushed down the organization to teams of managers who are fully responsible for their programs. In a large urban centre, programs have 100 to 150 beds each and can be defined according to population group (e.g., gender, ethnicity, age, geography), by disease or health problem (e.g., HIV, cancer, heart disease), by patient need (e.g., rehabilitation, continuing

care), by type of service (e.g., outpatients, home care), or by medical specialty (e.g., medicine, surgery). Most important, programs are multidisciplinary, self-contained units that are each unique or special in some way, with the capacity to become centres of excellence.

There is a movement (especially in provinces such as Alberta) to facilitate the creation of hyper-specialized hospitals that will function as "focused factories." Examples include the Shouldice Hospital in Toronto (for hernia treatment) and the Gimble Eye Centre in Calgary (for cataracts and corrective eye surgery). These hospitals are based on the notion that very high-volume and high-frequency procedures, such as hernia surgery, cataract surgery, coronary bypass surgery, and cancer radiation, are associated with better outcomes when done in a very specialized hospital that gets very good at doing those few select procedures. These types of hospitals can improve quality outcomes (they work at very high volumes under highly standardized routines and protocols) and have the potential to increase efficiency as a result. For example, in 2014, researchers were able to show that the Shouldice Hospital in Toronto is able to perform hernia treatment at a lower cost than other general hospitals (Medtronic, 2019).

Physician Organization in Hospitals. As discussed earlier, in most Canadian hospitals, physicians are not employees but users of hospital facilities on behalf of their patients. This arrangement complicates hospital administration because many of the people making vital decisions are not the institution's employees.

However, some radiologists, pathologists, and a few other specialists, such as ED physicians, are employed directly by the hospital. Since the early 2000s, Canadian hospitals have witnessed the emergence of the "hospitalist" as a new occupational category. A **hospitalist** is a physician (usually with a specialization in family medicine, internal medicine, or sometimes pediatrics) who may or may not be an employee of the hospital (most often on salary) and who manages the medical care for hospital inpatients who do not otherwise have a primary care physician. It is likely that hospitalists will become more common in the future.

Typically, a physician requests the privilege of admitting patients to a general hospital and expects to be responsible not only for their care but also for patients referred by other doctors. It is usually a subcommittee of the PAC that screens physicians' credentials, competencies, and resources consumption and advises the board, which has the final authority for approval. Admitting privileges are granted according to an impact analysis, which considers the potential number of patients who would be attracted to the hospital by the physician's specialized skills, the effect on hospital resources caused by the physician's activities, the ability of the physician's reputation to enhance the hospital's prestige, and the number of physicians already providing the same or similar services. The board may reject the application or grant full or partial privileges, perhaps with some conditions (e.g., a general practitioner may not be allowed to do any surgery).

When physicians become members of the medical staff, they undertake certain responsibilities to the hospital in addition to the right and responsibility of looking after any patients they admit. Medical staff members may be required to provide on-call services in rotation, serve on committees, maintain and give final approval to hospital medical records, and attend staff meetings; they must abide by the rules and regulations passed by the medical advisory committee or hospital board. The medical staff is expected to be self-governing and self-disciplining through peer review and a chief of staff, usually a respected senior doctor, for each medical and surgical discipline, who is responsible for ensuring the quality of care delivered.

The Role of Nurse Practitioners in the Hospital Environment. Nurse practitioners were originally introduced into the US health care system in the 1960s, primarily to support underserved areas. Since the early 2000s, a growing number of NPs have been established across the Canadian health care system as well, and in 2009, it was estimated that approximately half of NPs in Canada work in Ontario (Soeren, Hurlock-Chorostecki, & Reeves, 2011) (see Chapter 17). NPs are considered to be an advanced nursing practice role in Canada, along with clinical nurse specialists (CNSs) in the hospital. NPs work in a number of different roles (e.g., primary care, rehabilitation, public health), including in hospitals. Similar to physicians, NPs can order diagnostic tests and medications and, in some provinces such as Ontario, the legislation allows NPs to admit and discharge hospital inpatients as well (Registered Nurses Association of Ontario, n.d.). With their expertise, NPs are a critical member of the health care team in a hospital, with roles in leadership (e.g., organizing educational rounds for learners, evaluating hospital programs), consultation (e.g., making referrals to other providers), research, and,

of course, clinical care (as previously discussed) (Soeren et al., 2011). The payment structure for NPs is discussed in Chapter 15.

The Role of Midwives in the Hospital Environment. Midwives are regulated health professionals who offer comprehensive care to women and their babies during pregnancy, labour, birth, and the postnatal period. Midwives practise in homes, the community, hospitals, clinics, birth centres, and health units. Midwives offer a choice of place of birth and, in most provinces, have hospital privileges. The Canadian Midwifery Regulators Council (CMRC) regulates the profession of midwifery (see Chapter 17). More detailed information regarding the practice of midwifery in each province and territory can be found on the CMRC's website.

The Role of Nurses in the Hospital Environment. Registered nurses (RNs) in Canada practise across the five domains—administration, clinical care, education, policy, and research—in the hospital. Most often, RNs work in hospitals (64%) than in other work environments (CIHI, 2017c) and can have many different roles. In advanced practice, CNSs in the hospital provide expert nursing care and play a leading role in the development of clinical guidelines and protocols. They promote the use of evidence, provide expert support and consultation, and facilitate system change. There is a move across Canada to have master's-prepared nurses work in the CNS role in hospitals.

Current Challenges and Realities in Canadian Hospitals

By the 1990s, hospitals had emerged as the cornerstone of Medicare in Canada, as well as for many local economies. They are major employers and engines of economic growth, and they are key workplaces for specialists, particularly surgical specialists and super specialists. They also compete for equipment, areas of specialization, and renowned physicians. Yet there is still almost no direct public accountability with respect to how hospitals spend their funding, although they have also become very expensive organizations to run.

Despite cutbacks, hospitals remain the largest component of health budgets in all provinces. Significant health system restructuring is not possible without hospital restructuring, but because there is little new money to invest in hospitals, restructuring requires reallocating dollars. It is not clear if hospitals will remain sheltered by Medicare or whether they will move beyond acute care, for example, into continuing care or community-based care.

In addition, the debate about the efficiency and efficacy of a parallel system of private hospitals has resurfaced. Some clear examples of private sector health legislation in Canada are Alberta's *Health Care Protection Act*, which empowers RHAs to subcontract surgical procedures to private providers under certain conditions. In Ontario, there are five still-existent private hospitals that were grandfathered in under the 1971 *Private Hospitals Act* and continue to operate. However, the legislation that is in place bans the establishment of any new private hospitals and restricts the expansion and bed capacity of the five existent private hospitals.

Public accountability requires transparency in terms of the quality of health care delivered by hospitals. In 2013, the Canadian Institute for Health Information (CIHI), in collaboration with provincial governments, created national performance indicators for hospitals, with outcome measures that are compared provincially and nationally (see Chapter 15 for details).

Government health insurance plans cover basic hospital and medical services in all of the provinces and territories, but there are extreme variations with respect to the coverage of extended health services, whether in the home or in the community, that are paid for by provincial or private insurance or by the individual. Affluent provinces provide a larger range of services financed through public revenue (see Chapter 15).

Long-Term Residential Care

In 2017 to 2018, there were 1360 residential care facilities across Canada, with 207 000 residents. There has been a rapid expansion of long-term residential care over the past 30 years. Several factors have played a role in this expansion, including more women entering the workforce and therefore being unable to care for their elderly parents; the deinstitutionalization of psychiatric hospitals, causing older clients with dementia and other psychiatric illnesses to end up in general hospitals; and rising hospital care costs. Under the *Canada Health Act*, "adult residential care service" and "nursing home intermediate service" are part of "extended health care services"; as a result of such services not always being covered by the public health care system, the private for-profit nursing home industry came into existence to cover this type of care.

The delivery of services for long-term residential care varies greatly across Canada. Long-term residential care facilities offer different levels of care and may be freestanding or co-located with other types of care or hospitals. They serve diverse populations that need access to 24-hour nursing care, personal care, and other therapeutic and support services. Long-term residential care, usually offering the highest level of support, may be subsidized by publicly funded health care for those who meet general provincial or territorial eligibility criteria, agree to participate in a formal health assessment, and are assessed as having needs that can be met by the services. Each province or territory has different eligibility criteria. Additionally, individuals can access private pay residential care when government subsidy does not apply. The number of long-term residential care beds is limited, and waitlists are often long. Seniors residences typically provide less intensive services than do long-term residential care and are generally paid for out of pocket.

The shifting demographic to a greater proportion of the Canadian population being aged 65 years and older (see Chapter 6 for more detail) raises concerns about the future need for long-term residential care because age is a strong predictor of admission (Ronald et al., 2016). According to the 2016 Census, 6.8% of Canadians aged 65 years and older were living in a nursing home or residence for senior citizens (hereafter referred to as a seniors' residence); this proportion jumps to 30.0% among Canadians aged 85 years and older (Statistics Canada, 2016).

> **CRITICAL THINKING QUESTION 16.5:** Because many long-term residential care facilities in Canada are private and for profit, what kind of impact do you think this has on the care of residents?

OVERVIEW OF COMMUNITY HEALTH SERVICES

Community health services help individuals to live with dignity in the community outside of institutions, with the aim of keeping individuals in better health by taking into account their environment and social conditions. Community health services focus on health promotion and disease prevention and management, which are designed to improve the health and well-being of local residents, as well as to take pressure off the acute care health system.

When Canadians access health care, their first point of contact is with essential primary care services at the community level. Here, it is important to distinguish between primary care and **primary health care (PHC)**. These two concepts are often used interchangeably, causing confusing and misunderstanding. As discussed in Chapter 1 and earlier in this chapter, PHC focuses on promoting health, preventing illness, population health, and citizen participation. The PHC approach means being attentive to and addressing the many factors in the social, economic and physical environments that affect health—from diet, income, and schooling to relationships, housing, workplaces, culture and environmental quality, as indicated in the Introductory Chapter (Fig. 16.1). PHC is undertaken by a variety of players, including government, community-based organizations, and the health sector.

On the other hand, primary care (as introduced at the beginning of this chapter) is included *within* the definition of PHC and is "an integral component of an inclusive PHC strategy" (Tarlier, Johnson, & Whyte, 2003, p. 180). PC, or first-point-of-contact care, includes services provided at the first contact between the client and the health care professional. Primary care places emphasis on physical or mental health restoration at the level of the individual. It does not include health promotion at the community level. Physicians, dentists, chiropractors, pharmacists, NPs, midwives, optometrists, dietitians, and others generally provide primary care.

This following section has been subdivided into eight areas of community health services: primary care, ambulatory care, CHCs, public health services, home care services including palliative care, mental health services, cancer services, and services for special populations.

Primary Care (Office Practice)

Primary care office practices typically are led by either primary care NPs, family physicians, or both, with or without a range of other allied health care professionals.

Most physicians (including primary care physicians) in Canada practice medicine as solo practitioners (25%), in shared practices, or in group practices, either in hospital or in the community (75%). The remainder have a variety of other arrangements (CIHI, 2017c). Generally, a shared practice is distinguished from a group practice by the extent of patient sharing among the participating physicians. *Shared practices* are usually limited to two or more physicians who have completely separate practices but share office space, rent, and secretarial services. *Group practices* usually involve income distribution, formal contracts, shared patient records, shared practitioner responsibilities, and possible provision of care in one another's absence. Most group practices (80%) consist of physicians in the same discipline, such as family practitioners, but a smaller proportion consists of specialists from different disciplines. Most practitioners have their offices in the community. In urban centres with medical schools, practices of full-time teachers, called geographic full-time practitioners, are located in

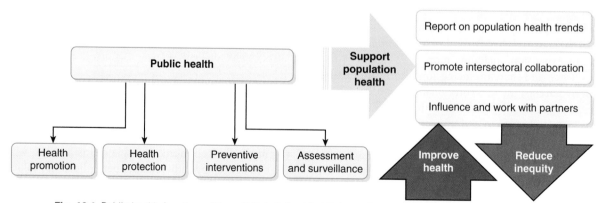

Fig. 16.1 Public health functions. (From British Columbia Ministry of Health. [2017]. *Promote, protect, prevent: our health begins here [B.C.'s Guiding Framework for Public Health]* (p. 9). Retrieved from https://www.health.gov.bc.ca/library/publications/year/2017/BC-guiding-framework-for-public-health-2017-update.pdf.)

the university hospitals and their affiliated clinics. With the implementation of primary care reforms, larger numbers of family physicians are increasingly joining the organized group practices.

In the 1990s, several provinces undertook initiatives that supported the expanded role for nonphysician primary care providers (see Clinical Example box), such as integrating midwifery services into the health care system. Midwifery practice is now legal in several provinces and is publicly financed in Quebec, Manitoba, Alberta, and British Columbia (see Chapter 17).

Support for the role of both community health nurses and NPs in primary care has also been growing. In 2018, for example, the government of British Columbia committed to hiring 200 NPs as a shift towards a team-based primary health care system (Government of British Columbia, 2018). NPs and community health nurses can also be found in remote rural communities. Nurse-run outpost clinics in Newfoundland and Labrador and in many remote and isolated Indigenous communities in the north, for example, have been a reality for many years (staffed by community health nurses as well as NPs), and NP–physician collaborations operate in many parts of the province. Such collaborations are also underway in other provinces, such as Saskatchewan. Because of the shortage of physicians in southern and urban areas, there is an increased demand for primary care provided by NPs. Urban centres and particularly specialized service sectors, such as cancer clinics, diabetic clinics, and EDs, are increasingly hiring NPs as well.

 CLINICAL EXAMPLE

Expanded Health Care Roles—The Health Bus

An example of an innovative clinic where roles have been expanded is the Health Bus in Saskatoon. This bus is staffed with NPs and paramedics and travels to underserved parts of the city and nearby Indigenous communities to offer health checks, chronic disease management, health education, wound care, flu shots, and referrals.

The Health Bus is a good example of bringing health care to individuals rather than individuals going to seek health care. For more information, visit https://www.saskatoonhealthregion.ca/locations_services/Services/Primary-Health/Pages/HealthBus.aspx.

Walk-in-Clinics

There has been a growing interest in walk-in clinics since they first began operating in 1984. Although there is no universally accepted definition of a **walk-in-clinic**, it is usually a freestanding group practice that offers extended hours for services (weekend and evening hours) and does not require an appointment. Walk-in-clinics are usually located in urban or suburban centres with large proportions of young families.

Although they are convenient for individuals, there is a concern that walk-in-clinics may provide lower quality care because of lack of continuity of care by a consistent health care provider or because they are more often staffed by recent graduates who might have less than adequate training (Chen et al., 2017). There is also some anecdotal evidence that people who see health care providers at walk-in-clinics after hours see their primary care practitioners for the same problem the next day.

The **urgent care centre** is a category of a walk-in clinic that is focused on the delivery of fulfillment care in a dedicated medical facility outside of the traditional ED. Urgent care centres operate from early morning to evening and on weekends and provide immediate care for ailments that are not serious enough to require an ED visit. Urgent care centres exist in most provinces. In 2018, British Columbia's government announced an annual $128 million funding increase for urgent care as an attempt to solve the lack of primary care providers in the province.

Ambulatory Care

Ambulatory care is a health care consultation, treatment, or intervention using medical technology or procedures to provide treatment for day admissions. Many of them are staffed by interdisciplinary health care teams consisting of professionals such as NPs, physicians, physiotherapists, occupational therapists, respiratory therapists, social workers, and so on. The underlying principle of ambulatory care relates to the fact that a significant proportion of inpatient care can be managed safely and appropriately on a same-day basis without admission to a hospital bed, which translates to cost savings within the health care system. Although not all admissions for such ambulatory care–sensitive conditions are avoidable, it is assumed that appropriate prior ambulatory care could prevent the onset of this type of illness or condition (e.g., complications of diabetes), control an acute episodic illness or condition, or manage a chronic disease or condition. Additionally, if a person with a long-term or chronic health problem such as asthma is able to obtain timely services in an ambulatory setting, her or his health status may improve, and the person is less likely to require costly hospital services. The Canadian Association of Ambulatory Care, a voluntary nonprofit organization developed for professionals working in various ambulatory care areas, provides a forum for networking opportunities with other health care professionals throughout their events and annual conference.

Integrating Chronic Care Models into Primary Care Services

As discussed in depth in Chapter 8, much of the burden of disease both in Canada and around the world is related to noncommunicable diseases (NCDs), which require ongoing, comprehensive care from a variety of health disciplines. Unfortunately, however, our current health care system, including primary care, is more oriented towards intermittent care for acute health issues (walk-in clinics are an example of care that is oriented to acute and episodic care). In response to this, the Chronic Care Model (CCM), rooted in primary care and prevention, was developed in the late 1990s to assist with shifting our delivery model to chronic care and making our system more conducive to caring for those with multiple and complex chronic NCDs. The vision of this model is creating evidence-informed interactions between "an informed, activated patient and a prepared, proactive practice team" (Improving Chronic Illness Care, 2019).

The Wagner CCM model consists of six key elements to improve care for chronic diseases, including self-management support (i.e., empowering clients to manage their own care journeys), redesigning delivery systems (to allow for effective, efficient care and enable self-management), decision support that is system wide (which speaks to basing decisions on data, evidence, and client preferences and characteristics), clinical information technology (to actually organize client data), linkages and mobilization to community resources (e.g., public health agencies, social supports), and health care system organization (to ensure that providers are delivering safe, high-quality care) (Improving Chronic Illness Care, 2019). Some of the types of primary care services described later (e.g., CHCs, team-based primary care) exemplify the key elements needed in a chronic care model.

> **EXERCISE 16.2 IMPROVING CARE FOR PATIENTS WITH CHRONIC DISEASES:** List one example of an intervention or activity that may be put into place under each of the six key elements for improving care for chronic diseases from Wagner's CCM model, as described in the text.

Community Health Centres

An integrated and high-quality community-based health system requires collaboration with community agencies, multisectoral partners, health care providers, and citizens. The Canadian model of CHCs provides an ideal place-based community setting to create locally driven solutions and address population health. According to the Canadian Association of Community Health Centres (CACHC), CHCs are multisector health and health care organizations that deliver integrated, people-centred services and programs that reflect the needs and priorities of the diverse communities they serve (CACHC, 2016).

A CHC has a voluntary board composed of members from the community. It receives an annual budget from the provincial government for specific health programs, and it provides a wide range of services, such as medical, dental, dietitians, social, and nursing by a multidisciplinary staff, all under one roof. All the professionals, including physicians, are on salary. In all provinces except Quebec, many of these centres are located in underserved areas or serve groups that are often not well served, such as poor individuals, older adults, Indigenous peoples, and immigrant groups. There are more than 700 CHCs in Canada that provide care to 2 million clients (CACHC, 2016).

An innovation ahead of its time, CHCs have been in existence in Canada since the 1920s as community clinics (Saskatchewan) and local community service centres (Quebec) and were formalized with federal recommendations in the 1972 Hastings Report (CACHC, 2016). Common features of all CHCs across Canada include the following:

1. They provide interprofessional primary care.
2. They integrate services and programs in primary care, health promotion, and community well-being.
3. Care is community centred.
4. Care actively addresses the social determinants of health.
5. Care demonstrates a commitment to health equity and social justice.

In Quebec, these centres are part of the regionalized health and social service system and are called **centres** locaux des services communautaires (local community service centres [CLSCs]), of which there are approximately 147. CLSCs integrate health and social services and emphasize prevention, health promotion, and provision of other personal services, including occupational health services, at one location; they are also required to provide services for extended hours in the evenings and on weekends.

New Models of Primary Health Care

In September 2000, Canada's premiers and the Prime Minister agreed that improvements to primary health care are crucial to the renewal of health services. The federal government established the $800 million, 4-year Primary Health Care Transition Fund (PHCTF) to accelerate the transition to new primary care models (Health Canada, 2002).

The PHCTF included a $240 million national component to support common approaches to primary health care reform and initiatives that include health of Indigenous populations; official language minorities; multiprovincial initiatives; and national partnerships with nurses, doctors, rural physicians, and other public health stakeholders. The fund was used to support pilot and demonstration projects, as well as research at the provincial or territorial and national levels. The 2002 Romanow report discussed the need for an overhauled approach to PHC, calling for comprehensive on-call care 24 hours a day, 7 days a week; interprofessional health care teams; and more emphasis on health promotion (Romanow, 2002).

Realizing the resistance of primary care physicians to joining the reform, the 2003 First Ministers Health Accord committed more funds toward the reform, with a stated goal that 50% of the population will have access to an appropriate health care providers, 24 hours a day, 7 days a week, within the next 8 years. Since 2002, provincial governments have invested more funding into primary health care through various practice care settings. For example, in British Columbia, primary care networks (PCNs) and patient medical homes (PMHs) have been developed. PCNs are a network of family practices (including traditional GP-owned family practices, community governed health centres, and health authority-delivered family practices) in a defined geography linked with each other and with other primary care services delivered by the health authority and other community-based organizations.

Patient medical homes (PMHs) are advanced primary care clinics that are defined by 12 attributes; key attributes of PMHs include the provision of timely access to comprehensive, coordinated primary care, which will require a focus on the following building blocks: engaged leadership, data-driven quality improvement, panel assessment and management, and team-based interprofessional care. Additionally, the Divisions of Family Practice were created in British Columbia through which groups of family physicians could address gaps in patient care and promote family medicine. Newfoundland and Labrador divided the province into 30 team areas to serve the entire population. While efforts are being made to create new models of PHC, the PCNs and PMH are primary care focused, which is only one aspect of reforming health care towards a PHC system.

> **CRITICAL THINKING QUESTION 16.6:** What are the benefits and challenges to having PHC models?

Primary Care Teams

An emerging trend in community health services is delivering care through team-based approaches underpinned by interprofessional practice. In Alberta, Primary Care Teams (PCTs) are situated within Primary Care Networks (PCNs). PCNs include doctors, nurses, dietitians, social workers, and pharmacists working together to meet primary health care needs in their communities. Approximately 80% of primary care physicians are registered in a PCN. Established in 2003 through the Primary Care Initiative, Alberta now has 41 PCNs involving more than 3 800 physicians and the full-time-equivalent of more than 1 000 health care providers. PCNs provide services to close to 3.6 million Albertans (Alberta Health, 2018). Similarly, in Ontario, **family health teams (FHTs)** are community-centred primary care organizations whose programs and services are geared to the population groups they serve to ensure that people receive the care they need in their communities. Each team is set up based on local health and community needs. FHTs include a team of family physicians, NPs, RNs, social workers, dietitians, and other professionals who work together to provide primary health care for their community. Since 2005, 184 FHTs have been operationalized in Ontario, with 68 FHTs serving rural communities and 42 FHTs serving northern communities (Ontario Ministry of Health and Long-Term Care, 2016). Additionally, Ontario's Primary Health Care Expert Advisory Committee has recommended a population-based model of integrated primary health care delivery, designed around **patient care groups (PCGs)**, which are fund-holding organizations that are accountable to the ministry. The entire population of the province and all primary care providers would be assigned to primary care fund-holding organizations (PCGs), based on geography. PCGs would contract with local primary care providers to deliver primary care services to the PCG's assigned population. However, given the lack of stakeholder consultation and engagement to date, the acceptability and feasibility of this model are as yet untested.

> **CRITICAL THINKING QUESTION 16.7:** What are the advantages and drawbacks of enrolling in a primary health care team?

PUBLIC HEALTH SERVICES

Public health encompasses "the organized efforts of society to keep people healthy and prevent injury, illness and premature death" (Government of Canada, 2008). Public health, as you can see by its definition, is broad-based and involves many sectors in society. Public health–specific agencies, however, tend to take on and lead this role. Their work involves investigating and identifying the causes of poor and good health. Acting on this information improves the health of the population by preventing disease, illness, and injury; protecting populations from health risks; and promoting healthy public policies, environments, and behaviours. Fig. 16.1 outlines public health functions, with an emphasis on supporting population health, improving health, and reducing inequities (British Columbia Ministry of Health, 2017).

Local Public Health Units and Departments

Public health is primarily considered to be a provincial and territorial responsibility under the constitution; however, responsibility for **health protection** (i.e., the actions to ensure that water, air, and food are safe; protection from environmental threats; and a having a regulatory framework in place to control infectious diseases) is less clear, with responsibilities being shared among federal and provincial and territorial governments. As discussed in Chapter 14, most provincial and territorial governments provide public health services. However, the federal government plays a leading role in the health promotion and protection of Indigenous populations, Canadian Forces personnel, veterans, Royal Canadian Mounted Police,

> ### BOX 16.2   The Role of First Nations and Inuit Health Branch
>
> Health Canada's First Nations and Inuit Health Branch (FNIHB) is often the lead agency responsible for the delivery of public health services for both on reserve First Nations communities, and Inuit communities, in partnership with these communities (although some Indigenous communities have also created their own independent organizations to lead the public health functions). Additionally, although the provinces and territories are mostly responsible for primary health care services, in some remote on-reserve communities where there isn't ready access to provincial and territorial or Indigenous-run and operated primary health care services, FNIHB also takes on that role in partnership with the local communities. Two examples of services offered by the Primary Health Care and Public Health Directorate include outbreak management and the provision of community nursing posts in remote communities (Government of Canada, 2013). When provincial and territorial public health agencies are in close proximity or available to on-reserve or Inuit communities, FNIHB and these provincial or territorial agencies are advised to work together to coordinate service provision and minimize confusion regarding the accessing of these services.

and inmates in federal penitentiaries. For a more detailed description regarding the provision of both community health and public health services for Indigenous people in Canada, refer to Box 16.2 and Chapter 7.

In Canada, government and nongovernment agencies, as well as the private sector, provide public health services. Public health units and departments are the primary providers of publicly funded statutory and nonstatutory programs and activities for disease prevention, health protection, and health promotion at the local or regional level in all provinces and territories. These activities fall within the five core functions: population health assessment, health surveillance, health promotion, disease and injury prevention, and health protection. Specific examples of activities that public health departments may take on include supporting breastfeeding, writing regular reports on health status of the community, home visitation programs, dental screening, outbreak management, follow-up of cases of reportable diseases, inspecting food premises, and coordinating community action on the opioid crisis.

Public health activities in all provinces and territories are governed by public health legislation and accompanying regulations and a variety of other acts specific to different functions, such as health protection and promotion, RHAs, occupational health and safety, and tobacco sales. Some jurisdictions also have public health standards to which regional or local public health bodies must adhere. At the ministry level, all provincial governments maintain central departments responsible for public health matters and have a chief medical health officer or equivalent. Most, but not all, have statutory powers related to communicable disease control (e.g., issuing quarantine orders, shutting down restaurants or other facilities that may pose a health hazard); other responsibilities include acting as a consultant or advisor to regional or local medical health officers, providing policy advice on population health promotion, and acting as spokespersons on public health issues. They are part of the government hierarchy, depending upon provincial or territorial structure.

Currently, public health services are, for the most part, the responsibility of regional or district health authorities. Provinces are divided geographically into health regions or health units. Health units (e.g., in Ontario) are semiautonomous, community-based delivery structures that form liaisons with local hospitals, medical practitioners, and voluntary health agencies and have their own buildings and staff. In many provinces, public heath services and functions are integrated into health care services and organized into RHAs. The province of Quebec is unique in that it has been divided into 18 regional boards of health and social services (Régies régionales de la santé et des services sociaux), each with a director of public health responsible for the assessment of the health needs of the population and the development of the most effective preventive interventions, surveillance, and control of communicable and NCDs; the director of public health also deals with real or perceived public health emergencies and health promotion and disease prevention, working closely with the CLSCs and other regional health and social services agencies. Most health units are now under the direction of RHBs that determine the overall direction of programs and policies, as well as the amount of public funding. The major portion of funding for local health units comes from the provincial government (through regional funding) with some funding from local governments. However, in Ontario, approximately 75% of the total funding of public health services comes from the provincial governments in the form of grants, with the remainder 25% from the local municipalities. With these financial arrangements, local governments retain autonomy in policy and program planning while following provincial guidelines. The lack of uniformity in services provided across the province is compensated by assessment and fulfillment of local needs. Additionally, many public health authorities in Ontario prefer the formal link with local municipalities because they have oversight and decision-making authority in many of the social determinants of health, including transport, the built environment, social policy, and so on. As such, it is easier to build healthy public policy in partnership with the municipalities.

Public health agencies, given their broad mandates and functions, are by nature multidisciplinary, with a range of different types of staff and professionals working together. For a more detailed description of the various types of professionals involved in public health at the local or regional level, see the Interprofessional Practice box.

INTERPROFESSIONAL PRACTICE
The Mix of Skills in a Public Health Agency

Public health at the local or regional level has responsibilities that vary from outbreak control to working with municipal planners on healthy built environment initiatives. As such, they require a diverse range of staff with all sorts of expertise in the health sector and beyond.

Public health nurses (Box 16.3) tend to make up the backbone of much of the public health workforce. They work very collaboratively with epidemiologists and data analysts, health educators or promoters, dietitians and nutritionists, physicians, research and policy analysts, public health investigators (described further in Chapter 11), and legal professionals, among others.

An outbreak investigation would require nurses and investigators, along with a data person, someone who is skilled in communications, and likely the law as well, in case it is a high-profile outbreak involving a private institution with its own policies and procedures.

Communications specialists also have an important role to play when it comes to health promotion and partnering with the media for positive health messaging or crisis messaging (in the case of major outbreaks, for example).

Increasingly more often, people with skills in fields like health economics and planning or urban design are also being brought into the local public health scene because they can help work on things such as evaluating health policies, analyzing the economics of health interventions to inform local governments, and developing healthy and active physical spaces for communities to enjoy.

BOX 16.3   Public Health Nurses

Public health nurses (PHNs) are often community health nurses who work specifically in a public health agency (e.g., for an RHA or public health unit). Typically, they are generalists with a baccalaureate degree in nursing, who have expertise in areas such as school health, communicable diseases, or health promotion. Their focus is the health of populations, and on health promotion, disease prevention, and assessing community assets and needs, to name a few. They are holistic in their approach and work with communities to foster agency and empowerment like other community health nurses. In traditional public health agency settings (e.g., health units), public health nurses may be involved in following up cases of sexually transmitted reportable infections (e.g., syphilis, HIV), planning and implementing breastfeeding support services, overseeing home visitation programs, and leading partnerships in the community (Canadian Public Health Association, 2010; Manitoba Health, 1998).

Functions of Local Public Health Units

Public health programs and services vary greatly in geographic area and population size served. Fig. 16.2 provides an overview of British Columbia's public health strategic framework as an example of how service can be organized and delivered.

The population count of local public health units could range from hundreds to more than 2 million, and catchment areas can vary from 15 to 1.5 million square kilometres. Programs also serve a variety of communities (most serve a combination of urban and rural populations). As already mentioned, the mandate of the local health units stems from the public health acts or regulations passed by the provincial legislature. For example, Ontario's Public Health Standards outline standards for public health services in general and lists the goals and objectives for specific programs. Local governments also pass health-related bylaws if the province so authorizes (e.g., bylaws regulating noise levels or smoking in public places). The extent of services provided depends on the province's public health act and the number of qualified personnel employed by each agency in relation to the population. Many rural agencies do not have enough personnel to employ a full complement of public health staff. In addition to mandated activities, RHAs have expanded into many new health fields outside their traditional role, especially in urban areas. Foremost among these are health promotion, mental health, services for people who are aged or have disabilities, and issues related to the physical environment.

In the following section, the functions of health units (communicable disease control, women's health and maternal and child health, health promotion, dental health, environmental health, population health assessment, and disease surveillance) are discussed.

Communicable Disease Control. The control of communicable disease continues to be a basic function of public health agencies, including regional or local health units. Their duties include disease surveillance (which can be supported by provincial public health technical and scientific agencies, such as Public Health Ontario and the British Columbia Centre for Disease Control [BCCDC]), the provision of consultation services to local physicians and hospitals, the supply of immunizing agents (e.g., vaccines), health education, and special epidemiological surveys and studies. Health units are granted authority to control communicable disease by legislation and regulations; they are also responsible for the investigation and management of outbreaks, such as food poisoning in nursing homes, measles in schools, and diarrhea in daycare centres. Most local health units operate sexually transmitted infection (STI) clinics, either by themselves or in conjunction with the local hospital; these clinics provide free diagnostic and treatment services at convenient hours. In some areas, these units pay private physicians to give free and anonymous treatment; also with their help, local health units are involved in case findings of STIs and other communicable diseases, follow-up of contacts, and health education programs for STIs. Local public health units provide contraceptive and family planning services as well. This is described in more detail in Chapter 10.

Women's Health and Maternal and Child Health. In recent years, maternal and child health divisions in public health units in many provinces have been renamed and their functions expanded to focus more on family and women's health. The divisions may have different names in different provinces, but they all have similar functions. Public health nurses employed by local health units carry out preventive health programs such as education and immunization of infants and children in clinics. The maternal and child health services may include classes for expectant parents, postnatal visits to all or high-risk new parents, advice on parenting, and visits to daycare centres. Whereas immunization of children is a statutory program in public health units in Alberta and Prince Edward Island, private physicians and health

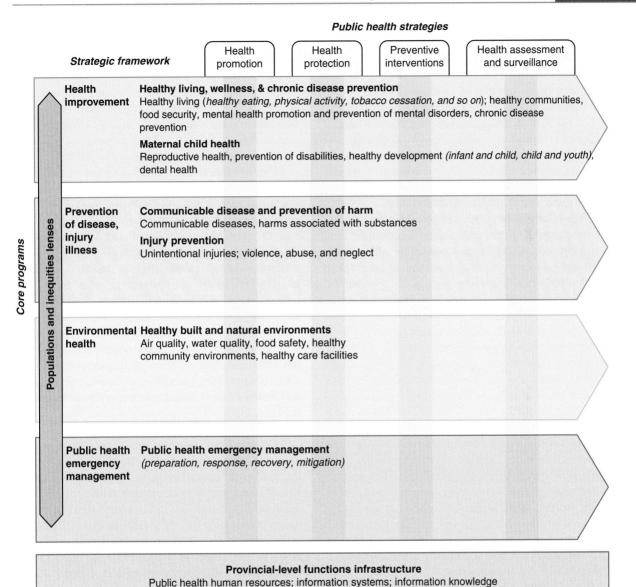

Fig. 16.2 Example of British Columbia's public health framework. (From British Columbia Ministry of Health. [2017]. *Promote, protect, prevent: our health begins here [BC's Guiding Framework for Public Health]* [p. 16]. Retrieved from https://www.health.gov.bc.ca/library/publications/year/2017/BC-guiding-framework-for-public-health-2017-update.pdf.)

units in other provinces share immunization responsibilities. Alberta also has comprehensive preschool surveillance programs (to monitor growth and development), which cover about 90% of children. In many provinces, health units provide health care services for school children; however, in others, the local education authority or private practitioners may provide this service. The type of school health services varies considerably across Canada, and the provision of services by larger city departments may differ from that found in a rural health unit. Vision screening tests and immunization programs have become standard practice in most local areas, but audiometric screening for hearing loss is discretionary in some areas. The public health nurse provides continuity for the health surveillance of school children and maintains contact with the parents and family doctor.

Health Promotion. Public health units increasingly emphasize health promotion, community development, and health advocacy. Health promotion as a separate discipline has been receiving growing recognition. Strategies include educational methods to improve knowledge and skills, encouragement of public participation in health practices conducive to healthy living, and public policies that create environments that support health. Many local health departments employ health promotion specialists. Their responsibility includes continually assessing the health needs of their community, coordinating local health promotion services, and consulting with personnel in the voluntary and civic organizations interested in health. **Public health nursing** (see Box 16.3) is involved in implementing and planning health promotion strategies. Public health nurses may also be involved in helping communities mobilize against a public health problem; for example, they can provide information on secondhand smoke and its effects on health, enabling citizens to bring about the necessary environmental changes through political or legislative processes. Nutrition consultants prepare reference and educational materials for professional health care personnel and for the public. Examples of health promotion programs include consulting with city planners on regional official plans to ensure a health-promoting urban design and advocating to various levels of government for positive health reforms such as the banning of sugar-sweetened beverages in public buildings or nonsmoking bylaws in public parks. Health promotion programs provide education in schools on smoking, alcohol, drugs, sex, healthy active living, positive mental health, and nutrition.

Dental Health. Public health initiatives such as fluoridation of municipal water supplies (described further in Chapter 11) and improved dental hygiene have successfully reduced dental caries in Canadian children. Public health now focuses on provision of dental treatment to underprivileged groups and older adults. Dental health divisions of provincial ministries, in collaboration with local health units, have sponsored the provision of dental care for children in remote areas. There are travelling clinics staffed by provincial dental teams in Manitoba, Nova Scotia, Ontario, and Prince Edward Island that visit rural and remote areas. These clinics deliver a considerable amount of emergency care for all age groups. A program to subsidize dental expenses in communities

that do not have a resident dentist has been developed in British Columbia; in rural Alberta, dentists who volunteer to supply services on a private practice basis for short periods are provided with dental equipment, office facilities, and living accommodations. In some provinces, the dental health division of the provincial health department administers school dental programs. This responsibility may be delegated either to the department of education or to the board of health, particularly in cities.

In all of these models, dentists or dental hygienists are employed to carry out functions such as case finding, education, prevention, and treatment. Such services are generally provided to preschool children or up to grade 1 or 2. Treatment services are offered primarily to children from lower income groups.

Environmental Health. **Public health inspectors** hired by local health units protect the public from physical, chemical, and biological hazards. This is carried out through the inspection of food-handling premises such as restaurants, butcher shops, and bakeries. Public health inspectors are responsible for community sanitation such as the maintenance of sanitary supplies of potable water, milk, and food; disposal of wastes; and the quality of recreational water. They also respond to public complaints and emergency situations such as spills of toxic chemicals. In some of the larger cities, indoor air pollution monitoring is carried out by public health units. A number of health units have hired environmental specialists to conduct environmental risk assessments and provide consultation for their staff. The role of the public health inspector in environmental health is addressed further in Chapter 11.

Population Health Assessment. Population health refers to the health of a population as measured by health status indicators, described in Chapter 4. The belief that social, economic, and environmental conditions have a great deal of influence over health has been integral to public health since the beginnings in the 18th century. Epidemiologists assess the health indicators for populations and subpopulations that are necessary for the linked functions of effective public health practice, health promotion, disease and injury prevention, and health protection.

Health Surveillance. Health surveillance is the tracking and forecasting of any health event or health determinant through the collection of data and its integration, analysis and interpretation into surveillance products, and the dissemination of those surveillance products to those who need to know. Similar to population health assessment, health surveillance capacity is an integral part of public health because it provides essential knowledge for the planning of effective interventions. It, too, is carried out by epidemiologists. Surveillance is described further in Chapter 2.

CRITICAL THINKING QUESTIONS 16.8:

1. Across the country, there has been a debate regarding how to best organize public health services: are they best placed within the structure of an RHA where there are formal linkages to the rest of the health care system, including hospitals and primary care services, or best placed in the structure of a local or regional municipal government that provides services such as transport, waste, water, social services, and so on? How does the public health system in your own province or territory work (which structure is it most aligned with), and what are the implications of this way of being organized for the overall health of your community?
2. What role do RNs play in organized public health services in your city, province, or territory?

HOME CARE SERVICES

As discussed in Chapter 15, home care in Canada is defined an array of services provided in home and community settings that encompasses health promotion and teaching, curative intervention, rehabilitation, support and maintenance, social adaptation and palliative end-of-life care, and integration and support for the family caregiver (Canadian Home Care Association [CHCA], 2013). Home care services comprise medical and support services provided in the home setting to meet the needs of individuals and their families and volunteer caregivers. Generally, a home care program substitutes for services provided by hospitals and long-term care facilities, serves as a maintenance function so clients can remain in their current environment rather than moving to a new and often more costly venue, and serves a prevention function by providing patient services and monitoring at additional short-run but lower-run costs (CHCA, 2013).

Most current health reform aims to strengthen and expand community- and home-based care. This shift away from hospital-based care is motivated in part by fiscal constraints (home care is less expensive than institutional care) and in part by the belief that services provided in the home effectively meet the needs and preferences of patients, especially among older adults.

Home care services play a key role in "aging in place" strategies by managing chronic disease, reducing hospital admissions, repeat ED visits, and associated wait times; and in ensuring quality end-of-life care (Accreditation Canada, 2015).

A History of Home Care in Canada

The roots of home care can be traced back to England in the mid-1800s when William Rathbone, a wealthy businessman and philanthropist, with the help of Florence Nightingale, established a school to train visiting nurses in helping the "sick poor" in their homes (Buhler-Wilkerson,1985). Until that point, it was often only wealthy people who were cared for at home, while the poor, homeless, or indigent were treated in hospitals.

As the home health nurse role evolved, it became inseparable from community health nursing, as each nurse provided the full continuum of nursing care, including health promotion and disease prevention, hands-on care to restore health, or palliative care (Community Health Nurses' Initiative Group, 2000). RNs have formed the backbone of home care services and have been instrumental in the development of interprofessional practice working as part of a team with social workers, physiotherapists, occupational therapists, respiratory therapists, and physicians.

In most provinces, provision of home care services began with smaller, urban programs run by agencies such as the Victorian Order of Nurses. As a result of rising hospital costs and pressure on hospital facilities, home care programs were developed mainly to relieve hospitals of the care of patients who only needed additional nursing services or physiotherapy. Some provinces developed comprehensive, government-oriented home care plans in the 1970s. In 1977, as a part of the Extended Program Financing services, legislation provided the first concrete financial support for home care programs (see Chapter 15). By the late 1990s, all provinces and territories had government home care directorates or divisions, although there is no common approach to funding and delivery. For example, Veterans Affairs Canada offers home care services to clients with wartime or special duty area service when the service is not available to them through provincial and territorial programs. Health Canada's Territorial region, created in 1998, is responsible for the delivery of various community-based programs to Indigenous people in the three territories.

There is now a growing body of literature internationally and in Canada which indicates that home care can be a cost-effective substitute for long-term facility care and acute care within an integrated system of health care. In 2012, more than 2 million Canadians were enrolled in home care programs across Canada. Greater demand for home care has resulted from a number of different factors, including:

- Improved technology that allows for the delivery of services in the community (e.g., home-based dialysis)
- Increase in outpatient surgery, earlier hospital discharges, and reduction in long-term and acute care hospital beds
- Patients' desire to have care delivered closer to home, whether it is in the community or in the home
- Increasing average life expectancy, particularly among the baby boomers
- Decreased availability of informal care-giving by family members because of changing family structure and work patterns (CHCA, 2013).

 CASE EXAMPLE

Robert's Need for Home Care

After reading the case example below, think about the benefits of home care for Robert and the health care system.

Robert, who is 82 years old, recently lost his wife of 60 years. "She's the one who took care of everything," he thought. He remembered how she paid the bills, took care of insurance, and asked all the questions at the doctor's office. As her health failed, she even insisted on getting caregivers to ease the burden on him. "I want a husband," she said, "not a nurse." Even though she was now gone, she could still make him smile.

But right now, Robert is having a hard time with his own health care. He recently had surgery and wasn't sure if he was supposed to feel better than he did or not. There were so many instructions that he couldn't be sure if he was doing all he was or wasn't supposed to. And then there were so many doctors! Each time he had a visit, there seemed to be more instructions that just confused him even more.

Robert again thought about his wife's caregivers and wondered if there wasn't some similar type of help for him. So, he called the discharge coordinator who had assured him before he left the hospital that he could call if he needed anything. After he explained what his difficulties were, she referred him to a local in-home care service.

He had a nice call with a nurse, who assured him that they could help get him to doctor's visits, sit with him

---

 CASE EXAMPLE—CONT'D

Robert's Need for Home Care

while the doctor explained what needed to happen, and then make sure that it all was coordinated with the plan of care he got when he left the hospital. She said his caregiver would help make sure his other doctors knew all the various aspects of his care. And if he needed, his caregiver would help him make lists so that he had clear instructions to follow for when she wasn't around.

"We want to help you get healthy and stay out of the hospital," she said. After hearing that, Robert started to worry less and looked forward to having someone to talk with again.

Source: Home Instead Senior Care. [2018]. *Gaining compliance of a plan of care*. Omaha, NE: Author. Retrieved from https://www.returninghomecare.com/home-care-scenarios/

Types of Home Care

Different basic forms of home care are described next.

Maintenance and Preventive Care

Home support services (e.g., homemaker, transportation, and Meals on Wheels programs) provide autonomy and mobility for those with assessed functional deficits. These services are not primarily medical and may be provided along with medical treatment. Although many people can remain at home without the help of these services for some time, early use of the services can prevent health decline and institutionalization.

Long-Term Care Substitution or Chronic Care Services

Long-term care substitution or chronic care services are provided to people with significant functional deficits, usually resulting from one or more medical conditions, who require these services to remain in their homes. Chronic care services are designed for people with stable conditions or designed to delay deterioration and eventual hospitalization.

Acute Care Substitution

Acute home care is usually provided after hospitalization to people who are unable to travel to outpatient facilities and is provided on a short-term basis according to need. It is designed to reduce the length of hospital stay and to assist the recovery process. People usually receive acute home care from 2 or 3 days to a maximum of 90 days.

Extra-Mural Hospital or Hospital Without Walls

Founded in 1981, this New Brunswick program was Canada's first government-funded home-hospital program. The mandate of the Extra-Mural Program (EMP) is to provide a broad range of home health care services to all residents for the purpose of promoting, maintaining, and restoring health within the context of their daily lives and to provide palliative services. Services include health education (i.e., chronic disease management, diabetes, COPD, complex medical needs such as postsurgery, stroke recovery, medication management, dementia, and end-of-life care, and a home oxygen program). Meals on Wheels, homemaking, and other support services can be purchased by the patient, who must be formally admitted by an attending physician who directs the medical care plan and authorizes discharge. Nursing services are available 24 hours a day, 7 days a week, and all other disciplines deliver services Monday to Friday. To be eligible, the patient must be acutely but not critically ill and must require one or more professional services such as nursing, occupational therapy, or physiotherapy. Twenty-three service delivery sites provide the delivery of EMP services to clients across the entire province. In 2018, the administration of service for EMP was privatized; however, eligible patients will continue to receive services free. This move by the government has prompted both criticism and accolades from health care providers and labour groups.

CRITICAL THINKING QUESTIONS 16.9

1. What are the benefits having the EMP privatized?
2. What are the drawbacks of having the EMP privatized?

Palliative Home Care

Palliative home care is provided to terminally ill patients such as those with terminal cancer. Palliative care is provided by a multidisciplinary team at home and is described in greater detail later in the Palliative Care section.

Delivery of Home Care

Two features characterize most home care programs: centralization of control of services within the program and ongoing coordination of services to meet the changing needs of the patient. In all provinces except Nova Scotia, the RHAs are responsible for administration of home care programs. There is also a substantial private sector component to home care with services financed directly by the patient or family.

All provinces offer a similar range of basic services: client assessment, case coordination, case management, nursing services, and home support (the latter including personal care, homemaking, Meals on Wheels, and respite services). Other services, such as rehabilitation services (e.g., physiotherapy, occupational therapy), oxygen therapy, respiratory therapy, and specialized nursing services are in development as part of home care in some provinces. Seven provinces (British Columbia, Alberta, Saskatchewan, Manitoba, Ontario, New Brunswick, Nova Scotia) have contracts for oxygen therapy services. Social work, speech therapy, and dietitian services are offered as part of some home care programs. There is a greater emphasis placed on applying a multidisciplinary approach to care in some jurisdictions. Overall service delivery models are undergoing review and/or change in some provinces (including British Columbia, Ontario, and Quebec) (see Real-World Example and Clinical Example boxes).

◤ REAL-WORLD EXAMPLE

Increasing the Accessibility of Home Care

Expanding home care is challenging, given the limited resources for home care services. However, a community paramedicine movement has expanded the roles of paramedics to provide health care in individuals homes or in extended care facilities. A good example of an innovative program to bring care closer to individuals is in Nova Scotia. Nova Scotia's Extended Care Paramedic nursing home program allows seniors to be treated at home instead of in the ED. The program has paramedics working along onsite nurses in long-term care homes to treat about 70% of seniors on scene instead of transferring them to the ED. This type of program has expanded to at least two other provinces (Alberta and Ontario), where paramedics make house calls.

Evaluation of these programs is showing to have a positive impact on participants. Agarwal et al. (2018) found that residents at facilities served by a paramedic nursing home program had a better quality of life, which resulted in a significant decrease in emergency ambulance calls. Residents said they were able to continue their regular activities and get more physical activity.

CLINICAL EXAMPLE

Rapid Response Nursing for Medically Complex or Frail Adult Clients

The transition from hospital to home is a vulnerable period for anyone but especially for those who have complex conditions, are frail, are at risk for adverse events, and are unable to navigate a system of poorly coordinated care in the postdischarge period.

Achieving seamless transitions between care settings is viewed as being crucial to high-quality care. Care transition interventions are seen as being effective care-coordinating mechanisms for reducing avoidable adverse events associated with the transition of the patient from the hospital to the home.

Comprehensive support for clients with complex medical issues is limited within traditional home care services, due to the number of clients they service each day. However, Ontario's Rapid Response Nursing service provides direct support between hospital discharge and home for some clients and families dealing with complex medical conditions. The goal is to support a successful discharge home, with prompt interventions to avoid any unnecessary returns to hospital and improve the client's confidence to remain safely at home. Within 24 to 48 hours, the nurse will conduct an initial home visit, with targeted short-term (2–3 weeks) intensive nursing interventions in the individual's home. Interventions may include medication teaching, discharge follow-up, and facilitating linkages with the client's home clinic or primary care provider, along with chronic disease education and management.

PALLIATIVE CARE

Palliative care is a relatively new field in Canada, which first emerged in 1974. Demand is increasing, not only for palliative care but also for having a "good death," and evidence suggests that most people prefer to die at home (Gomes et al., 2013).

In recent years, many provinces have responded to the need of palliative care programs within their jurisdiction; however, there is still a dearth of palliative care programs, particularly in rural settings and Indigenous communities, for children, and for those responding to the needs of cultural communities.

Palliative care (comfort care) or **end-of-life care** is a special kind of health care for individuals and families who are living with a life-threatening illness that is usually at an advanced stage. The goal for palliative

BOX 16.4   Did You Know? The Palliative Performance Scale

In palliative care, the **Palliative Performance Scale, Version 2 (PPS)** can indicate a progressive declining condition. The PPS is an excellent communication tool for quickly describing a person's current functional level that, along with good clinical judgement, can guide the care team in planning for appropriate care supports.

To view a full version of the PPS and guidelines, visit http://palliative.info/resource_material/PPSv2.pdf.

care is comfort and dignity for the person living with the illness, as well as the best quality of life for both this person and his or her family. An important objective of palliative care is relief of pain and other symptoms. Palliative care is planned to meet the physical needs as well as the psychological, social, cultural, emotional, and spiritual needs of each person and the family (Box 16.4). The goal is not to cure but to provide comfort and maintain the highest possible quality of life for as long as life remains. The focus is on compassionate specialized care for the living. **Terminal care** refers to care delivered at the end of life and reflects only a portion of all of palliative care. Palliative care may be delivered in hospice and home care settings or in hospitals.

Hospices are residential facilities—separate buildings or apartments where palliative care is provided in a home-like setting. Some people move into hospices to receive palliative care on a 24-hour basis. Because medical needs vary depending on the disease that is leading toward death, specialized palliative care programs exist for common conditions such as cancer. Specialized care giving is also needed if organic changes in the brain lead to coma and dementia.

Palliative care is well suited to an interdisciplinary team, often supplemented by volunteers, that provides support for the whole person and to those who are sharing the person's journey. Palliative care should involve psychological support, assistance in interpersonal skills, coordinated service delivery, symptom control, bereavement counselling, independent living, counselling in legal and financial issues, and counselling in matters of spirituality, lifestyle, culture, and religion. It can be given in the home or in an institutional setting. Acute care facilities, which are geared to diagnosis and treatment, do not usually have the environment, skills, and flexibility needed to provide support to terminally ill patients and their families. Some facilities may designate palliative care beds and employ a palliative care team that includes nurses, social workers, respiratory therapists, physicians, and spiritual counsellors. As noted in the home care section, palliative home care is finally recognized as part of the core services.

MENTAL HEALTH AND ADDICTION SERVICES

The most common reason why individuals need home care is to address mental health issues, with one in seven Canadians (14%) reporting receiving care as a result of depression, schizophrenia, or other mental illness (Sinha & Bleakney, 2015). Mental health services, broadly defined, comprise a mix of health, social, vocational, recreational, volunteer, occupational therapy, and educational services, as well as housing and income support. They include activities and objectives ranging from mental health promotion and the prevention of mental health problems to the treatment of acute psychiatric disorders and the support and rehabilitation of persons with severe and persistent psychiatric disorders and disabilities. The morbidity, mortality, and economic burden associated with mental illness and addictions are described in Chapter 9.

In Canada, the provincial and territorial governments have primary jurisdiction in the planning and delivery of mental health and addiction services. Most provinces have a separate branch or department dealing with mental health and addictions and are either part of the ministry of health or community services or an independent ministry. For detailed programs and services provided by the provinces, readers are advised to visit provincial government websites.

Among provincially operated health services, mental health and addiction services represent some of the largest administrative areas in terms of expenditure and employees. In every province, at least 88% (nationally, 96%) of the revenue for mental institutions comes from the provincial government or the provincial insurance plan. For the past 6 decades, the provision of mental health services has gradually shifted from institutions to community-based services. Depending upon the nature and the severity of illness, services are now provided by mental health institutions, psychiatric units of general hospitals, special hospitals, private

hospitals, clinics, mental health care centres, prisons, shelters, and private practitioners such as psychiatrists, family physicians, NPs, clinical psychologists, and social workers.

Community mental health facilities are now extended beyond specific mental health institutions to provide greater continuity of care, to deal with incipient breakdown, and to rehabilitate patients in the community. Psychiatric units in general hospitals contribute by integrating psychiatry with other medical care and making it available in the community. Hospital inpatient services in psychiatric units are paid for by all provincial hospital insurance plans. Some provinces have small regional psychiatric hospitals that facilitate patient access to treatment and complete integration of medical services. There are day centres across the country that allow patients to be hospitalized during the day and return home at night, as well as community mental health clinics (some provincially operated, others municipally) and psychiatric outpatient services.

Addiction services (sometimes referred to as substance use or misuse services) vary widely across Canada. Residential programs are common and can be not for profit or private, providing an array of services from medical detox to group and individual therapy. One of the challenges with addictions services and programs is that there are often long waiting lists, which is a major barrier and deterrent to seeking help because the motivation to change behaviour and the action to do so often only occurs within a narrow time period. By the time someone on the waitlist is called, the motivation to change their behaviour may have shifted. To address this issue, since around 2016, Ontario, Manitoba, and British Colombia have introduced Rapid Access Addiction Clinics to expedite the long waiting list for persons seeking addiction services.

Specialized mental health rehabilitation services, which assist former acute care patients to function optimally, are operated by mental health hospitals and community agencies. They include sheltered workshops that pay for work and provide training and houses where patients can live and continue to receive treatment while settling in jobs. At present, there is a large gap in available community services for mental health patients because of shortages of affordable housing, jobs, recreational facilities, and mental health workers.

> **CRITICAL THINKING QUESTION 16.10:** Mental health and addiction services have been moving into the community from acute care hospitals. What are some potential challenges related to this transition from hospital to community?

CANCER SERVICES

More than one in three Canadians will get cancer in their lifetime; most will be diagnosed in their middle and later years. According to the Canadian Cancer Society (CCS), in 2017, there were an estimated 206 200 new cancer diagnoses and 80 800 deaths from cancer (CCS, 2017). For more detail on types of cancer and mode of prevention program, see Chapter 8.

Special provincial agencies for cancer control, usually run by the health ministry or a separate cancer institute, carry out cancer detection and treatment, public education, and professional training and research in cooperation with local public health services, community nurses, physicians, and voluntary CCS branches (e.g., the Alberta Cancer Board, the British Columbia Cancer Agency). Although the provisions are not uniform, cancer programs in all provinces provide a range of free diagnostic and treatment services, both to outpatients and to inpatients. Hospital insurance benefits for cancer patients include diagnostic radiology, laboratory tests, and radiotherapy. A number of provinces, including British Columbia, Ontario, Quebec, New Brunswick, and Nova Scotia, have organized screening programs for breast cancer for women.

The lack of uniform provision of services, however, results in differences in community cancer services between provinces and between communities. This can result in a lack of coordination of treatment and less than optimal dissemination of cancer treatment knowledge and information in the major centres.

> **CRITICAL THINKING QUESTION 16.11:** In your city, province, or territory, what kind of services are available for a person who has breast or lung cancer?

SERVICES FOR SPECIFIC POPULATIONS

Social and support services are available in the community for people with special, multidisciplinary needs (e.g., seniors, people with mental or physical challenges) and vary depending on the location of the community and the nature and type of disability. Overall, whereas rural communities have sparse services, metropolitan areas offer a full range of services (see Chapter 6). People with rare or very severe disabilities have fewer resources available for their care in the community. Medical and institutional care, such as long-term care in hospitals, extended care, rehabilitation care, and nursing home care, as well as many assistive devices for daily living, are available through either government insurance or subsidies. Most communities have home care programs available for those with multiple needs. In addition, the provinces are increasingly establishing "one-stop" access centres (e.g., multiple service agencies) to evaluate, assess, coordinate, and provide (or contract for the provision of) a wide range of health, social, and support services to seniors or people with disabilities. There are two types of voluntary agencies that deal specifically with people with mental or physical challenges: agencies that exclusively deal with people with a specific disease or problem (e.g., the Multiple Sclerosis Society), and agencies that deal with specific groups with a disability (e.g., the Easter Seal Society, which deals with children with physical disabilities). Depending on the special needs of each individual, many voluntary agencies also provide a range of services, such as Meals on Wheels, visiting homemaker services, travelling clinics, provision of appliances and equipment, and wheelchairs. At the social services level, there are income maintenance programs, recreational programs, vocational rehabilitation services, special transportation services, and independent living accommodations available for individuals (see Chapter 12).

Indigenous populations have special constitutional issues where there are jurisdictional disputes; this topic is touched on in Box 16.2 and discussed more fully in Chapter 7.

VOLUNTARY HEALTH AGENCIES

Voluntary health agencies play an important part in shaping our health, welfare, and educational systems. These are nonprofit organizations led by boards of volunteers rather than under the direct control of the government. Their primary or major objectives are the promotion of health; the prevention of illness or disability; and the identification, treatment, or rehabilitation of people with a disease or disability; and raising funds for research. The CCS is a good example of an agency that fulfills many of these functions. Voluntary organizations differ in the nature of their membership: some are organized by citizens to provide service to others and are designated as citizen-member organizations; more recently, groups have been organized by patients and their relatives and their friends to provide services for themselves, and hence are designated patient-member organizations.

The *citizen-member organization* is the familiar form of philanthropy. Its members are interested in community service and thus are motivated to give time, thought, and money to accomplish an objective to promote the welfare of their community. *Patient-member organizations* are motivated by mutual aid. Those who have a disease for which there is no known cure or have a disability that causes them to be different from and even shunned by other people often become isolated and withdrawn or seek the company of fellow sufferers. They are faced with anxieties and frustration, from which they find some relief by uniting to fight their common enemy, the disease. The patients may be able to help themselves in specific ways (e.g., by organizing better treatment facilities), or they may hope to help people with the disease, including their families if the disease is hereditary. They gain support from the knowledge that they are not alone in facing their problems. Recently, some groups, such as HIV/AIDS groups, have taken on an advocacy role.

Voluntary organizations are financed to a considerable extent, if not wholly, by fundraising. The organization may conduct its own campaign for funds or be a member of a federated fund, such as United Way. Many of the agencies also receive public grants.

Objectives and Activities

Generally, the objectives and activities of many voluntary organizations include:

- *Education:* public education and dissemination of information to lay and professional people
- *Advocacy:* social action, sometimes specified, sometimes implied
- *Research:* collection of statistics, investigation of reported cures, surveys of resources and needs, encouragement and support for basic and clinical research
- *Direct patient services:* supply of diagnostic and treatment clinics, special equipment (e.g., wheelchairs,

crutches, colostomy bags, hoists, inhalation tents, prosthetic appliances), transportation and accommodation for patient and family, home treatment, therapies, vocational assessment and workshops; some take on official functions (e.g., the Children's Aid Society) and provide many services needed by society, including eye banks and first aid
- *Prevention:* the prevention and eradication of the disease or disability
- *Coordination of key players:* the coordination of public and private agencies with similar interests
- *Fundraising*
- *Provision of treatment guidelines,* such as with organization like the Diabetes Canada or Heart and Stroke Foundation of Canada

---

EXERCISE 16.3 RESEARCH DIFFERENT VOLUNTARY ORGANIZATIONS: Conduct an Internet search of several well-known voluntary organizations, such as Heart and Stroke Foundation of Canada, and do some research to find out who sits on their boards of directors. What are the backgrounds and expertise of board members? Do any of the board of directors hold influence that could direct the way the voluntary organization recommends treatment guidelines?

Role in Relation to Government

Voluntary agencies continually identify new areas of need and provide for those needs to the limit of their capacity. This capacity relates directly to the agency's ability to raise money, and in some cases, needs are only barely met. Nevertheless, the organizations often are able to impress upon the public's mind the importance of the services they provide and occasionally change the public's sensitivity to needs. In the past, with increasing affluence and heightened social conscience, governments recognized that many of these initiatives were universally needed for the care of citizens and hence funded or took over the responsibilities of many volunteer organizations' services. In recent years, however, this trend has reversed, and there is now increased reliance on the voluntary sector. In practice, the functions of voluntary organizations and the government in the health care field intermingle to such an extent that at times there is little differentiation in function, which may create tension between the government and voluntary organizations.

Scope of Work

Some examples of national voluntary organizations are presented here.

The Canadian Red Cross Society was established to furnish volunteer aid to the sick and wounded of armies in times of war, in accordance with the Geneva Convention, and in times of peace or war to carry on and assist in the improvement of health, the prevention of disease, and the mitigation of suffering throughout the world. Activities include veterans' services, international relief, emergency services, water safety services, Red Cross Youth, and Red Cross Corps. (As of 1997, the Canadian Red Cross is no longer involved in the provision of blood transfusion services in Canada.)

The Canadian Cancer Society was established in 1938 to coordinate individuals and agencies to reduce the mortality from cancer in Canada, to disseminate information on cancer, and to research activities about cancer.

Local volunteer groups include local chapters of larger organizations, as well as volunteer organizations that meet special needs in the community. These include volunteer groups working in hospitals, nursing homes, and crisis centres.

Voluntary agencies have adapted to the changing needs of society. For example, what was once known as the Canadian Tuberculosis Association has changed its name and mandate, with the decreasing incidence of tuberculosis, to the Canadian Tuberculosis and Respiratory Disease Association; its Ontario chapter calls itself the Ontario Lung Association and focuses on all lung diseases.

Voluntary health organizations fulfill an important role in shaping the health care system and in recent years have taken up the burden of many of the services previously provided by the governments.

> **EXERCISE 16.4 VOLUNTARY HEALTH AGENCIES:**
> In your local community, research two or three voluntary health agencies and compare them with what is described in this chapter. How are they different and the same as what is described in this section?

SELF-HELP GROUPS

People join together in groups for companionship, mutual assistance, and the exchange of problem-solving skills. The most obvious example of the self-help concept is the family, a small group in which socialization, identification, and support originate. Self-help efforts are also evident in collective enterprises such as food or housing cooperatives, tenants' associations, and civil rights groups. They are usually formed by peers who have come together for mutual assistance in satisfying a common need, overcoming a common personal concern or life-disrupting problem, and bringing about desired social or personal change. **Self-help groups** can be defined as small, autonomous, open groups that meet regularly (Romeder, 1989). They may provide material assistance, as well as emotional support; they are frequently cause oriented and promulgate an ideology or values through which members may attain an enhanced sense of personal identity. The primary activity of these groups is personal **mutual aid**, a form of social support that focuses on sharing experiences, information, and ways of coping. Group activities are voluntary and usually free. In some cases, there is already a national or international body of self-help groups focused on a given concern, and this may offer consultative and public relations support to new self-help groups or associations. Alcoholics Anonymous, established in 1935, has been the model for the development of other self-help groups (e.g., Narcotics Anonymous, Schizophrenics Anonymous).

For many people, with many types of difficulties, such groups can be very effective for coping with personal pressures. The major activities of these groups include group meetings, sponsorship of new members, educational activities for their members and the general public, and advocating for change. Apart from these general services, activities are as diverse as the groups themselves. They include home or hospital visits, hot lines, newsletters and brochures, public conferences, fairs, advocacy, recreational activities, and material aid (e.g., sitter services, transportation, exchange of goods). There are a number of support groups that help persons with specific health conditions, such as HIV, breast cancer, and prostate cancer.

With the development of the Internet, virtual (or online) support groups have also emerged. These online support groups promote mutual aid and exist for a range of conditions, including cancer and HIV/AIDS, for example. As is the case with some other types of support groups, online support groups often depend heavily on having diverse group members, with both people looking for support and advice in addition to people who can offer such support and advice. For many, these virtual communities are the primary source of support, and for others, they act as a supplemental form of support (e.g., in addition to in-person support or self-help groups) (Lin et al., 2015). One of the questions that emerges with a growing online presence is how connected a person might feel to a virtual group compared with an in-person group.

SUMMARY

Health care is delivered at the local level through a variety of services, including primary care, secondary care, hospital care, home care, public health services, mental health care, and public and private nursing homes. The funding sources for these services are diverse. Although basic hospital and medical services in every province and territory are provided through government health insurance plans, what is provided either through public or private insurance varies.

Today hospitals are the major centres for health care services. They provide inpatient services and services for ambulatory patients in outpatient clinics, EDs, and rehabilitation services. Hospitals are classified on the basis of the kind of service they provide and are paid by the provincial government. In most provinces, a regional board governs them. Hospitals usually have a chief executive officer, president, or administrator who is in charge of day-to-day operations and executes policies formulated by the regional board. Most providers with admitting and discharging privileges are considered users of hospitals via hospital privileges rather than employees of the hospital.

Primary care services are provided at the first contact between the patient and the health care professional and is usually provided by family physicians or primary care NPs, with or without a multidisciplinary team. Apart from physicians and NPs, a number of other health care professionals provide primary health care (including dentists, nurses, chiropractors, optometrists, podiatrists, and physiotherapists). Specialized practitioners using specialized resources usually deliver secondary care. Patients usually receive secondary care after referral from a primary care provider. Tertiary care requires very specialized facilities and professional skills.

Public health agencies form liaisons with local hospitals, health care practitioners, and voluntary health agencies. Their functions depend on the mandate set out by the provincial public health act and funding and include the control of communicable disease, maternal and child health services, health promotion, dental health, and environmental health.

In recent years, there has been increasing emphasis on home care. The services delivered by the home care programs range from nursing services to an array of health and social services. There are four basic models for home care: the maintenance and preventive model, the long-term care substitution model, the acute care substitution model, and palliative care model. Most provincial home care programs are funded by the provincial or territorial government; some charge user fees, often based on the ability to pay.

Mental health and addictions activities represent one of the largest administrative areas in terms of expenditure and employees. Community mental health facilities are reaching beyond mental health institutions to provide greater continuity of care, deal with incipient breakdown, and rehabilitate patients in the community. Currently, funding is not adequate to meet the needs of deinstitutionalized patients or individuals with addictions and substance use issues.

The availability of social and support services in the community for people with disabilities depends on the location of the community and the nature and type of disability. Most communities have home care programs available for people with disabilities.

Voluntary organizations have played and continue to play an important part in shaping our health, welfare, and educational systems. These nonprofit organizations operate under boards of volunteers, with the primary or major objectives being the promotion of health; the prevention of illness or disability; and the identification, treatment, or rehabilitation of people with disease or disability.

Self-help groups are small, autonomous, open (and sometimes solely virtual or online) groups that meet regularly. As a result of personal crisis or chronic problems, members share common experiences and meet each other as equals. The primary activity of these groups is personal mutual aid, a form of social support that focuses on the sharing of experiences, information, and ways of coping.

KEY WEBSITES

British Columbia Centre for Disease Control: www.bccdc.ca
This provincial organization provides technical public health support (including in the area of health promotion, prevention, policy and analytics) to governments and health authorities. Its goals are reducing communicable and NCDs, environmental health risks, and injury.

Canadian Association of Ambulatory Care (CAAC): http://www.canadianambulatorycare.com
This nonprofit organization was established in 2012. Its membership includes a wide range of health care providers that provide care in ambulatory settings, including physiotherapists, occupational therapists, management, nurses, and so on. The CAAC's main goal is to emphasize the type of work being done in ambulatory care settings, both in Canada and across the world.

Canadian Association of Community Health Centres: https://www.cachc.ca
This association represents and promotes the voice and interests of CHCs across the country. It is a network that emphasizes principles and values of health equity, social determinants of health, and maintaining medicare.

Canadian Public Health Association: https://cpha.ca
This federal organization works to improve public health education, research, policy, and practice across the country and globally. One of its main accomplishments is the publication of the *Canadian Journal of Public Health*. The organization's staff also write position statements and discussion documents for the enhancement of the Canadian public health community.

HealthCareCAN: http://www.healthcarecan.ca/who-we-are/about-healthcarecan
HealthCareCAN is the national voice of health care organizations and hospitals across Canada. They foster informed and continuous, results-oriented discovery and innovation across the continuum of health care. HealthCareCAN acts with others to enhance the health of the people of Canada, to build the capability for high quality care, and to help ensure value for money in publicly financed, health care programs.

Primary Health Care Teams: http://primaryhealthcareteams.ca
This website, led by the School of Public Administration at Dalhousie University, represents a forum for people interested in interdisciplinary primary health care teams. It is a place where people can promote research and share their experience and knowledge about how these teams work and are evaluated in the Canadian context.

REFERENCES

Accreditation Canada. (2015). *Home care in Canada: Advancing quality improvement and integrated care.* Retrieved from https://www.accreditation.ca/sites/default/files/home-care-in-canada-report.pdf.

Agarwal, G., Angeles, R., Pirrie, M., et al. (2018). Evaluation of a community paramedicine health promotion and lifestyle risk assessment program for older adults who live in social housing: A cluster randomized trial. *Canadian Medical Association Journal*, 190(21), E638–E647. https://doi.org/10.1503/cmaj.170740.

Alberta Health. (2018). *Primary care networks.* Retrieved from http://www.health.alberta.ca/services/primary-care-networks.html.

Archer, S. (2018). *Why we need academic health science centres.* Retrieved from https://theconversation.com/why-we-need-academic-health-science-centres-98696.

British Columbia Ministry of Health. (2017). *Promote, protect, prevent: Our health begins here [BC's Guiding Framework for Public Health].* Retrieved from https://www.health.gov.bc.ca/library/publications/year/2017/BC-guiding-framework-for-public-health-2017-update.pdf.

Buhler-Wilkerson, K. (1985). Public health nursing: In sickness or in health? *American Journal of Public Health*, 75(10), 1155–1161.

Canadian Association of Community Health Centres. (2016). *About community health centres.* Retrieved from https://www.cachc.ca/about-chcs/.

Canadian Cancer Society. (2017). *Canadian cancer statistics.* Retrieved from http://www.cancer.ca/en/cancr-information/cancer-101/canadian-cancer-statistics-publication/?region=on.

Canadian Home Care Association. (2013). *Portraits of home care in Cana*da. Retrieved from http://www.cdnhomecare.ca/content.php?doc=274.

Canadian Institute for Health Information. (2017a). *CMDB hospital beds staffed and in operation, 2015–2016*. Retrieved from https://www.cihi.ca/sites/default/files/document/beds-staffed-and-in-operation-2015-2016-en.xlsx.

Canadian Institute for Health Information. (2017b). *National health expenditure trends, 1975 to 2017*. Ottawa: Author.

Canadian Institute for Health Information. (2017c). *Canada's health care providers*. Retrieved from https://secure.cihi.ca/free_products/hctenglish.pdf.

Canadian Public Health Association. (2010). *Public health—community health nursing practice in Canada: Roles and activities*. Retrieved from https://www.cpha.ca/sites/default/files/assets/pubs/3-1bk04214.pdf.

Challacombe, L., & Broeckaert, L. (2016). *Service mapping: One approach to building strong programs*. Toronto: CATIE. Retrieved from https://www.catie.ca/en/pif/service-mapping-one-approach-building-strong-programs.

Chen, C., Chen, C., Hu, H., et al. (2017). Walk-in clinics versus physician offices and emergency rooms for urgent care and chronic disease management (Review). *Cochrane Database of Systematic Reviews* (2), CD011774. https://doi.org/10.1002/14651858.CD011774.pub2.

Community Health Nurses' Initiative Group of the Registered Nurses Association of Ontario. (2000). *Home health nursing: a position paper*. Ottawa: Victorian Order of Nurses Canada. Retrieved from http://www.von.ca/english/Education/chnig.htm

Community Toolbox. (2018). *Windshield and walking surveys*. Retrieved from https://ctb.ku.edu/en/table-of-contents/assessment/assessing-community-needs-and-resources/windshield-walking-surveys/main.

Gomes, B., Calanzani, N., Gysels, M., et al. (2013). Heterogeneity and changes in preferences for dying at home: A systematic review. *BMC Palliative Care, 12*(1), 7.

Government of British Columbia. (2018). *Creating new opportunities for nurse practitioners as part of team-based care system*. Retrieved from https://news.gov.bc.ca/releases/2018HLTH0034-000995.

Government of Canada. (2008). *Chapter 2: The Chief Public Health Officer's report on the state of public health in Canada 2008—what is public health?* Ottawa: Author. Retrieved from https://www.canada.ca/en/public-health/corporate/publications/chief-public-health-officer-reports-state-public-health-canada/report-on-state-public-health-canada-2008/chapter-2a.html

Government of Canada. (2013). *First Nations and Inuit Health Branch*. Retrieved from https://www.canada.ca/en/indigenous-services-canada/corporate/first-nations-inuit-health-branch.html.

Government of Ontario. (2017). *Ontario making 2,000 more beds and spaces for patients*. Retrieved from https://news.ontario.ca/mohltc/en/2017/10/ontario-making-2000-more-beds-and-spaces-for-patients-available-this-year.html.

Health Canada. (2002). *Primary Health Care Transition Fund: Frequently asked questions*. Retrieved from www.hc-sc.gc.ca/phctf-fassp/english/faq.html [Seminal].

Hibbard, J., & Smith, D. (2005). *Nursing leadership and management in Canada*. Toronto: Elsevier Canada. [Seminal Reference].

Improving Chronic Illness Care. (2019). *Steps for improvement models*. Retrieved from http://www.improvingchroniccare.org/index.php?p=1:_Models&s=363.

Kulig, J.C., Thomlinson, E., Curran, F., et al. (2003). *Rural and remote nursing practice: an analysis of policy documents. Documentary analysis final report: Policy analysis for the nature of rural and remote nursing practice in Canada. R03-2003*. Prince George, BC: Author. Retrieved from https://www.unbc.ca/sites/default/files/sections/rural-nursing/en/18-completereport.pdf [Seminal Reference].

Leatt, P., Pink, G., & Guerriere, M. (2000). Towards a Canadian model of integrated healthcare. *Healthcare Papers, 1*(2), 13–35.

Lin, T., Hsu, J. S., Cheng, H., et al. (2015). Exploring the relationship between receiving and offering online social support: a dual social support model. *Information & Management, 52*(3), 371–383. https://doi.org/10.1016/j.im.2015.01.003.

Manitoba Health. (1998). *The role of the public health nurse within the regional health authority*. Retrieved from https://www.gov.mb.ca/health/rha/docs/rolerha.pdf. [Seminal Reference].

Martin, E., Pomey, M. P., & Forest, P. G. (2006). *A cross-provincial comparison of health care policy reform in Canada*. Retrieved from https://www.queensu.ca/iigr/sites/webpublish.queensu.ca.iigrwww/files/files/Res/crossprov/QC-Regionalization.pdf [Seminal].

Medtronic. (2019). *Canada's shouldice hospital case study—aligning value*. Retrieved from https://www.medtronic.com/us-en/transforming-healthcare/aligning-value/perspective/case-studies/shouldice-hospital-canada.html.

Ministère de la Santé et des Services sociaux du Québec. (2017). *Rapports statistiques annuels*. Retrieved from http://www.informa.msss.gouv.qc.ca.

Organisation for Economic Co-operation and Development. (2017). *Health at a glance, 2017*. Paris: OECD Publishing. Retrieved from https://www.oecd-ilibrary.org/docserver/health_glance-2017 en.pdf?expires=1548648272&id=id&accname=guest&checksum=A328166CA038E0CD07E2B-3D3AA121330

Ontario Ministry of Health and Long-Term Care. (2016). *Family health teams.* Retrieved from http://www.health.gov.on.ca/en/pro/programs/fht/.

Registered Nurses Association of Ontario. (n.d.). *The hospital-based nurse practitioner: context, scope of practice and competencies.* Retrieved from http://nptoolkit.rnao.ca/why-nps-make-sense/scope-practice.

Romanow, R. (2002). *Building on values: the future of health care in Canada.* Ottawa: Commission on the Future of Health Care in Canada. [Seminal Reference].

Romeder, J. (1989). *The self-help way: Mutual aid and health.* Ottawa: Canadian Council on Social Development. [Seminal Reference].

Ronald, L. A., McGregor, M. J., Harrington, C., et al. (2016). Observational evidence of for-profit delivery and inferior nursing home care: when is there enough evidence for policy change? *PLoS Medicine, 13*(4), e1001995.

Sinha, M., & Bleakney, A. (2015). *Receiving care at home.* Retrieved from https://www150.statcan.gc.ca/n1/pub/89-652-x/89-652-x2014002-eng.htm#a8.

Soeren, M. V., Hurlock-Chorostecki, C., & Reeves, S. (2011). The role of nurse practitioners in hospital settings: implications for interprofessional practice. *Journal of Interprofessional Care, 25*(4), 245–251.

Statistics Canada. (2016). *Data tables, 2016 Census: Dwelling type, age and sex for the population in occupied dwellings—Canada, provinces and territories, Census Metropolitan Areas, and Census Agglomerations* (Catalogue no. 98-400-X2016021). Released May 3, 2017.

Tarlier, D. S., Johnson, J. L., & Whyte, N. B. (2003). Voices from the wilderness: an interpretive study describing the role and practice of outpost nurses. *Canadian Journal of Public Health/Revue Canadienne de Sante'e Publique, 94*(3), 180–184 [Seminal Reference].

University of Ottawa. (2017). *Primary care: definitions and historical developments.* Retrieved from http://www.med.uottawa.ca/sim/data/primary_care.htm.

17

Human Resources for Health

ⓔ Additional resources are available online at http://evolve.elsevier.com/Canada/Shah/publichealth/

LEARNING OBJECTIVES

- Understand what it means to have professional status, including self-regulation, standards of practice, and scope of practice.
- Differentiate between a profession and a discipline.
- Understand how different health care professions are regulated.
- Understand the future of regulatory trends.

- Examine the roles of specific regulated health professions who are directly involved with patient care.
- Examine the purpose of interprofessional practice in health care.
- Understand abuse by health care professionals.
- Explore the health of health care professionals.

CHAPTER OUTLINE

KEY TERMS

advocacy
autonomy
certified
controlled acts
complementary health care providers
delegated acts

exclusive professions
interprofessional practice (IPP)
licensed
profession
professionalism
reserved titles

INTRODUCTION

Adequate numbers of human resources for health are required in order for a health system to function optimally. *Human health resources* (HHRs) generally refers to individuals who provide health care or health services to the public, including physicians, nurses, and allied health professionals, such as medical laboratory technologists, pharmacists, psychologists, and physiotherapists, as well as family and volunteer caregivers. All of these people, in their unique ways, contribute to health and well-being of individuals. It is essential that readers understand the roles of some of the major players who provide health care, particularly as it pertains to working interprofessionally, including the roles of informal caregivers such as family members.

The document *Building the Public Health Workforce for the 21st Century: A Pan-Canadian Framework for Public Health Human Resources Planning* (Public Health Agency of Canada, 2005) notes that it is important to develop an interprofessional workforce with the public health skills and competencies to meet population health needs. Although an interprofessional structure makes up the public health workforce, the reality is that public health in Canada encompasses multiple health care providers who do not necessarily have a direct connection to each other, except through a common employer. The Canadian Public Health Association (CPHA) is undertaking a project called *Creating a Certified Public Health Professional Designation for Canada's Public Health Workforce;* its purposes are to pilot test and provide recommendations on the introduction of a national public health certification program and establish a framework for the implementation of a Certified Public Health Professional (CPHP) designation in Canada (CPHA, 2017).

A Canadian health care team typically includes a wide range of regulated, unregulated, informal, unionized, and nonunionized workers, as well as those working under various public and private funding arrangements, such as dentists, chiropractors, and volunteer caregivers. The largest group of unregulated health care providers,

however, consists of family members, friends, and community volunteers.

Health professions that are regulated by provincial or territorial legislation are required to follow common rules and, through health professional colleges, investigate complaints and set educational and practice standards for registered members. More than 30 health professions are now regulated by legislation in at least one province or territory. Most health care providers work in hospitals, but this is changing as the sites of care move from the hospital into the community to include community clinics and client homes.

Trends such as population growth, demographic and epidemiological transition, and aging of the health care workforce are increasing the demand for health and social care. With the aging of the baby boom generation, many of today's health care workers will retire early and will need to be replaced at a time of overall slowing in population and labour force growth. This will also have an impact on the number and types of immigrants we bring to our country in future. Additionally, this group of baby boomers will also require more HHRs to care for them because older people require more health services and have higher per capita health care expenditures.

Despite the increasing number of students being admitted into medical and nursing schools, there are projected shortages of health workers in coming years. A recent report from the Global Health Workforce Alliance and World Health Organization (WHO) estimated a deficit of 12.9 million skilled health professionals by 2035 (WHO, 2014). Shortages of health care professionals are the result of an aging workforce, low birth rates in high-income countries such as Canada, early retirement of skilled health care professionals, and extended life expectancies in the population (FitzGerald et al., 2013). To address fragmentation within the health system (see Chapter 16), there has been a push towards innovative strategies, with HHRs at the forefront. Interprofessional education and collaborative practice is believed to be a key step in moving the health system to a position of strength (WHO, 2010). As interprofessional health care teams understand how to optimize the skills of their members, share case management, and provide better health services to clients and communities, improvement in health outcomes also occurs.

This chapter presents a synopsis of the regulated occupations that are directly involved with patient care and describes what they do. We begin with a definition of profession and professionalism and explore a number of values that are often attributed to what it means to be a professional, including interprofessional practice (IPP). Understanding each professional's role, scope of practice, and regulation provides for better coordination of care and ultimately safe, effective, and efficient care. Informal caregivers and voluntary organizations, such as the Diabetes Canada and self-help groups, have been described in Chapter 16. Following the Health System Performance Measurement Framework presented in the Introduction to this book, we draw on the issue of governance as it relates to appropriate human resources, their regulation, and scope of practice. Without good governance, the human resources available will be insufficient, and the functioning of the health system will be negatively impacted. The last section of the chapter covers abuse perpetrated by health professionals and the health of health care workers.

PROFESSIONS AND PROFESSIONALISM

An industrializing society has been described as a professionalizing society. The rapid proliferation of knowledge in all fields of science and technology has, in recent decades, brought about the establishment of many new professions, some of which are in the health care field.

The word *professional* comes from the Latin root "to profess" or declare something, implying that when you adopt the values of a profession, you are publicly declaring something important to society about your place within it. A profession also conjures up a specific role with many functions. According to *Merriam-Webster's Dictionary*, the meaning of the word **profession** is "a calling requiring specialized knowledge and often long and intensive preparation" (*Merriam-Webster Dictionary*, 2018). Most definitions emphasize the public service or altruistic aspect of **professionalism**. However, although many groups have been accorded professional status, it could be argued that only a few of them could be described in terms of (1) specialized knowledge and skill, (2) autonomy, (3) service orientation, (4) advocacy,

> ### BOX 17.1 The Nursing Profession
>
> In nursing, the profession is often recognized as being comprised of three pillars: (1) regulation (protection of the public), (2) professional practice (development, advocacy, and the promotion of the profession), and (3) labour relations. These three pillars, according to Mildon (2018), can be pictured as a three-legged stool whereby it takes all three of those legs, or pillars, for the stool to remain strong. Professional practice, the union, and regulation provide a solid foundation for the profession. Weakening or advancing one of those pillars at the expense of another will not make the other pillars stronger but cause the stool to fall down.
>
> Manitoba is an example of one province that has embraced the three-pillar approach to registered nursing. Table 17.2 provides an example of the differences between the three pillars in Manitoba.

and (5) ethics and values. See Box 17.1 for a description of the nursing profession.

Specialized Knowledge and Skill

There is a specific body of detailed knowledge and complex skills, common and unique to the members of a profession, which require a lengthy period of training to acquire. Health care professionals must apply that knowledge and use theoretical or evidence-informed rationales for their practice, with the purpose of continually improving care and health outcomes for their clients. Additionally, being open-minded, having the desire to explore new knowledge, and being committed to lifelong learning are also attributes of being a professional.

Autonomy

Professions are self-regulating, which means they are governed by organizations made up of members of the profession. The professional college or council sets standards for the practice of the profession and enforces uniformity of practice. **Autonomy** includes working independently and exercising decision making within one's scope of practice, being aware of barriers and constraints that may interfere with one's autonomy, and seeking ways to remedy the situation. Members are free to practice independently in the manner of their choice (within the aforementioned prescribed limits) and judgement in the best interests of their patients and are relatively free of bureaucratic control. Even members who choose to be employed by institutions or corporations rather than practise privately generally have flexibility to create their own roles.

Service Orientation

Professionals deal directly with their clients, and their prime concern is to provide good service rather than to pursue self-gain. This does not necessarily imply altruism but simply that personal gain is secondary to service. The professional must be free of outside influence to be able to make unbiased decisions, with only the client's welfare in mind.

Accountability

The health care professional understands the meaning of self-regulation and its implications for practice and is guided by legislation, standards of practice, and a code of ethics to clarify one's scope of practice. Health care professionals are committed to work with clients to achieve desired outcomes and are actively engaged in advancing the quality of care. In a team-based approach, each health care professional becomes dependent on team members competently fulfilling their individual responsibilities, including effectively communicating with other team members. Team members are expected to bring, within their scope of practice, the relevant professional knowledge and skills to the provision of care. As a result, the team-based approach to patient care has generally led to greater individual accountability.

Advocacy

Advocacy for the public interest is a core professional responsibility (Saskatchewan Registered Nurses Association, n.d.). Health care professionals advocate, when necessary, on behalf of their clients in a way that respects the views of others and is likely to bring about meaningful change that will benefit their clients and the health care system (Canadian Medical Association [CMA], n.d.). Health care professionals are also involved in professional practice initiatives and activities to enhance health care and are knowledgeable about policies that impact on delivery of health care in order to advocate for their clients.

Ethics and Values

Health care professionals are bound by a code of ethics and must also be knowledgeable about ethical values and concepts in order to identify ethical concerns, issues, and dilemmas. Applying knowledge of professional ethics to make decisions and to act on those decisions is also part of professional practice.

Exercise 17.1

1. The terms *profession* and *discipline* are often used interchangeably in many practice-based health care professions such as nursing. What are the differences between these two terms?
2. The terms *profession* and *occupation* are also used interchangeably. What are the differences between these two terms?

CRITICAL THINKING QUESTION 17.1: Almost all health professionals follow the foundations of the principles of three pillars as outlined in the chapter. However, depending upon the need for union, within some of the professions, union functions and professional association functions are combined in a single organization.

What professional organizations also carry out functions of a union?

REGULATION OF HEALTH CARE PROFESSIONS

Regulation is intended to protect the public interest; however, it also accords certain benefits to the profession with respect to recognition, credibility, and political influence. In this section, we provide a definition of regulation, review scope and standards of practice, and provide two examples of health profession regulation in Quebec (*The Professional Code of Quebec*) and Ontario (*Regulated Health Professions Act [RHPA]* of Ontario) to demonstrate how health care professions are regulated in Canada.

The *Constitution Act* of 1867 gave provincial governments the responsibility for health care and, as a result, the legislation that regulates the activities of the various health care occupations is provincial. The province may choose to delegate its authority to another group, such as the profession, which is termed **self-regulation**. Regulation is "a process or activity in which government requires or proscribes certain activities or behaviour on the part of individuals and institutions. and does so through a continuing administrative process" (Regan, 1987, p.15). The laws enacted by the government will dictate the structure and procedures the governing body must adhere to in order to maintain their self-regulatory status. For a health profession to self-regulate, it needs to be designated as a profession under regulation by the government. It follows, then, that in Canada, there are 13 different groups of legislation (10 provincial and 3 territorial). Although they are generally similar, there are also important differences. The medical profession (and some other health care professions) in Canada had achieved autonomy before the introduction of universal medical insurance. Since then, provinces have enacted legislation to ensure greater public control of the professions. Provinces call this type of legislation the Health Professions Act.

Most health care professions that require a license to practice have defined their own distinct scope of practice and standards of practice. Scopes of practice set out the services that members of an occupation perform and the methods they must use. The *Scopes of Practice,* published by the CMA, for example, outlines the general principles and criteria, which have been endorsed both by the CPHA and the Canadian Nurses Association (CNA) (CMA, 2002).

There has been a move toward **task-based regulatory models** or a system of controlled acts. Within this approach, only tasks judged to carry serious risks of harm if performed incorrectly require a license. In 1993, Ontario became the first province to adopt a system of controlled acts. British Columbia and Alberta have since adopted similar frameworks.

Whereas **scope of practice** includes all the interventions that regulated health professionals are authorized, educated, and competent to perform, **standards of practice** set out the legal and professional requirements for practice. Standards guide the professional knowledge, skills, and judgement needed to practice safely. Ensuring that the standards of practice are met is a shared responsibility between the profession, employers, and the college. In the next two sections, Quebec and Ontario are highlighted as case examples for how professions are regulated. Each province varies in terms of its regulation of professions.

The Professional Code of Quebec

Quebec's *Professional Code,* enacted in 1973, places the regulation of all professions under one act (Government of Quebec, 1973). A total of 45 professions are listed by the Office des professions du Québec, with 22 of them in the health care field (Office des professions du Québec, 2002). The Code is unique in that it defines what a profession is and establishes formal criteria by which an occupation gains statutory recognition as a profession. Each recognized profession is governed by a professional order (previously called a professional corporation). The order is charged with the traditional functions of a licensing agency. It determines the qualifications necessary to enter practice, including setting the length of training, examines candidates' credentials, maintains a register of members of the profession, defines the scope of practice, regulates specialists' certificates, determines what acts may be delegated, collaborates with educational institutions, and handles disciplinary matters within the profession. Under each governing legislation, acts are given exclusively to a profession, which could delegate an act to other professions; these are known as **delegated acts**.

In addition, because the order is first and foremost concerned with the protection of the public, it is responsible for the ongoing supervision of the practice of its profession and is given broad powers to supervise the practices of individual members. This is a significant innovation. Traditionally, professional regulatory bodies have only disciplined members whose unethical, improper behaviour, or incompetence has been reported by third parties. The Code requires each professional order to maintain ongoing surveillance of the quality of individual practices and take corrective measures, such as requiring refresher training. In addition, it ensures that the administration of any given profession is not conducted exclusively by the members of that profession. Nonmembers are appointed by the Office des professions and are there to represent the government and to protect the interests of the public. The disciplinary committee of each order handles disciplinary matters. The committee is informed of and investigates every complaint made against a member. It consists of at least three members, is chaired by a lawyer with at least 10 years of practice, and is appointed by the government. Professionals conducting the inquiry of their order into any complaint, as well as those testifying before a discipline committee hearing, are immune from prosecution.

There are two types of professions in Quebec: exclusive professions and those with reserved titles. In **exclusive professions** (*professions d'exercice exclusif*), only members who belong to recognized orders may use the title and perform professional acts exclusive to them by law (e.g., nurses or doctors). In professions with **reserved titles** (*professions à titre réservé*), members belonging to the order have the exclusive use of the title, although they do not have the exclusive right to perform professional acts (e.g., social workers or psychologists) (Government of Quebec, 2016). The Code also establishes two overall supervisory and regulatory bodies. The Office des professions du Québec is a governmental agency composed of five members appointed by the Lieutenant Governor-in-Council (the provincial Cabinet). It is responsible for ensuring that each order properly carries out its duty to protect the public. It monitors the performance of each order and takes corrective action when necessary. For example, it may require an order to issue a new regulation or revise an old one, and, if the order fails to do so, the board may act in its place. The Office reports directly to Cabinet. The second body is the Conseil interprofessionnel du Québec, made up of representatives from each of the professions covered by the Code. It coordinates the activities of the professional orders and deals with general issues encountered by all professional orders. It has no power to regulate but can, of course, make recommendations to the Office des professions du Québec (Government of Quebec, 2016).

> **CRITICAL THINKING QUESTIONS 17.2:** What are the 22 health care professions that are regulated in Quebec?
>
> Compare the list with the list of your own province's regulated health care professionals. What are the similarities and differences between the two lists and the reasons for the differences? How does this difference impact the health care that a client receives?

The Regulated Health Professions Act of Ontario

Ontario's RHPA was passed in 1991 but was not proclaimed until December 31, 1993, to allow the newly recognized professions time to organize themselves (Government of Ontario, 1991). The RHPA replaced the *Health Disciplines Act* of 1974, which had regulated only the professions of medicine, nursing, dentistry, pharmacy, and optometry. It increased the number of professions under its jurisdiction, including seven not previously covered. At present, there are 26 regulatory colleges that regulate 29 distinct professions—more than 300 000 health care professionals in Ontario under the RHPA (Federation of Health Regulatory Colleges of Ontario, 2018).

The RHPA has been amended three times since passage—first in 1993 to include regulations and sanctions for sexual abuse by health care professionals (discussed later in this chapter) and then in 1996 by the Omnibus legislation (*Ontario Act 26*) to allow the RHPA to comply with changes to the *Ontario Drug Benefit Act* and the *Prescription Drug Cost Regulation Act*. Like Quebec's *Professional Code*, the RHPA was enacted to obtain greater public accountability in the regulation of the health care professions. In 2018, the Act was amended to include a new definition of patient for the purposes of the prohibition of sexual abuse provisions, as reflected in the *Protecting Patients Act* of 2017. Many consider the RHPA to be progressive legislation. A "template from which many future legislative efforts in health care will evolve" (Pooley, 1992, p. 161), the RHPA increases equity within the health care professions by reducing the role of the physician as gatekeeper and increasing direct patient access to a wider variety of professionals. It allows for the growth of emerging health care professions, which can apply for regulation to raise their status. It allows for flexibility in reform and for the delegation of acts among health care professionals. Regulation is a separate issue from funding, however; although 29 health care professions are officially recognized and regulated in the RHPA, they are not all funded by the provincial health insurance plan.

The most progressive aspect of the legislation is that professionals are licensed to perform various **controlled acts** or tasks that are judged to carry serious risk of harm if performed incorrectly or by an unqualified person. There are 14 controlled acts established by the RHPA, as follows:

- Communicating a diagnosis
- Performing a procedure on tissue below the dermis, below the surface of a mucous membrane, below the surface of the cornea, or below the surfaces of teeth, including scaling of teeth
- Setting or casting a fracture of a bone or dislocation of a joint
- Moving the joints of the spine beyond usual range of motion
- Administering a substance by injection or inhalation
- Applying or ordering a form of energy prescribed by regulations under the Act
- Putting an instrument, hand, or finger into a specified list of body orifices

- Prescribing, dispensing, selling, or compounding a drug as defined in the *Drug and Pharmacies Regulation Act*
- Prescribing or dispensing for vision or eye problems, contact lenses, or eyeglasses
- Prescribing a hearing aid
- Fitting or dispensing dental devices
- Managing labour or delivering a baby
- Administering an allergy challenge test
- Treating, by means of psychotherapy technique, delivered through a therapeutic relationship, an individual's serious disorder of thought, cognition, mood, emotional regulation, perception, or memory that may seriously impair the individual's judgement, insight, behaviour, communication, or social functioning

None of the regulated health care professions is authorized to perform all of these controlled acts (although physicians are authorized to perform 13 of the 14; only fitting or dispensing dental devices falls outside their practice), and some (e.g., dietitians, speech and language pathologists, occupational therapists) are not authorized to perform any of them. However, these controlled acts can sometimes be *delegated* to others or performed under the supervision of a licensed individual. Furthermore, the same controlled act can come under the purview of more than one profession. For example, physicians, physiotherapists, and chiropractors are all authorized to manipulate the joints of the spine. These multiple authorizations were legislated to help break the monopoly that medicine had over health care services and allow people a greater range of health care providers when making decisions concerning their personal health. Traditional Indigenous healers and Indigenous midwives are exempt from the RHPA. Uncontrolled acts are open to all, including unregulated workers.

In addition to the controlled acts, the RHPA also specifies the scope of practice for a profession. Section 30(1) says: "No person, other than a member treating or advising within the scope of practice of his or her profession, shall treat or advise a person with respect to his or her health in circumstances in which it is reasonably foreseeable that serious physical harm may result from the treatment or advice or from an omission from them" (Government of Ontario, 1991). The RHPA also outlines the generic terms for authorized acts or, in other words, the activities a regulated health care professional may undertake after being ordered to do so by a physician.

One exception is people who perform acts that maintain the activities of daily living, such as insulin injections or colostomy changes. In its present form, the RHPA does not prohibit such "controlled acts" from being carried out by someone who does not fall under the jurisdiction of the RHPA, such as an acupuncturist.

The RHPA is structured so that individual acts regarding each profession's scope of practice and licensed acts follow a general section on legal and procedural provisions, which pertain to all the professions included in the RHPA. This allows for legislation to be coordinated instead of the previous patchwork of legislation. It gives the minister of health broad powers to supervise the regulation of all 29 disciplines, increasing their accountability and protecting the interests of the public. The emphasis is on the public good rather than professional interests.

Each health care profession must constitute a college that is responsible for regulating the practice of its profession and governing its members in accordance with the RHPA (Government of Ontario, 1991). The College must maintain standards of entry, qualification, and practice and must establish and maintain standards of competence and ethics among its members. Each college must have a governing council that excludes members of health care professions. The Lieutenant Governor in Council appoints public members to the council. Meetings of council, except in prescribed circumstances, are open to the public. In addition, a standard system of committees and a uniform method of handling licensing, hearings, and discipline are established for all colleges.

The statutory committee structure for each of the 29 professions included in the legislation is identical. There must be an executive committee, a registration committee, a complaints committee, a discipline committee, a fitness to practice committee, a continuing competence committee, a quality assurance committee, and a patient relations committee. The actual membership and quorum are different for each committee.

The Health Disciplines Board established under the *Health Disciplines Act* continues as the Health Professions Board, an independent, appointed body of 12 to 20 members, none of whom is a health care professional, indicating greater participation by lay members in regulatory affairs. The Board acts as an appeals agency for decisions made by the complaints committees and the registration committees of each college. It does not hear appeals from the disciplinary committees; these are made directly to the Supreme Court of Ontario. The disciplinary committee chairperson can assign a panel of three to five members for a hearing, one of whom must be a member of the public.

The minister of health is the designated member of Cabinet who is responsible for administering the RHPA. The minister's duties are to ensure that the regulatory system works and to focus both on the professions (making sure that they are regulated and coordinated in the public interest and that standards of practice are kept) and on consumers (ensuring freedom of choice of health care provider and that consumers are treated fairly and sensitively). To this end, the minister may conduct investigations into the operations of institutions or practices; may require reports to be submitted by the colleges; reviews proposed changes in college regulations; and may request that a college make, amend, or revoke regulations. If the college fails to do so, the minister may act in the college's place (through Cabinet). In practice, however, these powers are rarely exercised. In Quebec, these functions are carried out by the Office des professions du Québec rather than directly by Cabinet.

At this point, a distinction should be made between licensing and certification. Certain health care professionals are required to be **licensed**; that is, they must hold a licence to practise their profession, and all others are prohibited from such practice. Other professions and occupations are **certified**. In some instances, certification is controlled by government regulations, in which case individuals are prohibited from using the relevant title or claiming to be qualified in the occupation unless they are appropriately certified and registered, such as a personal support worker. They are not necessarily prohibited from performing some functions of the occupation. In some occupations, certification (or registration) is granted by voluntary organizations. This type of certification has no legal status, but employers frequently hire only those who are certified by their national or provincial associations; an example is social workers, who are certified by the College of Social Workers.

Health Professions Regulatory Advisory Council

The Health Professions Regulatory Advisory Council (HPRAC) is an independent council, separate from both the Minister of Health and the professional colleges, and created by the RHPA to facilitate ongoing policy development concerning the health care professions.

Specifically, the duties of the HPRAC include advising the minister of health on matters relating to regulating new health care professionals or deregulating existing ones, including changes in scope of practice and licensed acts; suggesting amendments to the Act and related regulations; and providing advice and policy guidance on any matter referred to it by the minister of health. Additionally, the HPRAC exercises supervisory functions, ensuring that the health care professionals (through their colleges) maintain good patient relations and effective quality assurance programs. The HPRAC is made up of five to seven lay people appointed by the Lieutenant Governor in Council and excludes registered health care professionals and Ontario public servants.

The HPRAC also has a number of statutory evaluation responsibilities. It is required to report to the minister of health 5 years after proclamation of the RHPA on the effectiveness of each college with regard to complaints and discipline procedures, professional misconduct of a sexual nature, patient relations programs, and quality assurance programs.

Current Ministerial referrals include Applied Behaviour Analysis, Controlled Act of Psychotherapy, Regulation of Chiropody under the RHPA of 1991, Registered Nurse (RN) Prescribing, Regulation of Diagnostic Sonographers under the RHPA of 1991, Referral on Chiropody and Podiatry, and Regulation of Paramedics under the RHPA of 1991. See Box 17.2 to understand the nuances of a self-regulating profession, between protecting the public and having a position of prestige.

> **CRITICAL THINKING QUESTION 17.3:** Now that you have read how professions are regulated in Quebec and Ontario, compare and contract the differences between the two provinces.
>
> How are health professionals regulated in your province or territory?

MAJOR HEALTH CARE PROFESSIONS

Several of the major health care professions are described in this section, as well as their regulatory organizations in various provinces. Just over 2 million people, representing 12.1% of all workers, are in the health care and social services fields (Statistics Canada, 2016). About 65% of those directly provide health services, and 35% are in ancillary jobs. HHRs are unevenly

BOX 17.2 A Critical Perspective: A Position of Prestige or Protecting the Public?

Entry into professional practice requires difficult and lengthy training and is often seen as an obstacle for many potential candidates that restricts membership to an elite group. Self-regulation, particularly with regard to licensing authority, can be viewed as a means of establishing a monopoly (Friedson, 1970). The self-governing profession is charged with deciding who is qualified to practise and in what areas. The profession also sets the standards of technical competence and ethical and professional conduct to be followed by members. Licensed members of a profession practise under a protective cloak of presumed competence, whether or not they actually are competent. Professional self-regulating bodies, called College councils, comprise both public members and professional ones, the latter usually forming the majority. Public members are appointed by government via Orders-in-Council from the Lieutenant Governor. Incompetence or unethical behaviour can be difficult to address because members of the profession are reluctant to criticize or blow the whistle on one another, and members are elected by their peers into decision-making positions. Many question the power and prestige that has traditionally been enjoyed by the established professions, especially the dominant role played by medicine. Self-regulated professions have also been criticized for being passive. For example, traditionally, they have relied heavily on licensing rather than on oversight of the practice of those who are licensed.

The truth must lie somewhere between opposite views of professionalism. Although professions are private interest groups that occupy positions of power and prestige in society, their regulatory legislation encourages them to be responsive to public interests.

Critical Thinking Question

Oversight modernization of College councils is underway across Canada to continue to protect the public. What reforms within College councils could help to improve the issues associated with self-interest or perceived self-interest when it comes to disciplinary action of its members?

federal government's *Pan-Canadian Health Human Resource Strategy* stated that "appropriate planning and management of HHR are key to developing a health care workforce that has the right number and mix of health professionals to serve Canadians in all regions of the country" (Health Canada, 2013). Planning for the workforce that delivers health services is primarily the responsibility of individual provinces and territories.

According to Statistics Canada, about 1.2 million individuals provided direct health services to Canadians in 2016. Table 17.1 shows the number of health professionals in Canada for 2016. Regulated nurses make up 48% of health care professionals, and this percentage has been increasing since the early 1990s. Since World War II, the traditional health care professions of physicians, nurses, and dentists have expanded to include some 32 regulated health professions and more than 150 categories of health care occupations. Most are extensions of established health care professions (e.g., nursing assistants, Licensed Practical Nurses (LPNs), technicians, nurse practitioners [NPs], dental hygienists, dental technicians). Others have developed from some special body of knowledge (e.g., clinical psychologists). As these new occupations evolve, many of their practitioners try to achieve independent status as self-regulatory professions. As a self-regulated profession, individuals within the profession are responsible for acting professionally and being accountable for their own practice. Most provincial governments now regulate and license a number of the health professions.

Medicine

Physicians are required to be licensed in all provinces. Although each provincial college has its unique requirements for licensors, a certain standard of uniformity has been established. All provinces require the physician to pass the national examination of the Medical Council of Canada plus examination by the Royal College of Physicians and Surgeons of Canada for specialists and, for family practice, by the College of Family Physicians of Canada. The example of Ontario is used here because most provinces have similar structures. In Quebec, there are two licensing colleges for physicians—one for general practitioners and a separate one for specialists. In Ontario, the licensing agency is the College of Physicians and Surgeons of Ontario and is made up of the following bodies, as detailed in the province's RHPA.

distributed and mainly concentrated in large urban centres and in wealthy provinces such as Ontario, Quebec, Alberta, and British Columbia. HHRs are a critical factor in health policy planning across Canada. The

TABLE 17.1 Number of Active Health Human Resources in Canada, 2016

Health Occupations	Total	Ratio: Practitioner/Population
Total health occupations	1 256 185	
Professional occupations in nursing	317 905	1:111
• Nursing coordinators and supervisors	16 835	1:2 088
• Registered nurses and registered psychiatric nurses	301 065	1:117
Professional occupations in health (except nursing)	259 135	
• Physicians and dentists	112 925	
• Specialist physicians	42 035	1:836
• General practitioners and family physicians	51 945	1:677
• Dentists	18 945	1:1 856
• Optometrists	5 235	1:6 715
• Chiropractors	7 385	1:4 760
• Allied primary health practitioners	7 245	4 852
• Pharmacists	37 415	1:940
• Dietitians and nutritionists	11 880	1:2 959
• Therapy and assessment professionals	61 795	1:569
• Audiologists and speech-language pathologists	10 880	1:3 231
• Physiotherapists	24 195	1:1 453
• Occupational therapists	15 535	1:2 263
Medical technologists and technicians (except dental health)	151 935	
• Medical laboratory technologists	20 890	1:1 690
• Medical laboratory technicians and pathologists' assistants	23 365	1:1 505
• Medical radiation technologists	20 215	1:1 739
• Medical sonographers	5 290	1:6 645
Dental hygienists and dental therapists	26 720	1:1 316
Opticians	8 780	1:4 004
Practitioners of natural healing	8 960	1:3 923
Licensed practical nurses	72 765	1:483
Paramedical occupations	28 205	1:1 246
Massage therapists	32 795	1:1 072
Dental assistants	34 180	1:1 029
Nurse aides, orderlies, and patient service associates	258 995	1:136

Source: Statistics Canada. (2016). Census of Population (Statistics Canada Catalogue no. 98-400-X2016355). Retrieved from https://www12.statcan.gc.ca/census-recensement/2016/dp-pd/dt-td/Rp-eng.cfm?LANG=E&APATH=3&DETAIL=0&DIM=0&-FL=A&FREE=0&GC=0&GID=0&GK=0&GRP=1&PID=112123&PRID=10&PTYPE=109445&S=0&SHOWALL=0&SUB=0&Temporal=2017&THEME=124&VID=0&VNAMEE=&VNAMEF=.

Council of the College

The Council is the governing body of the College of Physicians and Surgeons. The RHPA stipulates that the Council consist of at least 32 and no more than 34 members. The Council is composed of 16 elected physicians, 3 academic physician representatives, and 13 to 15 members of the public who are appointed by government. The overall governing body and board of directors of the College is made up of 3 members appointed by the medical faculties of five universities in Ontario, 13 to 15 lay members appointed by the Lieutenant Governor in Council, and 16 members elected by the membership at large. The inclusion of large numbers of lay members in Council and on other committees indicates the public's desire for greater participation in the regulatory affairs of professional bodies. The Council's most important functions are the preparation of regulations for the profession as authorized by the Act and subject to approval by the Minister and the appointment of members to the Executive Committee; Registration Committee; Inquiries, Complaints and Reports Committee; Education Committee; Finance and Audit Committee; Governance

TABLE 17.2	Three Pillars of Registered Nursing		
	REGULATORY BODY	**PROFESSIONAL ASSOCIATION**	**UNION**
	College of Registered Nurses of Manitoba	**Association of Registered Nurses of Manitoba**	**Manitoba Nurses Union**
Purpose	To protect the public through quality registered nursing regulation	To provide a professional voice for registered nurses in Manitoba	To protect the rights of nurses and advocate for improvements in areas affecting the nursing profession and the delivery of safe patient care
Top three primary functions	1. Set standards for nursing education and practice 2. Support RNs in meeting the standards 3. Take action when the standards are not met	1. Promotes and supports excellence in all areas of nursing practice 2. Advocates for registered nurses and the health of people living in Manitoba 3. Provides professional development, mentorship, and networking opportunities for RNs	1. Negotiates collective agreements 2. Enforces collective agreements and ensures workplace standards are met 3. Advocates to protect and improve the health care system for nurses and patients
Membership required?	Yes	No	Only for union positions

RN, Registered nurse.
Source: College of Registered Nurses of Manitoba. (n.d.). *Three pillars of registered nursing.* Retrieved from https://www.crnm. mb.ca/uploads/ck/files/Three%20Pillars%20of%20Registered%20Nursing.pdf.

Committee; Outreach Committee; Patient Relations Committee; Premise Inspection Committee; Quality Assurance Committee; and Fitness to Practice Committee.

Dentistry

Dentists are required to be licensed in every province. Graduates of approved Canadian dental schools must successfully complete the National Dental Examining Board of Canada's (NDEB) Certification Process. NDEB Certification does not guarantee licensure. Dental Regulatory Authorities (DRAs) may require additional documentation, jurisprudence tests, and evidence of language proficiency before licensure.

Nursing

In Canada, there are several categories of regulated nursing: RN, NP, LPN/Registered Practical Nurse (RPN), and Registered Psychiatric Nurse (RPN). RNs perform many functions depending on their location, their employer, and their appointment. At present, there are 21 nursing specialties (CNA, 2018). An RN holds a 4-year baccalaureate degree in nursing from a Canadian university or its international equivalent. Nurses working in the hospital may perform general nursing care or may work in very specialized units, such as intensive care, coronary care, renal dialysis, or neurosurgical units. Public health nurses deal with the community in such matters as immunization and health education.

Many nurses hold administrative positions within hospitals or other institutions. In rural and remote communities, nurses work in a variety of settings, such as in community health centres and physician's offices (NPs), in hospitals and community health centres (RNs), in nursing homes or long-term care facilities (LPNs), and in mental health or crisis centres (RPNs). Midwives focus on providing care during pregnancy, birth, and for 6 weeks postpartum for mother and baby. In addition, physicians, chiropractors, private care institutions, and corporations may privately employ nurses.

An NP holds a master's degree or advanced diploma in nursing. In Ontario, successful completion of the Extended Class Registration Examination (ECRE) is required to allow RNs to practise as NPs with the designation as an RN in the Extended Class, called an RN (EC). Each province has different specialty certificates for NPs. For example, in Ontario, there are NP–Primary Health Care, NP–Pediatrics, NP–Adult, and NP–Anaesthesia. After becoming authorized RN (EC)s, these nurses can complete annual physical examinations, counsel patients, provide immunizations, monitor patients with critical conditions, and complete certain procedures (e.g., defibrillation). According to the Health Force Ontario website, they can perform certain acts that regular RNs cannot, such as ordering diagnostic tests (radiography, laboratory tests, ultrasonography), communicating diagnoses to patients, and prescribing certain drugs.

Licensed practical nurses and RPNs are essentially different names for the same role and provide care in a variety of settings. The term LPN is used in all provinces and territories except for Ontario, where the preferred term is RPN. LPNs and RPNs hold 2-year practical nursing diplomas from accredited colleges. After completion of their studies, they must complete the national licensing exam before they can practice.

Registered Practical Nurses in Ontario are not to be confused with Registered Psychiatric Nurses in British Columbia, Alberta, Saskatchewan, Manitoba, Nunavut, Northwest Territories, and Yukon. These nurses must complete psychiatric nursing college programs and register with a provincial regulatory body.

Quebec has a distinct and separate regulatory body for nurses called the Ordre des infirmiers et infirmières du Québec. In other provinces, regulation is delegated to professional organizations. In British Columbia, there are 26 regulated health professions, regulated by 20 self-governing bodies, known as "colleges," and one government-appointed licensing board. In 2018, the following nursing colleges joined together in to become the British Columbia College of Nursing Professionals (BCCNP):

- College of Licensed Practical Nurses of British Columbia (CLPNBC)
- College of Registered Nurses of British Columbia (CRNBC)
- College of Registered Psychiatric Nurses of British Columbia (CRPNBC)

The BCCNP is the college empowered under the *Health Professions Act* to regulate the practice of all three distinct professions. This includes LPNs, Registered Psychiatric Nurses, RNs, and NPs. Only BCCNP registrants are authorized to use the title "nurse" while practising their profession in British Columbia. However, there are some criticisms regarding the move towards one regulator without a democratic process of engaging nurses at all levels and the influence of American type nursing registration exams (Duncan & Whyte, 2018).

The increase in the status and importance of nursing in recent years is indicated by the fact that three provincial ministries of health (British Columbia, Alberta, and Manitoba) now have special ministerial positions for provincial nursing officers or provincial nursing advisory councils. In 2017, NP programs received increased attention, and new or amended provincial or territorial legislation allows for an expanded role for RNs as NPs in every province and territory. In 2017, there were 4 967 NPs in Canada (CNA, 2017).

Although medicine, dentistry, and nursing are three health care professions traditionally considered most important to the delivery of health services, chiropractic and midwifery are two health care professions in which consumer demand for alternative delivery modalities helped create pressure for official recognition.

Chiropractic

The practice of chiropractic is defined as "the assessment of conditions related to the spine, nervous system and joints, and the diagnosis, prevention and treatment, primarily by adjustment of . . . the spine and joints" (Pooley, 1992, p. 162). To receive the legitimacy and official recognition of being one of the regulated health care professions, the practice of chiropractic moved much closer to mainstream medicine. Originally, in its historic development, it was seen as a direct alternative to medicine and was associated more closely with naturopathy. This association, as well as the broader scope of practice associated with earlier years of chiropractic, has been downplayed in recent years as chiropractors have become regulated and have come to make up part of the primary health care delivery team.

Because chiropractors are considered to be one of the primary care providers, they do not require referrals from other physicians. This status, together with their position as one of the five health care professionals authorized to diagnose, has been allowed because of the current general-diagnosis training of chiropractors is similar to that of physicians in medical schools. Chiropractors are licensed in all provinces (Chiropractic in Canada, 2002).

Midwifery

The practice of midwifery is defined as "skilled, knowledgeable, and compassionate care for childbearing women, newborn infants and families across the continuum from pre-pregnancy, pregnancy, birth, post partum and the early weeks of life. Core characteristics include optimising normal biological, psychological, social, and cultural processes of reproduction and early life, timely prevention, and management of complications, consultation with and referral to other services, respecting women's individual circumstances and views, and working in partnership with women to strengthen women's own capabilities to care for themselves and their families" (Renfrew et al., 2014, p. 1130).

Although community midwives have been practising throughout Canada (especially in rural and northern regions) for more than a century, they received little official recognition from the state. This has slowly started to change, largely because of ongoing consumer pressure to receive nonmedical labour and delivery care. Midwives are officially recognized as primary health care professionals and are regulated in all provinces and territories except the Yukon and Prince Edward Island (Canadian Association of Midwives, 2018).

Services Provided by Health Care Professionals

Among the many health care professionals who provide primary care in their area of specialization are those described below. It is important to keep in mind that although some professions are listed under primary care, many are not covered by medicare, creating an inequity for those who cannot afford to pay out of pocket and who do not have extended health benefits for these services.

Nurses

Nursing is the largest health profession and accounts for one quarter of all health care providers in Canada. There are four regulated nursing groups: RNs, NPs, LPNs/RPNs (Ontario only), and Registered Psychiatric Nurses. In 2016, there were 421 093 regulated nurses who had an active licence to practice in Canada, and of them, 397 628 said they were employed in their profession. Most RNs work in hospitals, although the number employed in community health is gradually increasing. In 2016, there were 116 491 LPNs and 5 859 RPNs working in Canada. RPNs are licensed only in British Columbia, Alberta, Saskatchewan, and Manitoba (Canadian Institute for Health Information [CIHI], 2016). The supply of internationally educated nurses (IENs) has increased slightly from 2007 (6.7%, 23 764) to 2016 (8.1%, 33 789); the average annual growth over the same period declined to 4.0% in 2016, from a high of 8.2% in 2008 (CIHI, 2016). A number of credentialling barriers exist that delay IENs qualification to practice in Canada, resulting in a deskilling process (Higginbottom, 2011).

Whereas some nurses work together with a physician and provide primary care with a physician's supervision, others work independently in community health centres or occupational health services or in remote areas where no physicians are available. They are generally paid by salary. Despite increasing recognition of NPs in Canada, not every province recognizes this specialty. NPs are trained to provide primary care and are allowed to dispense certain drugs. Currently, new or amended provincial and territorial legislation allows for an expanded role for RNs as NPs in Newfoundland and Labrador, Nova Scotia, New Brunswick, Ontario, Manitoba, Saskatchewan, Alberta and Yukon. Other areas are working on implementing similar legislation (see Chapter 16).

Physicians

After nursing, medicine represents the second largest regulated health care profession. For the 10th year in a row, as described in CIHI's report *Physicians in Canada, 2016*, the number of physicians increased at a faster rate than the number of people in the population, resulting in more physicians per person than ever before—one physician for every 374 people. However, many of the physicians are based in urban settings, creating a gap in primary care for rural communities. It is much more difficult to recruit and retain physicians for rural and remote communities, often necessitating physicians from less rural communities to fly in for 1-week locums once a month. Based on the number of MD degrees awarded by Canadian universities, the number of physicians is likely to continue to grow (Office of Research and Information Services, Association of Faculties of Medicine of Canada, 2016). The proportion of recent physician graduates (10 years or less since graduation) rose from 16.2% in 2012 to 20.0% in 2016.

Throughout Canadian history, a sizable number of medical practitioners have been immigrants, coming earlier from the white Commonwealth countries such as Australia, New Zealand, South Africa, Great Britain, the United States, and Ireland; however, since Canada opened up immigration to nonwhite countries in 1964, there has been an influx of physicians from India, Philippines, Pakistan, and so on. There are multiple roadblocks before these foreign-trained physicians can be licensed in Canada, particularly for those coming from developing countries. Newfoundland (37%) and Saskatchewan (52%) have a sizable proportion of practitioners who are foreign trained (CMA, 2018).

Dentists

Primary dental services are provided mainly in the offices of dentists, with the support of dental hygienists. To some extent, local public health units or government-sponsored clinics also provide primary dental health services, usually to particular subpopulations such as seniors, street-entrenched youth, or immigrant children. Indigenous populations living in First Nations communities are provided with dental care by First Nation and Inuit Health Branch (see Chapter 7). More specialized dental care can be provided by dental surgeons in hospitals. Dentists are paid mainly by fee for service through private insurance or by the individual (see Chapter 15). The extent of funding from provincial health insurance plans varies across Canada for routine dental care. In some provinces, routine dental care is covered for children and seniors. Services provided by dental surgeons in hospital are covered by all provincial insurance plans. However, many of the procedures performed by dental surgeons are performed outside of the hospital setting and therefore are not paid for by the provincial insurance plans.

Chiropractors

Chiropractors usually specialize in the manipulation of joints and muscles to correct musculoskeletal and other disorders. Chiropractic services are mainly provided in offices and, to a limited extent, in clinics organized by workers' compensation boards. Chiropractors are usually paid on a fee-for-service basis through private insurance or out of pocket by individuals and partially by provincial government health insurance plans in British Columbia, Alberta, and Manitoba. Federal government populations (Royal Canadian Mounted Police, Veterans Affairs Canada, Canadian Forces, First Nations and Inuit, and Correctional Services of Canada) are also partially covered for services.

Podiatrists

The podiatrist usually deals with foot problems. Like chiropractors, most work in private offices, although some work in either public health units, community health centres, or general hospitals. Their payment mechanism is also similar to that of chiropractors. The provincial insurance plans of British Columbia, Alberta, Saskatchewan, and Ontario cover part of the cost of services provided by podiatrists.

Optometrists

Optometrists handle refractory errors and minor ailments of the eye. They usually work in private offices or alongside optical dispensing outlets. Most optometrists are paid on a fee-for-service basis with a variety of payment mechanisms, depending on who is receiving services. Newfoundland and Labrador and Prince Edward Island are the only provinces in Canada that do not cover any services provided by optometrists. Other provinces, such as British Columbia, Saskatchewan, Manitoba, and Ontario, cover some costs through their provincial insurance plans. Alberta and Nova Scotia cover optometrists' services to children and older adults, and Quebec covers services to the poor and to certain groups. The balance of the costs is covered by private insurance companies or directly by consumers.

Midwives

Midwives deal with normal pregnancy, labour, delivery, and postpartum care. As of 2000, midwives were officially recognized as primary health care professionals. Midwives usually work in small group practices and are generally paid a yearly salary or on a per-case basis. Their main source of income used to be payment from individual users of their services, but now Ontario, Quebec, Manitoba, and British Columbia publicly fund midwifery services.

Pharmacists

By law, pharmacists' practice includes dispensing prescription medications. Canada's licensed pharmacists are distributed among three major employment groups. Approximately four of every five pharmacists (80%) work in community pharmacies; another 15% work in hospital or institutional pharmacies; and the remainder work in situations that may not legally require licensed pharmacists, such as associations, pharmaceutical companies, and consulting firms. Pharmacists working in privately owned and operated drug stores receive a dispensing fee for filled prescriptions as part of their remuneration. Non-owner and institution-based pharmacists, such as those working in hospitals, are usually paid by salary. Recently, the scope of pharmacists' practice has been expanded in some provinces; for example, they are allowed to provide influenza vaccinations and to test for streptococcus B infection, paid for by the individual out of pocket or by their health insurance plan.

Other Health Care Professionals

Hospitals, home care, and public health units usually employ physiotherapists, occupational therapists, speech pathologists, audiologists, social workers, nutritionists, and clinical psychologists. A number of them are in private practice, and the costs of their services are covered by individuals or by private health insurance.

Complementary Health Care Providers

Complementary health care providers include massage therapists, acupuncturists, homeopaths or naturopaths, Feldenkrais or Alexander teachers, relaxation therapists, biofeedback teachers, rolfers, herbalists, reflexologists, spiritual healers, and religious healers. These practitioners usually work in solo practices and are paid by those individuals seeking such services.

As one can see, there is a range of primary health care services provided by different professionals. The entry point into the primary health care system depends upon various factors, such as the employment, economic status and education of consumers, place of residence, their health beliefs, the type of health insurance, and the availability and accessibility of services and professionals.

As one can see, there are multiple individuals providing first contact health care in Canada. In Chapter 16, we discussed the fragmentation of primary health care and the need for interprofessional primary care (primary care teams). For secondary care, many ambulatory health care programs discussed earlier, there are concentrated efforts of interprofessional teams providing care to persons with complex health problems.

> **CRITICAL THINKING QUESTION 17.4:** Are there any professions you think have been left out of the preceding discussion? If so, which profession, and why do you think it was not included?

INTERPROFESSIONAL PRACTICE

Although the major health professions can all work in isolation from each other, **interprofessional practice (IPP)** (also known as collaborative practice) has been touted as a promising solution for some of the biggest health human resource challenges facing the Canadian health care system. IPP is being explored by researchers and decision makers to better understand how it can positively impact wait times, healthy workplaces, rural and remote accessibility, and patient safety. IPP is a collaborative practice that occurs when health care providers work with people from within their own profession, with people outside their profession, and with patients and their families (Canadian Interprofessional Health Collaborative [CIHC], 2009).

Through a national consensus process, the CIHC developed the National Interprofessional Competency Framework (http://www.cihc.ca) outlining the competencies that are key to collaborative practice. These competencies comprise skills and knowledge that are important in daily interactions between health care providers, their patients and students. The Competency Framework has six competency domains: (1) Role Clarification, (2) Team Functioning, (3) Interprofessional Conflict Resolution, (4) Collaborative Leadership, (5) Patient/Client/Family/Community-Centred Care, and (6) Interprofessional Communication. Each competency shows various behaviours that, together, enact the competency to its fullest extent (CIHC, 2010).

The CIHC outlines the following benefits of collaborative practice:

- Using appropriate language when speaking to other health care providers or patients/families
- Understanding that all health care providers contribute to the team or collaborative unit
- Showing respect and building trust among team members
- Introducing new members of the team in a way that is welcoming and gives them the information they need in order to be a contributing member
- Turning to colleagues for answers
- Supporting each other when mistakes are made and celebrating together when success is achieved

When health care providers work collaboratively, they seek common goals and are able to analyze and address problems that may arise. They make better use of their skills and knowledge, and they are able to more effectively coordinate care according to patients' needs. As a result, patients should receive higher quality care (WHO, 2010). In addition to enhancing quality care, collaborative practice contributes to job satisfaction for the health care provider (Mulvale, Embrett, & Razavi, 2016). As addressed in Chapter 16, interprofessional or primary care teams are emerging across Canada in primary care clinics or networks to support the needs of populations with different chronic diseases that can be managed in the community.

Interprofessional Education

Traditionally, there has been a prevalent uniprofessional approach to the education of health care professionals because training in each profession is often done in isolation from fellow students in other health professions. This can lead to strong identification with one's own profession and a corresponding reluctance to engage with other professions (Stull & Blue, 2016). Moving beyond these "silos" and developing a new generation of health care professionals who are skilled in interprofessional work and collaboration is a trend that is on the rise. Medical, nursing, pharmacy, social work, dentistry, physiotherapy, and occupational therapy students are now often taking courses together, learning with, from, and about one another at some Canadian universities.

> **CRITICAL THINKING QUESTION 17.5:** If you were a health care provider on an interprofessional care team working at a primary care clinic, and the dietitian who was also part of the team used discipline-specific language that you did not understand, what would you do?

ABUSE BY HEALTH CARE PROFESSIONALS

Headlines such as "Nurse in Ontario facing 8 murder charges now accused of trying to harm 6 more patients," "Grande Prairie doctor suspended, charged over inappropriate examinations," "Victoria nurse barred from practice over sexual misconduct," and "Disgraced Calgary psychiatrist Aubrey Levin facing new abuse allegations" do not represent isolated incidents. In the past 15 years, 250 health care professionals across Canada have been disciplined for patient boundary offences by self-regulatory bodies. The term "boundary offences" encompasses a wide range of improper conduct, including sexual comments, inappropriate touching (often

under the guise of a physical examination), taking photographs or videos without a patient's knowledge, or sexual intercourse with a patient (without or with consent—if a patient can truly provide valid consent in this context). Abuse represents a transgression of the trust placed in a health care professional. Because of the position of power of the health care professional in relation to the patient, any suggestive or sexual behaviour or language in a clinical setting is deemed to be inappropriate.

In Ontario, a task force on the sexual abuse of patients (which was an independent body commissioned by the College of Physicians and Surgeons) made a series of recommendations after the review of evidence from patients who had reported sexual improprieties on the part of medical practitioners. These recommendations were reviewed and published by the Council of the College of Physicians and Surgeons in 1992 (Task Force on Sexual Abuse of Patients, 1991), which recommended that the RHPA be amended to include a new section regarding actions of professional misconduct of a sexual nature with different levels of offence and penalties, such as fines or revocation of licence for the more severe offences. In 2014, another task force was initiated by the Ontario Government, and it submitted a report titled *To Zero: Independent Report of the Minister's Task Force on the Prevention of Sexual Abuse of Patients and the Regulated Health Professions Act, 1991*. The government's actions, based on the task force's recommendations from this report, included the following:

- Add to the expanded list of acts that will result in the mandatory revocation of a regulated health professional's license.
- Remove the ability of a college to allow a regulated health professional to continue to practice on patients of one gender after an allegation or finding of sexual abuse.
- Increase fines for health professionals and organizations that fail to report a suspected case of patient sexual abuse to a college.
- Increase transparency by adding to what colleges must report on their public register and website.
- Clarify the time period after the end of a patient-provider relationship in which sexual relations are prohibited.
- Fund patient therapy and counselling from the moment a complaint of sexual abuse is made.

Sexual abuse in the RHPA is defined as sexual intercourse or other forms of physical sexual relations between the practitioner and the patient, touching of a sexual nature of the patient by the practitioner, or behaviour or remarks of a sexual nature toward the patient. However, the legislation also states that the words "sexual nature" do not include touching, behaviour, or remarks of a clinical nature that are appropriate to the service provided. The RHPA includes procedures for awarding financial compensation to patients who have been sexually abused by health care professionals to cover costs of counselling and treatment for sexual abuse; financial compensation is not foreseen by the RHPA for any other patient complaints.

CRITICAL THINKING QUESTIONS 17.6

1. How can sexual abuse by health care professionals be prevented? How does your province handle sexual abuse of patients by health care professionals? Describe the mechanism and penalty associated with it where the health care professional is found guilty.

2. In your province or territory, is there legislation that protects and mandates services for individuals who have been sexually abused? If so, do you think the legislation is effective? Why or why not?

FREEDOM OF INFORMATION AND ITS IMPACT ON PRACTICE

Access to information is a legal right to review documents that are not already in the public realm. *Freedom of information (FOI)* is intended to help make government institutions more accountable during a time when not only are they holding vast amounts of data and information, but technology gives unprecedented ability to identify, interrogate, and analyze the data and information effectively. FOI is now generally viewed as a standard tool for increasing transparency and reducing corruption and is widely perceived to be a basic right in any healthy, democratic system of government. FOI can be used to access records relating to hospitals, mental health institutions, prisons, the military, foreign policy, Crown corporations, state agencies, policy development, policing, and much more. The federal government introduced the *Pan-Canadian Health Information Privacy and Confidentiality Framework* in 2005 to protect patients' personal information without restricting health service providers' access to essential data.

As new and evolving models of care develop, such as primary care networks, integrated health networks, and specialty-related medical groups working in association and with institutional or provincial electronic health records, the sharing of personal health information is now broadened beyond what is customarily understood by a patient to be included in their circle of care. In patient-centric institutional or provincial electronic health records, personal health information from a broad range of sources and providers can be shared with and accessed by others. Adding further complexity is the potential for secondary uses of personal health information by persons or organizations beyond the circle of care. Legislation has been enacted in all provinces and territories regarding FOI and the protection of personal information or privacy.

CRITICAL THINKING QUESTION 17.7: How can nurse practitioners who are working as part of a primary care team ensure that they are following the legislation regarding what information is collected and how it is used in their province or territory?

THE HEALTH OF HEALTH CARE PROFESSIONALS

The health of health care providers receives relatively little attention, except for the vast array of results produced by the Nurses' Health Study from Harvard University (Nurses' Health Study, 2018), which are related more appropriately to the overall lives of nurses than to work-related issues. The relation of work and health is described in Chapter 12. The nature of jobs for health care workers include caring for people under stress, lifting patients, giving needles, stitching wounds, and working in a changing environment that can expose workers to specific health risks.

Health care workers are exposed to infectious diseases such as tuberculosis, HIV caused by needlestick injury, hepatitis B and C, and Norwalk-like viruses (see Chapter 7). They are also exposed to numerous irritants and chemicals, such as nitrous oxide and latex allergies.

In recent years, nurses have reported experiencing violence in forms of verbal abuse or physical abuse. Workplace violence, often underreported, is a pervasive and persistent issue in health care, which has a significant impact on the psychological health and safety of health care workers. Emergency departments (EDs) are on the front line for incidents of abuse and are places where nurses are routinely spat upon and sworn at during the shift (New Brunswick Nurses Union, 2017). In Nova Scotia during an 11-month period, 61 incidents of violence and threats were reported (Homson, 2017). In 2015, Abbotsford Regional Hospital ED in British Columbia, three quarters of ED staff said they had been physically assaulted while working in the previous year, with more than half saying they had experienced such abuse more than 20 times over a 12-month period (Olsen, 2017). In Saskatchewan, nearly three quarters of registered psychiatric nurses reported having experienced violence (physical, verbal, or both) during a 12-month period (Stadnyk, 2008). More than 4 000 incidents of workplace violence against Canadian nurses were reported between 2008 and 2013 (Roussy, 2016).

Larger hospitals have employee health services and assistance programs to deal with issues related to the health of their employees. Recently, professional associations, in collaboration with regulatory bodies, have developed anonymous treatment facilities dealing with health care workers having mental health or addiction problems. More than 500 000 Canadians, including many who work in health care, will not make it to work during any given week because of a mental health problem or mental illness (Mental Health Commission of Canada, 2018). Doctors have the highest suicide rate of any profession, with female physicians experiencing higher rates of depression than male physicians (T'Sarumi et al., 2018).

CRITICAL THINKING QUESTION 17.8: Depression among health care workers contributes to absenteeism and reduced productivity in the workplace and can put patient safety in jeopardy. What is one of the main issues that health care workers are facing when attempting to obtain the support and help that is needed for mental health issues such as depression?

FUTURE TRENDS AND ISSUES

Regulation of Health Care Professionals

The recent process of deprofessionalization has begun. Legislation aimed at obtaining greater public control of the self-regulating professions has been enacted. This process is certain to continue. This section presents some of the issues involved and trends that may be expected.

Because governments now pay most medical bills, they are likely to become more interested in the value they receive for taxpayers' money, not only in terms of quantity but also of quality. This could mean greater government involvement in the design of medical school curricula, in the licensing procedures of provincial colleges, and in the monitoring of individual practices. The result could be periodic re-examination for relicensure, enforced continuing education, and similar measures for ensuring the competence of licensed physicians and other health care providers. Professions have responded by introducing codes of ethical conduct, clearly stating their legal responsibilities; spelling out detailed knowledge of informed consent; and increasing awareness about the overall health care system, the role their own discipline plays in a larger context, and introduction of mandatory continuing education requirements. The Medical Council of Canada's *Objectives of the Considerations of the Legal, Ethical and Organizational Aspects of the Practice of Medicine,* which lists needed competencies in these areas, and the CNA *Code of Ethics for Registered Nurses,* point to the future direction in health sciences education (CNA, 2002; Medical Council of Canada, 1999).

Change is coming from within College councils. The College of Nurses of Ontario (CNO) is at the forefront of reforms. Starting in 2014, the CNO began to explore whether it could do a better job of serving the public and initiated a governance review, and a task force was subsequently established to look at best practices around the world, study the literature on regulatory governance, and document international trends. In 2016, the CNO's council endorsed *Governance Vision 2020,* in reference to the year it hopes the provincial government will pass legislation to eliminate of council elections, among several other recommendations (CNO, 2016). The CNO hopes to have a diversified workforce with at least 20% of nursing leaders being Indigenous and visible minorities and 10% being male. The British Columbia College of Nursing Professionals was created in 2018, joining several nursing colleges into one regulator.

The medical profession is certain to see increased government regulation as a threat to its freedom and autonomy. Quebec's Bill 114, which forced doctors to work in understaffed EDs, is an example of increased control by the government on the practice of medicine (Borsellino, 2002). Bill 114 was withdrawn, but Bill 142 was later introduced in; it in essence requires a detailed regional plan for the staffing requirement for each region that considers the need of population, hospitals, EDs, centre local de services communautaires, long-term care facilities, and so on, for both general practitioners and specialists (Quebec Assemblée Nationale, 2002). Under Bill 142, practitioners can be assigned to areas where shortages are envisioned, as part of their conditions to participate in health insurance plans. The profession has reacted by becoming more politicized by lobbying governments and enlisting the aid of the public. Union-like activities (e.g., withholding of services) will probably become more common. The profession is also likely to react by improving its own regulation and becoming more socially accountable to communities in which they practice. Stricter requirements for relicensure, continuing education, peer review, and evaluation of individual practices may be imposed to forestall government action in these areas. Some degree of confrontation seems inevitable, but it is to be hoped that those issues described will be resolved in a manner that will lead to better health care for Canadians and, in the long run, a stronger, if less autonomous, profession.

Ontario's RHPA also throws some light on the future direction of the regulation of health care professionals. The RHPA states that "the sole purpose of professional regulation is to advance and protect the public interest. The public is the intended beneficiary of regulation, not the members of the professions. Thus, the purpose of granting self-regulation to a profession is not to enhance its status or increase the earning power of its members by giving the profession a monopoly over the delivery of particular health services" (Government of Ontario, 1991).

Another major change is that an increasing number of health care occupations are demanding to be considered as professions and to participate in health insurance programs. This will create tension among the different health care providers. Definitions of health care professions will become restrictive, and professionals will be equated with individuals with specialized knowledge and skill but not necessarily those with responsibility, autonomy, or service orientation. Many more new problems will undoubtedly arise as both governments and consumers seek to have a greater voice in health care.

Human Health Resources

Current and emerging HHR trends have a significant impact on the health system and Canada has been experiencing HHR challenges in many professions for a number of years. The societal cost of producing trained health professionals is significant and can vary from $22 000 for a single RN to $97 753 for a single resident physician, which does not include the direct costs by the student, such as tuition (Official Language Community Development Bureau, 2008). These costs also do not include the value of gaining specialized skills and advanced training during a career. The loss of any health professional because of student or professional attrition or early retirement has an immense impact on the health system.

Student attrition has been attributed to personal reasons, family difficulties, and financial problems (Kukkonen, Suhonen, & Salminen, 2016), and professional attrition (within 2 years of graduating), especially in nursing, has been attributed to transition shock. **Transition shock** is the contrast between the relationships, roles, responsibilities, knowledge, and performance expectations required within the academic environment with those required in the professional practice setting (Duchscher & Windey, 2018). Within the first year of employment of professional practice, 35% to 50% of new nursing graduates can be expected to change their place of employment or exit the profession altogether (McMillan, 2018; MacKusick & Minick, 2010). In the coming years, growing workforce challenges will impact the health system. Cutting-edge recruitment practices, databases, and automated systems will be required to bring workforce planning and management to a new level beyond assumptions and guesswork. Predictive analytics driven by "big data"—which can accurately predict patient demand, staffing needs, and staff schedules up to 120 days in advance—are beginning to change workforce recruitment, engagement, and management. Providing effective scheduling and staffing to bolster quality patient care, safety, satisfaction, and financial efficiency are necessary advancements to support our health care system.

SUMMARY

This chapter examined the definition of profession and professionalism, discussed their regulation, listed and described the various health care professions (including complementary health care professionals), and discussed FOI as it relates to health care professionals. IPP and education were also introduced as an innovative way to strengthen the health care system. Additionally, abuse by health care professionals and the health of health care professionals was also explored. The chapter concluded with a synopsis of possible future trends in regulation and HHRs.

The concept of professionalism is very difficult to define; hence, most definitions consist of lists of characteristics commonly attributed to an established profession. These characteristics include specialized knowledge and skill, autonomy, service orientation, accountability, advocacy, and ethics and values.

Provinces have enacted legislation to ensure greater public control of the professions. The earliest and most significant changes occurred in the provinces of Quebec and Ontario. Quebec's *Professional Code* defines what a profession is and establishes formal criteria by which an occupation gains statutory recognition as a profession. Furthermore, each profession is governed by a professional order. This order maintains surveillance of the quality of individual practices and is empowered to take corrective measures. The Code also establishes two overall supervisory and regulatory bodies: the Office des professions du Québec and the Conseil interprofessionnel du Québec.

In Ontario, the RHPA was enacted in 1991. One of the major aspects of the new legislation is the expansion of the number of professions under its jurisdiction to 23. The RHPA was enacted to obtain greater public accountability in the regulation of the health care professions and is regarded as increasing equity among the health care professions, reducing the role of the physician as the gatekeeper and increasing direct access for the public to a wider variety of professionals. The most revolutionary aspect of the legislation is that the professions are not defined by the scope of practice, but professionals are licensed to perform various procedures, or controlled acts, that are potentially dangerous.

The RHPA gives the minister of health broad powers to supervise the regulation of the 29 disciplines included

and increases the accountability and protection of the interests of the public. The emphasis is on the public good rather than on professional interests.

Each health care profession is required to establish a College that is responsible for regulating the practice of the profession and to govern its members. Physicians are required to be licensed in all provinces by the College of Physicians and Surgeons. This licensing agency is made up of the council of the College, the executive committee, the registration committee, the complaints committee, the discipline committee, and the fitness to practice committee, the continuing competence committee, and the medical review committee. Dentists, like physicians, are required to be licensed in every province. As well, in Ontario, the dental profession is regulated in a manner similar to physicians under the RHPA. Nurses are also required to be licensed in all provinces (RNs, LPNs, RPNs [British Columbia], RPNs [Ontario]) and perform many functions depending on their location, their employer, and their appointment. Chiropractic and midwifery are two health care professions where public demand for alternative health care delivery modalities helped to create pressure for official recognition.

Abuse represents a transgression of the trust placed in a health care professional. The term "boundary offences" encompasses a wide range of conduct, including sexual comments, inappropriate touching (often under the guise of a physical examination), and taking photographs or videos without a patient's knowledge, or sexual intercourse with a patient (without or with consent—if a patient can truly provide valid consent in this context). Several task forces have been created to investigate abuse by health care professionals and has resulted in changes to legislations to better protect the public.

Legislation has been enacted in all provinces and territories regarding FOI and the protection of personal information or privacy. The federal government introduced the *Pan-Canadian Health Information Privacy and Confidentiality Framework* in 2005; it was designed to protect patients' personal information without restricting health service providers' access to essential data. As new and evolving models of care develop, the sharing of personal health information is now broadened beyond what is customarily understood by a patient to be included in their circle of care.

Different types of work in health care are associated with different types of job-related health risks. Nurses, personal support workers, physiotherapists, and laboratory workers are at high risk for back problems and other soft tissue sprains and strains. Job strain, creating stress, and burnout are more common among those who are at the lower end of the hierarchy, such as personal support workers, orderlies, and attendants; for nurses, it is less common, and for physicians, it is the least common. Health care providers are also exposed to infectious diseases such as tuberculosis, HIV caused by needlestick injury, hepatitis B and C, and Norwalk-like viruses, as well as exposed to numerous irritants and chemicals, such as nitrous oxide, and latex allergies. In recent years, nurses have reported experiencing violence in forms of verbal abuse or physical abuse, which is much more prevalent in long-term care facilities.

Future trends include the recent process of deprofessionalization. Legislation aimed at obtaining greater public control of the self-regulating professions has been enacted, and this process is certain to continue. The medical and nursing professions are certain to see increased government regulation as a threat to their freedom and autonomy. Reaction by the professions is likely to take two forms: the professions will become more politicized and may attempt to improve their own regulation, which can be seen through CNO's *Vision 2020*. In the coming years, growing workforce challenges will impact the health system. The loss of any health professional because of student or professional attrition or early retirement has an immense impact on the health system. Cutting-edge recruitment practices, databases, and automated systems will be required to bring workforce planning and management to a new level beyond assumptions and guesswork.

KEY WEBSITES

Canadian Chiropractor Association: https://www.chiropractic.ca
This site provides information about chiropractic services, resources, and research. There is also information about associations and regulatory bodies across Canada.

Canadian Interprofessional Health Collaborative (CIHC) framework: https://www.cihc.ca/files/CIHC_IP Competencies_Feb1210.pdffur4
This site provides information about the Canadian Interprofessional Health Collaborative Framework.

Canadian Medical Association: https://www.cma.ca/en/Pages/cma_default.aspx
This site provides information about the Canadian Medical Association for members and the general public about various health related issues and topics.

Canadian Nurses Association: https://www.cna-aiic.ca/en
This site provides information about nursing practice, professional development, certification, policy, and advocacy documents.

Canadian Pharmacists Association: https://www.pharmacists.ca
This site provides information about pharmacy across Canada, with a focus on information about drugs and therapeutic products, professional development, and advocacy work.

College of Nurses of Ontario: Vision 2020: http://www.cno.org/en/what-is-cno/councils-and-committees/council/governance-vision-2020
This site provides information about the College's *Vision 2020* and how the change will affect the governing of the College.

Nurses' Health Study. (2018): Publications: http://www.channing.harvard.edu/nhs/pub.htmlfur14

This site provides information about the history of the study, principal investigators, resources, and data about the study's findings.

Quebec's Professional Code: http://legisquebec.gouv.qc.ca/en/showdoc/cs/C-26fur16
This site provides information pertaining only to Quebec's *Professional Code*.

Regulated Health Professions Act (Ontario): https://www.ontario.ca/laws/statute/91r18
This site provides the text of the RHPA itself, which is available for download regarding the regulation of health professions in Ontario.

REFERENCES

Borsellino, M. (2002). Bill 114: how to rally MDs united in opposition. *Medical Post*, September 3.

Canadian Association of Midwives. (2018). *Midwifery across Canada*. Retrieved from https://canadianmidwives.org/midwifery-across-canada/#1467634074483-f50b550d-db87.

Canadian Institute for Heath Information. (2016). *Regulated nurses 2016 report*. Retrieved from https://www.cihi.ca/sites/default/files/document/regulated-nurses-2016-report-en-web.pdf.

Canadian Interprofessional Health Collaborative. (2009). *Fact sheet*. Vancouver, BC: Author.

Canadian Interprofessional Health Collaborative. (2010). *A national interprofessional competency framework*. Retrieved from http://www.cihc.ca/files/CIHC_IP Competencies_ Feb1210.pdf.

Canadian Medical Association. (2002). *Scopes of practice*. Retrieved from www.cma.ca/cma/common/displayPage. do?pageId=/staticContent/HTML/N0/l2/where_we_stand/2002/01-21.htm.

Canadian Medical Association. (2018). *Basic physician facts*. Retrieved from https://www.cma.ca/En/Pages/basic-physician-facts.aspx.

Canadian Medical Association (n.d.). *The evolving professional relationship between Canadian physicians and our health care system: where do we stand?* Retrieved from https://www.cma.ca/Assets/assets-library/document/en/advocacy/policy-research/CMA_Policy_The_evolving_professional_relationship_between_Canadian_physicians_and_our_health_care_system_PD12-04-e.pdf.

Canadian Nurses Association. (2002). *Code of ethics for registered nurses*. Ottawa. Retrieved from http://www.cna-nurses.ca/pages/ethics/ethicsframe.htm.

Canadian Nurses Association. (2017). *Nursing statistics*. Retrieved from https://cna-aiic.ca/en/nursing-practice/the-practice-of-nursing/health-human-resources/nursing-statistics.

Canadian Nurses Association. (2018). *Certification poster*. Retrieved from https://cna-aiic.ca/-/media/cna/page-content/pdf-en/certification-poster-en.pdf?la=en&hash=-FEADC697DD92DFF063C1405C4ACA5326A612099C.

Canadian Public Health Association. (2017). *Creating a certified public health professional designation for Canada's public health workforce*. Retrieved from https://www.cpha.ca/creating-certified-public-health-professional-designation-canadas-public-health-workforce-0.

Chiropractic in Canada. (2002). *Provincial licensing offices*. Retrieved from http://www.ccachiro.org.

College of Nurses of Ontario. (2016). *Governance vision 2020*. Retrieved from http://www.cno.org/en/what-is-cno/councils-and-committees/council/governance-vision-2020/.

Collège des médecins du Québec. (1995). *ALDO-Quebec: legislative, ethical, and organizational aspects of medical practice in Quebec*. Montreal: Collège des médecins du Québec.

Duchscher, J. B., & Windey, M. (2018). Stages of transition and transition shock. *Journal for Nurses in Professional Development*, 34(4), 228–232.

Duncan, S., & Whyte, N. (2018). British Columbia's one nursing regulator: a critical commentary on the amalgamation process. *Nursing Leadership*, 31(3), 24–33.

Federation of Health Regulatory Colleges of Ontario. (2018). *Quick facts about FHRCO members*. Retrieved from http://www.regulatedhealthprofessions.on.ca/.

FitzGerald, D., Keane, R. A., Reid, A., et al. (2013). Ageing, cognitive disorders and professional practice. *Age and Ageing*, 42(5), 608–614.

Friedson, E. (1970). *The profession of medicine*. New York: Dodds, Mead, and Co.

Government of Ontario. (1991). *Regulated Health Professions Act*. Retrieved from https://www.ontario.ca/laws/statute/91r18.

Government of Quebec. (2016). *The practice of a profession governed by a professional order*. Retrieved from https://www.immigration-quebec.gouv.qc.ca/publications/en/professions/guide-practise-profession.pdf.

Government of Quebec. (1973). *Professional code*. Retrieved from www.canlii.org/qc/sta/c26/whole.html. [Updated to 19 December 2001] (October 2002).

Health Canada. (2013). *Health human resources action plan*. Retrieved from http://publications.gc.ca/collections/collection_2014/sc-hc/H22-1-3-2013-eng.pdf.

Higginbottom, G. (2011). The transitioning experiences of internationally-educated nurses into a Canadian health care system: a focused ethnography. *BMC Nursing*, 10, 14. https://doi.org/10.1186/1472-6955-10-14.

Homson, A. (2017, January 20). Report calls for new safety measures in N.S. emergency rooms. *Canadian Press*. Retrieved from http://atlantic.ctvnews.ca/mobile/report-calls-for-new-safety-measures-in-n-s-emergency-rooms-1.324940028.

Kukkonen, P., Suhonen, R., & Salminen, L. (2016). Discontinued students in nursing education–who and why? *Nurse Education in Practice*, 17, 67–73.

MacKusick, C. I., & Minick, P. (2010). Why are nurses leaving? Findings from an initial qualitative study on nursing attrition. *Medsurg Nursing*, 19(6).

McMillan, K. (2018). *A critical organizational analysis of frontline nurses' experience of rapid and continuous change in an acute health care organization*. (Doctoral dissertation, Université d'Ottawa/University of Ottawa).

Medical Council of Canada. (1999). *Objectives of the considerations of the legal, ethical and organizational aspects of the practice of medicine*. Retrieved from http://www.mcc.ca/pdf/cleo_e.html (October 2002).

Mental Health Commission of Canada. (2018). *Canadian employees report workplace stress as primary cause of mental health concerns*. Retrieved from https://www.mentalhealthcommission.ca/English/news-article/13522/canadian-employees-report-workplace-stress-primary-cause-mental-health-concerns.

Merriam-Webster Dictionary. (2018). *Profession*. Retrieved from https://www.merriam-webster.com/dictionary/profession.

Mildon, B. (2018). Commentary: regulation and the nursing profession: a personal reflection. *Nursing Leadership*, 31(3), 34–41.

Mulvale, G., Embrett, M., & Razavi, S. D. (2016). "Gearing up" to improve interprofessional collaboration in primary care: a systematic review and conceptual framework. *BMC Family Practice*, 17(1), 83.

New Brunswick Nurses Union. (2017). *Blog: a shocking history of workplace violence*. Retrieved from https://www.nbnu.ca/blog/shocking-history-workplace-violence/29.

Nurses' Health Study. (2018). *Publications*. Retrieved from http://www.channing.harvard.edu/nhs/pub.html.

Office des professions du Québec. (2002). *Système professionnel Québécois: Conseil interprofessionnel du Québec*. Retrieved from www.opq.gouv.qc.ca/03systeme/conseil_interprofessionnel.htm. [Accessed October 2002].

Office of Research and Information Services, Association of Faculties of Medicine of Canada. (2016). Retrieved from https://afmc.ca.

Official Languages Community Development Bureau. (2008). *Overview of the cost of training health professionals: Health Canada*. Retrieved from http://publications.gc.ca/collections/collection_2009/sc-hc/H29-1-2009E.pdf.

Olsen, T. (2017). Most Abbotsford ER workers had been subject of physical violence in 2015: report. *Abbeynews*. Retrieved from http://www.abbynews.com/news/most-abbotsford-er-workers-had-been-subject-of-physical-violence-in-2015-report/30

Pooley, D. (1992). Regulated Health Professions Act, 1991: the new benchmark for future health care legislation. *Journal of Canadian Chiropractic Association*, 36(3), 161–164.

Public Health Agency of Canada. (2005). *Building the public health workforce for the 21st century: a pan-Canadian framework for public health human resources planning*. Ottawa: Author. Retrieved from http://publications.gc.ca/collections/collection_2008/phac-aspc/HP5-12-2005E.pdf.

Quebec, Assemblée Nationale. (2002). *An act to amend the Act respecting health services and social services as regards the medical activities, the distribution, and undertaking of physicians* (February 2003).

Regan, M. D. (1987). *Regulation: the politics of policy*. Boston: Little Brown.

Renfrew, M. J., McFadden, A., Bastos, M. H., et al. (2014). Midwifery and quality care: findings from a new evidence-informed framework for maternal and newborn care. *The Lancet*, 384(9948), 1129–1145.

Roussy, K. (2016). Workplace violence against health-care workers under-reported, largely ignored. *CBC News* (April 27, 2016). Retrieved from https://www.cbc.ca/news/health/violence-against-health-care-workers-1.3555241.

Saskatchewan Registered Nurses Association. (n.d.). *SRNA position statement: professional self-regulation*. Retrieved from http://www.srna.org.

Stadnyk, B. L. (2008). *Workplace violence isn't always physical: a one year experience of a group of registered psychiatric nurses*. Saskatchewan: Registered Psychiatric Nurses Association of Saskatchewan. Retrieved from https://www.rpnas.com/?s=workplace+violence.

Statistics Canada. (2016). *Labour in Canada: key results from the 2016 Census*. Retrieved from https://www150.statcan.gc.ca/n1/daily-quotidien/171129/dq171129b-eng.htm.

Stull, C. L., & Blue, C. M. (2016). Examining the influence of professional identity formation on the attitudes of students towards interprofessional collaboration. *Journal of Interprofessional Care*, 30, 90–96. https://doi.org/10.3109/13561820.2015.1066318.

T'Sarumi, O., Ashraf, A., Tanwar, D., et al. (2018). *Physician suicide: a silent epidemic*. Presentation: American Psychological Association Conference. Retrieved from https://www.google.com/url?sa=t&rct=j&q=&esrc=s&source=web&cd=4&cad=rja&uact=8&ved=0ahUKEwigtq7g2KjbAhVG2VMKHZt0D5UQFgg-2MAM&url=https%3A%2F%2Fwww.psychiatry.org%2FFile%2520Library%2FPsychiatrists%2FMeetings%2FAnnual-Meeting%2F2018%2Fvirtual-registration-bag%2FPoster-Proceedings.pdf&usg=AOvVaw-2SoK1qIV0YaZhItMDAaslz.

Task Force on Sexual Abuse of Patients. (1991). *The final report of the Task Force on Sexual Abuse of Patients*. Toronto: College of Physicians and Surgeons of Ontario.

World Health Organization. (2010). *Framework for action on interprofessional education & collaborative practice*. Retrieved from https://www.who.int/hrh/resources/framework_action/en/.

World Health Organization. (2014). *Global health workforce alliance annual report*. Retrieved from http://www.who.int/workforcealliance/knowledge/resources/ghwa_annual_report2014.pdf.

Looking Forward

LEARNING OBJECTIVES

- Develop an understanding of the historical reforms that have shaped our health system.
- Identify an equity-oriented health care system.

- Identify trends in health care and explain how they will impact our health system.
- Identify advancements in public health and how they will impact our health system.

CHAPTER OUTLINE

KEY TERMS

artificial intelligence (AI)
augmented reality (AR)
drones

virtual reality (VR)
wearable consumer devices

A health care system—even the best health care system in the world—will be only one of the ingredients that determine whether your life will be long or short, healthy or sick, full of fulfillment, or empty with despair.

    —Honorable Roy Romanow, Former Chair of the Commission on the Future of Health Care in Canada

As we look forward to the future and as our health care system evolves, new trends and advancements are on the horizon. Some of these innovations include changes in health care delivery systems, the implementation of new technology systems, and advancements in medicine. With these advancements, new questions also emerge that will need to be discussed and debated, such as: How are consumers' privacy and security being protected when using health care apps? Does a technology-based future support our health and well-being?

    In this final chapter, we outline a number of emerging trends and advancements not addressed in the previous chapters that will have an impact on our health as Canadians. Time will tell whether these impacts will be positive or not.

Looking ahead requires an appreciation of how far we have come.

Remember how far you've come, not how far you have to go. You are not where you want to be, but neither are you where you used to be.

—*Rick Warren*

We begin this chapter by reviewing a number of reforms that have contributed to reforming and advancing our health system.

TRANSFORMING HEALTH CARE: A HISTORICAL REVIEW

The Canadian health care system has seen a number of reforms, task forces, royal commissions, and inquiries across provinces and federally since its inception. The most notable ones across provinces were Seaton in British Columbia (British Columbia Royal Commission on Health Care and Costs, 1991), Mazankowski in Alberta (Premier's Advisory Council on Health, A Framework for Reform, 2001), Fyke (The Commission on Medicare, 2001) and Dagnone (2009) in Saskatchewan, Sinclair (The Ontario Health Services Restructuring Commission, 2001) and Drummond (The Commission on the Reform of Ontario's Public Services, 2012) in Ontario, and Clair (Commission d'étude sur les services de santé et les services sociaux, 2000) in Quebec. Federally, there have been the National Forum on Health (1997); the Romanow (2002) Commission on the Future of Health Care in Canada; the Kirby (2002) Senate Standing Committee on Social Affairs, Science and Technology; and the Naylor (2015) report, *Unleashing Innovation, Excellent Healthcare for Canada*. With a renewed federal interest in health care, an external review was undertaken of the eight federally funded pan-Canadian health organizations (PCHOs) (Forest & Martin, 2018). Recommendations included amalgamating several of the PCHOs into one organization, eliminating the Mental Health Commission of Canada, the Canadian Partnership Against Cancer, and the Canadian Centre on Substance Abuse and Addiction; having PCHOs play a role in reconciliation by paying more attention to Indigenous health care issues; and having less centralization in Ottawa, with more federal–provincial–territorial collaboration.

Across all reviews, common themes have emerged, specifically, the lack of an integrated and patient-centred health care system, the importance of efficiency and value for money in ensuring system sustainability, and the need to build a shared knowledge base and learn from it to improve services for patients and overall system management (Naylor, 2015). Proposed solutions also converged, including reforming the health care system to prioritize primary care and the broad determinants of health, reforming health human resources policies, and improving evaluation and research to allow for more effective decision making.

Although the task forces have not resulted in transformative change of the health care system, many reviews have paved the way for improvements in health care. A national pharmacare program is on the horizon (see Chapter 16), funding for home care and mental health were increased in the 2017 and 2018 federal budgets (see Chapter 16), a national immunization strategy has been created (see Chapter 10), and we have seen reduced consumption of tobacco (see Chapter 9) because of a number of health promotion interventions working together to create environments where the healthy choice becomes the easy choice. However, there is still much work to be done to strengthen Canada's health care system, including but not limited to increasing access to primary care, changing payment mechanisms for physicians, decreasing wait times for surgery, improving health data and information management capacity, creating integrated care and sharing budgets, and scaling up the use of digital technology. All of these improvements will go a long way towards transforming our health care system; however, conditions of everyday life—where we work, live, learn, and play—still have a greater impact on our health (Raphael, 2018).

Many scholars and community health care providers would argue that strengthening Canada's social safety net will not only produce cost savings for our health care system but also enhanced health for all Canadians. Implementing health promotion strategies as outlined in the Ottawa Charter can change the social, economic, and environmental conditions that determine health (see Chapter 1). Influencing positive change through intersectoral action can be an effective strategy because many factors that affect health lie outside the health sector. Involving a wide range of people, communities, government departments, researchers, not-for-profit, and business sectors to work in partnerships is required to create conditions for good health.

Working across sectors to improve health and reduce inequities is a complex process that is driven by addressing local community issues. Therefore, there is no "cookie cutter" approach for how to collaborate intersectorally. However, there are many examples across Canada where sectors have worked together to change the social and living conditions for populations and communities (e.g., see Real-World Example box about BC Healthy Communities). Tools have also been developed to support health care providers, researchers, and decision makers in working more collaboratively. For example, the Early Childhood Partnership Tool (http://ecst.cichprofile.ca) helps anyone working in the areas of early childhood to find ways to create intersectoral partnerships by answering four questions. The tool provides a customized summary of data, information, resources, and links, as well as ideas on how to create partnerships that will increase your impact on the overall health and well-being of young children and their families.

 REAL-WORLD EXAMPLE

British Columbia's Healthy Communities

BC Healthy Communities (https://bchealthycommunities.ca), a not-for-profit organization, supports communities in building their capacity to work across sectors for the development of healthy, thriving, and resilient communities. Working from the belief that improving health lies outside the health care system, BC Healthy Communities focuses on connectedness, livability, and equity in all their work.

Now that we have covered a few of the historical reviews, we can turn our attention ahead and discuss a number of advancements and trends that are creating momentum to transform our health system.

ADVANCEMENTS IN HEALTH CARE DELIVERY

Equity-Oriented Health Care

Historically, health care in Canada has been rooted in medicine, without actively engaging with the broad determinants of health that impact individuals' lives. Care services have also not been universally available or accessible to all social groups, which highlights the inequities that exist in our health care system. However, several reports and reviews have highlighted equity as a value and an aspiration of our health care system. We discuss a few of those reports next to demonstrate that an equity-oriented health system is building and gaining ground in Canada.

The 1997 National Forum on Health identified, through public consultations, the fundamental values of Canadians toward their health care system; these include equity and access; compassion; dignity and respect for all individuals; quality, efficiency, and effectiveness; personal responsibility for appropriate use of health resources; and public

participation in health system decision making (National Forum on Health, 1997). The Romanow Commission echoed similar sentiments from Canadians, including the notion that the health care system is premised on equity, fairness, and solidarity. It stated that "Canadians consider equal and timely access to medically necessary health care services on a basis of need as a right of citizenship, not a matter of privilege of status or wealth" (Romanow, 2002, p. xvi). Concerns regarding access to services have been particularly pronounced. The Kirby Commission recommended addressing timely access through a national health care guarantee. The Romanow Commission recommended a Canadian health covenant as a common declaration of Canadians' and their governments' commitment to a universally accessible, publicly funded health care system rather than establishing new rights that would be subject to legal interpretation and decisions by the courts.

Whereas the National Forum on Health emphasized personal responsibility for appropriate use of health resources, the Romanow Commission stressed mutual responsibility, acknowledging the balance between personal responsibility for health and mutual responsibility for the health care system. This includes the financial responsibility to contribute to the system within each individual's means. The commission also identified the values placed on the system's being a public resource, on patient-centred care, and on transparency and accountability. Unfortunately, nearly two decades later, the idea of a Canadian covenant has not taken root. However, advocacy groups seeking equity and civil society organizations that serve many socially and economically disadvantaged groups have been waving the equity flag and moving forward with an equity agenda (Ontario Ministry of Health and Long-Term Care, 2016).

We have known for many decades what determines our health. The Lalonde report (see Chapter 1) set the stage for the discussion and eventual adoption of the social determinants of health (SDHs). In 2005, the World Health Organization's (WHO's) Commission on the Social Determinants of Health emphasized that what determines our health lies outside of the health care system. It is the social, political, economic, and cultural conditions and the structural drivers of these conditions that determine our health. The SDHs go beyond individual behaviours and beyond individual genetic endowment. Achievement of health equity requires action on the SDHs and on the structural drivers of these determinants. Taking action to address health inequities is building momentum across Canada (see Real-World Example box about RentSafe).

REAL-WORLD EXAMPLE

Rentsafe

RentSafe is a collaborative initiative of tenants, all public health units across Ontario, legal aid clinics, the Canadian Environmental Law Association, community health organizations, including community health centres, and the Canadian Partnership for Children's Health and Environment. Working together, they are taking action to create healthier living conditions in low-income and marginalized communities and reducing housing-related health inequities (Canadian Partnership for Children's Health and Environment, 2018).

As we look forward, what would our health care system be like if we were able to achieve equity-oriented health care? Perhaps the health system would continually be working on reducing the burden of illness, injury, and disability and improving the health and functioning of Canadians. Equity at a population level would mean a focus on improving health status and continuing to do so with the goal of reducing the inequities among particular groups.

Taking action on health inequities requires that community health care providers, decision makers, and researchers to create poverty reduction strategies and programs with the goal of addressing the unequal distribution of resources. Many antipoverty programs focus on the individuals who live in poverty rather than on the structural inequalities in power and influence that *cause* Canadians to live in poverty (Raphael, 2018). Raising the profile of poverty as a life-threatening health issue within the general public and shifting the focus of government towards improving the living conditions of those living in poverty would be required in an equity-oriented approach (Raphael, 2018). One not-for-profit organization that addresses the structural inequalities in power is Canada Without Poverty (CWP) (see Real-World Example box).

 REAL-WORLD EXAMPLE

Canada Without Poverty

Canada Without Poverty (CWP) (http://www.cwp-csp.ca) is an organization that acts from the belief that poverty is a violation of human rights and that poverty elimination is a human rights obligation. CWP educates Canadians about the human and financial cost of poverty, participates in research to generate new knowledge about poverty, and identifies public policy solutions.

Equity in care would mean that we have universal access; institutions and health professionals would deliver care to underserved populations without barriers such as racism and discrimination, and individuals would be treated fairly and justly. At the individual level, equity would mean the availability of care and quality of services are based on individuals' particular needs and not based on personal characteristics that are unrelated to the patient's condition or to the reason for seeking care. In particular, the quality of care would not differ because of such characteristics as gender, race, age, ethnicity, income, education, disability, sexual orientation, or location of residence. In an equity-oriented health care system, individuals could access their own medical records online, medical paperwork would not exist, and we would not need to answer the same question(s) over and over again with different health care professionals.

Innovations to reorient our health system towards equity and improving the health of populations are taking shape. No Community Left Behind (http://nocommunityleftbehind.ca) is one strategy working at the neighbourhood level to keep people well—to enable them to live, work, and raise their families in a safe and prosperous environment. Through a community development process, community partners engage, addressing the SDHs and exploring opportunities for local development and adopting new ways to building stronger, healthier, and safer communities. Ensuring health equity is effectively considered and acted upon within planning, and policy development can be done by using a Health Equity Impact Assessment (HEIA) (http://www.health.gov.on.ca/en/pro/programs/heia/docs/template.pdf), a tool that walks users through the steps of identifying how a program, policy, or similar initiative will impact population groups in different ways. The goal is to maximize positive impacts and reduce negative impacts, for more equitable delivery programs, services, and policies.

Is an equity-oriented health system achievable? We have all the integral pieces to make it work; what is uncertain is whether there is sufficient political will that could glue all of the pieces together. At any moment (as we have seen south of our border), politics could overtake any moral commitment aimed at advancing an equity-oriented health care system.

TRENDS IN HEALTH CARE

Increased Drug Prices

With the implementation of the 2018 United States-Mexico-Canada Agreement (USMCA), the cost of drugs will increase. This is because of extending the minimum "data protection" period for an expensive class of drugs known as biologics. Canada used to provide 5 years of data protection. However, big pharmaceutical lobby groups in Canada and in the United States drove that number up to 8 years, and with the USMCA, the time period is now 8 years. Biologics are made from or in living organisms, including cells and tissues, and can be gene based. They tend to be more complex to manufacture than drugs that are made from chemicals and therefore cost more. Biologics are injectable medications that are used to treat various forms of arthritis, Crohn's disease and ulcerative colitis (inflammatory bowel conditions), multiple sclerosis, and a variety of other diseases. The data that are being protected include information about the effectiveness and safety of drugs that comes out of the clinical trials conducted by brand-name drug companies when they want approval to market a new drug. These data are the private property of the brand-name companies and can't be used by anyone else, including generic companies, for a specific period of time. This means cheaper generic versions of these drugs will not be available as quickly in Canada as they used to be, and prices will be higher on average. It would be costly for generic companies to do the original testing all over again. It would also be unethical because the results of the drug trials are already known, and when the data are no longer protected, generic companies use it to produce cheaper drugs. The resulting increased data protection period means it takes longer for generic medications to reach patients—this is a problem when generics are needed to keep drug plans affordable.

Community Violence

A significant trend that is on the rise in Canada is exposure to community violence. According to the WHO's conceptual framework, community violence is a form of interpersonal violence perpetrated by strangers or acquaintances other than family members or intimate partners (Krug etal., 2002). Box 18.1 discusses a common but underestimated form of community violence. Mass shootings are one example of community violence. In 2017, a mass shooting occurred at the Islamic Cultural Centre of Québec. The attack resulted in 6 homicides and 40 attempted murders. In 2018, another mass shooting in downtown Toronto injured 13 people and killed 2 girls aged 18 and 13 years. Community violence occurs often in public spaces, with intentional motives to cause harm. However, the ripple effect of the targeted violent attack impacts witnesses. In 2018, stray bullets from a gun

---

> **BOX 18.1   Exposure to Community Violence in a Line-up**
>
> Clients who line up on the street to wait for health care clinics, food banks, or homeless shelters to open are exposed to various forms of violence, including being intimidated by drug dealers, bullying by others in the lineup, or being assaulted.
>
> Cool Aid Community Health centre in Victoria, which serves clients who live on low incomes, recognized that clients who lined up to wait for the clinic to open were being exposed to various forms of violence. Additionally, the clinic receptionists witnessing these situations were negatively impacted because they felt responsible for the clients' well-being. To address the exposure to community violence, the centre changed its clinic opening procedures to allow people to wait indoors (Browne et al., 2015).

---

attack injured two girls while they were playing at their neighbourhood park in Toronto with their mother. Only weeks later, there was a targeted van attack in Toronto's north end, injuring 16 and killing 10 people. Community violence does not always hit the news media, so although it looks like these events are only occurring in metropolitan areas, Statistics Canada noted that violence related to guns is mainly occurring in cities with fewer than 100 000 people and occurred most often in Saskatchewan and Ontario in 2017 (Statistics Canada, 2017).

A public health approach to community violence casts a wide net in understanding and finding solutions. Exposure to community violence can be viewed as an SDH impacting preterm birth, low birth weight, stress, lower cognitive functioning, aggression, depression, anxiety, post-traumatic stress disorder, shortened life expectancy, shortened survival expectations, and greater risk-taking behaviours (Caruso, 2017).

Treating community violence like a contagious virus is a promising intervention that is demonstrating positive impacts in communities around the world. According to Dr. Slutkin, who began this work in treating community violence as a disease, there is evidence that violence behaves like a contagious and epidemic disease (Slutkin, 2013). Stopping the spread of violence includes tailoring interventions to its disease-like characteristics. Working at the community level, health workers from the community are hired and trained to map out areas of highest transmission and symptom manifestation, reach out and intervene with those displaying clinical signs to reduce further transmission using methods tailored to the infectious agent at play, detect close contacts and others with emergent symptoms or at highest risk of future contraction, and render all those at highest risk less symptomatic and likely to transmit. Outreach workers are also hired with the role of being violence interrupters who prevent violent events and retaliations, reduce risk among those most likely to become violent, and shift norms to discourage the use of violence. New protective behaviours and new norms are promoted and supported, and working with public safety regarding enforcement has significantly reduced community violence (Slutkin, 2013). This is how Cure Violence, a nonprofit organization in the United States, is reducing shootings and killings and creating safer neighbourhoods where mothers and children can go to the park to play without the worry of being exposed to violence..

ADVANCEMENTS IN PUBLIC HEALTH

Oral Anticancer Medications

The paradigm in cancer care is shifting from hospital to community because of the advent of novel oral anticancer agents. This approach offers numerous advantages, including increased patient convenience compared with conventional parenteral therapy. Other advantages include reducing costs by decreasing the utilization of valuable resources such as beds, infusion areas, and health care providers' time. It is also preferred by many patients because it reduces the need and risks of invasive devices such as central venous catheters, saves time, is easier to administer, and gives them a feeling of control of their medications (Boons etal., 2018). However, the expanding use of oral therapy creates a unique set of challenges to providing optimum patient care—managing adverse effects. These challenges are further compounded by the high cost of and restricted access to many oral anticancer agents. Patients' concerns include adherence, understanding complex schedules, different side effect profiles, and interactions with foods and other medications (Boons etal., 2018). Health care professionals, particularly pharmacists, are facing the challenges of updating their knowledge, reducing medication errors, safe handling, educating patients and their caregivers, and managing side effects (Mekdad & AlSayed, 2017).

New Technology
Augmented Reality and Virtual Reality

Augmented reality (AR) represents a form of intermediated reality in which a view of the real world is modified by a computer in some way (Barsom, Graafland, & Schijven, 2016). As a result, the technology functions to change our current perception of reality. The popular game Pokémon Go is an example of AR that turns a mobile device into a multimedia networked device that overlays digital data on real-world situations in real time. AR currently uses image recognition or geopositioning (location recognition) technologies to identify physical objects or places in the real world and then visually overlays digital information about these objects or places on a digital display in situ. These digitally augmented elements are superimposed on the real world through head-mounted eyewear, a glass transparent screen, or a camera display such as a smartphone or tablet computer screen.

Ranked as an emerging technology by the Horizon Report in 2016 (Johnson etal., 2016), AR has continued to develop rapidly and now represents an emerging technology. AR is distinct from virtual reality (VR) in that AR does not attempt to create a fully digital world that users can interact with but instead relies on the blending of digital (virtual) and physical (actual) domains.

The role of AR in health care is expanding rapidly, and many of the biggest medical and public health advances are yet to be seen with how images are displayed. AR is helping nurses find veins more easily by using a handheld scanner that projects over skin and shows nurses exactly where a patient's veins are located. The results of this technology have made finding veins on the first stick 3.5 times more likely, thereby saving patients from extra needle pokes and pain. Pharmaceutical companies are using AR to improve patient education. Patients can see how a drug works in three dimensions in front of their eyes instead of reading the description on the bottle. As mentioned, Pokémon Go and games like it encourage the user to be physically active, thus increasing the health benefits of using AR for gaming. Pokémon Go has been shown to encourage users to increase their physical activity by 1 437 steps a day on average, representing a 25% increase compared with their prior activity level (Althoff, White, & Horvitz, 2016). Although the game has lost much of its initial appeal and calls into question the sustainability of its potential for increased exercise, it has demonstrated the potential effects of behavioural stimuli (e.g., nudging—see Chapter 3) from using AR.

Virtual reality as a total immersion technology platform may help with the prevention of sexually transmitted infections through sexual health education and training, creating a safe experience in which users can do everything from practice using a condom to decline consenting to a sexual encounter (Ross, 2015). VR can also be used for injury prevention, for example, by providing a safe, controlled environment in which to teach children pedestrian safety by having them practise skills and by providing consistent feedback during practice and opportunities for repetition. VR for injury prevention can be applied to many public health issues, opening the door to new ways of learning that affect the brain differently than traditional education methods have.

Artificial Intelligence

There is new excitement among health care organizations, professionals, and researchers that machine learning algorithms can provide new ways of diagnosing disease, identify people at risk of illness, and direct resources. **Artificial Intelligence (AI)** can be defined simply as the ability of a computer or robot to perform tasks commonly associated with human beings. Siri and Alexa are common examples of AI. The term *artificial intelligence* is frequently applied to the process of developing systems endowed with the ability to reason and learn from experience.

Canada is emerging as a global leader in developing this technology, and has a number of academic institutions working with industry partners. The Montreal Institute for Learning Algorithms, the Alberta Machine Intelligence Institute, and the Vector Institute for Artificial Intelligence are a few of these innovative companies in Canada. The federal government support has been well received by technology experts with the Pan-Canadian Artificial Intelligence Strategy in 2017 and the AI-Powered Supply Chains Supercluster, which is expected to generate $16.5 billion in gross domestic product over the next 10 years (Government of Canada, 2018).

Artificial intelligence techniques known as deep learning have rapidly improved performance in image recognition, caption generation, and speech recognition (Tang etal., 2018). Deep learning is also being used to develop self-driving cars, which are fully autonomous cars with no steering wheel or ability for drivers to intervene. General Motors has planned to put such a car into production in 2019. Autopilot is also being used in a similar way; however, the technology relies on drivers intervening if anything unexpected happens. There are several public health benefits and harms to individuals and population health such as road casualties, environmental health, aging populations, noncommunicable

disease, land use, and labour markets that must be considered when forming new transportation policy (Crayton & Meier, 2017).

Artificial intelligence could be a powerful tool for public health because it can predict future events based on past data, for example, predicting the next flu outbreak. AI is being used to prevent suicides based on applying machine learning to electronic health records within a large medical database, using algorithms that accurately predict future suicide attempts; this has been promising (Walsh, Ribeiro, & Franklin, 2017).

Theoretically, AI can take a person's genome and recommend treatment options, while limiting or even eliminating side effects (Research Canada, 2018). In the United Kingdom, an AI-driven smartphone app has been developed to handle the task of triaging urgent but non–life-threatening conditions to Accident & Emergency (A&E). Instead of calling a phone number and talking to an operator, individuals are able to chat to an AI-powered "chatbot" to check symptoms instantly and get most appropriate advice on the course of action to be taken (O'Hear, 2016).

Drones

If you have ever seen one of the movies in the trilogy *The Hunger Games*, then you know about the usefulness of **drones:** unmanned aerial vehicles that have the ability to deliver packages and mobile applications that send commands to an externals source with a simple touch. What may have been fantasy in movies has become an everyday reality. The potential for drones in health care is almost limitless. A drone can be used for a reconnaissance mission in which aerial photography and a video feed of the scene of an accident or natural disaster can be taken to give first responders a better idea of the situation on the ground. Another use is delivery, where drones serve as the vehicle used to medical equipment, drugs, and food to medical personnel on the ground or to injured individuals, as happened in Haiti after an earthquake in 2010 or in Rwanda, where blood products are being delivered to health teams in places where roads are washed out. Drones are literally changing the way health care is being delivered, and there are unlimited types of packages that could be delivered. Drones may also be used as medical command using medical expertise in which, through their video sensors, they provide high-fidelity data and two-way communication between health care providers and first responders—or even between health care providers and bystanders or injured people on the scene.

Wearable Devices

Wearable consumer devices are becoming popular in health, with monitoring capabilities such as electrocardiogram, electromyogram, heart rate, body temperature, electrodermal activity, arterial oxygen saturation, blood pressure, and respiration rate, which can all be sent to your medical professional via a wireless network. Monitoring and recording real-time information about one's physiological condition and motion activities can facilitate timely diagnosis and treatment of chronic illnesses such as cardiopulmonary disease, asthma, and heart failure. This type of device is especially helpful for individuals who are located far from medical care facilities, allowing for continuous monitoring, storing, and sending medical data to health care professionals over distance. Tehrani and Andrew (2014) define wearable devices (sometimes called "wearables") in simpler terms, as electronic technologies or computers that are incorporated into items of clothing and accessories that can be worn comfortably on the body. The growth of wearable technology since 2015 has been remarkably fast. In 2016, the number of connected wearables was already at 325 million, with the number predicted to grow to an estimated 830 million in 2020 (Statista, 2017).

Privacy and security issues with wearable devices are concerns for many because these devices continuously collect user's personal health information in real time. Because of these types of concerns, it can be challenging to adopt this type of technology to monitor your health. *Privacy* can be defined as the desire of citizens to be given a degree of control over the collection and dissemination of their personal health information by health organizations and technology vendors (Belanger & Crossler, 2011). An individual's personal health information is more sensitive than other types of information, such as demographic information and general transaction information. Therefore health care wearables should be regarded as a high-privacy-concern product (Kenny & Connolly, 2016).

CONCLUDING THOUGHTS

We now go back to the questions posed at the beginning of this chapter: how are consumers' privacy and security being protected when using health care apps? Does a technology-based future support our health and well-being? We hope we have shed some light on these questions and offered information for further debate and discussion.

New advancements and technologies have the potential to revolutionize the future of public health and preventive health care. With these innovations, there is the potential that health care costs could be reduced and better outcomes for Canadians could be created. Strengthening our health care system through innovation can improve the health and well-being of all Canadians (Naylor, 2015). However, ethical implications must also be considered, such as the ethical collection, analysis, and sharing of health data.

Work still needs to be done in these areas, exploring, for example, some of the ethical difficulties in making decisions and policy recommendations on the basis of probabilistic, imperfect, and even flawed data. The WHO has also recognized these advancements as being challenging and is in the process of developing a report for Member States called *Governing Big Data and AI in Health: Ethical Considerations*. The report will describe the ethical issues and points to be considered by Member States as they develop national policies on Big Data and AI. In all the new excitement and momentum created by advancements in medicine, Dr. Fridsma, an expert in informatics and health information technology, has offered the following cautionary note: "Patients are more than collections of discrete data: We diagnose diseases, but patients experience illness. AI can't solve this" (WHO, 2018, p. 2). We must be mindful that there are limitations, too.

REFERENCES

Althoff, T., White, R. W., & Horvitz, E. (2016). Influence of Pokémon Go on physical activity: Study and implications. *Journal of Medical Internet Research*, *18*(12), e315. https://doi.org/10.2196/jmir.6759.

Barsom, E. Z., Graafland, M., & Schijven, M. P. (2016). Systematic review on the effectiveness of augmented reality applications in medical training. *Surgical Endoscopy*, *30*(10), 4174–4183.

Bélanger, F., & Crossler, R. E. (2011). Privacy in the digital age: A review of Information. Privacy research in information systems. *MIS Quarterly*, *35*(4), 1017–1041.

Boons, C. C., Timmers, L., van Schoor, N. M., etal. (2018). Patient satisfaction with information on oral anticancer agent use. *Cancer Medicine, 7*(1), 219–228.

British Columbia Royal Commission on Health Care and Costs. (1991). *Report of the British Columbia Royal Commission on health care and costs: Closer to home.* Victoria, BC: Government of British Columbia.

Browne, A. J., Varcoe, C., Ford-Gilboe, M., etal. (2015). EQUIP Healthcare: An overview of a multi-component intervention to enhance equity-oriented care in primary health care settings. *International Journal for Equity in Health, 14,* 152.

Canadian Partnership for Children's Health and Environment. (2018). *RentSafe.* Retrieved from http://www.healthyenvironmentforkids.ca/collections/rentsafe.

Caruso, G. D. (2017). *Public health and safety: The social determinants of health and criminal behavior.* United Kingdom: Researchers Links Books.

Commission d'étude sur les services de santé et les services sociaux. (2000). *Emerging solutions: Report and recommendations.* Quebec City: Government of Quebec.

The Commission on Medicare. (2001). *Caring for Medicare: Sustaining a quality system.* Regina: Government of Saskatchewan.

The Commission on the Reform of Ontario's Public Services. (2012). *Public services for Ontarians: A path to sustainability and excellence.* Toronto: Government of Ontario.

Crayton, T. J., & Meier, B. M. (2017). Autonomous vehicles: Developing a public health research agenda to frame the future of transportation policy. *Journal of Transport & Health, 6,* 245–252.

Dagnone, T. (2009). *For patients' sake: Patient first review. Commissioner's report to the saskatchewan minister of health.* Regina: Government of Saskatchewan.

Forest, P., & Martin, D. (2018). *Fit for purpose: Findings and recommendations of the external review of the Pan-Canadian Health Organizations: Summary report.* Retrieved from https://www.canada.ca/en/health-canada/services/health-care-system/reports-publications/health-care-system/findings-recommendations-external-review-pan-canadian-health-organization.html.

Government of Canada. (2018). *AI-powered supply chains supercluster (SCALE.AI).* Retrieved from https://www.ic.gc.ca/eic/site/093.nsf/eng/00009.html.

Johnson, L., Becker, S. A., Cummins, M., etal. (2016). *NMC horizon report: 2016 higher education* edition (pp. 1–50). Austin, TX: The New Media Consortium.

Kenny, G., & Connolly, R. (2016). Citizens' health information privacy concerns: Developing a framework. In *Blurring the boundaries through digital innovation* (pp. 131–143). New York: Springer.

Kirby, M. J. L. (2002). *The health of Canadians—The federal role. Vol. 6: Recommendations for reform.* Ottawa: Standing Senate Committee on Social Affairs, Science and Technology.

Krug, E. G., Mercy, J. A., Dahlberg, L. L., etal. (2002). The world report on violence and health. *The Lancet, 360*(9339), 1083–1088.

Mekdad, S. S., & AlSayed, A. D. (2017). Towards safety of oral anti-cancer agents, the need to educate our pharmacists. *Saudi Pharmaceutical Journal, 25*(1), 136–140.

National Forum on Health. (1997). *Canada health action: Building on the legacy, the final report of the National Forum on Health.* Ottawa: Government of Canada.

Naylor, D. (2015). *Unleashing innovation: Excellent healthcare for Canada: Report of the advisory panel on healthcare innovation.* Retrieved from https://www.canada.ca/en/health-canada/services/publications/health-system-services/report-advisory-panel-healthcare-innovation.html.

O'Hear, S. (2016). *Babylon Health partner with UK's NHS to replace telephone help line with AI powered chatbot.* Retrieved from https://techcrunch.com/2017/01/04/babylon-health-partners-with-uks-nhs-to-replace-telephone-helpline-with-ai-powered-chatbot/.

The Ontario Health Services Restructuring Commission (1996–2000). (2000). *A legacy report: Looking back, looking forward.* Toronto: Government of Ontario.

Ontario Ministry of Health and Long-Term Care. (2016). *Improving the odds: Championing health equity in Ontario.* Toronto: Government of Ontario. Retrieved from http://www.health.gov.on.ca/en/common/ministry/publications/reports/cmoh_18/default.aspx.

Premier's Advisory Council on Health. (2001). *A framework for reform.* Edmonton: Government of Alberta.

Raphael, D. (2018). The social determinants of health of under-served populations in Canada. In A. N. Arya, & T. Piggott (Eds.), *Under-served: Health determinants of indigenous, inner-city, and migrant populations in Canada* (pp. 23–38). Toronto: Canadian Scholars' Press.

Research Canada. (2018). *Artificial intelligence and machine learning: Reshaping health research and innovation.* Retrieved from https://rc-rc.ca/reshaping-health-research-innovation-artificial-intelligence-machine-learning/.

Romanow, R. (2002). *Commission on the Future of health care in Canada. building on values: The future of health care in Canada: Final report.* Ottawa: Government of Canada.

Ross, H. A. (2015). *Health Infor [M-ED]: Black college females discuss a virtual reality platform for sexual health education and training* (Master's Thesis dissertation). University of South Florida. Retrieved from https://scholarcommons.usf.edu/cgi/viewcontent.cgi?referer=https://scholar.google.ca/&httpsredir=1&article=6967&context=etd.

Slutkin, G. (2013). Violence is a contagious disease. In *Contagion of violence, forum on global violence prevention, workshop summary* (pp. 94–111). Washington, DC: Institute of Medicine and National Research Council. The National Academies Press.

Statista. (2017). *Statistics & facts on wearable technology*. Retrieved from https://www.statista.com/topics/1556/wearable-technology/.

Statistics Canada. (2017). *Police reported gun statistics*. Retrieved from https://www150.statcan.gc.ca/n1/pub/85-002-x/2018001/article/54974-eng.htm.

Tang, A., Tam, R., Cadrin-Chênevert, A., etal. (2018). Canadian association of radiologists white paper on artificial intelligence in radiology. *Canadian Association of Radiologists Journal, 69*(2), 120–135. https://doi.org/10.1016/j.carj.2018.02.002.

Tehrani, K., & Andrew, M. (2014). *Wearable technology and wearable devices: Everything you need to know. Wearable Devices Magazine*. Retrieved from http://www.WearableDevices.com.

Walsh, C. G., Ribeiro, J. D., & Franklin, J. C. (2017). Predicting risk of suicide attempts over time through machine learning. *Clinical Psychological Science, 5*(3), 457–469. https://doi.org/10.1177/2167702617691560.

World Health Organization (WHO). (2018). *Big data and artificial intelligence for achieving universal health coverage: An international consultation on ethics*. Retrieved from http://apps.who.int/iris/bitstream/handle/10665/275417/WHO-HMM-IER-REK-2018.2-eng.pdf.

INDEX

Note: Page numbers followed by "f" indicate figures, "t" indicate tables, and "b" indicate boxes.